Human Motivation

David C. McClelland
BOSTON UNIVERSITY

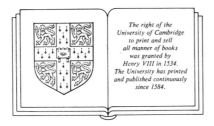

The right of the
University of Cambridge
to print and sell
all manner of books
was granted by
Henry VIII in 1534.
The University has printed
and published continuously
since 1584.

Cambridge University Press

Cambridge

New York, New Rochelle, Melbourne, Sydney

Published by the Press Syndicate of the University of Cambridge
The Pitt Building, Trumpington Street, Cambridge CB2 1RP
32 East 57th Street, New York, NY 10022, USA
10 Stamford Road, Oakleigh, Melbourne 3166, Australia

First published by Scott Foresman & Co. 1985
First published by Cambridge University Press 1987

Printed in the United States of America

Library of Congress Cataloging in Publication Data
McClelland, David Clarence.
  Human motivation.
  Bibliography: p. 609
  Includes index.
  1. Motivation (Psychology)   I. Title.
BF503.M42   1984   153.8   84–10540
ISBN 0 521 36951 7

Credit lines for copyrighted materials
appearing in this work are placed in
the Acknowledgments section at
the end of the book.

Preface

The psychology of motivation is a broad and loosely defined field. It covers everything from detailed investigations of the physiological mechanisms involved in animal drives to elaborate analyses of the unconscious motives behind abnormal or symptomatic acts in a person to factor analyses of the motives people assign to themselves to explain their behavior. Different textbooks and different courses have been organized around these different areas of investigation. In this book we will draw on all these sources of information and attempt to provide an integrated view of the field by narrowing somewhat the focus of attention.

The book emphasizes how motives differ from other determinants of action and how they relate to other motivation-type variables such as emotions, incentives, values, causal explanations, and conscious and unconscious intents. It examines how motives are acquired, where they come from, and on what they are based. Biological sources of human motives are reviewed, and this review introduces the topic of natural incentives, or what is sometimes called *intrinsic motivation*. Some selectivity is necessary in reviewing the large field of animal research on motivation in order to focus on biological sources of individual differences in human motive strength. Social sources of differences in motive strength are also considered, including everything from the way parents rear their children to educational interventions designed to change peoples' motives. Such studies contribute not only practical information on how to develop motives, but also theoretical information on the nature of motives and how they differ from other characteristics.

A major focus of the book is on how individual differences in the strength of human motives are to be measured. The emphasis is on measuring motives in associative thought or fantasy, a method that combines the sensitivity of Freud's clinical analyses of motivation with the rigor of experimental psychology, since the coding systems for human motives are derived from the effects on associative thought of experimental arousal of the motives in question. However, alternative methods of measuring human motive strength are also reviewed, and all methods are evaluated carefully in terms of acknowledged criteria for good measurement. What comes out of this analysis is the importance of distinguishing between more or less unconscious motives and conscious values as different determinants of behavior.

Four major motive systems—the achievement motive, the power motive, the affiliative motives, and the avoidance motives are examined in detail. The large body of research that has accumulated on how these motive systems affect behavior is carefully reviewed and evaluated. The text illuminates not only how motives serve to energize and orient behavior and to promote relevant types of learning; it also contains factual answers to such large questions as, Why do great civilizations rise and then decline? or, in motivational terms, What is the difference between the reasons for the commercial success of ancient Greece and the organizational triumph of the Roman Empire? Why are some kinds of people successful in business as managers while others are not? What have been the motivational characteristics of U.S. presidents, and how are those characteristics related to how they behaved in office? Why do nations make war? Can love really heal in the physical sense? The research that has been done on these motive systems not only provides information of theoretical importance; it also answers questions of great practical and social significance.

Since motives are treated as only one of the determinants of action, some of the usual topics in the field of motivation are discussed not in their own right, but as part of other matters. Take, for example, aggression or the aggressive drive or instinct, which is often a topic heading in books on motivation. In this book the usual subject matter for the topic of aggression is dealt with in two places—as a type of action characteristic of certain kinds of power-motivated people (Chapter 8) and as a type of action that suggests the existence of a natural incentive that yields pleasure from having impact (Chapter 5). Other such behavioral trends suggesting the presence of a motive, like pro-social or altruistic behavior, are similarly treated. Pro-social behavior appears as characteristic of people with a certain type of power motive (Chapter 8), and as indicating the presence of a natural incentive to get pleasure from being with people based on contact gratifications (Chapter 5) or from some kind of interpersonal exchange (Chapter 9).

I have benefited greatly not only from the contributions of generations of students and fellow workers in the field of motivation, but also from the specific advice of Charles Cofer, Dan McAdams, and Thomas Srull, who read and commented in detail on an early version of the manuscript. In addition, John W. Atkinson, David G. Winter, Abigail Stewart, David Buss, and Richard Patten have given me very useful feedback on particular chapters. Of course, none of these people should be held responsible for my mistakes. I also owe a special debt to the National Science Foundation, which provided me with the funds not only to complete parts of the research reported here, but also to spend a year free of other academic duties to concentrate on completing the manuscript. Finally, the book could never have been completed without the devoted, patient, and conscientious secretarial assistance of Kathleen McPherson and Samantha George, for which I am very grateful.

David C. McClelland

Foreword

More than most textbooks in psychology, this book reflects the work, the life, and the personality of its author. After forty prolific years of boldly original research and theorizing on the topic of human motivation, David McClelland has not produced a conservative, homogenized, and middle-of-the-road review of the literature. Like *Personality,* McClelland's classic textbook on personality psychology written over thirty years ago, this text takes some risks. First, the book does not aim to review all of the important literature on human motivation; rather, it seeks to explore in some detail a selected set of critical and intriguing motivational issues. Second, the book does not merely summarize theories, methods, and research findings pertaining to the scientific study of human motivation; rather, it attempts a theoretical synthesis of its own based on the author's particular perspective on human motivation—a perspective that has developed through a number of stages during the last forty years.

David Winter (1982)—a student and colleague of McClelland—has recently traced McClelland's intellectual biography as a psychologist through six stages. From his rigorous training within the behaviorist tradition of Clark Hull at Yale and his early research on verbal discrimination learning, McClelland moved to the study of thematic measurement of psychological motives (such as the achievement motive) in the late 1940s. The mid-1950s found him immersed in the almost audacious investigation of how human motives—reflected in such unlikely sources as children's readers and ancient urns—shape the economic development of entire cultures. By the mid-1960s McClelland and his colleagues were designing programs to facilitate the development of achievement motivation in businesspeople; whereas the late 1960s and 1970s witnessed a shift away from achievement to the study of the power motive and its myriad manifestations in such phenomena as risk-taking behavior, patterns of leadership in groups, alcohol consumption, and war. In the most recent stage, McClelland's work has moved into yet a new area: the relationship of psychological motives to physiological functioning, especially with respect to the body's immune systems and thus sickness and health.

Over the shifting course of McClelland's intellectual journey, a number of salient themes have been expressed again and again. As a student and colleague of McClelland for only a short while, I have come to perceive eight recurrent themes that aptly characterize his patented perspective on human motivation. The careful reader should discern these eight in the pages that follow:

1. *A fascination with Freud and the unconscious.* For McClelland, like Freud, the really important motives in human lives reside beneath the surface of everyday awareness. To understand motivation, therefore, the psychologist must tap into its subterranean source.

2. *A commitment to measurement and quantification of human motives.* Like Clark Hull and the behaviorists of his day, McClelland has little patience for things that cannot be measured and transformed into numbers. Given the well-known difficulties psychologists have encountered in measuring Freudian constructs, Themes 1 and 2 often exist in a dynamic tension in McClelland's work as he attempts to devise methods to measure what some psychologists have claimed is unmeasurable.

3. *An adherence to the measurement methodology of content analysis applied to open-ended responses such as the stories that people tell.* McClelland is a pioneer in the development of ways of interpreting the Thematic Apperception Test (TAT) so as to quantify motive trends that exist beneath the level of awareness. He has repeatedly argued that open-ended measures such as the TAT, dream analysis, and the coding of myths and stories are significantly more sensitive to unconscious motive trends than are self-report measures such as questionnaires and rating scales.

4. *An implied dimensional view of people.* McClelland is a "trait theorist" in the best sense of the term. He studies enduring and underlying dimensions of the personality which motivate (energize, direct, and select) behavior and experience. The three fundamental motive systems which he has identified and measured in human lives concern (a) achievement/success, (b) power/impact, and (c) affiliation/intimacy.

5. *An interest in individual differences.* McClelland tends to ask the question, 'How do people differ?' more often than do most motivational psychologists. Motivational differences are measured via thematic coding of open-ended responses, and the differences are often understood in terms of the three major motive systems.

6. *A preoccupation with major questions of human adaptation.* In his research and his theorizing, McClelland does not shy away from the big questions about human adaptation: Why do nations make war? Why are some people successful and others not? Can love really heal? This leads him into controversial, but fascinating, studies of healing, history, and mythology.

7. *A belief that motives can be changed.* McClelland and his colleagues have developed systematic programs for altering people's motivational profiles. The programs are seen as creative and cost-effective ways to help people

change the internal psychological needs which energize, direct, and select, their behavior. McClelland's methods have implications for psychological interventions in business, industry, government, and therapy.

8. *A concern about the welfare of society.* Like B. F. Skinner and Erik Erikson, McClelland has shown a keen appreciation for the intricate interplay of science and society through history. Laboratory findings are often couched in terms of their meanings for contemporary society and the imminent prospects of human happiness and misery, peace and war. In addressing the future welfare of humans living on earth, McClelland does not hesitate to scrutinize the motive patterns of entire nations and entire historical epochs.

McClelland's perspective on human motivation distinguishes this text from all others in the field. The author's creative blend of tough-minded empiricism and tender-minded humanism has given birth to a textbook on human motivation that should challenge, stimulate, and indeed motivate the student and the instructor alike.

Dan P. McAdams
Loyola University of Chicago

References

McClelland, D.C. *Personality.* New York: Holt, Rinehart and Winston, 1951.

Winter, D. G. David C. McClelland: An intellectual biography. In A. J. Stewart (Ed.), *Motivation and society.* San Francisco: Jossey-Bass, 1982.

Contents

Part 1

Background

1

Conscious and Unconscious Motives

• MOTIVES AS ONE OF THREE MAJOR DETERMINANTS OF BEHAVIOR

What is the subject matter of motivation? From the commonsense point of view, *motivation* refers on one hand to conscious intents, to such inner thoughts as, I wish I could play the piano, I want to be a doctor, and I am trying hard to solve this problem. On the other hand, looking at behaviors from the outside, *motivation* refers to inferences about conscious intents that we make from observing behaviors. Thus, if we see a young girl perform a connected series of acts such as walking into a room, drawing up the piano stool, getting out some music, opening the piano, and starting to play, we infer that she wants to play the piano. If she stops playing after a while, we infer that she no longer wants to play the piano. As Marshall Jones (1955) put it in introducing the annual volumes of the *Nebraska Symposium on Motivation*, the subject matter of motivation has to do with "how behavior gets started, is energized, is sustained, is directed, is stopped." Put another way, motivation has to do with the *why* of behavior, as contrasted with the *how* or the *what* of behavior. We can observe what the girl is doing, that is, playing the piano. Or we can observe how she is doing it, that is, what motor skills she is using to play the piano. Or we can try to determine why she is doing what she is doing.

Of course, when we make inferences from observing behavior about a person's intent, we can arrive at a conclusion about the intent that differs from what the person feels her or his intent was. We refer to people's perception of their wishes as *conscious intents,* and we infer that their wishes were *unconscious intents* if they differ from the report of conscious wishes or if people cannot report at all on their intents. The inferences we make about interests from observing behavior can be wrong; for example, we infer that the girl wants to play the piano, whereas the same acts would be consistent with her feeling that she is being compelled to practice.

It is very important to recognize at the outset that there are several kinds of answers to the question *why,* only some of which deal with the problem of motivation. A complete answer to the question *why* must include all the determinants of behavior, not just the motivational ones. To distinguish among the determinants of behavior, it is useful first to realize that any behavioral outcome is a function of determinants in both the person and the environment. Fritz Heider (1958) uses the example of a man rowing a boat across a lake to get to the other side. Getting to the other side (the behavioral outcome) may be determined partly by the individual who is rowing or partly by wind currents blowing on the boat. If the man did nothing and simply was blown across the lake, we ordinarily would make no inferences about his motivation—about his desire to get to the other side. On the other hand, if the day were perfectly calm and he rowed vigorously, we would attribute the behavioral outcome to his intent to go across the lake.

A number of recent experimental studies have dealt with the problem of *personal causation.* In general, we do not think of people as causing an outcome if we can find sufficient reason for the outcome in the external environment, as in the example of the wind blowing the boat across the lake (Deci, 1975). However, if there are no environmental pushes or if such pushes would work against a particular outcome, and if people have acted in ways that seem to produce the outcome, we are even more apt to attribute the outcome to their actions.

For a concrete example of this principle, consider an autobiographical statement made by Sigmund Freud (1910/1938), one of the most important contributors to the psychology of motivation, whose work will figure largely in this chapter and the next: "For psychoanalysis is my creation; for 10 years I was the only one occupied with it and all the annoyances which this new subject caused among my contemporaries has been hurled upon my head in the form of criticism." Freud is saying that all the environmental forces were acting against the creation of psychoanalysis. He got no help—only criticism—from his contemporaries. So it is proper to infer that he personally caused the creation of psychoanalysis, since he persisted in the face of criticism. Or as Weiner and Kukla (1970) have shown, "if one succeeds when others fail, or fails when others succeed, the outcomes are attributed to the person" (Weiner, 1980a). They found, for example, that if a person succeeded in performing a task at which only 10 percent of the people succeeded, judges overwhelmingly attributed the success to the person rather than to the characteristics of the task.

Once it has been decided that the person is responsible for an outcome, when do we attribute motivation to the person? As Heider has pointed out, common sense distinguishes between effort (the motivational factor) and ability. A behavioral outcome is jointly determined by a person's efforts and ability to perform the task. The outcome is also partly determined by the person's understanding of the situation. Jones and Davis (1965) use the example of Lee Harvey Oswald shooting President John F. Kennedy to illustrate how these three factors interact to produce an outcome. Before we can infer that Oswald intended or wanted to kill the President, we must know that he knew how to shoot a gun, that is, that he had the ability and had not accidentally pulled the trigger. We also need to know that he understood that the gun was loaded and that if he pulled the trigger a bullet might enter the President's head and kill him, as well as that this would somehow fit into his ideas of what ought to be. These ideas or expectations usually are referred to as *cognitive variables.*

Personal causation is made up of cognitions, skills, and motivations or intents. Any general theory of action or of personality must take into account a person's motives, skills or adaptive traits, and cognitions or schemas (McClelland, 1951). These three types of variables interact in complex ways, as later chapters will show, but the emphasis in this book is primarily on motivational variables. More careful definitions of the determinants of behavior will be given in later chapters. The purpose here is simply to give a general picture of the types of variables psychologists have used to explain behavior.

Once again let us turn to Freud's autobiography to see how these factors interact to produce an outcome in a concrete case. He said, "I had become a physician quite reluctantly, but was at that time impelled by a strong motive to help nervous patients, or at least to learn to understand something of their conditions. I had placed reliance on physical therapy and found myself helpless in the face of the disappointments with [it]" (Freud, 1910/1938). Freud made a statement about his motives—his desire to help nervous patients—and a statement about a technique or skill (physical therapy) he tried that is considered to be another separate determinant of his actions. More specifically, he tried to help a patient he called Dora. He knew of an event in her life that he believed had caused the outbreak of her illness but said, "I tried uncounted times to analyze the experience, but all that I could receive to my direct demands was the same scanty and broken description" (Freud, 1910/1938).

Only when he used his new technique of getting the patient to free associate backward from the scene itself to earlier experiences was he able to understand and solve the actual conflict. When he got to the root of the problem he discovered it was sexual: "The fact that a gross sexual . . . transference occurs in every treatment of a neurosis . . . has always seemed to me the most unshakeable proof that the forces of the neuroses originate in the sexual life" (Freud, 1910/1938). Freud was describing a third element that played an important part in his treatment of a patient—namely, his understanding of the situation or his sexual theory of the origins of the neuroses. In other words, his treatment or its behavioral outcome was a joint function of his motivation to help, a particular technique or skill he used (the free associative method), and his general understanding of the etiology of the neuroses.

As in this particular example, psychologists have shown that the personal determinants of a behavioral outcome can be broken down into motivational variables, skill or trait variables, and cognitive variables (beliefs, expectations, or understandings). A general theory of behavior must include the contribution of all three elements and their interactions, but this book will focus attention primarily on motivation.

• CONSCIOUS INTENTS

Consciously wanting something is an everyday experience. It will be called a conscious intent to have, to get, or to do something. What people tell themselves or others they want to do is closely related to what they will do, provided the intent refers to the here and now. If a man in a clothing store says he wants to buy a shirt, the chances are very good he actually will go to the shirt department and buy a shirt. If a woman in an automobile says she wants to get some gas, her statement of intent is excellent evidence that she will in fact buy gas and not a shirt. Psychological studies have shown that conscious intents in the here and now correlate about .95 with actions taken subsequently in the here and now (Ryan, 1970; Locke & Bryan, 1968). As a recent example of this well-known fact, consider a study reported by Smetana and Adler (1980). The investigators questioned a large number of women awaiting the results of a pregnancy test as to whether they did or did not intend to have an abortion if the test was positive. The stated advance intention of the fifty-nine women with positive tests correlated .96 with whether they had the abortion or not.

The reason such intents predict actions so well in the here and now is that they take into account not only motivation, but also the other determinants of action, as Chapter 6 will show. That is, the environmental determinant is present. The man is in the store; the abortion is available. Also, the skills necessary for performing an act like buying a shirt or going to see a doctor are available. So are the cognitive determinants of the act: the customer understands what a shirt or an abortion is for. Thus, conscious intents are not pure indications of the motivation involved. They are a product of the motivation (including its unconscious aspects, considered later in this chapter) and other determinants of action as well. Historically, however, intents have played an important role in the way psychologists have studied motivation.

Besides demonstrating the obvious point that conscious intents influence actual choices, early psychologists investigated the strength of conscious intents. Narziss Ach (1910) approached this problem by pitting an intent against a well-practiced habit. He had subjects learn a number of pairs of nonsense syllables that rhymed (for example, *dak-tak*). After the subjects had practiced learning these pairs for some time, he would introduce a new set; for example, he would ask the subjects to respond to the first nonsense syllable with its mirror image (*dak-kad*). He wanted to measure the strength of the new intent by discovering how many practice trials on the rhymed association task were necessary to break through the new set. That is, if the first, or rhyming, task had been practiced only a few times, it was easy to maintain the new intent (mirror image learning) without interference from the old one. As the number of practice trials on the first task increased, however, errors from that type of learning crept more readily into the new learning set, interfering with the intent to produce the mirror image of the first nonsense syllable.

Ach thought he was measuring the strength of will by pitting it against an old habit, but Lewin (1935) pointed out that there was an intent involved in the first task also, and that really a conflict existed between two intents. He took the position taken by this book: A habit (for example, an associative link between *A* and *B*) does not contain a motivational force of its own, as some association theorists have argued. Rather, an association is an aspect of the determination of a response that is conceptually distinct from the behavioral intent. Thus, in analyzing Ach's experiment, think in terms of a conflict between the old intent to say *dak-tak* and the new intent to say *dak-kad*.

Conflicts in Conscious Intents

Lewin's interest in the conflict of intents led him and his students to do a number of studies on motivational conflicts. He introduced a very elaborate system of notation for describing motivational forces in a psychological field, only a little of which is relevant here. Table 1.1 illustrates Lewin's contention that the intent, or psychological force, to perform an act was a product of two person variables (need and valence) divided by an environmental variable (psychological distance). *Need* meant the desire for some end state; *valence* meant the reward value of the end state; and *psychological distance* referred to all the difficulties involved in performing a task or in adopting the means necessary to get to the goal. Table 1.1 illustrates how this conceptual model explains the characteristics of different types of motivational conflicts.

Table 1.1.

LEWIN'S MODEL OF MOTIVATIONAL CONFLICTS (after Lewin, 1935)

$$\text{Force toward an action} = \frac{\text{Need} \times \text{Valence}}{\text{Psychological distance}}$$

Approach-approach conflict: deciding whether to stay home and write or go out to the opera.

$$\frac{\text{Needs fame (10)} \times \text{Fame from book (3)}}{\text{Psychological distance in difficulty in writing (6)}} = \frac{30}{6} = 5.$$

$$\frac{\text{Needs music (2)} \times \text{Enjoyment from opera (5)}}{\text{Psychological distance in going out to opera (2)}} = \frac{10}{2} = 5.$$

Avoidance-avoidance conflict: deciding whether to endure Jung's criticisms or the rejection of the scientific world.

$$\frac{\text{Needs scientific accuracy (10)} \times \text{Jung's critique } (-5)}{\text{Psychological distance in accepting Jung (5)}} = \frac{-50}{5} = -10.$$

$$\frac{\text{Needs acceptance of psychoanalysis (10)} \times \text{Anti-Semitic rejection } (-5)}{\text{Psychological distance in correcting Jung (5)}} = \frac{-50}{5}$$
$$= -10.$$

Approach-avoidance conflict: deciding whether to tell the truth or avoid Breuer's disapproval in writing up the Dora case.

$$\frac{\text{Needs scientific accuracy (6)} \times \text{Truth about Dora's sexuality (5)}}{\text{Psychological distance in writing up Dora case (5)}} = \frac{30}{5} = 6.$$

$$\frac{\text{Needs Breuer's friendship (5)} \times \text{Breuer's disapproval } (-6)}{\text{Psychological distance in writing up Dora case (5)}} = \frac{-30}{5} = -6.$$

An approach-approach conflict is unstable and easily solved. The traditional example of a donkey who starved because he was standing equidistant from two equally attractive piles of hay is incorrect. As a further example, suppose Freud is trying to decide whether to stay home and work on his book or go to an opera for the evening; both alternatives hold some attraction for him. If we assign appropriate weights to the variables in Lewin's formula, we can equalize the attractiveness of the two alternatives. On the one hand, he is an ambitious man who needs fame (let us assign that a value of 10) and knows that he will get some fame from publishing this book (3); however, there is considerable difficulty involved in writing (6), which somewhat reduces the overall attractiveness of this alternative. The formula determines the attractiveness of Freud's staying home and writing as $(10 \times 3)/6 = 5$.

On the other hand, Freud may need music (2) less than fame and enjoy the opera (5) somewhat more than writing, but the difficulty in going out to the opera (2) is much less than the difficulty in writing. This increases the attractiveness of this alternative, making its overall attractiveness the same as staying home and writing, or $(2 \times 5)/2 = 5$.

Note, however, that moving in one direction or the other toward either alternative immediately reduces the psychological distance, making that alternative more attractive and solving the conflict. If Freud puts on his coat in preparing to go out, he has reduced the psychological distance to the goal of going to the opera and is likely to continue in that direction. If he starts writing, however, the difficulty associated with that alternative is reduced, making it the likely choice for the evening. All the donkey has to do is accidentally move toward one pile of hay or the other for that choice to be more attractive.

An avoidance-avoidance conflict tends to be very stable. Early in the history of the psychoanalytic movement Freud was pleased to gain the support of an energetic young Swiss psychiatrist, Carl Jung. Freud was very sensitive to the scientific world's rejection of his sexual theories and felt some of the criticism was motivated by anti-Semitism, since all the early psychoanalysts were Viennese Jews. He felt that Jung, who was not Jewish, was a very important ally and arranged for him to be president of the Psychoanalytic Association. However, Jung soon began to differ with Freud and introduce ideas of his own. This put Freud into an avoidance-avoidance conflict. On the one hand, he was very upset by Jung's new ideas, which he felt were wrong and would undermine or dilute his most basic insights.

On the other hand, Freud wanted to avoid the criticism of the community by taking advantage of Jung's value as a non-Jewish supporter of psychoanalysis. As the formulas in Table 1.1 show, Freud's moving toward continuing to accept Jung would decrease the psychological distance in the first alternative, making the reality of Jung's deviationism even more painful. Thus, if he started to do this he would immediately back off, as this alternative would become more unpleasant than the other: $(10 \times -5)/5 = -50/5 = -10)$. On the other hand, if Freud moved toward correcting Jung or even removing him from the Psychoanalytic Association presidency, the reality of rejection by the scientific community would be even stronger. Having moved in this direction, Freud would find it even more unpleasant and would back off again to increase the psychological distance to this alternative. Thus, he would tend to vacillate, trying to avoid first one unpleasant alternative and then the other. This in fact happened over a number of years as Freud tried to resolve this avoidance-avoidance conflict. As Lewin pointed out, avoidance-avoidance conflicts are serious only if a person cannot escape simply by going out of the field and avoiding both. In this case Freud could not escape, because the action to be taken involved either correcting or accepting Jung.

An approach-avoidance conflict also has special characteristics. Consider the case of Freud's deciding whether to tell what he thought to be the truth about the sexual cause for Dora's neurosis or to avoid the disapproval of his mentor,

Josef Breuer, which he was certain would follow if he published his findings. Again, such a conflict is serious only if the same act or goal has both approach and avoidance aspects. If two different goals are involved, the person simply avoids the negative one and approaches the positive one. However, here the same act—writing up the Dora case for publication—would satisfy Freud's scientific needs (approach) but earn Breuer's disapproval, which in the end had less negative valence than his positive push to tell the truth about Dora's sexuality.

Other investigators have shown that as a conflicting goal in a situation like this is approached, the tendency to avoid its negative aspect grows stronger more rapidly than the tendency to approach its positive aspect. Figure 1.1 illustrates the different slope of approach and avoidance gradients. In the original study that demonstrated this difference, J. S. Brown (1948) placed some white rats in harness in a runway and measured the strength with which they pulled toward food or away from shock. One consequence of the difference in slopes is apparent in Figure 1.1. If the approach tendency is very strong, it will get a person very near the goal before he or she recoils in fear; this is not true if the approach tendency is weak. Thus, if a man is still strongly attached to a woman who has rejected him, he will do everything he can to get near her; just as he gets in her presence, however, he will pull back in fear. His fear reaction will be much stronger than it would be if he were not so attached to her, because in that case the fear would have blocked him from approaching her much sooner.

In reference to Figure 1.1, Miller (1951) says,

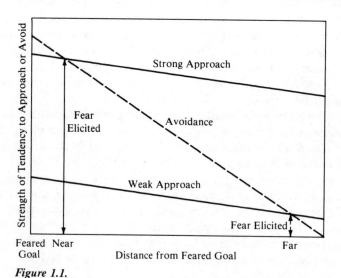

Figure 1.1.

Graphic Representation of an Approach-Avoidance Conflict and of the Effect of Increasing the Strength of the Motivation to Approach (Miller, 1951).

. . . When the point at which the gradients intersect is between the subject and the goal, approach is stronger than avoidance. Therefore, the subject moves toward the goal. When he passes the point of intersection, avoidance becomes stronger than approach; so he stops and turns back. Increasing the strength of the drive motivating approach raises the height of the entire gradient of approach. Since this causes the point of intersection to occur nearer the goal, the subject approaches nearer. Since this nearer point is higher on the gradient of avoidance, more fear is elicited.

These deductions hold only for the range within which the two gradients intersect. It is only for the sake of simplicity that the gradients are represented by straight lines in these diagrams. Similar deductions could be made on the basis of any curves that have a continuous negative slope which is steeper for avoidance than for approach at each point above the abscissa.

Another consequence of the difference in slopes is illustrated by the example of Freud's approach-avoidance conflict given in Table 1.1. Given the equal weights assigned the two tendencies in that case, it would be predicted that Freud would not have written up the Dora case. As he started to write up the Dora case, the threat of Breuer's disapproval would have grown stronger faster than would the positive pull toward explaining the truth about Dora.

Blocked Intent

Lewin and his students also were interested in what happened to an intent when it was interrupted, for it seemed to continue to influence behavior. For instance, Lewin had observed that if he intended to mail a letter, it would continue to "stay in his mind" even while he did other things until he actually had mailed the letter. One of his students, Zeigarnik (1927), showed that tasks that were interrupted tended to be better remembered than tasks that had been completed.

Other investigations dealt with what happens when an interrupted task cannot be resumed. Two possibilities are that the person either finds a substitute way of satisfying the intent or, if none is available, becomes frustrated and engages in disorganized or regressive behavior. For instance, in one study children were shown an attractive toy that was then covered up by a heavy shield with a handle on top. The children showed their intent to get at the toy by trying to lift the heavy cover off. If they could not succeed, they often complained or sat down, cried, and did nothing, showing signs of regression to maladaptive forms of behavior. If they were offered other toys, they might be satisfied with those as substitutes. Much work has been done on the conditions under which children will accept substitutes, regress, or show other forms of maladaptive behavior such as aggression when an intent is interrupted.

Conscious Goal Setting

Probably the most influential work carried out by the Lewin group involved the level of aspiration experiment (Lewin, Dembo, Festinger, & Sears, 1944). These studies deal with the effects of conscious goal setting on behavior. Subjects typically are given a task to perform in a limited period, for example, a page of arithmetic problems to solve in five minutes. At the end of five minutes the subjects observe or are told how many they have correctly solved and then are asked to state how many they are going to try to correctly solve in the next trial. The goal can be stated in terms of what they will "try for," the number they hope to solve, the minimum number they would be satisfied with, and so on. Then they work at the next page of problems, compare their performance with their goal, and set a new goal for the next trial.

Research questions have dealt with the factors that influence the goals set—in particular the discrepancy between the goal and past performance—and also with the effects of various kinds of goals on subsequent performance. It has long been known that conscious goals people set for themselves influence their level of performance. For example, Figure 1.2, based on some early work by Mace (1935), shows the effect on people's work output of trying to do their best versus trying to surpass a specific standard for performance set each day. Clearly the intent to do better improves performance, but intents that are tied to specific goals for improvement over past performance, as shown in the level of aspiration experiment, are even more effective in improving performance.

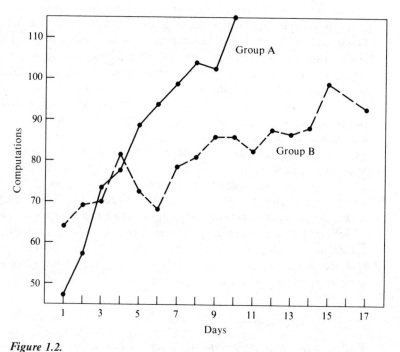

Figure 1.2.

Performance in Computation Under Two Instructions. Group A subjects (10) were instructed to surpass a specific standard prescribed for each day; group B subjects (10) were instructed to do their best to improve, with no specific standard (Mace, 1935, p. 21).

The relation of effort to performance has been confirmed in a different type of experiment: After failure, subjects are asked to explain their poor performance. If they attribute their failure to lack of effort, they are more likely to do better on the next trial (Weiner, Heckhausen, Meyer, & Cook, 1972). Locke and Bryan (1968) attempted to see whether conscious goals have an effect over a longer period of time. They asked college students what grades they hoped to get or would try for in the semester coming up and then correlated the goals set with the grades actually obtained. In general, the correlations were significant but low (around .30), indicating a slight tendency for students who aspired to higher grades to get higher grades. However, it is not possible to be sure that the intent was the causal factor here, because the ability the students had shown in previous school work undoubtedly influenced the goals they set for themselves. Thus, better students would tend both to set higher goals and do better the following semester; it is not possible to infer that the higher goals were responsible for better performance later on. However, Locke and Bryan realized this difficulty and controlled for the ability of the students (for example, for the grades they had obtained in previous semesters); thus, it may reasonably be concluded that trying for higher grades helps a little in getting better grades later in school.

Is Conscious Intent Necessary for Learning?

If conscious goal setting facilitates performance, can it be inferred that it is always necessary to produce performance? Must people always be motivated to some degree to do something before they will do it? This question has never been completely answered to everyone's satisfaction, and we will come across it again and again in different contexts throughout the book. For a time, association theorists argued that simple conditioned responses were obvious examples of learning without intent to learn. Suppose an experimenter sounds a tone just before delivering an air puff to the eye that elicits a blink. After a few trials the blink is conditioned to, or occurs in response to, the tone without the subject's "wanting" to blink. Other theorists pointed out that the blink avoids the unpleasant puff to the eye, so it seems reasonable to infer that it occurs in response to an intent—perhaps not very conscious—to avoid unpleasantness.

Early research on what was called *incidental learning* illustrates the complexity of this type of analysis. Incidental learning research was designed to answer the question of whether learning could occur without any intent to learn. Conscious goal setting or processing of material clearly facilitates performance, as has just been shown, if only because it gets people organized around doing things that will help them remember the material (Kintsch, 1977). But can learning occur incidentally when there is no conscious intent to learn? A typical experiment designed to investigate this problem was conducted by Jenkins (1933). He asked subjects to memorize a list of words read to them by an experimenter. After a number of repetitions he asked not only the subjects, but also the experimenter, to recall as many words as possible. The subjects who intended to learn the words recalled more than the experimenters, but the experimenters also recalled some words, apparently without any intent to remember them.

Many later, similar experiments conducted under a variety of conditions confirmed the two basic facts that conscious intents facilitate learning and that learning often occurs seemingly without conscious intent. Answering the question of whether learning could occur without any intent, however, was difficult, if not impossible, for it was not possible to prove there were no intents of any kind present in instances of incidental learning. When experimenters were asked to report what went on in their minds at the time, they often came up with intents that were not part of their instructions but that were sufficient to explain the learning that occurred. For example, the experimenters in the Jenkins study might have wanted to give meaning to the boring task they were involved in by forming the words into groups to make them easier to say, much as people group telephone numbers to remember them better.

Factors Underlying Conscious Intents

These experiments, like the conditioned blink experiment, raised the question of unconscious intents. Might not subjects be learning under the influence of a motive or intent of which they were unaware? A quite different tradition being established in psychology stressed the vital importance of unconscious intents on learning and memory.

However, this was not the only, or even the chief, difficulty with the psychology of conscious intents. The real problem lay in the fact that focusing on conscious intents did not sufficiently analyze the motivational processes involved. Intents, whether conscious or unconscious, are themselves the outcome of other motivational and nonmotivational variables, as was noted earlier. To focus on the outcome of these variables (the resultant intent) without even considering these variables is to engage in a kind of misplaced concreteness.

In performing a laboratory task, the subjects' motives may not be at all obvious. The experimenter asks the subjects to do something, and they set to work with a conscious intent to perform the task. Yet why do they comply and try hard? Some may want to please the experimenter. Some may want to prove to themselves that they are good learners. Some may fear looking foolish by not being able to perform at all. When the subjects are asked to set a goal (that is, to state their intent), they will be influenced (1) by these motive dispositions, (2) by the extent to which they perceive that doing well and performing the task satisfies these and other dispositions (the value of the task to them), (3) by the perceived difficulty of performing the task (or the skill they have shown in performing), and (4) by the fact that the task is there to be done (the environmental determinant).

The intent that results from such variables should not be confused with the most distinctively motivational aspect of the process, namely, the motive dispositions aroused in the situation. Intent as the outcome of all the determinants of behavior predicts choices in the here and now when the determinants are known and specifiable, but it has much less value for predicting long-range behavioral outcomes when the determinants are not so easy to specify. Thus, a student's statement that he or she intends to study right now will predict behavior fairly well; the same type of statement applied to "studying hard next year," however, should be greeted with some skepticism, because it is not known what attractive alternative courses of action the student will face, whether or not the courses taken will be interesting or not, and so on. Understanding such long-range trends requires paying more attention to stable motive dispositions, which lead to persisting in certain kinds of behavior (such as studying) in spite of a wide variation in the other determinants of action. The psychology of conscious intents in its early form now is largely of historical interest only.

• UNCONSCIOUS INTENTS

If we move out of the laboratory into the clinic and listen to people talking about themselves, the role of stable motive dispositions as determinants of immediate choices or intents becomes more obvious. At the same time, however, some of the motives reflected when people talk about themselves may be more obvious to others than to the people themselves; that is, they appear to be unconscious of them. Freud (1910/1938) commented on his own motives as follows:

> I sacrificed unhesitatingly my budding popularity as a physician and a growing practice in nervous diseases because I searched directly for the sexual origin of their neuroses . . . but the silence which followed my lectures, the void that formed about my person, and the insinuations directed at me, made me realize gradually that statements concerning the role of sexuality in the etiology of the neuroses cannot hope to be treated like other communications . . . but as my conviction of the general accuracy of my observations and the conclusions grew and grew, and as my faith in my own judgement and moral courage were by no means small . . . I was imbued with the conviction that it fell to my lot to discover particularly important connections, and was prepared to accept the fate which sometimes accompanies such discoveries.
>
> This fate I pictured to myself as follows: . . . science would take no notice of me during my lifetime. Some decades later, someone would surely stumble upon the same, now untimely things, compel their recognition and thus, bring me to honor as a forerunner, whose misfortune was inevitable. Meanwhile, I arrayed myself as comfortably as possible like Robinson Crusoe on my lonely island. When I look back to those lonely years, . . . it seems to me like a beautiful and heroic era.

Freud describes himself as having the conscious intent of discovering the sexual basis of neuroses in his patients in his daily practice. However, he explains his persistence despite the attacks of others as being due to two stable motivational dispositions in himself: a strong desire for fame as a scientific pioneer and a weak fear of rejection by his peers (or a strong belief in himself). Like most people, he has formed some clear ideas of his major motives in life. These dispositions not only are of an order of magnitude much greater than the temporary intents dealt with in the laboratory; they also are used to explain such intents, much as Freud explains his daily decisions in terms of his dispositions.

Can we believe him? Our conclusion that he has a strong need for fame already involves an inference that goes somewhat beyond what he says. He insists only that he desires to be scientifically correct, but we infer from the Robinson Crusoe image and his dream of postmortem fame that he truly wants greatness. His protests that he does not care what other people think of him are a little too frequent. We suspect that if he really did not care, he would not mention so often how much he is rejected. And it is Freud who taught us to be wary of believing what other people say about their motivational states or their motivational dispositions!

The major contributions of Freud's early work involved showing how the motives that influence what people do in everyday life are often unconscious. He was particularly ingenious in demonstrating that even the wildest thought sequences in dreams really were motivated by unconscious desires, which he could expose by the technique of psychoanalysis. Here is a simple example:

> "You are always saying that a dream is a wish fulfilled," begins an intelligent lady patient. "Now I shall tell you a dream in which the content is quite the opposite, in which a wish of mine is not fulfilled. How do you reconcile that with your theory? The dream was as follows: *I want to give a supper, but I have nothing available except some smoked salmon. I think I will go shopping, but I remember it is Sunday afternoon, when all the shops are closed. I then try to ring up a few caterers, but the telephone is out of order. Accordingly, I have to renounce my desire to give a supper.* (Freud, 1900/1938)

Freud explains that only she can find the explanation for the dream and that to do so, she should relax and say whatever comes into her mind about the dream. Her first associations have to do with the fact that her husband, who is a capable meat salesman, is growing too fat. He said he should undergo treatment for obesity, rise early, keep to a diet, and "above all, accept no more invitations to supper," which Freud points out contains the idea that her husband gets fat at other people's dinners. The woman then blocks a little in her associations and gives some irrelevant comments, which Freud attributes to unconscious suppression of what is about to come next. She then recalls a visit the day before to a thin female friend her husband admires greatly. "Fortunately this friend is very thin and lanky, and her husband likes full figures." But the friend has spoken to her about her desire to gain weight and asks Freud's patient, "When are you going to invite us again? You always have such good food."

Now the meaning of the dream is clear. The thought that runs in the patient's mind and determines the nature of the dream may be summarized as follows: "Of course I am to invite you to dinner so that you will get fat and be more pleasing to my husband! I would rather give no more dinners!" Why is the dream about smoked salmon? Smoked salmon is her friend's favorite dish. The dream is a simple expression of her wish not to make her friend plumper and more pleasing to her husband. The important point to note is that the patient was quite unaware of this intent when she related the dream, since she thought it disproved Freud's theory of dreams as wish fulfillments.

Forgetting a Proper Name Unintentionally

Freud also illustrated with many examples how conscious intents often do not bring about a desired result. In fact, the interest in his book *The Psychopathology of Everyday Life* (1901/1938) lies precisely in the fact that most people feel their conscious intents control everything they think, feel, and do. Let us examine an example drawn from Freud's own experience. Once when he was traveling by train in Yugoslavia, he fell into conversation with a stranger. They talked about visiting in Italy, and Freud asked if he by any chance had seen the famous frescoes of the Last Judgment in the dome of the cathedral in Orvieto executed by ———. Here Freud could not recall the name of the artist, Signorelli, although he knew it perfectly well and recognized it as soon as someone else mentioned it. Instead he recalled the names of two other artists, Botticelli and Boltraffio, the latter a painter who was much more obscure than Signorelli. In other words, the forgetting could not be attributed to a lack of knowledge. Therefore, it had to be attributed to intent. What unconscious intent could have interfered with the conscious intent to recall the name? To find out, Freud applied his usual technique of free associating to the situation in which he forgot the name.

He first recalled that just prior to the discussion of the frescoes of the Last Judgment in Orvieto, he had been discussing with the stranger the customs of the Turks living in Bosnia and Herzegovina, through which they were passing. Freud had related an anecdote told him by a physician friend about the Turks' being surprisingly resigned at the prospect of death. If the doctor had to tell them there was no hope for a man, they were apt to reply, "Sir, what can I say? I know that if he could be saved, you would save him." Freud next recalled that he also had remembered a second anecdote told him by the physician friend that involved the sexuality of Turks. In contrast to their resignation at the thought of dying, they were in utter despair over impotence. As one of them said to his physician, "For you know, sir, if that ceases, life no longer has any charm" (Freud, 1901/1938). Freud refrained from telling this anecdote to his companion "because I did not wish to touch upon such a delicate theme in conversation with a stranger." Freud inferred that these thoughts about death and sexuality were connected with another concern about death and sexuality that had been occupying his thoughts a good deal at the time, although it did not enter into his consciousness during this episode. These thoughts concerned the suicide of one of his patients in Trafoi over a sexual disturbance. Freud felt his anxiety over his failure as a physician influenced the chain of his associations for a reason that soon will become apparent.

Figure 1.3 shows how Freud explained his forgetting the name Signorelli. The key to this explanation lies in the fact that the first part of the artist's name —*Signor*—has the same meaning in Italian (sir) as the word *Herr* in German, the language Freud was speaking. The word *Herr* (*Signor*) cued off anxiety-

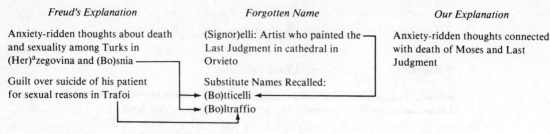

Freud's Explanation	*Forgotten Name*	*Our Explanation*
Anxiety-ridden thoughts about death and sexuality among Turks in (Her)ᵃzegovina and (Bo)snia	(Signor)elli: Artist who painted the Last Judgment in cathedral in Orvieto	Anxiety-ridden thoughts connected with death of Moses and Last Judgment
Guilt over suicide of his patient for sexual reasons in Trafoi	Substitute Names Recalled: (Bo)tticelli (Bo)ltraffio	

ᵃ*Herr* (sir) in German has the same meaning as *signor* in Italian.

Figure 1.3.

Associative Connections in Freud's Forgetting a Proper Name.

ridden thoughts about death and sexuality, since it was associated with *Her-zegovina*, in which the Turks lived and with two anecdotes, one relating to the death of a patient, and the other relating to sexuality among the Turks, which he had determined not to report.

Thus, Freud believed that his desire not to say something interfered with his desire to say something associated with it via the connection of both associations with anxiety over thoughts about death and sexuality. The substitute names of artists he thought of confirmed this analysis. The first syllable in both of them (*Bo*) refers to Bosnia, the other location in which the Turks lived. He regarded this as evidence that *Signor* had cued off thoughts about Turks, since the substitute names referred to another nonthreatening region associated with the Turks. The *elli* of *Botticelli* obviously came from the last part of *Signorelli,* and the last part of the obscure name *Boltraffio* he traced to his guilt over the suicide of his patient at Trafoi. He believed that forces of both conscious suppression and unconscious repression were involved. He consciously suppressed the intent to tell an anecdote about Turkish sexuality, but the screen name Boltraffio indicated to him that his thoughts about death and sexuality among the Turks also had touched on his guilt over the suicide of a patient in Trafoi.

Dozens of analyses of episodes like this convinced Freud and his followers in the psychoanalytic movement that unconscious intents had to be taken into account in explaining human behavior, particularly abnormal or unusual behavior. Laboratory psychologists simply ignored the evidence or explained it away as due to chance or associative interference. However, we must go further than Freud did in analyzing this phenomenon, because we have argued that momentary intents, whether conscious or unconscious, are themselves products of stable motive dispositions and other factors. Freud analyzes this episode entirely in terms of thoughts and feelings he had at the time, yet might not these in turn have been shaped by his dominant motive dispositions? Figure 1.3 also indicates that another explanation for Freud's forgetting the name Signorelli can be given based on a fuller knowledge of his life story.

Unconscious Motives in Freud

A further look into Freud's life and deepest convictions can illustrate his teaching that unconscious motives shape even the most ordinary acts, such as forgetting a name. It also can illustrate the methods he used in making such analyses. Freud was strongly committed to rationality, to the scientific method, and to making psychology into a natural science. Yet as David Bakan (1958) makes clear, the psychoanalytic approach Freud evolved had much in common with an ancient Jewish religious tradition that was anything but scientific and rational. This tradition involves mystical ideas about the nature of God and goes back at least to the first century A.D. By the eleventh century it was referred to as Kabbala, a mystical tradition of textual and oral communications involving the revelation of meanings hidden in the scriptures. The Kabbalists searched for hidden meanings. They found wisdom in explaining secrets just as Freud explained the secret meaning of dreams and symptomatic acts. Kabbalistic thinking played a role in messianic movements that swept the Jewish community in the seventeenth and eighteenth centuries. Charismatic leaders appeared and convinced many Jews that the messiah had come who would lead them out of the bonds of oppression and into a life of joy and union here and now with God.

The movements were branded as heretical by Orthodox Jewish rabbinical leaders, but the enthusiastic antirational tendencies they engendered survived in Chassidism, a movement that centered originally on Baal Shem-Tov, a man of magical healing powers and much folk wisdom, although technically he was an "ignoramus," that is, not trained in Jewish law and tradition. To nineteenth-century Viennese Jews of Freud's circle, Chassidism had a number of bad associations. It evoked thoughts of heresy, unseemly enthusiasm, the weird mystical ideas of uneducated people, and rejection of the scholarly rationality characteristic of Orthodox Judaism. It is small wonder that Freud wanted no connection made between what he was doing and the traditions of Jewish mysticism.

As noted already, however, the tradition emphasized, above all, penetrating secrets. So did Freud. The method used for discovering secret wisdom was described by a thirteenth-century Jewish mystic, Abraham Abulafia, as "skipping and jumping." By this he meant almost exactly what Freud meant by free associating on a text. In this way a person can penetrate beyond the outer meaning of a word of scripture (what Freud called the *manifest content*) to its inner meaning (Freud's *latent content*) much as one removes the shell of a nut to get at its kernel (Scholem, 1966).

The most important book in the mystical tradition came to be the *Zohar,* prepared in part by Moses de León in the thirteenth century. It conceived of the Torah (Jewish scripture) as a living organism. The Torah has a head, a body, a heart, a mouth, and so on (Scholem, 1966). Thus, the idea is clearly present that uncovering the truth about the Torah also uncovers the truth about man. Uncovering the truth about people by penetrating their thoughts and dreams is exactly what Freud thought he was doing. To Bakan it hardly seemed an accident that Freud chose the name Dora (pronounced like *Torah*) as the name for his earliest, most famous case for illustrating the method of his psychoanalysis.

Furthermore, the sexual metaphor is used throughout the *Zohar* for interpreting the ultimate meaning of life. "The soul, according to the Zohar, has an unquenchable yearning to be united with its source in God. This union is characteristically discussed in the metaphor of sex. . . . Thus human sexual relations become symbolic vehicles of divine acts. . . . Freud's use of the idiom of sexuality as the basic one for the expression of all the deeper and more profound problems of mankind is entirely in the spirit of the Kabbala" (D. Bakan, 1958). In this tradition, the ultimate form of secret knowledge is uncovering the fundamental sexuality of the universe. Mystical union with God is represented, again using the sexual metaphor, as union with the Holy Shekinah, or the female, maternal aspect of God (D. Bakan, 1958). The Hebrew word for "knowledge" used in this context also means "sexual knowledge," as is clear in the King James translation of the Hebrew biblical text when it states in Genesis that Adam "knew" his wife Eve, that is, "knew" her sexually.

Finally, the Jewish mystical tradition was antiestablishment, just as psychoanalysis was. It represented a revolt against patriarchal rabbinical authority; Freud, as an apostate Jew, often felt himself in a similar rebellious frame of mind. Although he remained identified with the Jewish community, he rejected Judaism as a religion. In fact, he conspicuously violated the First Commandment brought down by the father of Judaism, Moses, from the mountain: "The Lord thy God is a jealous god, thou shall have no other gods before me." Freud filled his consulting room with statues and other images of gods from many other religions. There is ample reason to believe, as Bakan points out, that Freud was somewhat ambivalent about his rebellion and that he specifically feared the wrath of Moses.

Freud describes at length his feelings when standing in front of the huge statue of Moses by Michelangelo in a church in Rome. Moses has returned from the mountain with the tablets containing the Commandments only to discover that the Jews are worshiping false gods. Looking at the seated Moses, Freud thinks to himself, "In his first transport of fury Moses desired to act, to spring up and take vengeance and forget the tablets (the Law) but he has overcome the temptation and he will now remain seated and still in his frozen wrath." Freud also says he felt "of the mob upon whom Moses' eye is turned." The text makes it clear that Freud felt he himself had some reason to fear the wrath of Moses.

What Freud does not mention is that as visitors enter the long, narrow church of San Pietro in Vinculi, where the statue of the seated Moses is placed at the back on the right side, they must pass on the left a vivid reminder of the death and destruction involved in the Last Judgment for all people. The entire wall is a huge collection of skeletons, skulls, and bones together with the Grim Reaper, which serves to remind the observer as vividly as possible of the Last Judgment. Was Freud to be punished for his revolt against Moses, the symbol of Orthodoxy—not just as an apostate Jew, but as a psychoanalyst arguing for freedom against the excesses "of the Mosaic type law which made for neurosis" (D. Bakan, 1958)?

The meaning of this deep-seated conflict in Freud's life is revealed by a visit to the Sistine Chapel, which contains some of the most famous paintings in

Rome. Certainly Freud knew about these paintings, as art and Rome had fascinated him from boyhood. The paintings suggest another reason why Freud forgot the name of the artist responsible for the frescoes of the Last Judgment in the cathedral in Orvieto. The dominant theme in the Sistine Chapel once again is the Last Judgment, represented in a huge mural painted by Michelangelo at the front end of the room. However, as a person enters the room through a small door at the rear, the first painting seen is the Death of Moses by Signorelli, the very painter whose name Freud forgot in connection with another representation of the Last Judgment. Furthermore, right next to this scene is one representing the punishment of the Cores (maidens), by Botticelli, whose name Freud thought of as a substitute for Signorelli.

Thus, it might be argued that the name Signorelli had a negative significance for Freud that went far beyond its casual link with some talk about Turks living in the neighborhood through which he was passing on a train. Signorelli also painted one of the most famous pictures of the death of Moses, who, Freud had argued, had been killed by apostate Jews like himself. In Freud's view that was why Moses had never seen the Promised Land. Thus, he had reason to fear the Last Judgment and to be anxious about any associations involving his profound revolt against religious Orthodoxy, as represented by Moses. Freud's theory of the Oedipus complex dealt with the guilt a son feels over his incestuous desires for his mother and his desire to kill his father. Symbolically Freud was worshiping false gods (that is, the Shekinah represented as female in the Jewish mystical tradition), killing Moses, and defying rational authority. No wonder the name of the renowned painter (Signorelli) of the scene representing the death of Moses had an unusually negative connotation for him—so much so that he was unable to recall it when thinking about the Last Judgment in another connection.

To return to Figure 1.3, another anxiety-ridden thought can be added that could have blocked Freud's ability to recall the name of the painter of the Last Judgment in the cathedral in Orvieto: Signorelli was associated with painting the death of Moses, which evoked Freud's anxiety over his rebellion against Mosaic authority.

So we have succeeded, using Freud's approach, in relating his momentary unconscious intent to avoid thinking of a name to a deeper, stable motive disposition in his life involving guilt and anxiety over his rebellion against established patriarchal authority.

Conclusions to Be Drawn from Freud's Approach to Motivational Analysis

What are we to make of this kind of motivational analysis? Has it any more than a historical interest as an explanation of one of the main traditions that has shaped modern motivational psychology? The following conclusions seem justifiable:

1. What people say about their motives should not be taken at face value. Even in ordinary life, but particularly in dreams and symptomatic acts, people often do not know what their motives are. When they do assign motives to their

acts, these motives, on further analysis, may turn out to be incorrect. Even Freud's motivational analyses should not be taken at face value: by examining his life a little further, we found a motivational explanation for his forgetting a name that was somewhat different from the explanation he was satisfied with.

2. Associative thought is extraordinarily fluid and easily influenced by conscious or unconscious motivational forces. What is striking about many of Freud's analyses is how quickly and automatically a thought or associative chain is deflected by a motivational influence, whether it leads the dreamer to imagine the telephone is out of order or leads Freud to forget the name of a famous painter. As Freud himself noted on another occasion, the overall impression that these observations create is that we are not complete masters in our own household. The mind functions quite easily and efficiently without our being in conscious control of it. And fantasy or free association, over which we exercise little control, reveals most obviously and easily motivational forces of which we may be unaware.

3. The ultimate motivation is not necessarily sexual, as Freud argued, although it is understandable why sexual motives were so important to him if he was drawing on Kabbalistic, mystical insights into the ultimate nature of man. Many others who associated with him early, like Carl Jung and Alfred Adler, insisted on the importance of other nonsexual motives, as Chapter 2 will discuss. In analyzing Freud's own life, we had to resort to power rather than sexual motivational dispositions. On the one hand, he showed a strong need for power in his dreams of fame and in his break with orthodox scientific and religious tradition; on the other hand, he clearly feared the power of others, from Moses to his scientific peers. The power motive will be discussed in Chapter 8.

4. The method of uncovering unconscious intents by analyzing free associations is not completely convincing. Whereas it often yields interesting explanations of otherwise puzzling behaviors, the chance exists that the explanation has been invented through free associations to please the psychoanalyst. What criteria are there for deciding whether an interpretation is correct? The ordinary ones are that the interpretation account for a number of otherwise inexplicable facts and that it satisfy the person who arrives at the interpretation. Thus, Freud was satisfied with his account of forgetting the name Signorelli, but we were not and pursued the matter further to locate a somewhat different explanation. We need a less-questionable method of establishing the truth about the influence of unconscious intents.

• EXPERIMENTAL STUDY OF UNCONSCIOUS MOTIVES

Experimental psychologists interested in the influence of unconscious intents have studied the effects of known unconscious intents on behavior, particularly fantasy. They then are not caught in the logically awkward position of trying to reason backward from effects to causes. For example, they have sometimes induced unconscious intents under hypnosis. A hypnotized woman is told that after she is awakened from the trance state she will meet and talk with another person she finds dull and uninteresting. She also is told she will have forgotten when she awakes whatever went on during hypnosis. She meets the stranger, starts talking with him, and after a while asks him to "shut the bore," thus displaying exactly the kind of slip of the tongue that Freud claimed unconscious intents produced.

Since whether the hypnotized person has really forgotten what she has been told can be questioned, the matter has been pursued further in experimental settings. Some overweight and normal weight undergraduates were asked to write imaginative stories in response to pictures shown on slides. One of the pictures showed two men and what was clearly a piece of steak, as was reported by nearly all subjects. However, one overweight subject who had reported in another situation that she was struggling hard to keep from overeating told a story about two men and a *snake* they had found on an island. There was no hint in the manifest content of the story that she had recognized the object in the slide as anything edible, but her fear of overeating had apparently led her to perceive a dangerous object that rhymed with the word *steak*.

Other studies have aroused intents experimentally to see whether their effects on fantasy are what Freud said they would be. Since Freud argued that sexual motivations were particularly likely to distort the associative flow, Clark (1955) arranged to have slides of nude pinup girls shown to a group of male undergraduates in a psychology class as part of a study they were told was to determine what features of the body were associated with attractiveness. Another control group of subjects was shown an equivalent number of slides of landscape scenes and buildings they were told were part of an investigation on factors affecting aesthetic judgment. Both groups of subjects then wrote imaginative stories based on pictures they were told were part of another study on creative imagination. All these stories were coded for the presence of manifest sexual imagery or for sex symbolism without knowledge of which group of slides the subjects had been exposed to. Manifest sexual imagery included references to sexual intercourse, kissing, dancing, fondling, or being in love.

Clark presumed the young men exposed to the nude slides would be more sexually aroused than those exposed to pictures of buildings. However, the amount of explicit or manifest sexual imagery in the stories from the aroused group was significantly *lower* than in the stories from the control group. This might be taken as evidence for Freud's position, namely, that unconscious sexual intents automatically elicit censorship, which tends to block out conscious thoughts about sex. Otherwise, why would young men who had just been made to think about sex subsequently think less often about sexual matters? Is it possible that they became bored or satiated with the subject? To be sure that this was not the case, and that they actually were more sexually aroused, it was necessary to conduct two further studies.

In one, the experiment was repeated by Clark (1955), but at a fraternity beer party rather than in the classroom. The nude slides or the landscape scenes were introduced accidentally by a stooge as something he owned and was showing to add to the fun of the party. Under party conditions the amount of sexual imagery in stories written after both the control and nude slides were shown was significantly higher than under classroom conditions. Apparently the alcohol and party setting together increased thoughts about sex, but the average amount of sexual imagery in the stories after seeing the nude slides was significantly higher than after seeing the landscape slides. This finding later was confirmed by Kalin, Kahn, and McClelland (1965) using an attractive female model as the sexually arousing stimulus in a controlled party setting. Sexual arousal of young males decreases the manifest sexual content of thought under conventional social conditions but increases it in party settings when alcohol is served. This confirms Freud's contention that unconscious (or even conscious) sexual intents often inhibit or disturb associative thought processes.

Freud also argued that the unconscious intents continue to operate by producing symptoms (screen names, apparently chance acts, and disguised wishes) from which can be inferred the presence of unconscious intent. This means that sexual arousal in the young men, while blocked from direct expression, would show itself through more thoughts of a disguised sexual nature. Therefore, Clark scored all the stories he obtained for sexual symbolism, using the criteria that by now are standard in the literature (see, for example, Gutheil, 1939; Hall, 1953). In general, sex symbols refer to objects that share key characteristics with sexual body parts (round objects = breasts; a long object = penis; a window or door as an entry point = vagina; and so on). In Clark's scoring, classic symbols had to be involved in some *action* that could be regarded as symbolically sexual. For example, if in response to a picture of a person silhouetted in a window, a person wrote "that this was a boy looking out of his dormitory *window*," this was not scored as symbolic. If the person described a thief *"climbing up* to go through the *window* in order to steal the *jewels* in the *house*," this was scored "as referring symbolically to sexual intercourse" (Clark, 1955).

Figure 1.4 plots the sexual symbolism score against the manifest sex score for young males under the sexually aroused and controlled conditions. Note first of all that the overall amount of sexual symbolism was considerably and significantly higher for the sexually aroused subjects than the control subjects. That is, the dotted line is higher than the solid line at every point in the two curves. This is what Freud would have predicted: sexual arousal not only blocks manifest expression, but it also promotes disguised expression of the intent. Note next that on the right side of the graph, if the manifest sex score is low, the sex symbolism score tends to be much higher in the aroused group. This also is consistent with Freud's interpretation of a blocked intent seeking an indirect expression.

However, one finding shown in the figure is not consistent with Freud's argument: subjects whose stories showed a great deal of manifest sexual content also included much sexual symbolism (the left side of the graph). This is consistent with a theory advocated by Hall (1953), who has maintained that "sexual symbolism in dreams is not a disguised expression of sex, the purpose of the disguise being to smuggle the content past the censor, but rather a means of representing as clearly as possible a particular conception of sexuality that the dreamer has in mind. One of several cogent reasons that Hall has for offering

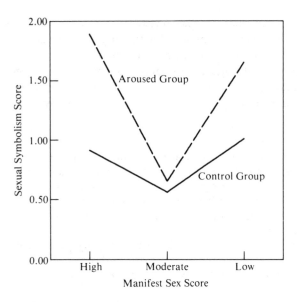

Figure 1.4.

Sexual Symbolism Score as a Function of Manifest Sex Score for the Aroused and Control Groups of the Nonalcohol Condition (Clark, 1955).

his alternative theory is that in his collection of dreams he often found both manifest and symbolic expressions of sexual activity in the same dream or in the same sequence of dreams" (Clark, 1955).

Why disguise sexual content if in the next moment it is revealed in manifest form? According to the results shown in Figure 1.4, both Freud and Hall appear to be correct. For some subjects sexual arousal apparently causes anxiety, which blocks manifest sex but allows disguised expression of the sexual arousal. For other subjects sexual arousal does not arouse anxiety, and the sexual drive expresses itself in both manifest and disguised or metaphoric terms. The general conclusion can be drawn, however, from Figure 1.4 that a sex symbolism score is a better indicator than overt sexual content of the presence of aroused sexual intents or motives for both types of people.

• ARE UNCONSCIOUS MOTIVES IMPORTANT?

These studies demonstrate that what Freud said did happen can happen. However, this is not the same as saying it happens very often. As a practical matter, need we worry about the way unconscious motives influence our everyday behavior, or can we assume that such phenomena occur only under very unusual circumstances? Gordon Allport (1953) was very concerned that the preoccupation with unconscious motives that developed in psychiatry following Freud might engender "a kind of contempt for the 'psychic surface' of life. The individual's conscious report is rejected as untrustworthy . . . the individual loses his right to be believed." Allport recognizes unconscious motives have to be taken into account for some people, particularly neurotic people, but generally speaking such motives can be ignored and what people say their motives are can be believed:

> The patient should be assumed insightful until he has proved otherwise. If you asked a hundred who go to the icebox for a snack why they did so, probably all would answer, "Because I was hungry." In 99 of these cases we may—no matter how deeply we explore—discover that this simple, conscious report is the whole truth. It can be taken at its face value. In the 100th case, however, our probing shows that we are dealing with a compulsive overeater, with an obese seeker after infantile security who, unlike the majority of cases, does not know what he is seeking—perhaps his mother's bosom—and not the leftover roast. In this case—and in a minority of all cases—I grant that we cannot take the evidence of his overt behavior, nor his account of it, at their face value.

Is Allport right that we can ignore unconscious motivations except for a few aberrant cases? Combs (1947) carried out a study that sheds some light on this issue. He had students write out full autobiographies and also write twenty stories to the pictures in Murray's Thematic Apperception Test (TAT). The idea behind the test is to sample fantasies or daydreams of the type Freud was interested in to find out what kinds of motives were on people's minds when they were not consciously reporting on their own desires. (See Chapters 2 and 6 for a fuller description of the TAT.) Combs then coded all the desires that appeared either in the TAT or the autobiography according to about twenty different categories. First he ranked the frequency with which various desires appeared in the autobiography and in the TAT stories. The correlation between these two rank orders was .74, indicating that there was considerable agreement between the direct and indirect measures as to the frequency with which various motives were mentioned.

Combs then observed whether a particular motive was mentioned by any given individual in the TAT stories alone, in the autobiography alone, or both. Table 1.2 illustrates some of his most important results. It shows that a number of desires were mentioned exclusively in the TAT. They included "to die" and "to atone," "to have sexual relations with," "to be accepted," and "to avoid blame." Allport clearly overestimated the frequency with which undesirable motives appear in consciousness. Even among normal people, a number of desires do not regularly appear in the conscious reports of motives. These desires do appear, however, in fantasies produced in the TAT. An area of overlap lies "in the milder, or expected desires of the average individual for security, response, recognition and pleasant occupation" (Combs, 1947). The TAT deals more often in "socially unacceptable and violent kinds of motivation." The autobiography, on the other hand, "emphasizes the socially acceptable, normal and expected more

Table 1.2.

NUMBER OF INDIVIDUALS SHOWING SIGNIFICANT DIFFERENCES FOR EACH ITEM OF THE DESIRES LIST IN ANALYSIS OF TAT AND AUTOBIOGRAPHY (after Combs, 1947)

Item	Appears in TAT Only	Appears in TAT and Autobiography	Appears in Autobiography Only	Number of Difference	In Favor Of
Sexual relation with	20	2	3	17	T
To die	17	0	0	17	T
To atone	17	1	0	17	T
To avoid struggle	16	3	0	16	T
To be with	15	4	2	13	T
To abandon	16	1	4	12	T
To avoid death	9	0	0	9	T
To protect	10	1	1	9	T
To know	12	9	3	9	T
To be consoled	17	4	8	9	T
To defy convention	8	1	0	8	T
To care for	17	4	10	7	T
To have sensuous experience	12	4	5	7	T
To have child	8	6	2	6	T
To punish	10	9	5	5	T
To control	12	6	7	5	T
To assist	12	6	7	5	T
To have means to	15	4	10	5	T
To believe in	12	3	8	4	T
To maintain relations with	14	9	10	4	T
To do as admired person wishes	15	7	11	4	T
To play	14	7	10	4	T
To do one's duty	12	9	10	2	T
To keep	9	0	6	2	T
To have mental peace	9	12	8	1	T
To be attractive to	11	9	10	1	T
To be safe	11	8	11	0	Neither
To maintain status quo	11	4	11	0	Neither
To belong	11	7	11	0	Neither
To avoid illness	4	1	6	2	B
To be married	9	9	11	2	B
To be loved	6	14	8	2	B
To be helped	9	8	11	2	B
To avoid restriction	9	12	11	2	B
To accomplish	10	11	13	3	B

Table 1.2. (Continued).

Item	Appears in TAT Only	Appears in TAT and Autobiography	Appears in Autobiography Only	Number of Difference	In Favor Of
To be respected	10	9	13	3	B
To avoid pain	4	1	7	3	B
To avoid blame	7	11	12	5	B
To be accepted	10	8	16	6	B
To overcome a handicap	7	2	15	8	B
Totals	456	227	286		

Note: Significance is defined here as any desire whose frequency for an individual is greater than the average frequency for the entire groups of subjects.

often than the TAT" (Combs, 1947). Any general theory of motivation must take both conscious and unconscious motives into account.

NOTES AND QUERIES

1. Philosophers always have divided the mind into several parts, just as we argued in this chapter that three different aspects of the mind must be taken into account in explaining behavior—motives, cognitions (understandings and beliefs about what is going on), and skills. One of the oldest controversies concerns the relative importance of motivation and reason. In the Middle Ages, church fathers argued that *nihil volitum nisi cognitum* (nothing is wanted unless it is understood). In other words, understanding, a cognitive variable, produces desires. The Freudian revolution seemed for a time to reverse the order of importance in insisting that cognitions were largely shaped by desires. Today psychology once again asserts the importance of reason, or the cognitive variables (Abelson, 1981). What is the best evidence for thinking that a motivational or dynamic component that is important in its own right as a determinant of behavior must be attributed to the mind?

2. Plato divided the mind into three parts: the desiring element, the reasoning element, and the spirited element (which became known as the *will* for other scholars). What has become of the will in our threefold division of the mind? Has it been left out, or is it an aspect of some other component? If strength of will cannot be measured the way Ach measured it, how can it be measured?

3. If setting a conscious goal reflects motivational and nonmotivational determinants of behavior, how can a pure measure of the motivational determinant alone be obtained? Why are dreams supposedly purer measures of motivational determinants?

4. When you first wake up, write out as completely as you can a dream you had that night. Later try free associating to it, as Freud suggested, to see if you arrive at a satisfactory explanation for why you dreamed as you did.

5. Make a list of some of the goals that are most important to you. Try to rank them in order from most important to least important. After you have completed the list of goals, write down different things you have spent time thinking about lately. Again rank them from those you have spent the most to the least time thinking about. Then try to match up what you have been thinking about with your goals. Is there a close fit? If there have been things you have been thinking about that do not seem related to your goals, can you explain your thoughts in terms of other goals? If certain goals are not related to any of your thoughts, what does that mean? For a reference on method, see Klinger, Barta, and Maxeiner (1980).

6. Laboratory studies of motivation seem dull compared with the analyses of motive trends in people's lives like the analysis of Freud's motives. Some psychologists focus entirely on the experimental, and others on the clinical, psychodynamic approach to motivation. What are some of the advantages and disadvantages of each approach?

7. Just because people write imaginative stories that contain more references to socially undesirable motives than their autobiographies do, does that mean people actually are influenced more often by such motives? How can you tell that the motives a person attributes to someone in a story also characterize the person writing the story? Freud's female patient accepted his interpretation of the motivation behind her dream, but is acceptability a safe criterion for establishing the truth of an interpretation? What other criteria are there for establishing that the motive attributed to a character in a story also belongs to the person writing the story?

8. Write some stories to pictures of the type used in the TAT. Try to determine if the concerns the characters have in the stories are in any way related to your concerns. Be careful not to be misled by superficial differences between your life and the lives you describe in the stories. For example, a woman wrote a story about a young man who led an irresponsible, dissolute life in which he wasted his inheritance. She felt this story in no way related to her because (1) it was about a man and she was a woman; and (2) she was not leading a dissolute life: quite the contrary, she felt she was leading a careful, well-controlled life, so how could his motivations be hers? When she was asked if she were concerned about waste, however, her face lit up and she replied, "But of course. That is what I worry about above everything else."

   When you write the stories, put aside analytic thoughts, relax, and write spontaneously whatever comes into your mind. Obviously, if you worry about what your writing will reveal or attempt to control what you write about, your stories will not give you a very accurate picture of what you are concerned about. Save the stories you have written. You will have opportunities to analyze them later, after methods of coding such stories have been explained in subsequent chapters.

2

Motives in the Personality Tradition

Students of personality have been primarily interested in motivational dispositions in the individual. They have asked, What motives are there? How many are there? What are the most important motives? How do we know what motives a person has? This chapter's goal is to provide an overview of the answers to such questions that motivational theorists have given and, in particular, to consider how motives might be measured in people. Let us begin with the phenomena that have led theorists to assign motive dispositions to people.

• MOTIVES AS REASONS FOR
WHAT PEOPLE SPEND THEIR TIME DOING

To a considerable extent there is a theory of motivation to go with every field of human endeavor. We observe that people do various things frequently and infer that therefore they must want to do them. People eat; therefore, they must want to eat. Some people do well in school, so we infer they have a need for academic success. Children play; therefore, they must have a need to play. Some people save; therefore, there must be a saving drive. People in business often work hard, and since business is organized around making a profit, economic theorists from the time of Karl Marx to the present have assumed they work because of the profit motive. In fact, a modern theorist like John Kenneth Galbraith (1967) has not hesitated to write a chapter in a book on economics entitled "The General Theory of Motivation" based on his observations of the various goals of economic enterprise.

Similarly, those who study politics infer that people have a desire to dominate one another, since they often fight political battles or actual wars in which people kill one another. By way of contrast, those who observe family life find there is a need to nurture and protect human beings.

What are we to make of all of this confusion? Is it possible to bring any order out of chaos and arrive at a list of a few basic human motives? Some theorists always have been skeptical about such a possibility. In thinking about the problem, U.S. personality theorist Abraham Maslow (1954), for example, concluded that "we should give up the attempt once and for all to make atomistic lists of drives or needs. . . . If we wished, we could have such a list of drives containing anywhere from one to one million drives, depending entirely on the specificity of analysis."

Anthropologists have been particularly likely to take this point of view, since they have observed that different cultures value different things, and therefore that what people want obviously varies from culture to culture. They reason that it would be impossible to discover a set of motives of importance that applied to all cultures. Some clinicians working with individuals have felt the same way. Each person appears to have a uniquely different set of motivational needs. Why not just spend time discovering them and stop worrying about whether or not they are similar to those discovered in other individuals? As U.S. personality theorist Gordon Allport (1937) was fond of saying, there are no simple sovereign motives common to all men. Each person is unique, just as each culture is unique.

Before we give up altogether trying to find motives of general significance, let us examine more critically the process of identifying motives that has just been described. First, to say that because people do something they must want to do it is little more than animistic thinking. It is like saying that because a plant grows it wants to grow, or because the apple falls it wants to fall. As Heckhausen (1980) and others have long argued, such a naming process is tautologous. It adds nothing of scientific value to our understanding of what is going on unless we have some independent way of measuring the alleged motive behind the behavior.

Second, we must remember, as Chapter 1 pointed out, that motives are only one determinant of behavior. If we consider a particular behavioral outcome such as eating, the hunger drive is only one of the reasons that explain it. People also eat because they know how to eat (the skill or habit determinant) and because it is time to eat or they think it is good for them to eat (the value determinant). In fact, they may eat for these reasons when they are not hungry at all. Thus, we cannot automatically infer a motive to perform an act from the performance of the act itself. Above all, we cannot infer exactly what general motive lies behind performing the act, since the same act can be motivated by several different drives. Thus, if students study hard in college, we do not know whether it is because they want to please their parents, because they want to do a good job, or because they want to earn social recognition. To infer simply that they have a "studying motive" is to commit the "naming" fallacy, which if pursued would create a long list of motives so specific they would have little value in explaining a wide variety of behavioral phenomena.

If we keep in mind that along with motives, values also influence behavior, we can escape the conclusion that there can be no general motives, since cultures differ so much in what they consider important. It is primarily cultures that influence values, and it is still possible to think in terms of a general human motive, such as the need for achievement—for doing something better (see Chapter 7)—which is expressed differently depending on variations in what the culture values. For example, mainland U.S. citizens appear to be more oriented toward individualistic success or achievement compared with native Hawaiians, who appear to value interpersonal relations more (Gallimore, 1981). Thus, it is possible that the achievement motive might be more engaged for Hawaiians in a collaborative situation than it would be for other U.S. citizens. Thus, some of the proliferation of motive concepts derives from a confusion between values and motives. What people value is in no way simply related to their motives, as will be shown later.

As another example of this fact, consider the so-called profit motive. Karl Marx argued over one hundred years ago in the *Communist Manifesto* that it was the profit motive that drove the capitalist class around the world seeking its advantage. Modern U.S. business executives agree it is the profit motive that drives their behavior. All this means is that such people *believe* the profit motive drives their behavior. That is, they *value* making a profit. It does not follow that profit actually is what motivates them to energetic entrepreneurial behavior. A belief in the profit motive certainly helps determine behavior. It may make business executives decide they are in favor of a tax cut to stimulate business.

However, it is fairly easy to demonstrate that it cannot be profit that motivates the sustained energetic behavior of business executives for two simple reasons. First, as Andrew Carnegie discovered somewhat to his surprise years ago, business executives often continue to work as hard as ever long after they have made as much money as they can possibly use. Something other than profit must be driving them. Second, there is no profit for the individual business executive in the Communist system as it has developed in the Soviet Union, yet many Soviet business executives behave just as energetically as their Western counterparts. The emphasis on profit, therefore, represents a kind of misplaced concreteness that easily can be shown not to be a very good way of describing what motivates business executives. Many of the motives that have been attributed to people in everyday life turn out to represent the naming fallacy, misplaced concreteness, or a confusion between what people value or believe in and the motives that energize their behavior.

McDougall's Classification of Motives

An early attempt was made by psychologist William McDougall (1908, 1932) to avoid these difficulties and separate motives from other human characteristics. He argued that certain behavioral tendencies (that is, propensities) were inherited, instinctive, and "common to men of every race and age." He defined an *instinct* as consisting of (1) a tendency toward selective perception of certain stimuli (a hungry person perceives food objects more readily than other objects), (2) a corresponding emotional excitement experienced on perceiving the object (the root of the instinct), and (3) the activation of a tendency to seek a goal. McDougall (1908) said, "Every instance of instinctive behavior involves a knowing of some thing or object, a feeling in regard to it, and a striving towards or away from the object." Put simply, his idea was that certain actions or objects innately give rise to emotional excitement, which leads to goal-directed activities. These goal-directed activities could be called *motives,* although he called them *instincts* or *propensities.* Other activities or objects did not create emotional excitement and hence did not qualify as motives.

McDougall went further and tried to identify the main instinctive propensities that drive normal behavior. Some typical examples from his last list of eighteen propensities (McDougall, 1932) are summarized in Table 2.1. His emphasis on the instinctive basis of all motives occurred during a historical period in academic psychology, when the behaviorist view was dominant and stated that nearly all human characteristics are learned and not based on inherited or innate tendencies. Therefore, McDougall had little influence at the time. Most psychologists, while willing to admit that a few physiological needs, such as hunger, were innate, felt that more complex motives, such as the need for submission or

---

Table 2.1.

SOME INSTINCTIVE PROPENSITIES (MOTIVES) IDENTIFIED BY McDOUGALL (1932)

---

1. Food-seeking propensity: to seek (and perhaps store) food.
2. Disgust propensity: to reject and avoid certain noxious substances.
3. Sex propensity: to court and mate.
4. Fear propensity: to flee; to cower in response to violent impressions that inflict or threaten pain or injury.
5. Curiosity propensity: to explore strange places and things.
6. Protective and parental propensity: to feed, protect, and shelter the young.
7. Gregarious propensity: to remain in company with fellows and, if isolated, to seek that company.
8. Self-assertive propensity: to domineer, to lead, to assert oneself over, or display oneself before one's fellows.
9. Submissive propensity: to defer, to obey, to follow, or to submit in the presence of others who display superior powers. . . .

13. Acquisitive propensity: to acquire, possess, and defend whatever is found useful and attractive. . . .

---

acquisition, were acquired and not innate in everyone. It was not until much later, when ethologists introduced the notion of "sign stimuli" or natural incentives (see Chapters 4 and 5), that some of McDougall's ideas came back into vogue. On the other hand, he did provide a beginning taxonomy of human motives based on normal behavior that influenced later students of human motives like Henry A. Murray and Raymond Cattell, whose contributions will be described later in this chapter. McDougall's descriptions of the characteristics of motives have continued to be part of their definition ever since.

• MOTIVES AS REASONS FOR ABNORMAL BEHAVIOR

Another approach to discovering basic motives has been to pay attention to what leads people to behave in unusual or abnormal ways. This makes sense if behavior is jointly determined by motives, skills or habits, and values or cognitive schemas. Suppose a hypothetical student suddenly stops studying—an unusual or abnormal act for her. We know that two of the determinants of studying behavior are in place: she knows how to study (she has been studying), and she values it. Thus, we infer that something has happened to her motivation and try to find out what motive is responsible for her not doing what she would normally do.

The most systematic theories of human motivation, in fact, have been developed by clinicians who have tried to determine why people behave in abnormal ways. These clinicians have had ample opportunity to build and check such theories in the course of psychotherapy as they listened to the waking and dreaming thoughts of patients hour after hour and day after day, sometimes for years. To a surprising extent clinicians have tended to agree that there are a few basic human motives, although they have not always agreed on just what they are. This approach has the obvious advantage of paying close attention to what people actually are thinking and doing, but it also has the important disadvantage of using data that are drawn almost exclusively from the minds of people who are disturbed enough to need psychotherapy. Thus, it is not surprising that the motives clinicians have discovered tend to be negative. They are conceived as powerful urges that, if not controlled or moderated, can produce mental and behavioral disorders such as depression, psychosis, and neurosis.

The Freudian Motivational Trilogy: Sex, Aggression, and Anxiety

Freud concluded on the basis of his studies of dreams and free associations, as described in Chapter 1, that the major human needs were—to oversimplify a bit—to obtain sexual satisfaction (in the broadest sense); to express aggression; and to reduce the anxiety and suffering that result from conflicts involving the first two drives, from conflicts of those drives with the demands of society, or from threats to survival. Freud viewed all three of these motives negatively as potentially producing suffering or illness. In this respect he was following a tradition set more than two thousand years earlier in the West by Plato. In Book 9 of *The Republic,* Plato has Socrates speak of the unnecessary pleasures and desires that

> . . . are active during sleep . . . when the rest of the soul, the reasoning, gentle, and ruling part of it is asleep. Then the bestial and savage part, when it has had its fill of food or wine, begins to leap about, pushes sleep aside and tries to go and gratify its instincts. You know how in such a state it will dare everything, as though it were freed and released from all shame and discernment. It does not shrink from attempting incestual intercourse in its dream, with a mother or with any man, god or beast. It is ready for any deed of blood.

Like Freud, Plato identified the major motives observable in dreams as involving sex (including incest) and aggression, and he also labeled them as unlawful or disruptive in the sense that they would fall short of "no extreme of folly or shamelessness." He contended earlier that these unlawful desires were "probably innate in everyone" and that they could be "disciplined by law and by the better desires with the assistance of reason." Freud did not really believe that there are any "better desires," but he did agree that the instinctual, unlawful desires that he consigned to the unconscious id had to be controlled either by society (law) or by reason. In fact, he spoke of psychoanalysis, the instrument he devised, as the means for the progressive conquest of the id through reason (Freud, 1927a).

Bad Desires and Good Desires

The distinction between bad or unlawful desires leading to sickness or sin and good desires is present in various religious traditions that emphasize that the good desires are the means of controlling or disciplining the bad desires. In Christian writings the sins related to excessive sexual or aggressive desires are mentioned prominently, but so is the virtue of loving kindness, as in St. Paul's famous passage on charity in his second letter to the Corinthians. Or, as Thomas put it in his epistle, "God is love and he who abides in love abides in God, and God abides in him." In Dante's dramatization of Christian theology in *The Divine Comedy,* the sins deriving from the unlawful desires are vividly described in the *Inferno.* Reason in the form of Dante's guide, Vergil, helps Dante understand how bad desires lead to sin and punishment as Vergil leads him through hell and purgatory, but Dante sees that he can only attain heaven and overcome these unlawful desires through the divine gift of grace, which confers the virtues of loving kindness, peace, and harmony with all.

In Buddhism the scenario is similar, although the concepts are different. To Buddha the most obvious fact of life was suffering. He viewed desires as the cause of suffering and therefore concluded that desires should be abandoned as soon as possible. He proposed as a method of disposing of desires the disciplined technique of meditation, which after years of practice enables a person to live without desires—or at least without unlawful or ordinary desires. This mode of coping with bad desires functions much as reason functioned for Plato, Dante, or Freud. However, in folk Buddhism, as Gombrich (1971) has pointed out, the desire to be loving and kind has become a virtue to be practiced as a means of eradicating some of the more unlawful and selfish desires, just as it is in Christianity. Even in the theology of Buddhist meditation, loving kindness is a desirable stage on the way to giving up all desires. In Buddhism, therefore, the desire to get rid of desires is a good desire that continuously motivates monks as they pursue arduous meditation practices. In fact, Buddha's last words were said to be something like "strive on mindfully." Clearly, there are good desires in this religious tradition as well as in the Christian tradition.

Freud did not believe in good desires such as kindness, perhaps because his patients, being ill, were unable to show them, or perhaps because of his general pessimism about human nature. In fact, he interpreted loving kindness as really representing other self-serving motives. Take, for example, the loving kindness Christians believe Jesus showed in dying on the cross to help sinners attain salvation. Freud (1918/1938) explained this understanding of the Crucifixion as a manifestation of deeper unconscious motives in all of us. He started with the assumption that all little boys wish to sleep with their mothers, are jealous of their fathers, hate their fathers, wish to kill them, but feel guilty over this wish because they also love their fathers. Their guilt over their incestuous and aggressive wishes normally leads them to want to atone in some way, and in the end they do so by identifying as closely with their father as possible. Thus, the appeal of Jesus' death on the cross is precisely that a son like themselves is killed as a means of atoning for their hidden, unconscious incestuous and aggressive desires. Jesus' Crucifixion helps males get rid of their guilt. Thus, people interpret his act as representing loving kindness, but in fact it is perceived as such only because of their own guilt. In this situation, as in so many others Freud wrote about, the master motives turn out to be sex, aggression, and anxiety or guilt.

Jung's View of Motivation

Other clinicians working at first within the Freudian tradition disagreed about the major forces that guided human behavior. Carl Jung, a Swiss physician of Protestant background, was an early follower of Freud. As Chapter 1 mentioned, Jung was welcomed by Freud because he was eager to extend the influence of psychoanalysis beyond the largely Jewish circle of analysts that clustered around him in the early days in Vienna. Jung also studied the dreams of his patients; however, he tended not to interpret them in terms of sexual urges, but instead to see them as representative of universal themes or archetypes.

For instance, in Jung's (1961) autobiography he describes a powerful dream he had as a young boy of going underground and seeing a giant phallus sticking straight up from a throne. As he gazed at it, he heard his mother's voice say, "That is the man eater," which he associated with a prayer she had taught him to say before he went to bed every night. The prayer spoke of being protected by, taken in by, or "eaten" by Lord Jesus to protect him from Satan, who wanted to devour him. A Freudian might want to interpret Jung's vision as an oedipal dream in which he is identifying with or admiring the phallus, which he wishes he could use on his mother. However, she warns him of its dangers, because it represents the father—both admired and feared—who will, like Lord Jesus, take him in or eat him. Jung enlarges rather than reduces the meaning of the vision and sees it as reflecting the conflict between the loving Lord Jesus (seen as above ground in the sunshine) and the underground Lord Jesus associated with death and dying. Jung was well aware from associating with his father, a pastor, that at funerals and in the cemetery the dead were seen as being taken in or protected by the Lord Jesus.

Thus, sex for Jung becomes not the root motive, but a means of dramatizing the real motivational conflict over loving and fearing the Jesus figure, which in turn can be traced to a universal image, or archetype, involving father figures. Dreams were used by Jung not so much to diagnose basic human motives as to enlarge the patient's understanding for therapeutic purposes. Thus, Jung has little to say directly about what the basic human motives are except to argue that every individual has a fundamental instinctive drive to push toward individuation or self-realization, a theme that recurs in the writings of other therapists as well.

Basic Motives and Later Psychoanalytic Theorists

Of the many psychoanalysts who came after Freud, space permits us to mention only a few who made distinctive motivational contributions. Alfred Adler (1917) was another of Freud's early disciples who eventually broke with him because he came to see the power drive as more central than the sexual drive. Adler felt that all children developed a striving for superiority because they all experienced the weakness of being small and less capable than adults. Thus, everyone is motivated primarily by the desire to compensate for weakness, to become stronger and more important in the eyes of others. This evolves into "social interest," a legitimate motive in its own right, according to Adler. The search for superiority in this form is similar to the drive for self-realization as described by Jung and others.

Freud always resisted yielding the primacy of the sexual instinct to other drives, as was advocated by Jung, Adler, and others, for several reasons. As Chapter 1 pointed out, Freud appears to have drawn much of his inspiration for psychoanalysis from the Chassidic tradition, which expresses the ultimate meaning of life in sexual terms. Even more important, the theory of sex was one of Freud's critical links with biology and the theoretical orthodoxy of nineteenth-century natural science. To cast it aside, as he told Jung, was to slide into "the black tide of mud of the occult" (that is, antiscience). The sexual instinct was to be understood developmentally as a recapitulation of phylogeny, and recapitulation theory held a prominent position among Darwinians—those developing the theory of evolution—at the turn of the century (Sulloway, 1979). According to the theory, the stages of development of the sexual instinct in the individual are the same as the stages of its development in the history of humankind.

Despite his insistence on the primacy of the sexual drive, Freud also recognized the great importance of the aggressive instinct and the drive for power. When Freud wrote about his own motives in the history of the psychoanalytic movement, it is clear from the quotations in Chapter 1 that he seemed often to be motivated primarily by a drive for power or glory that would not brook competition from others so far as his views on the ultimate nature of human beings were concerned.

Later therapists in the psychoanalytic tradition, such as Karen Horney and Harry Stack Sullivan, emphasized the importance of the other basic motive in the Freudian trilogy, anxiety. Horney (1945) felt basic anxiety comes from "the feeling a child has of being isolated and helpless in a potentially hostile world. A wide range of adverse factors in the environment can produce this insecurity in a child: direct or indirect domination, indifference, erratic behavior, disparaging attitudes, too much admiration or the absence of it." As a result of this basic insecurity, children develop motives either to move toward people (to gain protection, warmth, and support), to move away from people (to be self-sufficient or unassailable), or to move against people (to show they are more powerful than other people or to pay them back for past unjustices). At the root of all motives, however, lies anxiety.

In Sullivan's (1953) view anxiety derives from basic physical needs such as food or oxygen, but more importantly from a tension transmitted empathically from mother to child. The infant develops a "self-system" as a response, which exists as an "organization of experiences" designed to minimize anxiety. Anxiety is not the only motive for Sullivan, although it is the first. The need for interpersonal intimacy arises developmentally in preadolescence as a motive powerful enough to preempt anxiety, and impel the organism to transcend the self-system, risk anxiety, and seek "chumship" in order not to experience loneliness, which is worse than anxiety. Note that the new motive is another form of insecurity. Sullivan's and Horney's views happened to coincide with those arrived at out of the animal behavior tradition (described in Chapter 3), in which anxiety and anxiety reduction came to be viewed as the master motive.

• MOTIVES AS REASONS FOR CREATIVITY AND GROWTH

In contrast to the psychoanalysts, who focused on the negative motives that lead to illness because they inevitably conflict with one another or society's demands, American psychotherapist Carl Rogers (1942) found evidence in his patients of a basically constructive motive—the drive to become self-actualized. According to Rogers (1951), "the organism has one basic tendency in striving—to actualize, maintain, and enhance the experiencing organism." This rush toward self-actualization is instinctive and present in everyone, much as Jung and Adler had suggested. Rogers also felt two other important needs are acquired in growing up. One is the need for positive regard from others or, more simply, the need for love and acceptance by others. It develops from the fact that children learn that some things they do are approved and others are disapproved by significant others. They come to want the satisfaction that comes from approval. They also consistently act to defend themselves against disapproval, which indicates they are developing another need—the need for positive self-regard. Notice that all three of Rogers' needs are positive—the need for growth, for love, and for self-respect.

Thus, Rogers was taking a step in the direction advocated by Abraham Maslow (1954, 1967, 1968), who pointed out that there was a bias in the basic motives attributed to human beings that resulted from the fact that the people being studied were nearly all sick or unhappy. Thus, the motives discovered seemed predominantly negative. Maslow argued that the picture should be balanced by just as careful study of very healthy people. He too felt there is a basic "impulse toward growth" in all human beings, which is perhaps weak and relatively easily frustrated, but nevertheless is in every individual. He found strong evidence for the existence of such a drive toward growth in unusually active and healthy people he studied, such as Eleanor Roosevelt, Abraham Lincoln, and Albert Einstein. Maslow did not deny that there are negative needs, but as Plato did, he distinguished between negative, or "deficit," needs such as those for being loved and for self-respect and what he later came to call the "metaneeds," which were what Plato would have called the "better desires"—namely, those for justice, goodness, beauty, and order.

The best-known contribution of Maslow (1954) to motive theory is his classification of human needs in a hierarchy running from basic physiological needs to self-actualization needs (Table 2.2). The classification was a response to the problem so cogently stated by Allport, who argued that whereas it might be ac-

Table 2.2.

MASLOW'S HIERARCHY OF NEEDS (after Maslow, 1954)

Lower, or Deficit, Needs	**1.** Physiological needs (need for food, water, and sex): homeostatic and organic.
	2. Safety needs (need for security and protection from pain, fear, anxiety, and disorder); need for order, lawfulness, and discipline.
	3. Need for belongingness and love (need for love, tenderness, and togetherness).
	4. Esteem needs (need for achievement, respect, and approval).
Higher, or Growth, Needs	**5.** Self-actualization needs (need for self-fulfillment, for realizing one's potential, for understanding and insight).

curate to describe an infant as primarily motivated by physiological needs such as hunger and the relief of discomfort and anxiety, it certainly is inaccurate to think of mature adults as motivated primarily by such needs, even in the most derived or symbolic form. Allport (1937) argued for the "functional autonomy of motives," meaning that higher motives, such as the need for self-esteem, develop later in life independently of the lower physiological needs.

Maslow solved the problem by including both kinds of needs in his hierarchy and insisting that higher needs can emerge only as lower needs are satisfied. He used the image of primitive people to explain this. To survive, primitive people had to first satisfy their physiological needs—for food, water, and sex (to insure survival of the race). As they met these needs enough to survive, their next concern was for safety—from the saber-toothed tiger or from the elements (heat, cold, and floods). Therefore, primitive people lived in caves or built shelters. As their security needs were satisfied, they were free to establish tender relationships with fellow human beings. As they were assured of love, they were able to work on satisfying needs for achievement and self-esteem. Underlying this development, however—even in primitive people—was a push toward growth, individuality, or self-actualization. People do not rest content as their lower needs are satisfied but always are pushing on to higher things. Even if all the lower needs are satisfied,

> . . . we may still often (if not always) expect that a new discontent and restlessness will soon develop, unless the individual is doing what *he,* individually, is fitted for. A musician must make music, an artist must paint, a poet must write, if he is to be ultimately at peace with himself. What a man *can* be, he *must* be. This need we may call self-actualization. . . . It refers to man's desire for self-fulfillment, namely, to the tendency for him to become actualized in what he is potentially. (Maslow, 1954)

Lower needs are characterized by deficits—such as the lack of food and water—which push the organism to become active and to seek substances that will bring the organism back into homeostatic balance. Higher needs are less urgent and pull rather than push the person toward positive goals. They develop later in life than lower needs, but they also are "instinctoid"—that is, inborn in everyone. However, they are weaker and can be prevented from developing by the urgency of working to satisfy lower needs. Needs affect behavior only when they are unsatisfied. As they are satisfied, the person is free to pursue higher needs. Satisfying lower needs removes tension and gives peace and satisfaction. Satisfying higher needs leads more directly to joy and a feeling of personal accomplishment.

From his study of outstanding creative individuals presumably functioning at higher levels in his hierarchy, Maslow concluded that being able to satisfy lower needs and seek self-actualization leads to greater biological efficiency (sleeping better, eating better, longer life, and less sickness) and many desirable human traits such as spontaneity, reality orientation, spirituality, ability to distinguish between means and ends, creativity, autonomy, and democratic values. His theory gained wide acceptance in the mid–twentieth century because it fit in well with the liberal view that poor and oppressed peoples were prevented from functioning at higher levels because poverty and oppression forced them to spend their time trying to satisfy physiological (for example, food) and safety (for example, housing) needs, leaving them no time or energy to develop self-respect or their own potential. His theory was a major force in the development of the humanistic psychology movement in the United States, which stressed the primacy of the higher needs he had defined as opposed to the lower needs that, if unsatisfied, could lead to mental illness and despair.

Maslow's view can be criticized on the grounds that he picked creative individuals to study who showed the characteristics he thought such people should have. For example, he did not choose to study Richard Wagner, a creative musician who showed almost none of the characteristics Maslow valued. In his theorizing he also tended to neglect the nature of the environmental conditions that arouse the various needs in the hierarchy. Nor did he undertake the empirical investigations necessary to show that the needs really do form a hierarchy. Others have looked into this matter, as Chapter 10 will show, but what is most important about Maslow is that he gave psychologists a positive way of thinking about motives to contrast with the negative view deriving from the psychoanalysts, who learned about motives primarily from studying patients in need of therapy.

• MEASURING HUMAN MOTIVES

The motivational theorists so far mentioned provided psychology with a conceptual framework in terms of which to think about basic human motives, as well as a language of human motivation, so to speak. None of them, however, made a systematic attempt to measure the motives they thought were important. Thus, to a certain extent, they are guilty of the naming fallacy mentioned earlier. They observed that people thought and acted in certain ways and inferred that therefore they must have wanted to think and act in those ways. The only way to escape such a fallacy is by measuring the motives in question.

An early attempt at measuring human motives was made by W. H. Sheldon (1942), who was primarily interested in the varieties of human physique, which he called *somatotypes*. He had concluded that human bodies could be rated on three basic characteristics—namely, the extent to which fat predominated, or endomorphy; the extent to which muscle predominated, or mesomorphy; and the extent to which skin predominated, or ectomorphy. He then argued that certain temperament traits (which are in part motivational) derive from each of these characteristics of the body. Sheldon developed temperament rating scales, which included motivational variables. Thus, the viscerotonia scale, which was associated with endomorphy, contained items like "love of physical comfort" and "sociophilia," or love of being with people. The somatotonia scale, which was associated with mesomorphy, included items like "love of physical adventure," "love of dominating," and "lust for power." The cerebrotonia scale, which was associated with ectomorphy, contained items like "love of privacy" and "sociophobia," or dislike of being with people.

The motive measurements are very crude, but they do represent attempts to be more specific about some of the motives clinicians had talked about. And Sheldon identified two of the motive types that have cropped up again and again in psychological literature, namely, the contrast between those who love risk and physical adventure (somatotonics) and those who love privacy (cerebrotonics). The former also have been called *extraverts* and the latter, *introverts,* following a distinction first popularized by Jung and later forming a major orientation in the work of the British psychologist H. J. Eysenck (1947). The distinction appeared again in the work of Zuckerman (1974), who has measured the extent to which people seek excitement and sensation, as extraverts do, or seek to avoid it, as introverts do. The work on extraversion-introversion will be discussed again in later chapters, although its place in the psychology of motivation is not clear because it has been conceived primarily as a trait—a consistent way of behaving—rather than as a difference in motivational orientation.

Such theorists have attempted to delimit the bewildering variety of possible human motives by anchoring them to a more limited set of biological characteristics. This strategy was pursued vigorously by those who concentrated on animal motivation, as the next chapter will show.

Murray's Study of Motives

A systematic approach to measuring human motives was introduced by Henry A. Murray (1938) at Harvard University, who sought ways of assessing the motives clinicians had found to be important. His method was eclectic: he set out to measure in a variety of ways any and all of the motives previous theorists had felt to be important. This method had several advantages from the point of view of advancing knowledge of human motives.

First, Murray primarily was interested in understanding and measuring human motives as contrasted with other aspects of personality such as traits, habits, or skills. Thus, he realized that whereas investigators could look for consistency from one act to the next so far as a trait like assertiveness was concerned, motives often would find quite different behavioral outlets in different people. For example, a desire for power might be satisfied by a person's watching sex and aggression movies on television, arguing with other people, or joining organizations to feel more powerful as part of a larger group. The people who often argued, however, would not necessarily be more likely to watch sex and aggression programs on television or join organizations, so any attempt to build a measure of a "need for Power" by adding together such activities would be likely to fail. This simple fact is well known to clinicians, who often see symptoms as alternative manifestations of basic needs, but it has not been well understood by personality theorists, who keep looking for consistency in the behavioral manifestations of motives. As Murray pointed out, motives are necessary to explain inconsistencies in personality and traits are necessary to explain consistencies.

Second, because Murray saw motives as expressing themselves in a variety of alternative ways, he stressed that their manifestations should be studied in every possible way—through autobiographies, through behaviors in laboratory experiments, through reveries associated with music, through dreams, and through questionnaires about sentiments and attitudes—but above all through a special instrument he devised and called the Thematic Apperception Test (TAT). Of all the measurement techniques Murray and his collaborators invented, this is the one that caught on, particularly in clinical psychology. In effect, it is a method of systematically collecting the kind of free associations Freud and his successors had used to draw inferences about motives in their clinical work. In the TAT, subjects are asked to tell imaginative stories after viewing a series of twenty pictures suggestive of key emotional complexes in the life of the individuals, such as the relationship of father to son or mother to daughter. The first ten pictures represent typical dramas from normal life (for example, father-son or mother-son relationships) and the second ten, more fantastic scenes to elicit more deeply repressed unconscious associations. The resulting "daydreams" are subjected to the same kind of analysis carried out by psychoanalysts, which will be illustrated later in the chapter.

The third advantage of Murray's method was that the subjects in his research were small groups of college undergraduates who were studied intensively over the entire four years they were in college. Thus, he collected as much material as psychotherapists often collect, but on relatively normal individuals, so the bias toward seeing motives as leading to illness could be avoided. Furthermore, he gathered enough material over time to study consistencies and inconsistencies in motives and the extent to which they were changed, aroused, or weakened by events that occurred during the four years. However, there is some bias in the fact that the subjects were all male and quite intelligent and articulate compared with the general run of individuals.

Fourth, to measure motives properly, Murray realized he had to begin by carefully defining each of the motives he was trying to measure. He gathered together a diagnostic council of experts representing a variety of motivational traditions to decide what the main motives were and how they should be defined and measured. Perhaps his greatest contribution, in addition to the TAT, is a vocabulary of human motives that has shaped work in the field ever since. Table

2.3 lists some of the most important needs he measured, together with their definitions.

Obviously, Murray's approach does not reduce all human needs to one basic motive force (such as Jung's, Rogers', or Maslow's drives for self-realization), or to two or three basic motive forces (such as Freud's sex, aggression, and anxiety needs). Murray also does not fall into the opposite difficulty of listing so many needs that working with all of them becomes impractical. Science is an economizing enterprise. Its purpose is to explain as much as possible of the bewildering variety of events with as few basic constructs and laws as possible. In this respect the field of human motivation is no different: the goal is to find the fewest motives that will account for the most human behavior. Obviously no set of human motives can account for everything a particular individual thinks or does. Only three motives in Murray's list have been the subject of extensive investigation since his time: the need for achievement, the need for affiliation, and the need for power (or dominance), as later chapters of this book will describe.

The fifth advantage to Murray's method was that his council of experts solved the problem of measuring the strength of an individual's need in all its manifestations by asking each judge to rate the need based on all information available, and then by having the ratings discussed in a group to arrive at a final rating that would represent a synthesis of the viewpoints of all the judges. This procedure gave the council greater confidence that it was arriving at the truth about a person's needs, but as a measurement technique it has important drawbacks. A difficulty with this procedure lies in the group process by which the final rating is reached. One judge may have been more influential than another in arriving at the final rating; it does not follow, however, that this judge was necessarily nearer the truth, nor does it follow that the opinion of a group of judges is better than the opinion of the "best" judge by some outside criterion. Another difficulty lies in the fact that it is impossible to reconstruct exactly what thoughts or actions the judges were using in arriving at their ratings. It is not even possible to be sure that most, or even any, of the judges were closely following the motive definitions in making their judgments. Methods of dealing with these difficulties through more precise coding definitions have been developed (see Chapter 6).

Cattell's Identification of Motives Through Factor Analysis

Like Murray, Raymond Cattell (1957, 1965) has sought to identify and measure the major human motives. He too recognized that motives were only one of the determinants of behavior (along with abilities and temperament traits), and he too obtained many different presumed indicators of different motives. However, instead of using human judges to synthesize them all into a numerical rating for the strength of a particular motive in a person, as Murray had done, Cattell employed factor analysis to arrive at a final score for a motive for a person. Factor analysis is essentially a statistical method for extracting the factors that account for covariation among various measures.

Table 2.3.

ILLUSTRATIVE LIST OF MURRAY'S NEEDS (Hall & Lindzey, 1957, after Murray, 1938)

Need	Brief Definition
Abasement	To submit passively to external force. To accept injury, blame, criticism, or punishment. To surrender. To become resigned to fate. To admit inferiority, error, wrongdoing, or defeat. To confess and atone. To blame, belittle, or mutilate the self. To seek and enjoy pain, punishment, illness, and misfortune.
Achievement	To accomplish something difficult. To master, manipulate, or organize physical objects, human beings, or ideas. To do this as rapidly and as independently as possible. To overcome obstacles and attain a high standard. To excel oneself. To rival and surpass others. To increase self-regard by the successful exercise of talent.
Affiliation	To draw near and enjoyably cooperate or reciprocate with an allied other (an other who resembles the subject or who likes the subject). To please and win affection of a cathected object. To adhere and remain loyal to a friend.
Aggression	To overcome opposition forcefully. To fight. To revenge an injury. To attack, injure, or kill another. To oppose forcefully or punish another.
Autonomy	To get free, shake off restraint, break out of confinement. To resist coercion and restriction. To avoid or quit activities prescribed by domineering authorities. To be independent and free to act according to impulse. To be unattached, irresponsible. To defy convention.
Counteraction	To master or make up for a failure by restriving. To obliterate a humiliation by resumed action. To overcome weaknesses, to repress fear. To efface a dishonor by action. To search for obstacles and difficulties to overcome. To maintain self-respect and pride on a high level.
Defendance	To defend the self against assault, criticism, and blame. To conceal or justify a misdeed, failure, or humiliation. To vindicate the ego.
Deference	To admire and support a superior. To praise, honor, or eulogize. To yield eagerly to the influence of an allied other. To emulate an exemplar. To conform to custom.
Dominance	To control one's human environment. To influence or direct the behavior of others by suggestion, seduction, persuasion, or command. To dissuade, restrain, or prohibit.
Exhibition	To make an impression. To be seen and heard. To excite, amaze, fascinate, entertain, shock, intrigue, amuse, or entice others.
Harmavoidance	To avoid pain, physical injury, illness, and death. To escape from a dangerous situation. To take precautionary measures.
Infavoidance	To avoid humiliation. To quit embarrassing situations or to avoid conditions that may lead to belittlement: the scorn, derision, or indifference of others. To refrain from action because of the fear of failure.
Nurturance	To give sympathy and gratify the needs of a helpless object: an infant or any object that is weak, disabled, tired, inexperienced, infirm, defeated, humiliated, lonely, dejected, sick, mentally confused. To assist an object in danger. To feed, help, support, console, protect, comfort, nurse, heal.
Order	To put things in order. To achieve cleanliness, arrangement, organization, balance, neatness, tidiness, and precision.

Table 2.3. *(Continued).*

Need	Brief Definition
Play	To act for "fun" without further purpose. To like to laugh and make jokes. To seek enjoyable relaxation of stress. To participate in games, sports, dancing, drinking parties, cards.
Rejection	To separate oneself from a negatively cathected object. To exclude, abandon, expel, or remain indifferent to an inferior object. To snub or jilt an object.
Sentience	To seek and enjoy sensuous impressions.
Sex	To form and further an erotic relationship. To have sexual intercourse.
Succorance	To have one's needs gratified by the sympathetic aid of an allied object. To be nursed, supported, sustained, surrounded, protected, loved, advised, guided, indulged, forgiven, consoled. To remain close to a devoted protector. To always have a supporter.
Understanding	To ask or answer general questions. To be interested in theory. To speculate, formulate, analyze, and generalize.

An example of how Cattell worked will make it easier to understand his method. He started with the supposition, just as McDougall and Murray had, that there might be a motive disposition for affiliating with others, which he labeled *Gregariousness*. One way to find out if people are strong in such a motive is to ask them to introspect on their desires in the area by answering yes or no to statements such as "I want to belong to a sociable club or team of people with congenial interests." But Cattell realized that such self-reports are influenced by response sets—sentiments or other factors that have nothing directly to do with the motive in question. Thus, he also sought a number of other indicators of Gregariousness such as the knowledge people had about clubs available in the area, how many clubs the people would join or had joined, and the emotional response of the people (as reflected in imperceptible sweating affecting the galvanic skin response) when presented with a stimulus phrase such as "Today too many people are joining clubs."

The next question to be answered by factor analysis is whether all of these different indicators covary, or "hang together." That is, do people who say they want to join clubs also react emotionally to the statement that too many people are joining clubs? Cattell argues that it can be concluded that there is a motive called *gregariousness* only when such a series of indicators related to a common goal can be shown to covary, preferably by the objective method of factor analysis, which is based on the statistical intercorrelation of indicators. He defines a *motive* (or *Erg*, in his terminology) in part as starting "various courses of action (equivalents) which cease more completely at a certain common, definite, consummatory goal activity than at any other. The common goal character is demonstrable by, among other methods, a factor-analytic proof of functional unity in attitude-action courses that can be perceived (or demonstrated) by the psychologist to lead to a common goal" (Cattell, 1957).

Cattell has carried out dozens of factor analytic studies on dozens of such indicators in thousands of subjects in an effort to define the major motive dispositions and find objective measures of them. He has arrived at a list similar to Murray's and McDougall's and includes such Ergs (motive energizers) as curiosity, sex, gregariousness, protection, self-assertion, security, hunger, anger, and disgust. His method appeared to be particularly promising, because it provided an objective, statistical method of "proving" the existence of a motive and of combining different indicators into a single factor score for the motive, as contrasted with Murray's intuitive method of attaining these same goals.

However, the approach also has its drawbacks. First, what comes out of a factor analysis depends entirely on what measures are put into it, which in turn depends on the psychologists' judgment as to what is relevant or important to measure; this in turn depends on their intuitive understanding of the field. The results may show whether the psychologists' intuitive understanding was correct, but they do not guarantee that they put in everything of importance. Second, factor analytic results for different samples of subjects from whom the same measures are obtained often reveal differences as to what indicators define an Erg that can be reconciled only in a speculative, intuitive, or superficial way. Third, and most important, the factor analytic score is a composite of many different indicators that can be classified as belonging under a common label only in a very loose way. Statistical precision may lead to conceptual confusion: How could this behavioral indicator that loads high on the Gregariousness factor really indicate a desire to affiliate with people? And why does this other indicator, which ought to indicate Gregariousness, fail to load on the factor?

Cattell has dealt with such questions in imaginative ways but has failed to convince many psychologists that factor analysis provides the ideal way of solving such problems. Instead, as we shall see, the trend has been toward more careful conceptual and measurement definitions of a few motives that then are studied in detail rather than toward construction of the overall picture of all motives and other personality variables sought by Murray and Cattell in different ways.

• STAGES IN MOTIVATIONAL DEVELOPMENT

So far we have reviewed motives identified by personality theorists and some preliminary attempts to measure them. However, such an overview leaves out how personality theorists have identified the presence of motives in a concrete case. Generally they have been most convincing in doing so when they have analyzed fantasies, dreams, or more generally, thought processes. To give a better idea of how this approach works in practice, considerable space will be devoted to illustrating how it can be used to make inferences about a person's motives. The context will be one of explaining more about the Freudian view of stages in motivational development, since this has had a wide impact on the field, particularly as it has been elaborated by Erik Erikson (1963).

Freud concluded not only that there were a few basic human motives, but also that one of them, the sexual drive, developed in certain stages. In observing how the sexual instinct manifested itself, he followed the strategy of linking stages of development to biological events. He noted first of all that the most striking character of sexual activity is "that the impulse is not directed to other persons but that the child gratifies himself on his own body" (Freud, 1905/1938). He observed that "the first and most important activity in a child's life, the sucking from the mother's breast (or its substitute)" (Freud, 1905/1938), has acquainted the child with the pleasure to be obtained from the lips, which Freud referred to as the *oral erogenous zone.* Sucking and getting food are normally combined, but sucking becomes pleasurable in its own right: in Freud's view the sexual instinct gratifies itself first in the region of the mouth, or the oral zone. In more general psychological terms, the oral stage represents a period of dependency in which gratification comes from intake—from taking something in from the outside.

Next, according to Freud, children begin to get gratification from the anal zone—from holding on to and letting go of feces. This provides pleasure in the simple biological sense, but it also represents a period in which children learn self-control. They are now becoming independent in the sense that they alone can control whether they hold on or let go.

In the third stage, children discover the pleasure to be obtained from manipulating the genitals. In more general terms, they are learning to get pleasure from assertiveness, from actually doing something active to produce pleasure. In psychoanalytic theory this period is referred to as the *phallic stage* to distinguish it from the later, truly genital stage, which derives pleasure from the sexual intercourse between a man and a woman and is characterized by mutuality.

Stages Reflected in a Freudian Dream

Using this elementary introduction to Freud's conception of psychosexual stages, let us look at the method used by clinicians to analyze two dream sequences to see how it enables them to make inferences about motivational stages, particularly as they have been described more fully by Erikson (1963). The purpose of such an exercise is not only to give a better idea of stages in motivational development, but also to give a concrete demonstration of the modes of analysis typically used to arrive at motivational inferences from fantasy material.

The first sequence consists of two dreams reported by Freud, which were later analyzed in some detail by Erikson (1964), who also made use of Freud's associations to the dreams. The following is Freud's first dream, as described by Erikson (1964):

> I went into a kitchen in search of (*um mir geben zu lassen*) some pudding. Three women were standing in it, one of them was the hostess (*Wirtin*) of the inn and was twisting (*drehen*) something about in her hand, as though she was making *Knodel* (dumplings). She answered that I must wait till she was ready. (These were not definite spoken words.) I felt impatient and went off with a sense of injury (*beleidigt*— insulted).

Obviously, the dream has to do with the oral stage, with being fed. The English translation, Erikson points out, is misleading, because what the German states is not that Freud goes actively in "search of" food, but that he goes into the kitchen in order for someone to give him some food. He is dependent on others to be fed. The fact that the dream has to do with being fed is not surprising, since Freud had it after going to bed without his supper; the way in which the oral crisis is described, however, is of key importance.

Before interpreting it further, let us review Freud's associations to it. First, he remembers a novel he read when he was thirteen years old (incidentally, this is a critical point in a Jewish boy's life when he has his Bar Mitzvah representing his initiation into Jewish manhood) in which the hero went mad, calling out the names of three women who had been responsible both for his greatest joys and sorrows. Freud then recalls the three Fates, who in Greek mythology were responsible for spinning people's destiny. Finally he realizes that the hostess is his mother: "love and hunger, he reflects, meet at a woman's breast" (Erikson, 1964). His associations so far have to do with women controlling people's fate.

He next recalls an incident that further illustrates that men do not have control over their fate with women. He recalls that a man he was with noticed how attractive his former wet nurse was and remarked that it was too bad he had not been big enough to take advantage of his opportunities at the time.

Finally, Freud recalls an episode when he was six years old; his mother was trying to illustrate for him the meaning of the biblical passage "dust thou art to dust returneth." She rubbed her hands together vigorously until the skin peeled off in little black rolls to convince him of the truth of the statement. As Erikson (1964) notes, "here it is important to see that the very *origin of man,* and, in fact, the origin of living matter is at stake, and that the mother, the source of life-giving food and of hope-giving love, herself demonstrates the fact that her very body is created of dead matter, of earth and of dirt" (p. 182). Freud's disillusionment with women seems to be complete.

Now we are in a better position to interpret this dream in terms of the characteristics of the oral stage as they have been outlined by Erikson in Table 2.4. In his search for food, the dreamer goes to the kitchen, where the food is provided, and meets women, who normally provide him with food. Then he is told he must wait. In the oral stage that is all the baby can do—wait initially for the mother to provide nourishment somewhat magically. Whether the mother provides nourishment and love in a predictable manner or not causes the development of the sense of trust or mistrust that characterizes the psychosocial equivalent of the oral psychosexual stage, according to Erikson. As he puts it elsewhere, "it is clear then that the optimum total situation implied in the baby's readiness to get what it is given is his mutual regulation with the mother who will permit him to develop and coordinate his means of getting as she develops and coordinates her means of giving" (Erikson, 1963). The ability of the growing child to develop trust and hope depends on this mutual coordination.

If the coordination fails in some critical sense, the child distorts reality in an attempt to get basic oral gratification and becomes either *delusional,* as in some types of schizophrenia; *addictive,* an attempt to get oral gratification

Table 2.4.

CHARACTERISTICS ASSOCIATED WITH PSYCHOSEXUAL STAGES (after Erikson, 1964)

Psychosexual Stage	*Organ Mode*	*Psychosocial Stage*	*Rudiment of Ego Strength*	*Related Psychopathological Mechanisms*	*Related Elements of Social Order*
I. Oral-sensory-cutaneous	Incorporative	Basic trust versus mistrust	Hope	Psychotic, addictive	Cosmic order
II. Muscular-anal-urethral	Retentive-eliminative	Autonomy versus shame and doubt	Will	Compulsive, impulsive	Law and order
III. Phallic-locomotor	Intrusive	Initiative versus guilt	Purpose	Inhibitive, hysterical, phobic	Ideal prototype

through drugs; or *depressed,* as when mistrust develops to such a degree that a person gives up trying to adapt. Thus, from a psychoanalytic point of view, traumas at the oral stage are the most serious in that they cause the most fundamental breaks with reality, leading to such major disorders as schizophrenia and depression.

What about Freud's reaction in the dream and his associations to it? He does not want to wait, goes off with a sense of injury, and in his associations makes it very clear that men cannot depend on women, who are "too perishable, too mortal, and too dangerous" (Erikson, 1964).

Instead, in the next part of the dream he turns away from women toward men and toward establishing his own identity. The second part of the dream is as follows:

> In the second part of the dream one lone man appears, and no women. After some altercations, a stranger and the dreamer become "quite friendly with each other"—which "ends the dream." (Erikson, 1964)

In associating to this dream Freud first thinks of a number of names of men reminiscent of food. This reminds him of his own name, which has inspired some crude jokes. As Erikson points out, in German the two most obvious related names are *Freudenhaus* (house of joy, or whorehouse) and *Freudenmädchen* (girl of joy, or prostitute). Again, Freud seems to be casting aspersions on women with his name. As Erikson (1964) sums it up, "If your own mother is made of earth or dirt, or worse, and if your own name is like a curse, you cannot trust mother, origin, or fate: you must create your own greatness and, indeed, all the dreamer's associations concerning men converge on the great Vienna Institute of Physiology in which, so the dreamer says, he spent the happi-est hours of his student days" (p. 183). Freud recalls a poem by Goethe about yearning daily evermore for the "breasts of wisdom," or knowledge, which, since it is related to the real world, gives people power to control what happens to them. This differs from the oral period, in which they can only wait.

Freud then remembers cocaine, a substance he had introduced for anesthetic purposes before its addictive powers were known. This suggests there are also dangers in incautious intake. Thus, the role of mistrust is precisely to warn the growing child against taking everything in heedlessly, but obviously the danger of too much mistrust is that it inhibits taking anything in at all. Thus, Freud feels the dream reminds him that he should take advantage of opportunities even though there may be some drawbacks in doing so, as in the case of co-caine. As Erikson (1964) sums it up,

> . . . the second part of the dream, then, emphasizes the turn from dependence to self-help, from women to men, from perishable to eternal substances, and ends with a friendly affiliation with a man with a pointed beard—a paternal teacher figure. . . . If the first part of this dream, evoked by hunger, goes back to the actuality of the first stage of life, the second part leads (as I think all successful dreams do) forward again; for it obviously promises to the sulky dreamer autonomy from women and participation in the world of intellectual skills.

To return to the stage model presented in Table 2.4, Freud has thought himself forward in his dream from Stage I, where the issues have to do with waiting and taking in, to Stage II, where the person has progressed to issues of autonomy and self-help. Failures in development at Stage II lead to compulsive or impulsive disorders. People either become too willful in holding on or at-tempting to control everything in an obsessive-compulsive way, or they give up and act always on impulse, or they alternate between the two modalities. Erik-son also makes the point that just becaue Freud is thinking in his dream about the issues of the oral stage, it should not be inferred that he has in any way "re-gressed." Instead, his hunger reminds him of one of life's major themes and the way he has successfully dealt with it by moving from dependence to autonomy, or from Stage I to Stage II.

Stages Reflected in a Murderer's Dream

There are other examples of progression through stages in a dream. In his book *In Cold Blood,* Truman Capote (1965) gives a vivid account of the lives of two young men with criminal records, Perry Smith and Dick Hickok, who brutally murdered a farmer and his family. What caught the attention of the press and Capote was the fact that the murder, particularly the first murder of Mr. Clut-ter, the farmer, seemed to be entirely without a motive. Perry and Dick had broken into the farm at night in the hopes of stealing some money, but they had found none. They had no intention of harming the family, but having wakened the people and tied everyone up, they hung around for several hours trying to decide what to do. In attempting to explain what then happened, Perry said in his confession after he was caught, "I didn't want to harm the man. I thought he was a very nice gentlemen. Soft-spoken. I thought so right up to the moment I cut his throat." Even the psychiatrists from the Menninger Clinic who examined Perry could not really find a motive for the murder. They noted that he had a history of impulsive acts of violence and concluded that somehow something in the situation had elicited a similar act.

Fortunately from the point of view of motivational analysis, Capote provides a very detailed record of Perry's dreams and associations. What follows is a dream Perry reports to Dick:

> As long as you live, there's always something waiting, and even if it's bad, and you know it's bad, what can you do? You can't stop living. Like my dream. Since I was a kid I've had this same dream, where I'm in Africa. A jungle. I'm moving through the trees toward a tree standing all alone. Jesus, it smells bad, that tree; it kind of makes me sick, the way it stinks. Only it's beautiful to look at—it has blue leaves and diamonds hanging everywhere. Diamonds like oranges. That's why I'm there—to pick myself a bushel of diamonds. But I know the minute I try to, the minute I reach up, a snake is gonna fall on me. A snake that guards the tree. This fat son of a bitch living in the branches. I know this beforehand, see? And Jesus, I don't know how to fight the snake. But I figure, well, I'll take my chances. What it comes down to is I want the diamonds more than I'm afraid of the snake. So I go to pick one, I have the diamond in my hand, I'm pulling at it, when the snake lands on top of me. We wrestle around, but he's a slippery sonofabitch and I can't get a hold, he's crushing me, you can hear my legs cracking. Now comes the part it makes me sweat even to think about. See, he starts to swallow me. Feet first. Like going down in quicksand. (Capote, 1965, p. 92)*

From Freudian analyses of dreams and the experimental studies of sex symbolism reviewed in Chapter 1, we know sexual thoughts and desires often disguise themselves in dreams. The method of disguise involves replacing the sexual objects or desires with other objects or desires that have similar attributes. Thus, to decode the first part of Perry's dream, we must ask what has all the strange attributes he describes. That is, what is it (1) that is enormously valuable ("beautiful," "diamonds") that Perry wants desperately ("more than I am afraid of the snake"); (2) that is in a strange place (Africa, jungle); (3) that smells bad ("makes me sick, the way it stinks"); (4) that is round and attractive and hanging "like oranges"; and (5) that if he takes it a snake falls on him and starts to swallow him.

It is not difficult to decipher this in terms of the standard oedipal triangle. Perry is reaching in his dream for his mother's breasts (which are seen as enormously valuable to him, round and hanging, to be plucked and taken like a treasure; this already makes us think he desperately needs them or his mother's love). The whole scene takes place in a jungle, which normally represents the unconscious in dreams. And this valuable prize is guarded by a snake that falls

*From IN COLD BLOOD by Truman Capote. Copyright © 1965 by Truman Capote. Reprinted by permission of Random House, Inc. and Hamish Hamilton Ltd.

on him when he reaches for it. The snake can readily be seen as the father figure, which punishes Perry for his incestuous wishes.

Some details in the dream, however, make sense only if we know a little more about Perry's life history. Why should the tree smell bad and make him sick? Perry's mother was a full-blooded American Indian and his father Irish. They were at first expert rodeo performers ("Tex and Flo"), and Perry's happiest early childhood memories were of his mother as "a lean Cherokee girl riding a wild horse, a bucking bronco." Unfortunately, they had to retire because of ailments, and his mother "took to whiskey," left her husband, abandoned her children, and became so promiscuous that she would sleep with any man who would drink and dance with her beforehand. Perry had what he called "odious" childhood memories of watching his mother sleeping with strange men. When she drank she often got sick, so in the end she "strangled to death on her own vomit." Hence the bad smell in Perry's dream reinforces our belief that it is really about his mother.

Perry loved his father and, when he was young, often tried to run away from his slovenly mother to be with him. However, they also fought. Describing one such battle, Perry says, "Dad, though, he's slippery, a smart wrestler." Again, the fact that he uses the same imagery to describe the snake reinforces our interpretation of the snake as a father figure. Notice, however, that the snake is swallowing him and crushing his legs. Perry had in fact broken his legs in a motorcycle accident some years earlier, an event that had a profound effect on his image of himself as "a real man," which had always been shaky.

If we refer back to Table 2.4, we can see that, in terms of motivational stage theory, this part of the dream has to do with taking initiative, with acting on the world in Stage III fashion. However, Perry knows ahead of time that this initiative will fail, and in fact it does fail and he is crushed for making the attempt—crushed at least symbolically in the phallic region. Even more important is the image of being sucked down into quicksand, which suggests going even deeper into the unconscious, or regressing back to an earlier stage.

The account of Perry's dream continues:

Dick said, "So? The snake swallows you? Or what?"

"Never mind. It's not important." (But it was! The finale was of great importance, a source of private joy.) He'd once told it to his friend Willie-Jay; he had described to him the towering bird, the yellow "sort of parrot." Of course, Willie-Jay was different—delicate-minded, "a saint." He'd understand. But Dick? Dick might laugh. And that Perry could not abide; anyone's ridiculing the parrot, which had first flown into his dreams when he was seven years old, a hated, hating half-breed child living in a California orphanage run by nuns—shrouded disciplinarians who whipped him for wetting his bed. It was after one of these beatings, one he could never forget ("She woke me up. She had a flashlight, and she hit me with it. Hit me and hit me. And when the flashlight broke, she went on hitting me in the dark.") that the parrot appeared, arrived while he slept, a bird "taller than Jesus, yellow like a sunflower," a warrior-angel who blinded nuns with its beak, fed upon their eyes, slaughtered them as they "pleaded for mercy," then so gently lifted him, enfolded him, winged him away to "paradise."

As the years went by, the particular torments from which the bird delivered him altered; others—older children, his father, a faithless girl, a sergeant he'd known in the Army—replaced the nuns, but the parrot remained, a hovering avenger. Thus, the snake, that custodian of the diamond-bearing tree, never finished devouring him but was itself always devoured. And afterward the blessed ascent! Ascension to a paradise that in one version was merely "a feeling," a sense of power, of unassailable superiority—sensations that in another version were transposed into "a real place." Like out of a movie. Maybe that's where I *did* see it—remembered it from a movie. Because where else would I have seen a garden like that? With white marble steps? Fountains? And away down below, if you go to the edge of the garden, you can see the ocean, terrific! Like around Carmel, California. The best thing, though—Well, it's a long, long table. You never imagined so much food. Oysters. Turkey. Hot dogs. Fruit you could make into a million fruit cups, and, listen—it's every bit *free*. I mean, I don't have to be afraid to touch it. I can eat as much as I want, and it won't cost a cent. That's how I know where I am."*

The next part of the dream confirms this impression. It has to do with Stage II, the retentive-eliminative stage. Perry had wet his bed for years and had been punished severely for it in the orphanage. The adjustments related to Stage II, therefore, also had not been properly resolved. In fact, he was both compulsive and impulsive. On one hand, he was obsessively neat and clean, and one of the things he disliked most about his companion in crime was that he was sloppy. On the other hand, as the psychiatrist had noted, there were instances in his life in which he had suddenly "let go," just as he had let go in wetting his bed.

What happens next? Once more a problem at a given stage in development is resolved by regressing to an earlier stage. The wonderful parrot bird comes, avenges him on the nuns who persecuted him, and lifts him to an oral paradise. In his dream he revels in all the wonderful kinds of food available. And there is no waiting, as there is in Freud's dream. "It's every bit *free*. . . . I can eat as much as I want, and it won't cost a cent." Perry has regressed from Stage III to Stage II, and then back to Stage I, where he rests totally happy in the kind of loving support, symbolized in terms of food, that he never got in real life. Instead of thinking himself forward up the developmental scale, as Freud did, he thinks his way backward to a dream of escaping to paradise.

There were hard feelings between Perry and Dick. Perry originally had teamed up with Dick because he had doubts about his own ability to be tough and strong and thought Dick was the image of the strong man. However, he found that Dick was weak: "Just then it made my stomach turn to think that I had ever admired him, lapped up all that brag . . . I meant to make him admit that he was a phony and a coward." Perry had given a knife to Dick, trying to persuade him to kill Mr. Clutter so that there would be no witnesses. Dick, however, would not or could not do it. So Perry took the knife and later said, "But I didn't realize what I had done till I heard the sound. Like somebody drowning. Screaming under water."

What happened before the murder is very like the sequence in Perry's

*From IN COLD BLOOD by Truman Capote. Copyright © 1965 by Truman Capote. Reprinted by permission of Random House, Inc. and Hamish Hamilton Ltd.

dream. He is faced with the crisis of taking initiative. He has doubts about his ability to take initiative, just as in the dream. He tries to get Dick to take the initiative and fails. What is the way out of this crisis? Unfortunately for Mr. Clutter, the situation suggests a possibility very like the escape route Perry has always followed in his dream: regressing to a Stage II mode of action, which is associated with ultimate escape to an oral paradise. Mr. Clutter is tightly bound and his mouth taped shut. This suggests a Stage II crisis (holding on versus letting go) Perry has resolved in the past by suddenly letting go, which he does this time by cutting Mr. Clutter's throat in a peculiarly liquid way. To his unconscious mind (since he did not consciously intend to harm Mr. Clutter) it seems the only, as well as the habitual, way out of a crisis in order to escape to the oral paradise or find the sunken treasure, dreams of which had led him to plan the robbery in the first place. Thus, the dream sequence provides a clue to explaining what happened in real life, which was so puzzling to Perry himself and to all those associated with the murder.

Implications of the Dream Analyses

Several conclusions can be drawn from our interpretation of Freud's and Perry's dream sequences:

1. They vividly illustrate several sources of pleasure or concern that seem to be quite general, at least in thought patterns. They can be conceived of as general goals: (a) to receive or take in food, love, and support; (b) to be autonomous and regulate one's own behavior; and (c) to take initiative or be successfully assertive. The next, or genital, stage is not illustrated by the dream sequences or listed in Table 2.4, although Erikson (1963) elaborated on it, along with later developments in the life cycle. Its goal is mutuality or generativity.

2. These general goals appear to be arranged in a developmental sequence. Freud arrived at them by tying them to sources of erogenous satisfaction on the body surface that seem to be the focus of attention at progressively later periods in the child's life. As Erikson has generalized this idea and as we observed the sequences in these dreams, progression or regression occurs from one stage to the next in adults without reference to the parts of the body on which they are presumably based. Freud thought forward from the oral stage to the stage of autonomy, and Perry thought backward from the stage of initiative to the stage of autonomy to the stage of oral dependency.

3. Psychological health and psychopathology appear to depend on how successfully a person negotiates these stages one after the other. Perry had not successfully negotiated the oral crisis involving, in Erikson's (1963) terms, "the mutual regulation with the maternal source of supply." His yearning for his mother's breast, so vividly portrayed in his dream, may not have been so much sexual as it was a desire for love and support. However, the disruption was not so great that he became psychotic. He did progress somewhat through to the stage of autonomy, but here too he ran into problems, as he did when he made tentative attempts to achieve the assertive goals of Stage III. He was half crippled at every stage, so to speak, and tended to resolve his problems by regress-

ing back to a goal of an earlier stage. Freud, on the other hand, successfully negotiated the oral crisis and moved on to the stage of autonomy.

4. These developmental stage goals and how they are negotiated appear to have very wide effects on the personality—not only in the realm of psychopathology, but also in the realm of a person's whole outlook on life. Thus, Erikson relates the stages to such virtues as hope, will, and purpose and to such elements of the social order as a person's philosophy of life, the importance of law and order, or ideal prototypes (see Table 2.4). And in both Freud's and Perry's cases, but particularly in Perry's we were able to show that the sequence of thoughts about these issues is related to what the men actually did in the real world.

• OTHER VIEWS OF DEVELOPMENTAL STAGES

The psychoanalysts have not been the only ones to describe goals characteristic of different periods in the life of the growing child. Even Jean Piaget's description of cognitive stages in development can be understood in motivational terms. In discussing how children play a game like marbles, Piaget (1932) identifies first a stage of conformity, in which the children are busy learning how to play the game. Their goal at this stage is to play the game correctly according to the rules, that is, to conform. When they are very young they cannot even comprehend that the game could be played differently. This corresponds in Freudian terms to Stage I—the intake stage—in which children are totally dependent on others for support (Freud) or information (Piaget). Obviously the two theorists place the intake stage at different ages—emotional intake in the first year of life (Freud) and information intake at the age of five or six, when children play games (Piaget). That is, the stage goals are functionally equivalent and occur roughly in the same sequence, but not at the same age.

Next, according to Piaget, as children mature cognitively, they begin to realize that the rules of the game can be changed. They no longer are bound by what others tell them the rules are but begin to invent rules of their own or challenge the rules. In Freudian terms they are now at Stages II and III, having become autonomous and assertive in their own right.

Finally, according to Piaget, they become intellectually capable of empathy —of understanding the viewpoint of another player in the game rather than just their own viewpoint. Once they are able to assume the role of another, they want to. They then are able to design or play games that take their own and other viewpoints into account. In Freudian terms they are in Erikson's fourth stage, which is characterized by mutuality.

The Freudians used the sequence of pleasure in erogenous zones and relations to parents to define the developmental stage goals, whereas Piaget used characteristics of intellectual development to define very similar stage goals. More recently, other scholars such as Loevinger (1976) and Kohlberg (1969) also have defined and measured stages of conformity, autonomy, and mutuality that parallel somewhat the Freud-Erikson stage sequence, although there also are important differences. Thus, the Freud-Erikson sequence obviously has great appeal as a model of the hierarchy of goals pursued in conceptions of the maturing process.

In fact, parallels also exist in the world's principal religions, all of which describe first a stage of people's being good by conforming to standards set by others because they do not know any better. But this does not represent ideal maturity, because people must freely choose to be good on their own. They must question the rules and become somewhat autonomous and assertive until they have developed enough to choose the good voluntarily and knowledgeably. This period of self-development eventually leads to the highest level of maturity, in which the goal is to "lose the self," the sense of which has been so laboriously gained, in the service of others. The progression is from conformity to self-realization to altruism. Once again the agreement on developmental stage goals is considerable, although the basis for arriving at them is quite different.

• CHECKING THE VALIDITY OF THE MOTIVATIONAL STAGE THEORY

How do we know that the mode of analysis used in Erikson's interpretation of Freud's dream or our interpretation of Perry's dream has yielded valid findings? How can we be sure Perry's dream really is about his mother and father? Maybe he just likes diamonds and oranges and dislikes snakes. Academic psychologists have always been extremely suspicious of this way of measuring and identifying motives, because there does not seem to be any way to find out whether an interpretation really is correct. If there is no way a hypothetical interpretation can be falsified or proved wrong, it is not a genuine scientific hypothesis. Could not someone else come along and interpret Perry's dream in some other way that was equally plausible? How then could we decide between the two interpretations?

Academic psychologists initially reacted to this dilemma in one of two ways. They either left this kind of analysis wholly outside the field of scientific psychology, or they attempted to design experiments in the laboratory that would check some of the hypotheses in a falsifiable way. This section will review some of these recent experiments, but first let us consider a third alternative, which argues that the experiments are unnecessary.

Hermeneutics

In recent years scholars have argued that a careful distinction must be made between understanding the meaning of a text, a dream, or a life, and proving by independent investigation that the interpretation is really correct. In their view, understanding comes about through the correct application of hermeneutics, the science of interpretation, which involves fitting pieces of information together into a meaningful whole, much as a person would fit pieces into a jigsaw puzzle

(Radnitzky, 1973; Steele, 1979). In Steele's words, "analysis is complete when the circle of meaning is constructed, when the puzzle is finished. Meaning resides in the articulation of the parts with each other and the whole. . . . The puzzle fitting together precisely is vital, for any incompleteness creates doubt. . . . The original text of the dream—its solution, the latent meaning—exists solely as a product of interpretation; just as the analysand's life story with its gaps filled in and its distortions corrected is a product of the analytic encounter."

Understanding is a product of the analyst's personality and view of the world as determined by the particular historical period in which he or she lives. It is also the product of the exchange between the analyst and the text as the analyst tries out various interpretations and corrects them. This is even more true of the therapeutic encounter in psychoanalysis, in which understanding is the product of a dialogue between the analyst and the analysand: "Reality comes to reside in the ever expanding circle of meaning between analysand and analyst" (Steele, 1979). Thus, Freud (cited in Steele, 1973) used the method of hermeneutics in interpreting dreams and life histories, but he was very worried about its subjectivity: " 'Interpret!' A nasty word! I dislike the sound of it; it robs me of all certainty. If everything depends on my interpretation, who can guarantee that I interpret right?"

In Steele's view, therefore, Freud made the mistake of trying to bolster his interpretations by appeals to "objective" facts of biology and history outside those obtained by the hermeneutic method. Objective facts, if they lie outside the circle of meaning, are irrelevant. Thus, it does not matter that a patient remembers a childhood event that turns out never to have occurred. It is the memory of the event that is relevant to understanding. The soundness or credibility of an interpretation of a dream text or a life depends on the same criteria used in evaluating the credibility of an interpretation of facts obtained in a series of experiments.

In each case there are a number of events a theory is constructed to explain. In both instances, whether the theory is good or not depends on whether the rules of logic or reasoning are carefully followed. Is the interpretation internally consistent? Does it maximize understanding the parts in terms of the whole? Does it account for all the facts—in this case, the images in the dream? Is there an alternative explanation that will fit all the facts as well? If something is inconsistent with the interpretation, does the interpreter shift his or her stance and explain it away?

The analysis of Perry's dream is a crude example of hermeneutics. It attempts to account for a number of images in the early part of the dream sequences—the diamonds, the fact that the dream is in a jungle, the oranges, the snake swallowing him feet first, and so on. However, things are left out. Why are they oranges and not apples, which could symbolize breasts just as well? Is it because of his mother's bronzed, yellowish skin as a full-blooded American Indian? Even more significant, what explains the tree that is "standing alone"? Or the parrot? Why is it yellow?

Obviously, a much more detailed *explication de texte* could be made, and it would be made by someone engaged in a serious application of the science of hermeneutics. Such a thorough investigation should result in a convincing demonstration that the interpretation given, and only that interpretation, could account for all the images in the dream sequence.

As has been noted, advocates of hermeneutics argue that the appeal to facts outside the text to validate an interpretation is unnecessary. Thus, it would not be proper to go beyond the text to bring in the fact that Perry's mother often vomited to account for some of the dream imagery. Even more important, we should not attempt to predict actual behavior from interpretations of a textual sequence, as we attempted to do in going from Perry's dream to his murder of Mr. Clutter. To these theorists that would be simply to confuse two different "texts," so to speak (the dream sequence and the murder sequence), each of which would have its own interpretation. However, there seems to be no powerful reason for leaving out any source of information in attempting to arrive at correct scientific inferences. Thus, it does seem to lend credibility to the interpretation of Perry's dream sequence to bring in facts about his mother, his father, and the murder he committed apparently without a motive.

Experimental Studies of the Psychoanalytic Theory of Motivational Stages

Experimentally oriented psychologists never have been satisfied with hermeneutical demonstrations of psychosexual or psychosocial stages of motivational development as outlined in Table 2.4. They have felt that gifted interpreters could make sense out of almost any dream sequence and could manage to find, if they were creative enough, the particular kind of sense they were expecting to find. Therefore, efforts have been made to check the theory by other, more conventional methods.

However, extensive reviews of these studies by Sears (1943) and Kline (1981) have not led to convincing proof by these methods that motives exist and develop as the Freudians have argued. As Silverman (1976) pointed out, most of the studies have attempted to discover whether certain types of unconscious wishes are more common among those who have a personality disorder, which, according to psychoanalytic theory, derives from the conflicts in those unconscious wishes. For example, psychoanalysts have argued that male homosexuals have a strong incestuous wish to sleep with their mothers, which is accompanied by castration anxiety (like Perry's fear of having his legs broken). They deal with this by denial, so they lose all sexual interest in the opposite sex. But it has been difficult to show that incest wishes and castration anxiety are more common in male homosexuals than in male heterosexuals. In fact, psychoanalytic theory does not unequivocally state that there should be a difference. Rather, it argues that while incest wishes and castration anxiety are universal, they have a peculiarly strong *motivating* impact on male homosexuals.

To return to Erikson's analysis of psychosocial stages, everyone goes through an oral period, but how a person negotiates the period affects how strong the motives deriving from that period will continue to be throughout the individual's life-span. Freud dreamed about oral wishes and so did Perry, but we must conclude that the oral wishes had a much stronger motivational impact on Perry than they did on Freud, who dreamed about leaving them behind rather than returning to them.

The most systematic attempt to put Freudian motivational theory to the experimental test has been made by Silverman (1976). He has designed a procedure that makes it theoretically possible to check the specificity of the link between conflicts characteristic of a motivational stage and adult personality disorders associated in psychoanalytic theory with those conflicts. His method presents visual stimuli so rapidly that they cannot be recognized, and it shows that the stimuli that evoke the stage conflicts supposedly characteristic of different disorders affect only people with those disorders, and not others. The method permits so much greater precision in the conclusions drawn than other approaches that it is worth reviewing in some detail. Some examples will show how it works in practice.

Psychoanalysts have argued that disturbances in the oral stage of motive development can lead to serious distortions of reality, and particularly to schizophrenia, as we pointed out in discussing Table 2.4. More specifically, schizophrenia often develops out of the second part of the oral stage, in which the infant learns to take "pleasure in biting *on* hard things, and biting *through* things and in biting pieces *off* things" (Erikson, 1963). This is the beginning of the child's understanding of the difference between good (being close to Mommy) and evil (losing Mommy as she withdraws in anger from the biting). As Erikson (1963) puts it so strikingly,

> Our clinical work indicates that this point in the individual's early history can be the origin of an evil dividedness, where anger against the gnawing teeth, and anger against the withdrawing mother, and anger with one's own impotent anger all lead to a forceful experience of sadistic and masochistic confusion leaving the general impression that once upon a time one destroyed one's unity with a maternal matrix. This earliest catastrophe in the individual's relation to himself and to the world is probably the ontogenetic contribution to the Biblical saga of paradise, where the first people on earth forfeited forever the right to pluck without effort what had been put at their disposal; they bit into the forbidden apple, and made God angry. (1963)

So Silverman argued that the oral aggressive wish should be particularly disturbing to schizophrenics. He aroused the wish unconsciously by presenting oral aggressive stimuli in a tachistoscope so fast (for four milliseconds) that subjects could not consciously report what they saw. He knew from prior research that stimuli presented for this exposure time in fact did register and have effects, even though they could not be consciously reported.

Silverman (1976) measured the effect of such an unconsciously arousing stimulus by coding the thoughts of the subjects after its exposure for pathology ("illogical, loose, or unrealistic thinking," called *primary process thinking*). One of the oral aggressive stimuli he used was the phrase *Cannibal eats person,* a Stage I stimulus (see Table 2.4). He found that thought pathology, or primary process thinking, was greater among schizophrenics after being exposed to this stimulus than after being exposed to control stimuli such as the phrase *people are walking* or a picture of a man reading a newspaper. Furthermore, the difference in the pathology of thought did not occur if the *cannibal eats person* stimulus was presented slowly enough so that the schizophrenics could recognize it. In other words, the wish had to be *unconsciously* aroused to disturb thought, as psychoanalysts would argue.

Perhaps it is not oral aggressive wishes that disturb schizophrenics, but rather any aggressive wish. To find out, Silverman tested another group of schizophrenics, using the arousing stimulus phrase *murderer stabs victim,* a Stage III (intrusive) stimulus. It did not increase primary process thinking in schizophrenics.

As was noted, the oral aggressive wish provokes anxiety precisely because it is associated with the mother's withdrawal, and so Silverman also presented subliminally the stimulus phrase *I am losing Mommy.* This increased thought pathology in schizophrenics, as it should have if the oral aggressive wish were associated in the schizophrenic's mind with the mother's withdrawal. The phrase *destroy Mother* with a picture of someone about to stab an elderly woman had the same effect. Furthermore, the opposite phrase *Mommy and I are one* reduced pathological thinking in schizophrenics, presumably because it reduced the anxiety connected with the basic oral aggressive wish by suggesting an unending source of oral supplies, such as Perry dreamed of.

Silverman demonstrated the specificity of the motivational issue involved by showing that the stimulus phrase *Daddy and I are one* did not reduce primary process thinking in schizophrenics. The advantage of this mode of studying the motivational complexes involved is that it permits testing and falsifying all sorts of alternative formulations of the motivational stage conflicts involved.

Table 2.5 summarizes the findings for thought disorder in schizophrenics, who are the victims of Stage I conflicts, and compares the effects of similar and different stimuli on the reactions of people who have negotiated in an unusual way Stage II (stutterers) or Stage III (homosexuals). The table shows how Silverman can carefully check the specificity of the hypotheses in regard to the relationships involved by varying the stimulus inputs and determining their effects on people with different types of problems.

The extent to which alternative hypotheses to explain the results can and have been checked is much greater than in other research of this type. For comparison, consider the results obtained with stutterers, who, according to psychoanalytic theory, have a disorder associated with not negotiating the second, or anal, psychosexual stage successfully. That is, their key conflict represents "wishes and inhibitions relating to the expelling and retaining of feces" (Silverman, Klinger, Lustbader, Farrell, & Martin, 1972; Silverman, Bronstein, & Mendelsohn, 1976). They stutter precisely because they are in conflict as to whether to let go (that is, speak) or hold on (that is, not speak). Therefore, Silverman aroused motivational conflicts in various ways associated with Stage I (for example, by a picture of a lion roaring), with Stage II by a picture of a dog defecating or the phrase *go shit* with an accompanying picture, and with Stage III by the phrase *fuck Mommy* with a picture suggesting sexual intercourse. He examined stuttering behavior after very rapid exposure to these stimuli and

Table 2.5.

EFFECTS OF AROUSING MOTIVES CHARACTERISTIC OF STAGE CONFLICTS IN INDIVIDUALS WITH DISORDERS ATTRIBUTED TO THOSE STAGES (after Silverman, 1976; Silverman, Bronstein, & Mendelsohn, 1976; Silverman, Klinger, Lustbader, Farrell, & Martin, 1972; Silverman, Kwawer, Wolitsky, & Coran, 1973)

Examples of Stimuli Rapidly Presented[a]	Type of Disorder and Measure Used		
	Schizophrenia, Stage I (Oral Conflicts): Thought Disorder Reaction	Stuttering, Stage II (Anal Conflicts): Stuttering Reaction	Homosexuality, Stage III (Phallic Conflicts): Sexual Feelings Reaction
Stage I: Oral			
Cannibal eats person or picture of lion roaring			
Unrecognized	Increased	Weak increase	
Recognized[a]	No change	No change	
I am losing Mommy	Increased		
Destroy Mother[b]	Increased		
Mommy and I are one	Decreased		No change
Recognized[a]	No change		
Daddy and I are one	No change		
Stage II: Anal			
Go shit[b] or picture of dog defecating		Increased	
Stage III: Phallic			
Murderer stabs victim	No change		
Fuck Mommy[b]	No change	No change	Increased homosexual and decreased heterosexual feelings (no effect on heterosexuals)
Control stimuli (for example, *People are walking* and pictures of a man reading)	No change	No change	No change

[a]Stimulus was presented in a tachistoscope too rapidly (for four milliseconds) to be recognized, except where indicated.

[b]Phrase was accompanied by picture showing the action; both were subliminal.

other neutral stimuli. As Table 2.5 makes clear, the stimuli suggesting Stage II conflicts increased stuttering most significantly in stutterers.

To return to what motivates male homosexuals, who negotiate the third, or phallic, stage of motive development in an unusual way, Silverman, Kwawer, Wolitzky, and Coran (1973) presented to them the stimulus *fuck Mommy* subliminally, sometimes with an additional suggestive picture to increase the anxiety they supposedly feel over their particularly strong, guilt-ridden incest wishes. The investigators found the stimulus increased homosexual and decreased heterosexual feelings among male homosexuals as reflected in self-ratings, but it had no effect on heterosexuals. Thus, Silverman (1976) concludes he was able to demonstrate "that this kind of sexual orientation involves (in part) a flight from incest." That is, among male homosexuals the anxiety about incest with the mother has generalized to all women, and the sexual urge is diverted to men. However, the same phrase had no effect on thought pathology among schizophrenics or on stuttering in stutterers, indicating that the incest conflict was particularly crucial for male homosexuals.

So far Silverman's experimental approach has been applied only to the links between the unconscious motive conflicts that presumably are connected with certain types of psychopathology according to psychoanalytic theory. This approach has made considerable progress in demonstrating the specificity of some of these links, although some still are skeptical about Silverman's results and claim they cannot be replicated (Allen & Condon, 1982; Heilbrun, 1982).

The psychopathological implications of motivational stage theory represent only one of its aspects. What also needs to be studied using a technique like Silverman's is whether there is a hierarchy of stages, as the theory claims. That is, if there is blocking or frustration at a higher stage, will there be a tendency to regress to the next lower stage in thought among those with behavior disorders like Perry, and not among normal individuals? If a motivational conflict representing Stage II, for example, is presented to normal people, will they be more likely to think themselves through to Stage III, as Freud did, demonstrating their greater maturity? Furthermore, we need to know much more about characteristics of normal individuals that are not so extreme as to be psychopathological, but that might represent only mildly unresolved motivational conflicts representative of a particular stage. Above all, we must have some way of measuring the extent to which individuals possess motivational orientations characteristic of various motivational stages. A technique for doing this has been invented by Stewart (1973) and will be discussed in Chapter 8.

• CONTRIBUTIONS OF THE PERSONALITY TRADITION

Most people tend to explain everything others do in terms of motives invented on the spot. Psychologists studying personality have progressed well beyond this "naming fallacy" by identifying a limited list of key human motives and generally distinguishing them from other personal characteristics such as traits and abilities. Above all they have provided a vocabulary of adult human motives in terms of which to describe individual lives. Those who were required by their occupation as therapists to make sense out of disordered lives have made the greatest contribution to describing the motives and motive conflicts that account for what people do or fail to do. They have not agreed entirely on what the key motives are, but there has been a widespread consensus that these motives often are unconscious and not known to the individual, and that any final short list of human motives certainly would have to include needs for aggression or power, for love (or sexuality in the broadest sense), for relief from anxiety and insecurity, and for some kind of mastery or self-actualization.

The major limitation of personality theory has been its inability to measure the motives in question, which has made it difficult (if not impossible) to test rival theories and clarify relationships among motives and presumably connected behaviors or symptoms. Both Murray and Cattell launched major research programs designed to remedy this shortcoming. They invented many ways of measuring a wide variety of motives and then tried to integrate the information collected about a person's motives through either a diagnostic council of judges or factor analysis. Neither integrative approach succeeded completely in providing definitions of motives that were conceptually clear in the measurement sense. However, the efforts of Murray and Cattell created a much better understanding of the measurement problems involved and made further advances possible.

The most successful method of assessing motives in clinical settings has involved the analysis of dreams, free associations, or fantasies. It is believed this is true because certain key motives, such as sexual and aggressive urges, are rejected as bad; continue to function out of consciousness; and show up only in dreams and fantasies, which are not as subject to censorship as conscious thoughts. As Chapter 6 will discuss, motives are also best measured in dreams because other determinants of behavior are less influential in shaping fantasies, so they give clearer indications of motivational—and only motivational—reasons for what a person is doing. Whatever the reason, the analysis of fantasy has provided the most convincing evidence of the existence of key human motives and the best theory currently available about the stages in their development, as outlined by Freud and expanded by Erikson.

Efforts to check the validity of the information on motives obtained through analysis of fantasy had been made with limited success until recent investigations by Silverman improved the methods employed. Whatever the outcome of these validity checks, it seems likely, in view of the experience of personality theorists, that the best way to measure human motives will involve some use of fantasy material.

NOTES AND QUERIES

1. To arrive at a short list of the most important motives, most theorists (McDougall, Freud, Sheldon, and Maslow) try to link certain behavioral trends to inherited or innate biological characteristics. Is there any other way to determine what the most powerful and pervasive human motives are likely to be?

2. Motives are defined by most theorists in terms of behavioral trends. McDougall speaks of persons' domineering, avoiding, or seeking the company of their fellows; Murray, of influencing or submitting passively to others, or drawing near to others; and Cattell, of acting gregariously. However, in Chapter 1 we repeatedly pointed to the dangers of trying to infer motives

from behavioral trends, since other factors play a role in determining actions. Is there any alternative way to define motives? Could they be defined in terms of end states—that is, states of being—rather than in terms of the means of getting to the end states? Try to make a list of end states.

3. Murray's definitions of needs contain many elements. How could we be sure all the elements listed belong under a given need? For example, "to excel oneself" and "to rival and surpass others" are part of the definition of the need for Achievement. How can we tell whether these characteristics go with another need for Achievement characteristic like "to accomplish something difficult" rather than, for example, with the need for Exhibition, defined in part as "to be seen and heard"?

4. The following is a list of the attitude items that load high on one of the motivational factors ("Ergs") Cattell (1957) has identified by statistical intercorrelation of a large number of such items. Try explaining as consistently as you can why each item would indicate a need or wish for something. Try to formulate a definition of the motive in question that would include all these items.

	Loading
I like to take an active part in sports and activities.	.5
I would rather spend free time with people than by myself.	.4
I have no wish to disagree with authorities.	.3
I do not enjoy hunting and fishing.	.3

What are some of the difficulties in trying to infer motives from attitudes?

5. Academic psychologists have been very critical of the kinds of psychoanalytic interpretations of dream sequences discussed in this and the preceding chapter. For example, Eysenck (1965) concludes, "As has often been pointed out, the complexities of psychoanalytic reasoning effectively preclude any scientific testing of these theories." Do you agree? What reasons are there for agreeing or disagreeing with Eysenck?

6. Research has demonstrated that there is little relationship between people's attitudes toward authority figures and the way they write about authority figures in imaginative stories produced for the TAT (Burwen & Campbell, 1957). Psychologists have concluded (see Mischel, 1968) either that TAT stories give no information of value about people or that people are just too inconsistent to characterize. What other inference might be drawn from this fact? Think, for example, of the way Perry thought of his father in real life and in his dream.

7. Do you think Silverman's work demonstrates that adult psychopathology is derived from early traumas in psychosexual development? What other explanation can you give for the fact that a phrase such as *go shit*—uniquely, out of all the emotional phrases used—when presented too rapidly to be recognized, increases stuttering in stutterers? How would you determine if childhood traumas were actually involved? Perry was exposed to some rather severe toilet training. Why did he not stutter?

8. A comparison of Freud's and Perry's dream sequences suggests that people's thinking themselves forward or backward through psychosexual stages might indicate greater or less maturity. Can you think of a way in which a measure of a person's maturity might be obtained in this way? You might want to consult Stewart's method of measuring the Freud-Erikson stages, as described in Chapter 8.

9. In commenting on the interpretation of dream sequences like Perry's, Eysenck (1957b) remarks that "while it may be interesting at times, it has not produced a single fact which could be regarded as having scientific validity. Everything is surmise, conjecture, and interpretation; judgements are made in terms of what is reasonable and fitting. This is not the method of science . . . [in which] you state a definite hypothesis, make certain deductions from the hypothesis, and then proceed to carry out experiments to prove or disprove your theory. This is the scientific method, and that is precisely what is missing in all the work." What is the difference between the scientific and the hermeneutic method? Is there a difference between checking a hypothesis against a fact (for example, a dream image) and against the result of an experiment?

3

Motivation in the Behaviorist Tradition

• THORNDIKE'S STUDIES OF ANIMAL MOTIVATION

At the very moment Freud was discovering the motives behind the dreams of his patients in Vienna, psychologists in the United States were pursuing a radically different approach to understanding motivation. They felt that reports of inner states of mind were unreliable and therefore could never form the basis of an objective science of psychology patterned after the natural sciences. The idea is nicely expressed in a recent physiology textbook (Vander, Sherman, & Luciano, 1975): "Conscious experiences are difficult to investigate because they can be known only by verbal report. Such studies lack objectivity . . . in an attempt to bypass these difficulties scientists have studied the behavioral correlates of mental phenomena in other animals."

It was this line of reasoning that led the U.S. psychologist Edward L. Thorndike to begin studies of motivation and learning in kittens, dogs, and chickens in the 1890s. He placed animals in boxes made out of orange crate slats with a door that opened when a string was pulled or a button inside was turned from the vertical to the horizontal position. Thorndike (1899) summarized his observations as follows:

> A kitten, three to six months old, if put in this box when hungry, a bit of fish being left outside, reacts as follows: it tries to squeeze through between the bars, claws at the bars, and at loose things in and out of the box, reaches its paws out between the bars, and bites at its confining walls. Some one of these promiscuous clawings, squeezings, and bitings turns round the wooden button and the kitten gains freedom and food. By repeating the experience, the animal gradually comes to omit all the useless clawings, etc., and to manifest only the particular impulse (e.g., to claw hard at the top of the button with the paw, or to push against one side of it with the nose) which has resulted successfully. It turns the button round without delay whenever put in the box.
>
> There need be no such congruity between act and result. If we confine a cat and open the door and let it out to get food only when it scratches itself, we shall after enough trials find the cat scratching itself the minute it is put in the box.

Several aspects of this procedure commended themselves to psychologists interested in building a science of behavior. It was objective: anyone could observe what the cat was doing, and in time its actions even could be recorded mechanically. It was potentially quantitative: the number of hours the animal had gone without food could be recorded, as could the number of minutes the animal took to get out of the box. It was experimental: the number of hours the animal went without food could be varied, as could the size of the food reward or the nature of the response required to get out of the box. Above all, this procedure led to results that could be interpreted without recourse to such seemingly vague concepts as purpose and reason, which tended to be invoked when human beings were involved.

At this time in the United States, psychologists were beginning to define psychology as the study of such behavior, that is, of concrete observable and recordable acts rather than inner wishes, thoughts, and expectations, which they did not know how to measure objectively. Thus, it seemed perfectly natural to study animals, which could show the same type of acts as humans could but under more controlled conditions. Psychologists further assumed that whatever principles were found to govern the behavior of lower animals would apply to humans.

Thorndike was interested in the effect of hunger on the activities of animals in the box. He used the term *impulse* to describe what hunger led the animals to do in preference to terms like *motive* or *desire,* which he felt implied the subjective or conscious experiences he was trying to ignore for the moment. This practice has been followed by psychologists in the behaviorist tradition ever since, except they later substituted the word *drive* for *impulse.*

Thorndike (1899) observed first of all that a hungry animal was much more active than one that was not hungry. In his words, a hungry cat "will claw and bite and squeeze incessantly." He stated that the starting point for the kitten was "discomfort from confinement or lack of food" and that this discomfort was relieved when the kitten got out of the box.

Whereas Thorndike correctly reported that "discomfort from confinement" was more characteristic of cats than other animals put in the box, this type of drive was not investigated further by the early behaviorists. They focused on the hunger drive, because it produced similar effects across species; they wanted to establish the most general laws they could, ignoring species' differences, particularly because they might raise the fundamental issue of whether the human species might differ in important ways from the animal species being studied.

The fact that getting to the food reward led the animal to make the correct response to get out of the box more and more quickly was formulated by Thorndike (1911) into what he called the *Law of Effect,* which he stated as follows:

> Of several responses made to the same situation, those which are accompanied or closely followed by satisfaction to the animal will, other things being equal, be more firmly connected with the situation, so that, when it recurs, they will be more likely to recur; those which are accompanied or closely followed by discomfort to the animal will, other things being equal, have their connections with that situation weakened, so that, when it recurs, they will be less likely to occur. The greater the satisfaction or discomfort, the greater the strengthening or weakening of the bond.

Thorndike is particularly careful to avoid referring to such subjective states as "feelings of pleasure" or attributing intelligence to the animal or the idea that a response will lead to satisfaction. Thus, he defines a satisfying state of affairs as "one which the animal does nothing to avoid, often doing such things as attain and preserve it. By a discomforting or annoying state of affairs is meant one which the animal commonly avoids and abandons" (Thorndike, 1911). Inferences about satisfaction or dissatisfaction are made according to the actions the animal takes. Furthermore, the automatic nature of the strengthening of the response is made clear by the example of the kitten learning to make a response like scratching itself, which does not in the real world lead to opening the door.

This emphasizes the fact that the animal's learning the response occurs automatically, without its necessarily understanding a connection between the response and the reward.

So far Thorndike has identified two functions of drive: it *energizes* behavior and *selects out* certain responses that lead to reward; that is, it causes learning. Another function of drive is also easily observable. The animals in the box typically spend more time on the side on which the food is placed. Their biting, squeezings, and clawings are not purely random. They are *oriented* toward the goal, or food reward. Thus, the early behaviorists observed that drive has three important functions: it energizes, orients, and selects behavior.

No one has seriously questioned these functions (see Melton, 1941), although they have inspired much discussion about the terms to be used to describe what Thorndike and the early behaviorists discovered. Some have been so impressed by the similarity between animal drives and human motives that they use the terms more or less interchangeably, as we shall in this book. Others have elaborated further what Thorndike refers to as a satisfying state of affairs. It is described as *rewarding* or *reinforcing* from the objective point of view, since it rewards or reinforces the response that leads to it. From the subjective point of view, it is commonly called an *incentive,* since the anticipation of it leads to making the appropriate response.

Later work stressed that the directive, or orienting, function of drive shows up as much in increased sensory or perceptual sensitivity to certain stimuli as it does in a more focused set of activities. Some scholars, however, felt that this directive function of drive should be attributed to its cue characteristics, or to the associations it evokes, rather than to drive itself (see Farber, 1954).

Finally, B. F. Skinner (1938) and his followers believed it was not at all necessary to talk about drives in the organism, since the learning to get out of the box that Thorndike observed could be explained solely in terms of the rewards or reinforcers provided the animal under various conditions. As we take up these matters, however, remember that Thorndike's observations are as true today as when he first made them: drives or motives serve to energize, to orient, and to select behavior.

Drives as a Means of Insuring Survival

In the functional behaviorist tradition, drives were closely linked to biological needs, because they led the organism to learn to do things it needed to do to survive. Obviously, an organism needs such things as food, air, and water to live. Thus, it is adaptive if the lack of these substances causes disturbances in the body that lead to activities that will remove the disturbances. Drives were thought to be like thermostats that turn on the furnace when the temperature gets too low. Early studies seemed to show this was the way the hunger drive, in particular, functions. For example, Richter (1927) demonstrated that when rats were hungry they turned an activity wheel many more times than when they were satiated. Furthermore, if they were allowed to eat whenever they wanted to, they were much more apt to eat when they were most active. Hunger was associated with activity, which was associated with eating, which decreased the activity.

Warden (1931) and a group at Columbia University designed an obstruction box to measure the strength of various biologically based drives. The animal was placed in a starting box and had to cross an electrified grid to get to what was needed. The strength of the drive was measured by the number of crossings an animal would make when the grid was electrified at a certain level of shock. The researchers plotted the number of crossings against days of food or water deprivation. They found that maximum strength of drive, as measured by the number of crossings, occurred after one or two days of food and water deprivation and then tended to fall off as the animal got weaker. See illustrative data for the white rat in Figure 3.1. Furthermore, as the figure shows, the strength of the rats' drive to get food and water was somewhat higher than the drive of a male rat to cross the grid to get to a female rat in heat. The strongest drive of all was for a mother rat to cross to get to her young. It was reasoned that the sexual and maternal drives obviously were important, because without them the species would not have survived.

Earlier it had been discovered that stomach contractions actually increased as people went without food for some hours (Cannon & Washburn, 1912). Air-filled balloons that subjects swallowed clearly showed evidence of such contractions. This finding was historically very important; it suggested that biological

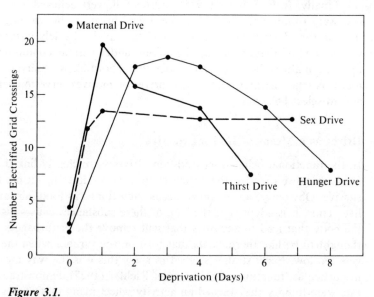

Figure 3.1.

Effect of Increasing Drive Strength on Willingness of White Rats to Endure Pain to Get to Various Goal Objects (after Zimbardo, 1979, after Warden, 1931).

needs might create strong sensations inside the body, which could be the basis for the discomforts that activities were designed to remove. Later research showed that stomach contractions are not the main factor governing the tendency to eat. Blood sugar level is much more important (see Mayer, 1955; Thompson & Campbell, 1977). If it falls below a certain level people feel hungry and eat more; if it rises above a certain level they feel full and eat less. It is difficult to imagine what sensory end organ would be strongly stimulated by a decreased blood sugar level, but this discovery had not been made at the time the behaviorist model of drive was constructed. Thus, many behaviorists concluded that drive could be conceived as strong sensations of the sort derived from the hunger cramps that developed from going without food.

• HULL'S MODEL OF HOW DRIVES FACILITATE ADAPTATION OR LEARNING

Most psychologists, following Thorndike's lead, devoted their attention to trying to understand how drives facilitated learning ultimately in the interest of survival. Like Thorndike, they wanted to describe the process in a completely objective way without recourse to terms suggesting subjective states of mind, such as *feelings, hopes, fears,* and *purposes.* Edward Tolman (1932) used such terms but was careful to objectify their meaning. For example, he felt *purpose* could be defined simply by observing behavior in an animal that *persisted until* some end state was reached.

Clark Hull (1943) tried to go even further and delete such terms as *purpose* altogether from a scientific vocabulary by demonstrating that what was called *purpose* could be explained in purely mechanical stimulus-response terms. He thought it was best for psychologists to think of an organism—whether human or animal—as a machine, and he conceived of himself as an engineer trying to create "a truly self-maintaining robot" (Hull, 1943). In this way Hull could avoid using vague mental states of mind to resolve difficulties in explaining behavior, for "the temptation to introduce an entelechy, soul, spirit, or demon into a robot is slight." Therefore, as a model for the organism, he created in his fancy a motorized machine that ran about on little wheels. It contained an oil tank and a proboscis—something like a flexible gas pump hose or an elephant's trunk—that could move about freely. He equipped the robot with a liquid level indicator that, when the oil fuel supply got below a certain point, would activate the machine, and particularly the proboscis, so both would move about much more vigorously.

Hull imagined the robot was moving about in a landscape where there were little pools of oil in various places. He reasoned that by chance (not by forethought!), in waving about, the proboscis might come in contact with one of these pools of oil. When it did so, because of a mechanism built into it, it would automatically start sucking up the oil into the tank until the liquid level indicator rose and turned off the mechanism causing the increased activity. Hull then equipped his robot with a memory device that after this experience would lead it more quickly to a pool of oil the next time its fuel supply ran low. This device corresponded to Thorndike's Law of Effect. It simply insured that whatever response the robot was making when it sucked up oil was more likely to occur the next time it ran low on fuel.

What was important to Hull was that no one could conceive of a robot saying to itself, "Aha, I see when I am running out of fuel I'd better look around for some pools of oil so that I can replenish my supply." The whole process was conceived in purely objective, mechanical terms. Hull wanted psychology to be a natural science, like nineteenth-century physics. Thus, his task as a psychologist was to identify the key variables in psychology analogous to such variables as mass, velocity, and time in the physics of his day and to state the empirical relationships among these variables in quantitative form, just as the laws of physics were stated.

Hull's approach appealed greatly to many psychologists in the 1930s and 1940s. It was objective. It was quantitative. It promised to develop a natural science like the other natural sciences that had so successfully improved the understanding of the physical world. Above all, it appeared to explain some very complex mental phenomena in terms of a few simple concepts and their precisely stated relationships. The task of psychology was reduced to manageable size: it consisted of working out the basic principles of behavior and then applying them to explain all sorts of complex phenomena, from psychotherapy to human aggression and war. It is not feasible, nor is it any longer appropriate, to describe Hull's principles and their application in any detail. It is important, however, to understand how his model of motivation worked, for it has influenced thinking about the problem ever since.

Figure 3.2 presents a simplified version of the model as it was developed at Yale University by Hull and others associated with him, including Miller and Dollard (1941), Mowrer (1950), and Spence (1956). It represents in mechanical or objective terms what goes on in a motivational sequence, such as when a woman walks down the street, feels hungry, sees a restaurant, enters, and eats. As she walks along she is exposed to certain cues, or stimuli, in the environment, such as the sights of various storefronts and other pedestrians, or the sight and sound of automobiles in the street. These cues are represented by the symbols S_1, S_2, and so on. Now suppose her "hunger stat," analogous to a thermostat, is tripped off. This provides a new source of stimulation corresponding perhaps to hunger pangs, which are internal and represented by the symbol S_D, for *drive stimulus.* It is also represented by an increase in the line at the bottom of Figure 3.2 representing an increased drive tension. The woman also is making responses (represented as R_1, R_2, and so on) as she proceeds down the street: she is walking, looking at storefronts, and so on.

Suppose she sees a restaurant (S_2) at the moment her drive increases. There now is a new stimulus complex ($S_2 + S_D$); in the past it was associated with responses such as entering a restaurant and eating that have led to drive reduction, which has strengthened these responses. Therefore, on this occasion the $S_2 + S_D$ complex evokes entering the restaurant (R_3), which in turn leads to eating (defined as R_g, or the *goal response,* since it leads to a reduction in the

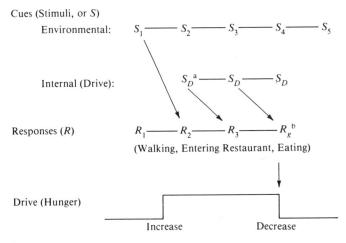

Cues (Stimuli, or *S*)

Environmental: $S_1 \text{———} S_2 \text{———} S_3 \text{———} S_4 \text{———} S_5$

Internal (Drive): $S_D{}^a \text{———} S_D \text{———} S_D$

Responses (*R*) $R_1 \text{———} R_2 \text{———} R_3 \text{———} R_g{}^b$

(Walking, Entering Restaurant, Eating)

Drive (Hunger)

Increase · · · · · Decrease

^aS_D = Drive stimulus (hunger).
^bR_g = Goal response.

Figure 3.2.

How Cues, Responses, Drive, and Drive Reduction (Reward) Combine to Produce Behavior Motivated by Hunger.

drive). Drive reduction automatically reinforces the connections between the stimuli and responses in this sequence, so that the next time the cue complex of hunger plus sight of restaurant occurs, the response of entering and eating will occur more promptly and efficiently. Note that the complex behavior of a human being has been explained without recourse to any concepts other than those used to explain the behavior of Hull's self-maintaining robot.

Furthermore, the model can explain such a purely mentalistic concept as *purpose* in mechanical terms. Note that the drive stimulus (S_D) is associated with the goal response (R_g), which is regularly followed by drive reduction. Therefore, the bond between S_D and R_g is strengthened; every time S_D occurs it should tend to evoke R_g. However, it cannot elicit the full response of eating, since no food is present. Therefore, it elicits a fractional anticipatory response—namely, salivating (r_g)—rather than R_g, the full goal response. This notion came from Ivan Pavlov's conditioning experiments with dogs, in which he found that a bell associated with feeding a little later would, in time, evoke salivation before the food actually was presented.

Furthermore, since every response produces some sensations, the anticipatory salivary response (r_g) also produces its own stimulation, s_g, that is, $r_g \rightarrow s_g$. This third type of stimulation combines with S_2 and with S_D (sight of the restaurant) in the model in Figure 3.2 to make up the total stimulus complex that leads to the responses of entering the restaurant and eating. It is crucial here to observe that the hunger drive (S_D) evokes a *fractional anticipatory goal response* with its attendant stimulation (s_g) that moves forward from the end of the sequence to the beginning and becomes a determinant of what follows. In commonsense terms, a man thinks about eating and the relief of his hunger pangs that goes with eating. Therefore, he enters a restaurant to eat; that is his *purpose*. In the behaviorist model, however, there is no need to invoke a mentalistic concept like purpose: it is represented by the fractional anticipatory goal response, which is set up automatically from previous experiences with eating and which also automatically moves forward in the stimulus-response sequence to the beginning whenever S_D occurs.

Drive as a Strong Stimulus

Miller and Dollard (1941) most explicitly generalized the model of drive built on hunger pangs. They state the following:

> A drive is a strong stimulus which impels action. Any stimulus can become a drive if it is made strong enough. The stronger the stimulus, the more drive function it possesses. The faint murmur of distant music has but little primary drive function; the infernal blare of the neighbor's radio has considerably more. While any stimulus may become strong enough to act as a drive, certain special classes of stimuli seem to be the primary basis for the greater proportion of motivation. These might be called the primary or innate drives. One of these is pain. Pain can reach stabbing heights of greater strength than thirst, the pangs of extreme hunger, and the sore weight of fatigue which are other examples of powerful innate drives. The bitter sting of cold and the insistent goading of sex are further examples. (Miller & Dollard, 1941)

Note that they say that a person in all such instances seeks relief from stimulation or discomfort. There is no such thing as an interest in pleasure per se. Even what looks like pleasure seeking really is motivated by the desire for tension reduction. For example, people ride roller coasters to get what they call "pleasure," but they simply are inducing tension to get more satisfaction from reducing it. Even the pleasure from something like tickling derives not from the sensations as they are induced, but from their dying away or fading out afterward. Such interpretations may seem farfetched in light of many human experiences, but they were essential to a theory that maintained drives could only derive from strong stimulation.

Drives also can be acquired. The most important acquired drive in the Miller and Dollard model is fear or anxiety. Pain is a strong drive stimulus that leads to many activities, some of which are associated with escaping the pain. In time, therefore, any cues associated with the pain get connected with the sensations and responses associated with it, so that in time the cues have the ability to elicit what accompanies the pain before the pain actually occurs. Since the effects of the pain are strong, what the cue elicits serves as a new type of strong stimulus or a secondary, or learned, drive, commonly called *anxiety*.

An experiment reported by Miller (1948) illustrates the way this happens. Miller placed rats in a white compartment, the floor of which was a grid that could be electrified. The rats were given a series of brief electric shocks every five seconds in the compartment; a door then was opened, which allowed them to escape into another compartment painted black. After the rats had been shocked a few times in the white compartment, most quickly learned to escape from it into the black compartment as soon as they were placed in the apparatus. Notice, however, that the white compartment had no drive stimulus value in the beginning. It acquired drive value because it was associated with the pain of electric shock. The evidence for this fact was that after experiencing shock, the rats would run out of the white compartment even when they were not shocked. The only way this could be explained was to assume they were escaping an acquired strong stimulus that derived from the learned anticipation of strong shock sensations.

Next Miller put a barrier between the white and the black compartments that could be let down only if the rats managed to turn a wheel that dropped the door between the two compartments. Would the fear of the white compartment—the secondary, or acquired, drive—be sufficient to motivate the rats to learn a new habit, namely, wheel turning to escape the fear? Figure 3.3 shows the results. Note that the animals were learning to turn the wheel more and more quickly as they got out of the white box that way in successive trials. Since they no longer were getting shocked, the only way this result could be explained in terms of the model is that there was a new acquired drive—namely, fear or anxiety—responsible for the learning.

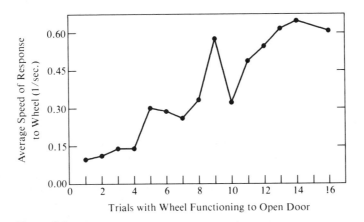

Figure 3.3.

Rats' Learning the First New Habit, Turning the Wheel, During Trials Without Primary Drive. This figure shows the progressive increase in the average speed with which animals ran up to the wheel and turned it enough to drop the door into the nonshock compartment during the sixteen trials when they no longer received shock in the first compartment (Miller, 1948).

From such an analysis it was but a short step to the inference that anxiety could well be the master motive in human behavior (Mowrer, 1950), since human beings are subjected to so many discomforts they might wish to avoid before they occur. Thus, in this model it is fear that drives people to accumulate money in order to avoid the discomforts that come from lack of money. It is fear that leads people to associate with and seek the approval of others because of the suffering they must endure if others punish and disapprove. Freudian theory also emphasized the importance of anxiety as a master motive, and this was just beginning to be widely understood, if not entirely accepted, at about this time in the United States. Thus, the behaviorists were particularly gratified to think they had found an objective means of showing how and why anxiety was so important in human life.

Does Animal Learning Occur in the Absence of Drive?

Some psychologists associated with E. C. Tolman at the University of California at Berkeley in the 1920s had reported a phenomenon that seemed to throw into question Thorndike's Law of Effect and the model of learning constructed by Hull and his associates. Rats were first allowed to explore a maze without food reward. After they had explored the maze on several days, food was placed in the goal box. Almost immediately the rats showed great improvement in getting from the starting box to the goal where the food was. They ran the maze more quickly, making fewer errors. As Figure 3.4 shows, "Group I was given a food reward on every trial. In Group II, the food reward was not introduced until the seventh day (at point *Z*). In Group III the food reward was not introduced until the third day (at point *X*). Both Group II and Group III showed a substantial decrease in errors after the first rewarded trial" (Weiner, 1980a).

Apparently the rats were learning something even when they were not being rewarded. They showed signs of what was called *latent learning.* How could this be, according to the model of learning that stated associations were formed by rewards or reductions in drive? Tolman concluded that the Law of Effect referred to performance rather than to learning. In other words, the animals had learned "what went with what"—which turns in the maze led where—through sheer contiguity. Neither reward nor drive reduction was necessary for this kind of learning. Instead, rewards determined how the rats used the information they had acquired to get from the start to the goal.

However, the mechanism of acquired drive allowed the Hullians to explain this apparent contradiction in terms of their model. They only needed to assume that rats did not like surprises, that strange or unfamiliar stimuli would produce discomfort, and that to reduce such discomfort the rats would learn their way around the maze. This was the explanation given for *exploratory drive;* its evidence was the tendency of rats when put in a maze to explore all its aspects (W. I. Walker, 1959). In this view, novel stimuli would serve as mild drive stimuli, which the rat would learn to reduce by exploring the maze. The explanation for latent learning, then, was that the learning had occurred in the service of the exploratory drive rather than the hunger drive, and when hunger and food re-

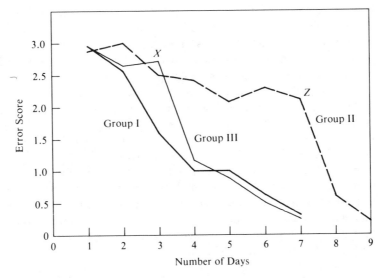

Figure 3.4.

Latent Learning Phenomenon. Errors made by rats in running a maze when food was available from the start (Group I) or introduced at Points *X* and *Z* (Groups II and III) (Weiner, 1980a, after Blodgett, 1929).

ward were introduced the learning simply transferred to another drive stimulus (see Montgomery & Segall, 1955). The argument is involved, but it seemed reasonable and saved the Hullian model from what could have been a fatal objection.

Cue Characteristics

In the behaviorist model, as Figure 3.2 illustrates, cues, or environmental stimuli, determine where and when a response will be made. For a hungry woman, the sight of a restaurant trips off the response of entering it to eat. In the same way, a dinner bell elicits going into the dining room, and a factory whistle evokes the response of leaving work. Cues also determine which response will be made, since they get associated with the particular response that happens to reduce a drive. Our hypothetical hungry woman enters the restaurant when she sees it. She does not throw a rock through the window, because entering has been associated with satisfying the hunger drive and throwing a rock has not. However, if cues are responsible for directing or channeling behavior, how can we say that drives *direct* or orient behavior?

Some have argued that, strictly speaking, drives do not direct behavior (see Farber, 1954), although the cues associated with them, like any other stimuli, have the capacity to direct behavior. Different drives have different cue values. The sensations produced by thirst are quite different from those produced by hunger. These unique sensations produced by different drives may get uniquely associated with different means of reducing each drive—by drinking in the case of thirst and eating in the case of hunger.

The stimulus characteristics of drives were particularly emphasized by Estes (1958), who analyzed data showing that response strength varied as a function of the relationship between drive level during training and during testing. Suppose rats were trained to go down a runway to get food after ten hours of food deprivation. Now suppose the rats are deprived of food for twenty hours and placed in the same runway, but this time without any food at the end. How long will the rats continue to run? How long before the running response is extinguished altogether? Oddly enough, the rats will not run as many times as they would have if the hours of deprivation were the same as those under which they had been trained, even though they are hungrier during testing. Estes' (1958) explanation is that "changing the level of deprivation between training and test has the effect of dropping out some of the drive cues that had become conditioned during training." This means the running response will be less strongly evoked during testing, because responses learned to one type of cue do not occur as strongly to different, although similar, cues.

Hull called this phenomenon the *stimulus generalization gradient.* It is well known in conditioning studies that if, for example, the salivary response of a dog is conditioned to a sound, so that every time the sound occurs the dog salivates, a change in the sound—for example, replacing it with one of a different pitch or lesser intensity—will evoke a weaker salivary response. The response generalizes to other stimuli similar to the one to which it was conditioned, but the capacity of stimuli to evoke the response declines regularly the more dissimilar they are to the original conditioned stimulus. In other words, there is some transfer of learning to different stimulus situations, and this principle applies to the transfer of learning across drive stimulus situations. The same principle of transfer of learning was invoked to explain latent learning in the maze discussed in the previous section. In that case, the learning associated with the exploratory drive stimulus was supposed to have transferred to the hunger drive stimulus.

It was also generally believed that stronger drives tended to flatten the stimulus generalization gradient (see Miller, 1948). That is, the stronger the drive, the greater the tendency to respond to stimuli a little different from the original conditioned stimulus. Rosenbaum (1953) showed that experimentally induced anxiety tended to increase stimulus generalization. A school phobia illustrates the principle. As one child gets closer to school, he gets more and more afraid until, by the time he is a block away, he is too frightened to go any further. However, if another child has an even stronger phobia, she might respond to stimuli present three blocks away from the school just as strongly as the first child did to stimuli one block away. In extreme cases she might not even leave the house. Looked at in another way, the anxiety drive appears to be sensitizing the children to more and more cues related to the cue originally connected with it (the school). They perceive even streets far away from the school as school related. Perceptual sensitization was not particularly studied by the behaviorists, because they focused more on action than perception.

Response Characteristics

In the model presented in Figure 3.2, a response must occur before it can be "stamped in," or learned. Scared children cannot be rewarded for entering the school if they are so afraid they never make the response of entering the school. Where do these responses come from? Some are innate, such as when a rat jumps up as electric shock is applied to its feet. Others occur randomly if they are part of the animal's repertoire, as when a cat is first placed in one of Thorndike's boxes.

Especially important is what Hull called the *habit family hierarchy*. That is, an animal or person normally enters a situation with some responses much more likely to be evoked than others because of past experience in similar situations. These responses are conceived as being arranged in a rank order in which the strongest one occurs first, then the next strongest, and so on. Reward changes the rank order of responses in this situation. The cat may respond first by trying to stick its paw through the slats, but this response is not rewarded; eventually the response of turning the button, which is rewarded, assumes the highest place in the habit family hierarchy in the box situation. It is important to remember, however, that a reward increases the likelihood of recurrence of any response associated with it, no matter how irrelevant it actually may be to producing the reward. Thus, the cat may learn to scratch itself, even though scratching did not directly open the door.

The behaviorists recognized that so far as people were concerned, many of the important responses were not overt actions and therefore could not be observed. People obviously think as well as act; they have ideas and expectations. They use language to try out responses before performing them visibly. The behaviorists cut themselves off from studying such responses directly, largely by working with animals, which could not talk. That was justified on two grounds: First, it prevented psychologists from using poorly defined mentalistic concepts, as Hull had argued. Second, it was assumed that it was easier to work out the principles of behavior with overt acts and that these same principles then could be applied to any kind of behavior, including covert or symbolic acts such as thoughts.

Reward Characteristics

Rewards were defined as anything that reduces a drive, but the behaviorists recognized that many objects or situations could be shown to have reward value in the sense of facilitating learning even though just what drive or drives they were reducing was not always clear. Thus, a child might collect stamps or marbles, and it would be difficult to determine just what strong stimuli these objects were reducing. Perhaps the child had been teased for not having had any marbles and collected them to reduce the acquired anxiety drive resulting from teasing. Once it had been determined that marbles were important to the child, however, they could be used reliably to get him or her to learn things. This line of reasoning led Skinner (1953) and his associates to discard the notion of drive altogether and to argue that it was sufficient simply to list what would serve as a reward or reinforcer for various types of learned behavior.

According to Hullian theory, objects could acquire reward value by being associated with primary drive reduction. They were called *secondary,* or *acquired, rewards* to contrast them with *primary rewards,* like food, that were innately rewarding. An early and very influential experiment by Wolfe (1936) illustrated how objects could acquire secondary reward value, even for animals. He taught chimpanzees to use poker chips to get food. When they inserted a chip in a vending machine, it would provide them with a piece of banana or a grape. The chimps even learned that chips of different color had different value: a blue chip might produce five grapes and a white chip, only one. Wolfe demonstrated that the chimps would work almost as hard to get the chips as they would to get food rewards, even if the rewards were delayed after the chimps put the chips in the vending machine to get food. How hard the chimps would work depended on the value of the chips and on how many chips they already had. Furthermore, they hoarded chips and competed to pick them up if a number were thrown into a cage where two chimps were present. In other words, the chips had definitely acquired a reward value they did not have before they were associated with producing food, which resulted in primary drive reduction.

The analogy with the way humans work for and collect money was inescapable. Miller and Dollard (1941) put it this way:

> During the course of his socialization, the individual learns that the possession of money is the means of gratifying many different needs and that the lack of money is a signal that he may have to bear the uncomfortable goading of many undesirable desires. Some of the drives upon which the desire for money is based are primary drives, such as hunger and cold. Others may be secondary, such as anxiety. Because of the number of different drives supporting the need for money, it is a rare occasion when the individual is without any primary motivation to summate with and activate his need for money."

Secondary rewards even generalize from the situation in which they are learned to another situation. Estes (1949) demonstrated that a sound associated with drinking had a reinforcing effect even when rats were hungry but not thirsty. In this way, lucky charms acquire reward value. A person might have been wearing something when almost hit by a car, so that it is associated in his or her mind with escape from pain. Thus, the person wears the same item on any threatening occasion to reduce the anxiety that arises.

The Incentive Variable

In the first set of principles published by Hull (1943), excitatory potential, or the tendency to act, was a joint function of drive strength and habit strength, or the number of hours of food deprivation and the number of practice trials in running a maze. However, it was apparent from the very beginning that size of reward also affected the tendency to make a response, even though drive was held constant. This point is made dramatically in Figure 3.5. In this experiment, the strength of the tendency to act was measured by the speed with which rats traversed a runway to get to food. They ran much faster to get sixteen pellets of food than to get one pellet of food and ran still faster to get 256 pellets of food, even though in all these conditions the hours of food deprivation were held constant. Furthermore, if the amount of food reward shifted part of the way through the experiment, so those formerly getting 256 pellets now received only sixteen, speed of running declined sharply. However, the speed increased if the amount of the food reward went from one to sixteen pellets.

To take into account the influence of the size of the incentive on response strength, Hull added a variable to his equation, generally labeled K (incentive). In his revised principles (Hull, 1952) it read as follows:

$$\text{Excitatory potential} = \text{Drive} \times \text{Habit strength} \times \text{Incentive},$$

$$\text{or } {_S}E_R = D \times {_S}H_R \times K.$$

That is, on the basis of the data then available, Hull thought it likely that the incentive value (K) would multiply with the product of habit strength (${_S}H_R$)

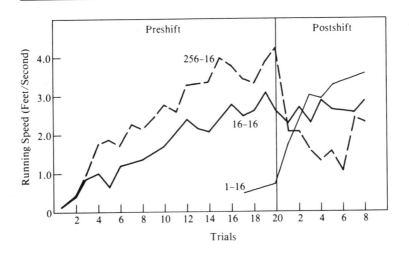

Figure 3.5.

Speed of Running in a Long Runway as a Function of Amount of Reinforcement. For the first nineteen trials different groups were given 1, 16, or 256 pellets of food (acquisition data for the one-pellet group are not presented); after trial twenty, all subjects were given sixteen pellets (Weiner, 1980a, after Crespi, 1942).

and drive (*D*) for much the same reason as he thought these two variables would multiply with each other to determine response strength. If any of the variables in the equation is reduced to zero, there should be no excitatory potential ($_SE_R$) for the behavior in question. If the animal has zero drive, it will not run, no matter how practiced it is or how huge the reward. It also will not be able to run a maze without error—no matter how strong its drive or the incentive—if it has had no practice, indicating zero habit strength. Likewise, no matter what the level of drive and habit strength, if there is no reward or incentive, there should be no action.

Kenneth Spence (1956, 1958a, 1958b) disagreed. He was a major exponent of the view that incentive value had to be added to the equation, but felt that it summated with drive as follows:

$$_SE_R = (D + K) \times _SH_R.$$

Spence felt this was a more likely way for the two variables to combine because he conceived of the influence of *K* as occurring largely through the fractional anticipatory goal response mechanism ($r_g - s_g$) discussed earlier. A large food reward would produce an $r_g - s_g$ distinctively different from the one produced by a smaller food reward. The different kinds of $r_g - s_g$ would move forward in time and combine additively with the drive stimuli present from the drive state, and the sum of the two sets of stimuli would multiply with habit strength to produce excitatory potential. Research investigations never conclusively settled the question of which of these two formulations was more nearly correct.

• EXCITATORY POTENTIAL IN BEHAVIOR THEORY AND THE MEANING OF THE TERM *MOTIVATION*

Hull and Spence referred to the product of habit, drive, and incentive as "excitatory potential," which is analogous to what Thorndike called the "impulse to act." Several recent texts (Atkinson & Birch, 1978; Klein, 1982; Weiner, 1980a) have dropped this terminology and substituted the word *motivation* for *excitatory potential.* Thus, in their terminology, anything that increases the tendency to act can be described as a motivator or as increasing motivation. In this sense, habits increase motivation, as do expectations and motives or drives. For example, suppose we are trying to find out what "moves" a person to go into a restaurant at 6:00 P.M. At least three factors contribute to the tendency to perform this act: the fact that the person usually eats at this time and place (habit), the fact that the person expects that food is likely to be present in the restaurant (expectancy), and the fact that the person is hungry.

Atkinson and Weiner refer to habits and expectancies as increasing "motivation" to perform the act, as "moving" the person to perform it. We will use the term *motivation* only to refer to the aroused motive, that is, to hunger in the example just given. This is because to describe a habit as a motivator or as contributing to motivation not only departs from traditional usage; it also contradicts common sense and introduces conceptual confusion, particularly in studying human motives. At that level we must distinguish between a motive—conceived as an individual disposition or trait (the general tendency to be hungry all the time)—and motivation—conceived as a motive disposition aroused at a particular moment in time (how hungry the person is here and now). If the term *motivation* already has been used to describe any factor that moves a person to act, it is no longer available to describe an aroused motive. For all these reasons, we will use the term *motivation* to describe an aroused motive and such terms as *excitatory potential* or the *impulse* or *tendency to act* to describe the effect of the sum total of all determinants of action, following Hull's example. (See Tables 6.1 and 12.2 in Chapters 6 and 12, respectively.)

Excitatory Potential for Operants More Indicative of Motivation

Hull built his model of motivated behavior by starting from the conditioning experiment in which a stimulus is associated with a response followed by a reward. This meant he used, as measures of response strength, latency (the time between stimulus and response), the amplitude of the response, the regularity of response to the stimulus, or the resistance to extinction (the number of times a response occurs on presentation of the stimulus when the reward is not present). Skinner (1938), however, pointed out that there are many responses that occur naturally for which a stimulus cannot readily be identified; for these responses, he said, such measures of response strength are unavailable. He called these responses *operants*. They appear to occur spontaneously, and the measure of their response strength is simply frequency of occurrence rather than latency or other such measures of the strength of a stimulus-response connection. Skinner focused attention on observing the rate with which a rat would press a bar to get food in a small box; in this case the "stimulus" that evokes bar pressing is not easily identifiable. He found that the frequency of the bar-pressing response was readily influenced by variables of the incentive type or reinforcers and the schedule with which they were provided to the rat. Thus, for Skinner, variables of the motivational type were particularly important in influencing the strength of operant behaviors. In fact, Skinner (1966) flatly stated that "operant behavior is essentially the field of purpose." The distinction between respondents, where a stimulus can be identified, and operants, where it cannot, is important, and we will return to it in Chapter 13. It appears that the response probability of an operant is a more sensitive indicator of motive strength than are the measures of respondent response strength, such as latency, amplitude, and resistance to extinction.

• THE BEHAVIORIST MODEL OF MOTIVATION APPLIED TO HUMANS BY SPENCE AND OTHERS

Behaviorists since Thorndike had studied animals exclusively to get the simplest, most objective picture possible of how motivation influenced learning. Having developed a model of motivation from studying other animals, they tried to apply it to human behavior. One way to do this was simply to assume complex human motives had to be explained in terms of the principles they had established (Korman, 1974). The way behaviorists accounted for the desire for money, as described earlier, is a good example of how they proceeded. Money is a secondary reward that has acquired its value because of its association with many different kinds of drive reduction. Unfortunately, there was no real way to check this assertion, nor was there any attempt to study the "money drive" as it functioned in human behavior. It was enough simply to show how it could fit into the model of motivation that had been constructed (see J. S. Brown, 1961).

This was obviously unsatisfactory, because it left human motives altogether unstudied. Then Kenneth Spence and his associates, particularly Janet Taylor Spence, to their great credit, undertook a whole series of investigations using human subjects; the investigations were designed to test directly the applicability of the model to human motives. In one group of studies they investigated the conditioned eye blink (Spence, 1958b). In the experiment a sound is followed after a brief interval by an air puff to the eye, which elicits an eye blink because the puff is aversive. After a few trials the sound evokes the eye blink before the puff occurs, and the eyelid response is said to be *conditioned.* A conditioned eyelid response is one that occurs to the sound cue before the aversive air puff is applied.

Kenneth Spence and his associates were interested in two motivational influences on the curve of acquisition of the conditioned eyelid response. The first was the intensity of the air puff, which corresponded to variations in induced drive strength. They reasoned that if the air puff were stronger, the drive stimulus and the anxiety conditioned to it also would be stronger, and the conditioned eyelid response should be learned faster because the drive was stronger. This is exactly what happened, as Figure 3.6 shows. Note that the pair of learning curves for the stronger air puff is above the pair of curves for the weaker air puff throughout the learning trials. That is, the stronger air puff elicited a higher percent of conditioned responses throughout than the weaker air puff.

Notice also that the curves tend to draw apart, as they should if drive and habit strength are multiplying, as Hull and Spence claimed. A little arithmetic will show why this should be so. In the following numerical example it is assumed that the weaker air puff has a D value of 1 and the stronger air puff, a D value of 2, and that habit strength (H) has the value of the trial number indicating the number of times the conditioning has been carried out. If we multiply $D \times H$, the difference in the predicted response strengths on the second trial would be $1 \times 2 = 2$ versus $2 \times 2 = 4$. On the tenth trial, however, the relative values would be $1 \times 10 = 10$ versus $2 \times 10 = 20$. The difference between 10 and 20 is much greater than the distance between 2 and 4, which is exactly the way in which the curves draw apart in Figure 3.6. If the two factors (D and H) simply summed rather than multiplied, the curves would stay a constant distance apart throughout their entire course.

Spence and his associates also were the first to be interested in studying individual differences in the strength of a motive. Once again they worked with the anxiety motive, and Taylor developed a self-report measure of symptoms of

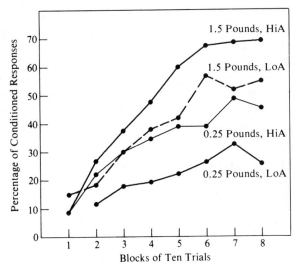

S_c = Conditioned stimulus (light, 1.5 footcandles).

S_u = Unconditioned stimulus (air puff).

$S_c - S_u$ = 450 milliseconds.

Figure 3.6.

Performance in Eyelid Conditioning as a Function of Test Anxiety Score (A) and Intensity of Unconditioned Stimulus (Air Puff to Eye) (after Spence, 1958b).

manifest anxiety, the Taylor Manifest Anxiety Scale (MAS). In other words, they recognized that not only could anxiety be increased experimentally, but also that individuals might vary as a result of their life histories in the extent to which they had developed a generalized type of anxiety drive. The scale score consisted of the extent to which individuals agreed with items like "I worry quite a bit over possible misfortunes." Spence and his associates divided their subjects into those who agreed very much with items like this and those who agreed very little with them. The learning curves for those scoring very high (the high anxiety, or HiA, subjects) and for those scoring very low (the low anxiety, or LoA, subjects) are shown separately in Figure 3.6.

It is evident that this type of drive also interacts with habit strength over the course of learning in the same way induced anxiety (from the air puff) does. The high anxiety subjects conditioned more rapidly than the low anxiety subjects at both levels of induced anxiety, represented by weaker or stronger air puffs. The strength of the air puff can be conceived of as an index of aversive *incentive* in the situation, since it can be assumed that the eye blink is learned to avoid the unpleasant puff, and the stronger the puff, the greater the drive reduction from avoiding it and the stronger the incentive to blink. If so, the curves should give some indication as to whether drive (D) and incentive (K) multiply (as Hull thought) or add together (as Spence thought) in multiplying with habit strength (H) as represented by the number of practice trials. If they multiply, the curves for the high anxiety subjects, for example, at two incentive levels should be much farther apart and show greater separation with increasing H than if D and K summate. Unfortunately, the results are ambiguous: The curves do not seem as far apart as Hull's assumptions would suggest they should be. Thus, Spence's model may seem more reasonable, but there is no way to judge for certain how far apart the curves should be.

How a Strong Drive Can Interfere with Performance on Complex Tasks

In the conditioned eyelid experiment, one response is clearly dominant, namely, the eye blink. In more complex learning situations, however, many responses are potentially relevant. In some cases the response most likely to occur (the one highest in the habit family hierarchy) may be the wrong one for solving a problem. Yet according to the behaviorist model, drive should facilitate the appearance of the strongest response, even if it is the wrong one. It follows that increases in drive strength might delay learning of complex tasks because they would increase the likelihood of making a wrong or irrelevant response at the beginning of learning.

Haner and Brown (1955) carried out a very simple experiment that demonstrated how increasing drive could make it more likely that an irrelevant response would occur. They had subjects play a game in which the objective was to place thirty-six marbles in small, round holes in a board in a limited period of time. The experimenter signaled when the time was up by pushing a lever, which dropped all the marbles down below the board. The strength of drive was manipulated by indicating that the time was up after various numbers of marbles had been put in place. That is, it was assumed that frustration would be greater if the time were up after the subjects had put nearly all the marbles in place (thirty-two out of thirty-six) than if they had put only half of them in place (eighteen out of thirty-six). In drive theory, frustration is an important source of tension, or drive strength. After the trial was ended by dropping the marbles below, the subject had to push a plunger to get ready for the next trial. As frustration or drive strength increased from the subjects' being interrupted nearer and nearer the goal, they tended to push the plunger more and more vigorously. However, vigor of plunger pushing is in no way related to doing better at the task, and under certain conditions such responses might interfere with solving a complex problem.

An experiment in learning paired associates was conducted to test this hypothesis (Spence, Farber, & McFann, 1956). Subjects were presented with a word like *barren,* to which they had to learn to say a response word whenever *barren* recurred. In one experiment the response words were highly associated with the stimulus words. For example, *fruitless* was the response to be associated with *barren.* In such instances the correct response would be assumed to be fairly high in the subject's habit family hierarchy and likely to occur in any case. In another experiment the response words were totally unrelated to the stimulus words. Now a word like *grouchy* would have to be associated with *barren.* In this instance, more dominant responses to *barren,* like *fruitless* or *arid,* would be incorrect; according to theory, however, greater drive strength should strengthen them, just as it strengthens all responses that tend to occur in the situation, so learning should be slowed. Thus, the prediction was that greater drive strength should facilitate the learning of highly associated pairs where the dominant responses were appropriate, but it should inhibit the learning of unassociated pairs where the dominant responses were incorrect.

The measure of drive strength was whether the subject scored very high or very low on the Taylor MAS. Some of the early results confirm the prediction made by the theory, as Figure 3.7 shows. The high anxiety, or high *D,* subjects learn the highly associated pairs faster than the low anxiety subjects, but they learn the unassociated pairs less quickly than those low in anxiety.

Sarason, Mendler, and Craighill (1952) obtained similar results in a different test situation and explained them a little differently. They asked subjects to place digits under associated symbols, with either of two sets of instructions. In one case they told the subjects that they could not be expected to finish substituting all the digits for symbols in the time allotted, and in the other they told the subjects that the average college student should find it fairly easy to complete the test within the time limit given. They also divided the subjects into those who scored high or low on self-reports of the amount of anxiety experienced in testing situations. As the results in Table 3.1 shows, the highly anxious subjects did

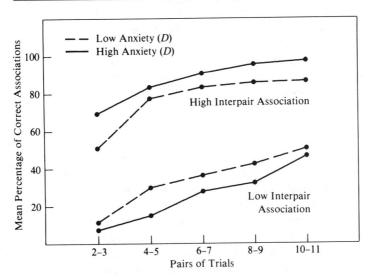

Figure 3.7.

Paired Associate Learning as a Function of Anxiety or Drive Level and Degree of Interpair Association (after Atkinson & Birch, 1978, after Spence, Farber, & McFann, 1956).

Table 3.1.

EFFECT OF INDUCED PRESSURE ON PERFORMANCE FOR SUBJECTS HIGH AND LOW IN TEST ANXIETY (data from Sarason, Mandler, & Craighill, 1952)

	Mean Number of Digit Symbol Substitutions Made on Trial One			
Subject Classification	*When Expected to Finish (A)*	*When Not Expected to Finish (B)*	*Difference (A − B)*	*p difference*[a]
Subjects high in anxiety	28.7	29.8	−1.1	.09
Subjects low in anxiety	32.7	29.8	+3.1	.003

[a]Probability of the difference occurring by chance.

less well under the pressure of being expected to finish, and they made fewer substitutions than when they were not expected to finish. The subjects low in anxiety performed better when expected to finish than when not expected to finish.

To explain this difference, the authors again draw on the principle that a stronger drive strengthens all responses more. In the case of the high anxiety subjects, the increased drive strength induced by performance pressure strengthens task-irrelevant responses (for example, interfering thoughts about doing badly) that frequently have been evoked in the past for these subjects. Therefore, their performance is poorer when they are expected to finish. In contrast, for the low anxiety subjects an increase in drive strength evokes task-relevant responses that have led to success in the past. So they perform better when they are expected to finish.

In this case the responses strengthened by drive are in the subject rather than in the material to be learned, as they were in the Spence studies. Other research has shown that highly anxious subjects generally do worse when faced with complicated or difficult tasks. For example, Tennyson and Woolley (1971), using the Spielberger measure of the state of anxiety at the moment (Spielberger, Gorsuch, & Lushene, 1970), found that high anxiety subjects made many more errors on a difficult task than did low anxiety subjects. The task was deciding whether a line of poetry illustrated trochaic meter or not; it was arranged so some of the identifications were very easy and others were difficult. In the easy identifications, the high anxiety subjects did better than the low anxiety subjects because of their higher drive level. However, when drive was pushed still higher, by requiring the subjects to work on a difficult task, it facilitated the appearance of task-irrelevant responses (for example, worries about how well they were doing), which interfered with performance. This suggests that task demands can first facilitate performance and then, as they increase still further, interfere with performance—a phenomenon known as the Yerkes-Dodson law, which will be discussed in Chapter 6.

Interference Effects Due to More Experiences of Failure

Weiner (1966) noticed an obvious fact about the Spence experiments that also would explain Tennyson and Woolley's results. Generally speaking, the tasks at which the highly anxious subjects did more poorly were more difficult, and the ones at which they did better were easier (see Figure 3.7). On more difficult tasks, subjects experience more failure as they go along, and perhaps it is the experience of failure that makes highly anxious subjects do worse rather than the effect of increased drive on irrelevant responses.

Weiner designed an experiment to test this hypothesis. He employed the same sets of paired associates used in the Spence experiments, but he severed the connection between experiences of success and failure and task difficulty as follows:

> Subjects learning an easy list of paired associates were told that they were performing poorly relative to others. In this manner the easy task was paired with a failure experience. Subjects learning a difficult paired associates task were told that they were doing well relative to others, thus pairing the difficult task with a success experience. If the differential reactions to success and failure experiences are the essential determinants of behavior in this situation, then on the easy task highly anxious subjects experiencing failure should perform *worse* than subjects low in anxiety experiencing failure. On the difficult task, highly anxious subjects experiencing success should perform *better* than subjects low in anxiety experiencing success. The experimental design consequently provides a definitive test of the alternative explanation of the Spence et al. data. (Weiner, 1966)

Weiner's results, as shown in Table 3.2 and confirmed in a subsequent experiment, conform to his prediction. Subjects high in anxiety do better than subjects low in anxiety after success, even on the difficult paired associate task. This was the same task on which they did worse when they were given no information as to how well they were doing and inferred they were not doing very well because they kept failing at it (see Figure 3.7).

This finding is very important, but it does not resolve all questions arising from this type of research. Spence (1958a) reports that with certain types of more difficult tasks, the more anxious subjects do better, contrary to Weiner's prediction, although this result could not be regularly obtained. If we do not accept the Hull-Spence explanation of why high anxiety subjects do better on easy tasks or on those in which the dominant response is correct, how is this fact to be explained? One possibility is that failure increases task-irrelevant responses in high anxiety subjects and success quiets them. This would explain why highly anxious subjects do better on easy tasks at which they are successful than on difficult tasks at which they fail; however, it would not explain why the highly

Table 3.2.

**MEAN NUMBER OF TRIALS TO SUCCESSFUL LEARNING OF PAIRED
ASSOCIATES (after Weiner, 1966)**

Subject Classification	Easy List (Failure)	Difficult List (Success)
Subjects high in anxiety (H)	9.55	14.85
Subjects low in anxiety (L)	7.08	20.10
Difference ($H - L$)	2.46	−5.25
	$p < .10$	$p < .10$

Note: Low score indicates faster learning. Subjects high in anxiety do better than subjects low in anxiety after success, even on a difficult task, but they do worse even on an easy task if it is associated with failure.

anxious subjects do better than less anxious subjects on easy tasks, since less anxious people should have no task-irrelevant responses to interfere with their performance. We are led to infer, as Atkinson and Birch (1978) argue, that other motives must be higher for the highly anxious subjects. Perhaps subjects high in anxiety have a stronger need for social approval than subjects low in anxiety, which leads them to do better when they are not bothered by task-irrelevant responses.

Later research has tended to emphasize the importance of other motives present in performance situations. For example, Tables 3.1 and 3.2 might bring up the question of why the subjects low in anxiety do better after being put under pressure. Atkinson argues that the only way to understand this is in terms of knowing something about the achievement motivation of the subjects (see Chapter 7). This is because challenges increase performance among subjects high in achievement motivation, particularly if they are also low in anxiety. Atkinson reinterprets the results of these experiments in terms of the joint effects of the fear of failure, as measured by test anxiety, and the achievement motive, as Chapter 7 will show. Subjects low in anxiety are often high in achievement motivation, so setting challenging or explicit goals for them may improve their performance for a reason quite unrelated to the drive level of anxiety. Certainly other motives in a situation need to be taken into account, but no one can question the importance of the attempt Spence and his associates made to apply the behaviorist model of motivation to individual differences in motive strength at the human level.

How the Presence of Others May Increase Drive and Interfere with Performance on Complex Tasks

Just as the line of investigation started by Spence had begun to run its course, Zajonc (1965) came up with a human application of the behaviorist model of motivation in a quite different area. He reviewed a considerable body of research evidence that showed that the presence of another member of a species often increases response strength. For example, if a chicken is allowed to eat its fill until it stops eating, and then another chicken is introduced and starts eating the common food supply, the first chicken will begin to eat again. It looks as if the second chicken has increased the hunger drive level of the first chicken. The phenomenon is generally known as *social facilitation.* Zajonc found evidence that social facilitation improves performance of simple tasks but can decrease performance of more complex tasks. He saw this as another application of Hull's model, since the presence of another, if it increases drive, should facilitate performance if there is a simple dominant response and should inhibit performance if there are many competing responses that would be strengthened by the increased drive.

Zajonc and Sales (1966) designed the following experiment to test the hypothesis. They flashed nonsense syllables briefly on a screen, which they told the subjects were Turkish words that the subjects were to learn to pronounce when they saw them. A given word was presented one, two, four, eight, or sixteen times. In short, some words were seen and pronounced much more often than others. Interspersed among the presentations were some blurs, which the subjects were told were words they could not see very well but were to guess at anyway. These were called *pseudorecognition trials.* The average number of words that had been exposed different numbers of times that were called out in the pseudorecognition trials is plotted in Figure 3.8. As the general upward slope of the curves indicates, the subjects were more likely to call out words to the blurs they had seen more often.

Some of the subjects performed this task alone, and others while two other students watched them—in what was called the *audience condition.* If we suppose that adding two watchers increases drive, the two curves would seem to conform to the prediction made from Hull's model. The subjects under conditions of high drive (audience condition) produced more of the dominant responses (those exposed sixteen times) than did the subjects with lower drives (alone condition). However, the reverse is true for the infrequently exposed words, where there is no clearly dominant response. It is assumed here that high drive would make it more likely that subjects would respond with any word high in their hierarchy, so they would be less apt to respond with a word that had been seen only once than a subject performing alone at a condition of lower drive.

However, more complications arose as others joined in investigating this application of the Hull model. Cottrell, Wack, Sekerak, and Rittle (1968) showed that it was not just the presence of others that produced this effect, but rather what Cottrell called *evaluation apprehension*—the expectation that the audience would evaluate performance. He repeated the Zajonc and Sales experiment using "Turkish" words, except that the two others present were blindfolded, and the subjects were told they were sitting there to adapt their eyes to the dark. Under these conditions the curve obtained was exactly parallel to that obtained for subjects when they were alone.

Cottrell et al. (1968) also used the paired associate technique used by

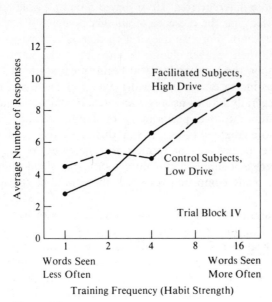

Figure 3.8.

Average Number of Responses of Different Frequency Classes in Separate Trial Blocks of the Pseudorecognition Series (after Zajonc & Sales, 1966).

Spence and others to test the application of the model for the anxiety drive, and they obtained the same results. That is, the presence of an audience tended to improve performance on the paired associates of high association value where there was a dominant response, and it impaired performance on the low association pairs where there was no dominant response. Cottrell (1972) argues that "through experience the individual learns to anticipate subsequent positive or negative outcomes whenever others are merely present and not overtly doing anything that has motivational significance for him. It is these anticipations, elicited by the presence of others, that increase the individual's drive level." In other words, Cottrell agrees that drive level is increased by an audience and produces the effects expected from the Hull model, but he is defining the nature of the drive differently from the way Zajonc defined it.

Geen and Gange (1977) have reviewed these experiments and showed that all kinds of influences can result from the presence of others, depending on the nature of the situation. Others may simply provide more information on what to do. Goldfish swimming in a group learn a response faster than when swimming alone. Others may increase competitiveness, or fear that the other person will take what one wants. An audience may increase fear of disapproval, which leads subjects to make more conventional—and also more common or dominant—responses. The presence of others simply may distract people so they can concentrate less on the task. It clearly is too simple to think of the mere presence of another as having a universal effect on drive level.

• REINTERPRETING THE BEHAVIORIST STUDIES OF HUMAN MOTIVATION IN TERMS OF WHAT GOES ON IN PEOPLE'S MINDS

A serious limitation of studies in the behaviorist tradition is that they cut themselves off from determining what is going on in the subjects' minds during an experiment. That is why the behaviorists started working with animals in the first place. Instead, as different conditions produced different effects, they were forced to *infer* what was going on in the subjects' minds, whether animal or human. If a satiated chicken starts eating again when a second chicken eats its food, the experimenter may *infer* that the hunger drive is aroused in the first chicken or that it "feels" more competitive. However, there is no way to be sure what is going on in the chicken's mind, although experimenters can carry out further experiments designed to test whether it is the competitive urge or hunger that is aroused.

The research on the audience effect in humans has been carried out according to the animal model; it tries to *infer* what is happening in subjects' minds from studying their behaviors in different situations. Compared with using animals, however, using human subjects has an important advantage: it is entirely possible to find out what is going on in their minds. Fortunately, Kawamura-Reynolds (1977) has carried out an experiment that does just that. She first demonstrated that the subjects in her experiment showed the standard effect supposedly caused by the increase in drive due to an audience; that is, subjects in the audience condition (higher drive) learned difficult paired associates of low association value (with no appropriate dominant responses) more slowly than they did in the alone condition (lower drive). The explanation, according to the behaviorist model, is that the increased drive due to the audience strengthens task-irrelevant associations when there is no dominant association, so the subjects take longer to learn the difficult associations.

Kawamura-Reynolds then did something different. After the subjects had learned the associations, she had them write imaginative stories to pictures, using a technique fully described in Chapter 6. This procedure was to find out what the subjects had on their minds or were thinking about in the alone and audience conditions. She used six picture cues: Three were designed to evoke standard or dominant responses in everyone. One had to do with thirst and drinking; one, with hunger and eating; and one, with art and aesthetic activity. Three other pictures were ambiguous and designed to evoke stories relating to achievement or affiliation. Kawamura-Reynolds' first prediction was that if the behaviorist model was correct, and the audience had increased nonspecific drive, it should increase the likelihood of *simple,* dominant responses being made in the audience condition compared with the alone condition. She obtained this result, as Table 3.3 shows. More of the subjects in the audience condition gave

Table 3.3.

NUMBER OF SUBJECTS SHOWING DOMINANT IMAGINATIVE THEMES IN RESPONSE TO THREE STRONGLY CUED PICTURES AND STRONG NEED FOR AFFILIATION RELATIVE TO NEED FOR ACHIEVEMENT IN RESPONSE TO THREE WEAKLY CUED OR AMBIGUOUS PICTURES (after Atkinson & Birch, 1978, after Kawamura-Reynolds, 1977)

Dominant Themes	Strongly Cued Pictures		Need for Affiliation Relative to Need for Achievement	Ambiguous Pictures	
	Audience	Alone		Audience	Alone
One or more	25	17	High	22	14
None	11	19	Low	14	22
	$\chi^2 = 3.66^a$			$\chi^2 = 3.52^b$	

[a]$p < .03$ in the direction predicted by drive theory.

[b]$p < .04$ in the direction predicted by cognitive theory of instigating force and dynamics of action.

more conventional or dominant themes, such as a drinking story to a thirst cue, than subjects in the alone condition.

However, Kawamura-Reynolds, following Cottrell's argument, also had predicted that the presence of the audience would evoke evaluation apprehension, which would show up in the stories as a greater concern for affiliation, as contrasted with a concern for achievement (both scored according to the standard procedures described in Chapter 6). That is, it has been established that subjects with a stronger need for Affiliation (abbreviated *n* Affiliation) generally have a greater need to be liked and approved of. Thus, if the audience in fact increases the need for approval or evaluation apprehension, as Cottrell argues, it should show up as an increased need for Affiliation. This is what Kawamura-Reynolds found, as the right side of Table 3.3 illustrates. More subjects in the audience condition than in the alone condition had a higher *n* Affiliation score relative to their need for Achievement (*n* Achievement) score. Furthermore, she found that it was the subjects who were relatively higher in their affiliation concern who produced more dominant or conventional responses to the strongly cued pictures. In other words, it may be the specific motive aroused by the audience—rather than a nonspecific drive—that on one hand produces more conventional or dominant responses in simple situations and on the other produces anxiety that interferes with performance in complex situations.

What is important about this study is that it introduces a methodology that enables experimenters to check directly their inferences about what is going on in subjects' minds. This should greatly speed up understanding of situations like these, in contrast to what can be gained from dozens of experiments in the behaviorist tradition aimed at trying to pin down inferences about what subjects are thinking or wanting.

• A COMPARISON OF THE PSYCHOANALYTIC AND BEHAVIORIST CONTRIBUTIONS TO THE STUDY OF MOTIVATION

Similarities

It is useful to compare Freud and Hull as representatives of the psychoanalytic and behaviorist traditions in psychology, respectively, because their characteristics strongly influenced these traditions and in the end epitomized them. On the surface they seem very different—Freud the cultured product of European civilization who saw wealthy patients in his Viennese consulting room, and Hull the American son of an illiterate father who ran white rats in mazes in New Haven, Connecticut. As far as the science of psychology was concerned, however, they basically agreed. Both were strongly antireligious and felt psychology could never become a natural science unless it got rid of such obviously absurd notions as God, the soul, sin, and loving kindness. They were both thoroughgoing determinists, believing that the scientific study of people could be modeled after nineteenth-century physics and that they could explain the notion of "free will" in purely mechanistic terms. They both opposed studying conscious experience, although for different reasons—Hull because he thought such study would lead inevitably into mentalistic or religious concepts, and Freud because he was fascinated by the power of unconscious processes.

Both Freud and Hull believed psychology could become a quantitative science, as physics was, and that it should be based on physiological processes, although neither used physiological information directly in their work. Both were close reasoners and scorned sloppy thinking; Freud's analyses of clinical cases read like the careful unraveling of a complicated plot in a detective story in the Sherlock Holmes tradition. Hull's model for thinking was geometry, with its axioms, propositions, and careful derivations. Both intensely disliked armchair speculation because it involved loose thinking, was often moralistic, and was not based on observable behavioral facts.

Darwin's theory of evolution greatly influenced both Freud's and Hull's thinking about motivation. They concluded that organisms were endowed with motives to help them survive. The hunger motive enabled the individual to survive, and the sexual instinct enabled the race to survive. Freud and Hull came up with surprisingly similar conceptions of how drives affected the organism: they energized behavior. Hull spoke of hunger activating the organism and Freud of the energy provided by the libido, or sexual drive. They both believed drives were tension inducing or disturbing and that reward or pleasure was primarily relief from tension. Drives also had aims (Freud) or goals (Hull), which focused behavior in one direction or another. Finally, drives were responsible for fixation of symptoms (Freud) or learning (Hull). Since Freud was not particularly interested in problem solving, he did not emphasize learning very much; he thought of symptoms as fixated (Hull would say *learned*) responses produced by a strong drive.

It is small wonder, in view of these similarities, that Freud's contributions to psychology have always been more acceptable to the behaviorists than, for example, Jung's. Jung did not share many of these values. He was overtly religious; he was not averse to speculation, particularly about mystical as opposed to mechanical matters; and he was not so thoroughgoing a determinist.

Differences

Freud and Hull both were empirically oriented toward behavioral facts and observations, but in quite different ways. Hull emphasized the experiment and what could be learned about motivation by systematically varying external experimental conditions. Freud focused on the case study, on the pattern of motivation that would explain a number of symptomatic behaviors in an individual. This approach lent itself to the study of individual differences in motives much more than did the experimental approach. However, an adequate study of motivation involves an understanding of how the person (Freud's orientation) and the situation (Hull's orientation) interact to produce behavior.

Another difference was in the relative emphasis they gave to induction and deduction. Freud was obsessed with factual observations—with inferring the motivational meaning of particular dream contents or symptomatic acts. By induction he arrived at generalizations from all these observations and interpretations, but since he incessantly made new critical observations, his generalizations kept changing; therefore, it is difficult to find "the" Freudian system. He kept changing his mind as he got new and better insights from further clinical studies. This led to great creativity and originality. Freud's books have been continuously mined by psychologists ever since he wrote them for ideas on what is important to investigate in psychology.

In contrast, Hull developed a tight, logically related, simple system of principles that could be used to explain the most complex aspects of behavior, much as a few laws in physics explain many complex natural phenomena. Once these principles had been established, the only task left for psychology was to apply them. Facts that did not fit the principles were a nuisance; they seldom led to new insights or ideas. Instead, they were "explained away" by some more elaborate deduction from the basic principles. What Hull gained in systematic thinking, therefore, he lost in originality, and what Freud gained in originality, he lost in systematic thinking. Good science requires both approaches and a balance between induction and deduction, as well as between adhering to a system and being open to new ideas.

Hull was interested in objective, observable acts and Freud, in symptoms, thoughts, and dreams. The acts of particular interest to behaviorists were those that produced learning or solved problems, whereas maladaptive acts, symptoms, or drives interested Freud. As was just noted, trying to carry out motivational studies of action in the behaviorist tradition without knowledge of dreams or what people are thinking about is like trying to paste up wallpaper with one hand tied behind your back. There is no reason to exclude the kinds of behaviors Freud was interested in from experimental studies of motivation. They have been excluded out of ignorance about how thinking can be studied objectively and out of fear that such an approach would reintroduce mentalistic, subjective, or spiritual concepts. Fortunately, recent studies of cognitive factors in human psychology have begun to correct this behaviorist bias.

However, the Freudian emphasis on dreams and symptoms led to a neglect of the human adaptive capacities. Later psychoanalysts attempted to overcome this deficit with a study of the ego, although for the most part without the benefit of the knowledge U.S. psychologists had accumulated about the learning process.

• LIMITATIONS OF THE BEHAVIORIST MODEL

Hull's view of drive was attacked early and effectively by those who demonstrated that motivation did not always involve tension reduction. Sheffield and Roby (1950) showed that a nonnutritive sweet taste from saccharin had reward value for rats. That is, the rats would learn to get the sweet taste even though saccharin could not reduce tension or the hunger drive. Sheffield, Wolff, and Backer (1951) reported that male rats would cross an electric grid to copulate with a receptive female even though they were always interrupted before orgasm so there was no drive reduction. Harlow, Harlow, and Meyer (1950) found that rhesus monkeys would work to disentangle a mechanical puzzle even in the absence of primary drive reduction. It was difficult to imagine what kind of secondary reward in the situation could account for their persistent attempts to disentangle the puzzle. In fact, the introduction of food reward for working the puzzle correctly interfered with the monkeys' performance. Furthermore, at about this time, Olds (1955) was beginning his very important series of studies showing that there appeared to be "pleasure centers" in the brain: rats would press a bar to get a slight electrical stimulation in some portions of the brain and not others. All these experiments and many others pointed to the existence of many sources of motivation other than those related to stimulus or drive reduction. They will be discussed in the next two chapters.

Another criticism of the Hullian theory of drive was that it excessively focused on survival needs, such as hunger, thirst, and pain avoidance. Thus, materialistic needs were primary, and all other so-called higher needs were secondary, derived from, and presumably less urgent than primary drives. Even humanistically oriented psychologists like Maslow and Allport, as noted in Chapter 2, bought the notion that materialistic biological needs are primary, although they then declared that the higher needs were independent of their biological origins.

The idea is not new. The sixteenth-century French satirist François Rabelais, in his *Fourth Book of the Heroic Deeds and Sayings of Pantagruel,* made the point vividly in picturing Sir Gaster (that is, Sir Stomach) as the ruler of the world, or

> . . . foremost master of arts in the world. . . . Into whatever company he may go, there can be no discussion there of first rank or preference; for he always goes before all others, even though they be kings, emperors, or the Pope himself. . . . To serve him, all the world is busy, all the world labors; and as recompense, he does this for the world: he invents for it all arts, all machines, all trades, all implements, and all refinements. . . . He invented water-mills, wind-mills, hand-mills and myriad other contrivances, to grind his grain and reduce it to flour, invented yeast to ferment the dough and salt to give it flavor. . . . If a sea or river stood in the way of its transportation, he invented boats, galleys and ships.

Is the stomach the master of all arts? Do material needs take precedence over all others, which in the end derive from them? The behaviorist position implied that biological needs were primary.

Even the prima facie case for such a proposition is not as strong as one might think in view of its wide acceptance. Certainly in history individuals and groups have often acted in ways that were quite contrary to the satisfaction of their material wants. Martyrs have gone to the stake for principles. Christians were willing to be eaten by lions rather than deny their Christianity. Whole nations have embarked on idealistic adventures that have deprived them of material pleasures. A miscalculation in U.S. foreign policy at the time of the Bay of Pigs disaster in Cuba was based in part on the assumption that material incentives would take precedence over more idealistic social values. It was known at the time that the Cuban people were suffering from severe shortages of food and other material goods under the Communist Castro government. It was therefore assumed by U.S. policy makers, many of whom had been taught in psychology courses that the hunger drive was primary, that the Cubans would be ready to revolt against an oppressive regime that was not satisfying their material wants, and that an invasion from the outside was all that was needed to touch off the revolt. History proved these assumptions incorrect. The Cuban people were undoubtedly in physical need. Other incentives and motives proved more important to them, however, and they did not join in the attempt to overthrow the government. At the very least it would have to be concluded that the case for the primacy of material wants is not proved.

This viewpoint could well be mistaken; motives could develop around biological needs in the same way they develop in general out of certain built-in tendencies to approach and avoid certain experiences. This viewpoint is elaborated in the next two chapters, which maintain that all motives, including hunger, are learned out of experiences with certain natural incentives. Some motives may be stronger than others for a variety of reasons, but there is no convincing evidence that motives based on biological survival need take precedence over all others in human adults.

The final major limitation of the behaviorist model of drive has already been referred to several times: its approach to human motivation, as opposed to animal motivation, was scholastic rather than empirical, except for the flurries of research started by Spence and Zajonc summarized earlier. The approach was scholastic in the sense that explanations for human desires and needs, such as the desire for money, were simply derived from basic principles and never actually studied (J. S. Brown, 1961). Once a researcher had shown that the need for money could be explained by the fact that money was likely to be associated with the reduction of various primary and secondary drives, there was nothing more to be done. Such a conclusion was not a hypothesis that could be realistically tested in any way; thus, it was not a scientific hypothesis, but instead was a scholastic deduction from first principles.

It is ironic that a movement that was begun to eliminate mentalistic concepts ended up attributing mental states to people that could not be checked empirically. Behaviorists like Hull, Spence, or Skinner often use mentalistic concepts or refer to inner states of mind to explain what they mean. They apologize for doing so and defend themselves by saying they must use such terms instead of more objective ones to be understood easily. What they fail to recognize is that in the meantime methods have been developed for coding and counting thought contents, and these methods are just as objective as those used in observing overt actions. These methods, as illustrated by the Kawamura-Reynolds experiment, are explained in Chapter 6 and throughout this book. They clearly must be used to supplement the behaviorist contribution.

The concepts in the behaviorist model were too limited in scope, but that should not blind us to its contributions. It demonstrated the great importance of the motivational experiment, which must be used to test alternative hypotheses. The behaviorist model discouraged psychologists from using vague, ill-defined concepts to explain what is going on. It taught them that relationships among well-defined variables must be explicitly and carefully stated so they can be checked for their validity through observation and experiment.

NOTES AND QUERIES

1. The behaviorist model objectified purpose through the concept of the fractional anticipatory goal response. After a rat had been fed in a maze, it was supposed to start salivating when it was put back in the maze, indicating that it was already anticipating eating as much as it could with no food present. The increased salivation could be interpreted as a sign that it was "thinking about eating." Does this seem equivalent to "wanting to eat"? No one actually checked to see if rats did salivate more in this way. What would be the implications of finding or not finding that they salivated more when they were put back in a maze after being fed in it?

2. How would you measure the strength of the "money motive" in humans? How would you determine whether such a motive is based on relief of tensions, discomforts, and anxieties, or on something else? How would the motive in question be identified in people at a time before they began using money?

3. The behaviorist model explained that rats' latent learning of maze pathways (see Figure 3.4) was actually the result of learning in the service of the exploratory drive. Thus, the effort to show that learning could occur where no motivation was present appeared to fail, just as similar examples of incidental learning were explained away as being due to motives human subjects themselves brought to laboratory experiments (see Chapter 1). Can you think of a way of testing whether learning can occur in the absence of motivation? If motivation must always be present to explain learning, is it a falsifiable hypothesis that motivation is necessary for learning? If the hypothesis is not falsifiable, is it a scientific hypothesis? What is the difference between stating that motivation facilitates learning and stating that motivation is necessary for learning?

4. Is it necessary to assume that drives are based on strong stimuli and rewards on stimulus reduction or tension reduction? What else could drives be built on?

5. The chapter argues that acquired, or secondary, rewards in humans often appear to be much stronger than the primary rewards on which they are based. This is seldom if ever true in animals. For example, no matter how much experience Wolfe's chimpanzees had with token rewards, they still preferred and worked harder for grapes and pieces of banana than for the tokens. Why then would Christians allow themselves to be eaten by lions, giving up all primary rewards from going on living in favor of secondary, or acquired, rewards from sticking to their beliefs? Can you think of circumstances that might make acquired rewards stronger than primary rewards (see McClelland, 1942)?

6. Why should behavior occurring in the absence of an identifiable stimulus (that is, operant behavior) reflect more sensitively motivation or purpose than behavior occurring in response to a stimulus?

7. According to the way *motivate* is used in this book, is the term properly used in the sentence "One way to motivate people to cooperate is to increase communication among them"? If not, how would you rephrase the sentence to reflect the terminology adopted here?

8. Sometimes people cannot recall the name of someone they know very well no matter how hard they try. Then somewhat later, when they no longer are trying to recall it, the name pops into their head. How can this phenomenon be explained by the behaviorist model of how drive multiplies with response strength to produce a response? If you do not like its explanation, how would you explain the phenomenon?

9. Do you think subjects high in anxiety drive would be more likely than subjects low in anxiety drive to forget names, as described in the previous question? Why or why not?

10. Why do you think subjects low in anxiety do not do as well on easy tasks as subjects high in anxiety? How does your answer fit with various theoretical positions?

11. Do you perform better or worse when someone is watching you? Does it matter what you are doing? How do your reactions fit with various explanations given in the chapter for audience effects?

12. Why, in your opinion, should subjects high in the need for Affiliation or for social approval have given more dominant or conventional responses than those low in this need to highly cued pictures in the Kawamura-Reynolds experiment (see Table 3.3)? What if subjects high in the need for Achievement also had given more such responses than those low in the need for Achievement? What would the implications of such a result be for the Atkinson versus the Spence explanation of the results of this experiment?

13. Why do you think so much hostility existed between psychology and religion in the early part of the twentieth century? How do religious views of motivation differ from psychological views of motivation?

14. Chapter 1 argued that Freud's cultural heritage influenced his view of human motivation. Make a case for the hypothesis that Hull's background also shaped his view of human motivation.

15. One of the main objections to the behaviorist model of motivation was that it was too simplistic in defining satisfactions and in assuming that people's behavior was wholly determined by the pleasure principle or reward and punishment. Gordon Allport (1946), for example, summarizes these objections with the following example: "What happens in normal human learning, beyond the infant stage, is that experiences of satisfaction serve as *indicators,* which, valuable as they are to the individual, are not dynamically decisive. If I am trying to become a writer and am downcast by a rejection slip, I *may* thereupon cease the style of work I was attempting . . . yet I *may* be so sure of myself (in my ego-structure) that I will persist in the face of bad news." Allport is arguing that rewards and punishments do not seem to control behavior very closely among human adults the way they do among Thorndike's kittens or Hull's rats. Why not? What does Allport mean by *ego-structure?* Could personal motive dispositions of the type discussed in Chapter 2 be part of the ego structure and explain why individuals react differently to bad and good news, as well as why what they do is less controlled by such external events?

Part 2

The Nature of Human Motives

4

Emotions as Indicators of Natural Incentives

• EARLY ATTEMPTS TO FIND
A BIOLOGICAL BASIS FOR MOTIVES

Motives as we experience them are bewilderingly complex. We want to graduate from college. We would like to be respected by others. We want to be loved. We would like to get married. We would like some excitement in our lives. Or perhaps we would just like to be able to study harder. Where do these motives come from? Are they instinctive, as McDougall, Freud, and Maslow argued (see Chapter 2)? Are they simply the product of our learning to satisfy certain biological needs like hunger, as the behaviorist model argued (see Chapter 3)? Do we learn to want these things because our society teaches us that we should want them? Or are there some deeper drives guiding human action that shape society?

Initially many theorists like McDougall had found it easy simply to reason that certain fundamental urges were biologically built in, or instinctive. The behaviorists, however, were skeptical. They felt such a hypothesis was vague and impossible to test empirically. How could one prove that a drive for power, for example, was instinctive rather than built on social learning? Since the behaviorists were oriented entirely toward overt behavior (rather than inner "urges"), they not unreasonably asked what were the fixed *action patterns,* shown by all human infants (prior to learning), that would signal the presence of an innate power need. They recognized that lower animals showed such fixed action patterns, which therefore could be called *instincts* and could be used to explain the way birds build nests or cats pounce on mice. However, human beings show little evidence of such fixed action patterns. All they can do at birth is sneeze, vomit, suck, and display a few other innate reflex responses. Where is the drive for power or for love to be found in such simple innate responses? More complex motives had to be the product of learning, or so these theorists argued.

As Chapter 3 showed, learning theorists found in the so-called primary drives like hunger and thirst a biological base on which all the more complex motives could be built through learning. In the simplest version of the theory they argued that the only innate biological given was strong stimulation or tension and the innate satisfaction that comes from reducing it. The idea was appealing in its great simplicity: The organism started out in life with a few biological sources of tension such as hunger pangs, pain, and various types of strong stimulation, relief from any of which was automatically rewarding. The organism acquired more complex drives and rewards through association with these primary determinants of action.

As we have seen, however, this solution to the problem was too simple. It led to derivations of secondary, more complex motives that were theoretical and difficult to confirm through actual observation and experiment. Above all, it failed to account for the fact that organisms often seek stimulation as well as stimulation reduction. Various attempts were made to shore up the stimulus- or tension-reduction theory and restore its obvious appeal. For example, Fiske and Maddi (1961) argued that it was better to think of the organism as seeking certain optimal levels of activation. If it was below the optimal level at any point, it would seek stimulation. If it was above the optimal level, it would seek stimulation reduction. There was nothing wrong with the idea as such, except it was too general and did not predict with enough precision in advance what stimulation children or adults would seek in a given situation.

Tomkins (1962) also tried to expand the notion of stimulus intensity to cover what he called "the density of neural firing." In this biologically based model it was not only the intensity of stimulation that mattered, but also the rate of increase or decrease of stimulation and the number of different sources of stimulation. Thus, if the rate of increase was very fast, the person would react with *startle*. A somewhat slower rate of increase combined with a lack of recognition of the source of stimulation would give rise to fear, and a still slower and less dense increase in stimulation would give rise to interest-surprise. A sudden reduction in dense firing would give rise to joy-happiness-pleasure. Thus, changes in a few aspects of stimulation as represented by neural firing could generate quite different emotions, and for Tomkins different emotions were the basis of different motives.

One difficulty with both these theories is that they deal in terms of a "conceptual nervous system." It has been hard to identify activities in the brain and nervous system that correspond to what the theories refer to, and therefore they have been hard to test.

• SIGN STIMULI IN ETHOLOGY AS A BASIS FOR NATURAL INCENTIVES

What directed attention away from such overly general theories was the progress being made by ethologists like Lorenz (1952) and Tinbergen (1951) in identifying the sign stimuli that released instinctive behaviors in lower animals. For example, it had long been known that male sticklebacks (a kind of fish) often will attack other male sticklebacks in the springtime. From this it was inferred that sticklebacks have an aggressive "instinct." However, Tinbergen showed conclusively that it was certain sign stimuli—namely, the red belly of the other sticklebacks, which appeared only at certain times of the year—that released the attack response. By making dummies of a fish in various sizes, shapes, and colors, Tinbergen showed it was particularly the red belly that elicited the attack response. He and other ethologists reported dozens of similar instances in which particular responses like following, attacking, pecking, and so forth were released by very specific sign stimuli.

Note the important shift in emphasis here from what had been the focus of attention in earlier instinct theory. Then it was the instinctive behavior that was of primary interest. Now the focus was on perception and on the sign stimuli that released the behavior. Although the ethologists paid attention to action patterns displayed, they described more the variation in the acts preparatory to the consummatory act. For instance, the sight of the red belly of the male stickleback releases aggressive behaviors that vary in speed, direction, and form as the other male attacks.

Earlier instinct theory had been rejected as inapplicable to humans on the grounds that humans did not display fixed invariant patterns of behavior, as lower animals did. Now, however, the question arose as to whether humans might not be affected by sign stimuli in more subtle ways, just like lower animals. That is, human beings may be "turned on" innately by certain sign stimuli, which they experience just the way the male stickleback does when "turned on" by seeing the red belly of another male stickleback. However, the nature of the behavior the "turn on" elicits in humans may be less specific or more variable than it is for other species. In fact, it may be something like affective, or emotional, arousal in humans, which through learning leads to the adoption of specific behaviors to sustain a positive emotional state or dissipate a negative one. Also, the nature of the sign stimulus itself may be much less specific in humans than in lower animals, being more like a pattern or sequence of stimuli or response-produced sensations. In fact, it is easy to imagine human beings seeking out these "turn on" sign stimuli through a flexible variety of behaviors rather than through a fixed invariant pattern of responding being released by a general type of sign stimulus. For the sake of convenience, let us refer to these possible "turn on" sign stimuli as *natural incentives* and review some of the reasons for thinking they exist.

• THE CASE FOR NATURAL INCENTIVES IN HUMANS

Sensory Incentives

It has long been realized that certain sensations are innately pleasant and sought, whereas others are unpleasant and avoided. For example, Engel (see Woodworth, 1938) published curves showing that practically all concentrations of sweet solutions are considered pleasant, whereas sour, salty, and bitter solutions are considered pleasant in weak concentrations and unpleasant in strong concentrations, as shown in Figure 4.1. As the widespread use of perfume testifies, certain smells are pleasant and others unpleasant. In fact, some smells and tastes are so unpleasant they lead to the facial expression of disgust, which seems part of a general nausea response preliminary to getting rid of an offending substance.

Certain types of colors, sounds, and physical contact seem to be innately pleasing, whereas others are displeasing. For instance, softness and smoothness are more pleasant than stiffness, roughness, and coarseness (Berlyne, 1967). Aside from these qualitative differences, psychologists beginning with Wundt (1874) have long noted that as stimulus intensity in any modality increases from low to moderate levels the effect is pleasant, whereas if it increases to still higher levels the effect is unpleasant. Thus, tones and lights of moderate intensity generally are sought out over tones and lights of great intensity or very low intensity. A typical result confirming this curve is shown in Figure 4.2, which was obtained after asking subjects to judge the pleasantness of a spot of light as it

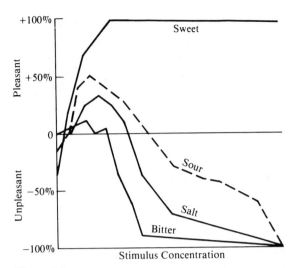

Figure 4.1.

Preponderance of "Pleasant" or "Unpleasant" Judgments in Relation to the Concentration of a Sapid Solution. The ordinate gives the percentage of "pleasant" minus the percentage of "unpleasant" judgments. The abscissa is proportional to the concentration, the full length of the baseline standing for 40 percent cane sugar, 10 percent salt, and 0.004 percent quinine sulfate, all by weight (Engel, cited in Woodworth, 1938).

varied in intensity. The subjects observed the spot in the center of a translucent eggcup fixed to one eye. The illumination of the eggcup total field, or "Ganzfeld," was set either fairly low or fairly high, so the eye could be adapted to low or high illuminations. When the eye was adapted to a low level of illumination, increases of intensity of the spot were at first judged pleasant and then unpleasant, just as the Wundt curve predicted. However, when the eye was adapted to a bright light, any intensity of the spot less than this adaptation level was judged pleasant. Thus, the shape of the hedonic curve to increasing stimulus intensity depends on the adaptation level of the sense organ, as well as the upper and lower physiological limits of its sensitivity.

Intense stimulation can lead to pain sensations, particularly if it involves sensory end organs in the skin or on internal body surfaces. Thus, extremes of heat and cold produce painful sensations, as do electric shock to the skin, muscle cramps, or bladder distension. Pain can be regarded as a natural negative incentive in the sense that it usually evokes vigorous behavior designed to escape from the pain. Learning occurs very quickly in response to this incentive. A child quickly learns that touching lighted electric bulbs leads to pain and avoids touching them in the future to reduce the anxiety or fear associated with thinking about doing it (an anticipatory goal response, in the language of Chapter 3).

Such phenomena led early theorists such as Miller and Dollard (1941) and

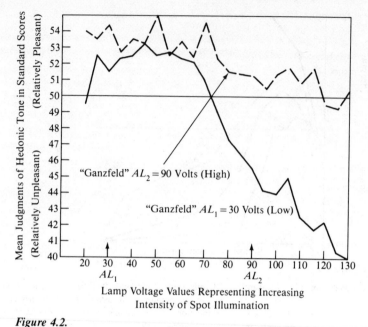

Figure 4.2.

Hedonic Tone Judgments for Discrepancies in Spot Illumination Above and Below Low (AL_1) and High (AL_2) "Ganzfeld" Illuminations. A red light was used; ten subjects made four judgments at each lamp voltage value (Alpert, 1953, cited in McClelland, Atkinson, Clark, & Lowell, 1953).

Mowrer (1950) to conclude that all motives were based on the need for pain avoidance or tension reduction. No one doubts that some motives are built on these negative incentives, but there is ample evidence that not all motives depend on them. For example, McMurray (1950) reported the case of a girl who apparently developed quite normally without ever having felt any pain. How could she develop into a normal adult if pain reduction is the fundamental basis of all motivation?

An important recent discovery for motivation theory is that the body contains a natural mechanism for moderating the effects of excessive pain. The brain can release a number of endogenous opiates or morphinelike substances, which produce analgesia and sensations of warmth and pleasure. This can be demonstrated by the use of naloxone, a drug that blocks the action of endogenous opiates. After the administration of naloxone, subjects report much greater pain from strong stimuli, indicating that the morphinelike substances are no longer moderating or counteracting its effects. Thus, it appears that pain not only acts as a negative incentive, but also releases substances that can serve as positive incentives, namely, the endogenous opiates (Olson, Olson, Kastin, & Coy, 1980).

Opponent Process Theory

Richard Solomon (1980) has accumulated evidence showing not only that pain often is followed by pleasure, but also that pleasure often is followed by pain. From these observations he has developed a theory that "for some reason the brains of all mammals are organized to oppose or suppress many types of emotional arousals or hedonic processes, whether they are pleasurable or aversive, whether they have been generated by a positive or negative reinforcer" (Solomon, 1980). That is, either a positive or negative affective process automatically sets in motion its opponent process. In other words, Solomon has identified another source of natural incentives in the way in which affective experiences automatically influence each other.

Table 4.1 illustrates the way these opponent processes develop over time after repeated exposure. In the sauna-bathing example at the top of the table, bathers feel nothing in particular before the first experience, during it they feel very uncomfortable from the heat, and afterward they feel relief. After repeating the unpleasant experience, perhaps because they believe it is good for their health, the picture changes. Bathers find the experience quite exciting, and they feel exhilarated or very good afterward. It is as if the repeated experience of heat in time more dependably elicits the endogenous opiates that give a strong feeling of being "high" afterward, much like the feeling an injection of morphine would produce. Many have suggested that a rather painful experience like jogging also produces a high after a time, perhaps also because of the release of endogenous opiates.

Solomon's opponent process theory also works the other way. As shown by the example at the bottom of Table 4.1, a duckling quickly gets imprinted on its

---

Table 4.1.

CHANGES IN AFFECT BEFORE, DURING, AND AFTER EACH STIMULATION FOR THE FIRST FEW AND AFTER MANY EXPERIENCES (after Solomon, 1980)

Period	*Affect During First Few*	*Affect After Many*
Sauna bathing		
Before	Resting state	Resting state
During	Pain, burning	Hot, exciting
After	Relief	Exhilaration
	Resting state	Resting state
Social attachment in ducklings		
Before	Contentment	Some distress
During	Excitement	Following
After	Distress	Intense distress
	Contentment	Some distress

mother or a moving mother surrogate soon after birth. In the duckling's first contacts with the mother surrogate, it shows no special emotion before contact, some excitement during contact, and some distress followed by a return to its normal state after contact. After a number of contacts, however, the duckling shows some distress beforehand in the absence of the mother surrogate, following behavior when the sign stimulus is present, and intense distress after the sign stimulus has disappeared. In other words, the positive affect associated with contact and following the mother surrogate builds up its opponent process in time—namely, strong negative affect, which occurs when the stimulus disappears. That negative affect, however, was not present before the experience of positive attachment. As Solomon (1980) points out, "this new motivational problem would never arise for the ducklings if they never saw a mother surrogate."

The opponent process theory can be used to explain many unusual motivational phenomena, such as drug addiction. Why do people get addicted to a drug like heroin, which produces a strong positive "rush" after several experiences? According to the theory, the repeated positive experiences build up the negative opponent process so strongly that the intense distress following withdrawal of the drug forces the person, like the duckling searching for the mother surrogate, to seek the drug that will remove the distress—and also cause an even greater distress after its removal in an intensifying vicious circle. Solomon's theory also explains in the same way the intense distress of lovers who are separated from each other. Their many positive experiences together have built up a strong negative opponent process, which erupts as soon as they are no longer in each other's presence.

Why do people engage in sport parachute jumping, which produces strong anxiety in the first few jumps? According to Solomon's theory, the anxiety automatically builds up a positive opponent process, which gives the jumper an increasingly positive rush during and after the jump. Solomon's theory provides a ready explanation for some phenomena that are otherwise difficult to explain. For example, it accounts for the fascination that the thrills and chills of amusement parks have for children and even adults. People are purposely undergoing frightening experiences they ought to avoid, but in fact undertake because they feel exhilarated afterward. This exhilaration is far more than just the tension relief suggested by earlier drive theory. It represents positive pleasure, which seems to come automatically from the frightening affective experience.

Solomon's theory is too new to have been thoroughly checked. It remains to be seen whether all positive or negative affective experiences automatically produce their opposites afterward. One difficulty with the theory is that whereas Solomon has produced curves showing how the opponent processes theoretically affect each other, it is as yet not clear what brain or other physiological mechanisms underlie the curves. Once these mechanisms have been identified, it will be possible to check whether these curves have an empirical basis. The one possible physiological mechanism involved, which has already been mentioned, is that in time negative affect, or pain, increases the release of endogenous opiates, which produce pleasure. However, this would occur whether the pain were removed or not, whereas the opponent process theory indicates the greatest pleasure occurs after the removal of the negative affect. No similar mechanism has been suggested for explaining the way in which positive experience might automatically release or build up some physiological substance—perhaps another neurohormone—associated with negative affect.

Whatever the final judgment on Solomon's theory, it calls attention dramatically to the fact that there appear to be strong positive and negative natural incentives that influence behavior in important ways.

Intrinsically Satisfying Activities

There is another, very simple basis for believing in natural incentives. Psychologists have long noted that animals and human beings often do things for "intrinsic" reasons. Monkeys like to spend their time looking through a window at a monkey in another cage, at a toy train, or even at another part of the laboratory (Butler, 1954). Children spend an enormous amount of time just "playing." Deci (1975) has accumulated much evidence showing that offering people extrinsic rewards such as food or money for doing these intrinsically interesting things often decreases their tendency to do them. He had subjects spend time putting together a three-dimensional spatial relations puzzle (much like Rubik's cube) into various configurations. The subjects enjoyed doing it and, in fact, would return to playing with the puzzle when they had free time. However, if he paid them a dollar for each puzzle correctly solved, they would not return to the activity when they were free to do what they liked and were no longer being paid.

Lest we infer that the subjects reasoned there was no point in doing the puzzles if they were no longer going to be paid, it is worth remembering that Harlow, Harlow, and Meyer (1950) reported exactly parallel results for monkeys in a study done a generation earlier. Monkeys, like people, enjoy manipulating things. But when Harlow's monkeys were given a food reward for correctly putting together a mechanical puzzle, they abandoned playing with the puzzle on their own. Extrinsic rewards seem to interfere with intrinsically satisfying activity. Thus, it is hard to argue that liking to manipulate things is somehow based on the satisfaction of primary drives like hunger. Yet these studies do not make much progress toward identifying what experiences are intrinsically satisfying. They simply call attention to the fact that some undoubtedly are.

Language learning is another vivid example of what appears to be an intrinsically satisfying activity guided in some way by natural incentives. R. Brown (1973) noted that while it is clear all children learn to talk in a way that approximates what they hear older people around them saying, no one really knows why they improve their speech. At first it was assumed that children's speech was shaped by rewards and punishments from parents or others. If children speak incorrectly, they will not be understood, and therefore they will correct their speech so they can be understood. Or if they speak incorrectly their parents will correct them. This is a typical "application" of the behaviorist model of motivation. However, actual observational studies show that parents, in fact, do not correct grammatical mistakes very often and that children are understood perfectly well even when they speak without the use of such words as the article *the*. Almost no one bothers to correct children if they do not use *the,* as in *get ball.* However, all children in time learn to use *the* if adults around them use it. The inference seems inescapable that it is not selection pressure from the environment that improves the speech of children, but some as yet unidentified "natural incentives" or "turn ons" that are intrinsically satisfying when the children match their response to the one they hear.

Csikszentmihalyi (1975) has studied in some depth what he calls *autotelic activities*—things that are enjoyable in themselves. In his words, "in a world supposedly ruled by the pursuit of money, power, prestige, and pleasure it is surprising to find certain people who sacrifice all those goals for no apparent reason: people who risk their lives climbing rocks, who devote their lives to art, who spend their energies playing chess" (Csikszentmihalyi, 1975). He extensively interviewed and observed people who devoted a good deal of time to rock climbing, dancing, playing chess, and playing basketball and found that it did not seem reasonable to conclude that they spent their time that way for ulterior reasons related to primary drives or basic personality needs. Instead, they found aspects of the activities themselves enjoyable.

Even more persuasive is Csikszentmihalyi's study of "microflow" activities, or little things people seem to enjoy doing when they are not doing anything in particular. He found that people spend much time humming, whistling, or singing to themselves; watching people or things; chewing; walking; touching, rubbing, or fiddling with objects; playing a musical instrument; doodling; or simply browsing, shopping, or joking with others. While some of these activities some of the time undoubtedly are in the service of major motives, much of the time they seem to be "incentive driven" in the sense that some experiences attained this way are innately satisfying. Csikszentmihalyi does not make much progress toward identifying what these natural incentives are, but his work points strongly to the conclusion that such natural incentives do exist.

• EMOTIONS AS INDICATORS OF NATURAL INCENTIVES

Phylogenetic Basis for Emotions

In the course of evolution, the human brain evolved slowly from lower forms. In particular, the human forebrain, or neocortex, underwent great expansion as man evolved out of lower primates and mammals. This is the part of the brain associated with thinking, reasoning, and imagining. However, the older, more primitive parts of the brain still exist encapsulated, so to speak, in the cortex. Paul MacLean refers to what he calls the *triune brain,* because there are three brains in one in humans—namely, the oldest, or reptilian, brain; the next oldest, or paleomammalian brain; and the large, late-developing neomammalian brain, which includes the neocortex (see Figure 4.3). The limbic system, or early mammalian brain, mediates the affective states, or emotional experiences of desire, anger, fear, sorrow, joy, and affection (MacLean, 1975).

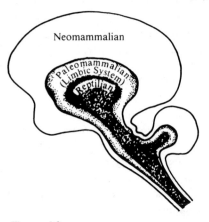

Figure 4.3.

Evolutionary Human Brain Expansion in Hierarchic Fashion in Three Basic Patterns: Reptilian, Paleomammalian, and Neomammalian (MacLean, 1975).

Therefore, it makes sense to think of our affective experiences as representing a more primitive level of brain function that can be modified and modulated enormously by cognitive events taking place in the cortex of the brain. In lower animals with lesser cortical development, specific sign stimuli release specific behaviors via the older brain centers. In humans, releasing stimuli are more variable and more modified by the cortex; however, the affective core—to use a phrase employed by McDougall long ago (1908)—remains a key to understanding what human beings find satisfying or not. In short, emotions, as well as motives built on them, appear to be mediated by a different and older part of the brain than are cognitions or associations.

Unfortunately, at present it is not possible to be much more specific about how this happens. One possibility is that there are certain natural incentives (or sign stimuli) in humans that give rise to affective states in the older brain system; these in turn get connected with specific actions but do not lead automatically to them, as older instinct theory contended. Another possibility is that the natural incentives themselves must be defined in much more general and changing terms than is common when describing lower animals. We will return to this matter later.

Emotions as Primary and Universal

Emotions are more primitive than cognitions in the sense that they are mediated by the older portions of the brain. They are universal—everyone experiences emotions—inescapable, and at times very intense. They act like amplifiers, as

Tomkins (1962) has pointed out. Certain body requirements, such as the need for oxygen, are normally met easily without the involvement of affect or emotion: the accumulation of carbon dioxide in the lungs automatically leads a person to breathe more rapidly and take in more oxygen, thus bringing the body into homeostatic balance, much as Hull's model of a mechanical robot assumed. However, the effect of hunger is different: It does not automatically lead to the eating response that relieves the hunger. Furthermore, if an infant is not fed, the hunger cues lead to widespread signs of emotional upset and distress, which amplify the effect of the hunger per se. Evidence for this conclusion is readily obtained simply by picking up and holding a crying baby, which can reduce the emotional distress without reducing the hunger.

In Tomkins' view, affect promotes motivation in several ways. It amplifies biological signals, but even in the absence of such signals (1) affect increases the variety of the consummatory responses that will serve to reduce or increase motivation, and (2) affect engages the learning capacity of the organism in finding ways of reducing or increasing motivation. That is, breathing is the automatic, unlearned consummatory response to the lack of oxygen: no other response will do, and no learning is necessary to teach the organism to make the response. However, when affect is aroused—whether it be distress or happiness—the organism is energized to reduce or enhance it *in various ways* at various times and places, and its learning capacity will be engaged in finding these instrumental activities.

Whereas for a time psychologists overlooked the primary, compelling aspect of affect in their concern for cognitive variables like memory, expectations, and attitudes, Zajonc (1980) recently summarized evidence that affective judgments like pleasant-unpleasant or good-bad are more "primary" than cognitive judgments like seen before–not seen before. Affective judgments are more effortless, inescapable, immediate, irrevocable, and difficult to verbalize, although they are easy to communicate and understand. It is as if the older part of the brain is responding more quickly or immediately before the newer, cognitively oriented part of the brain has time to function. For example, under some conditions people say they like stimuli better to which they have been exposed previously. (See the discussion in Chapter 5 on the variety incentive.) That is, they like "old" stimuli better than "new" ones. Zajonc (1980) reports a number of studies that show old stimuli are liked better than new ones even when they are not yet recognized as having been seen before. Recognition is less sensitive to previous repetitions than affect is. Thus, the affective response of like-dislike precedes and is more "primary" than the cognitive recognition response of seen before–not seen before.

The universality and "demanding character" of emotions suggest they may be innate responses to certain natural incentives or sign stimuli. Unfortunately, not much progress has been made in defining just what "elicitors" give rise to different emotions. Some feel there are unlearned elicitors (Eibl-Eibesfeldt, 1970), such as the sign stimuli in lower animals; others have argued that sign stimuli are not as specific in humans as in lower animals and that social learning produces the main elicitors for various emotions (Ekman, 1972; Tomkins, 1962). This summary by Klinger (1977) is typical: "The emotions are 'primary' in the sense that they are unlearned reactions to certain basic kinds of situations. For instance, anger may be an unlearned reaction to interference with a goal-directed sequence of behavior. However, people learn a wide variety of new situations are equivalent to the basic situations for which the primary emotional reactions are programmed. They then respond to these new situations as well." A possible sign stimulus or natural incentive is mentioned ("interference with goal-directed sequence of behavior"), along with the indication that it can change with experience. This is about as far as theorists have been able to go in identifying precisely what the natural incentives or sign stimuli are for different types of emotions.

However, extensive studies of the facial expression of emotions suggest there are a limited number of basic, or primary, emotions, at least as reflected in facial expressions, and that each is uniquely associated with a particular set of evoking situations (or sign stimuli). The evidence for these conclusions comes from a series of photographic studies of facial expressions of infants in the United States and other cultures (Ekman, 1972; Izard, 1979). While experts do not completely agree, there is a general consensus that at least six different emotions can be distinguished in all babies from all cultures, indicating that the emotions are innate. They are joy-happiness-pleasure, sadness-distress, anger-excitement, disgust, fear, and interest-surprise (see Figure 4.4). Furthermore, these facial expressions are readily recognized by members of a culture very different from the one to which the person expressing the emotion belongs. People in the United States can recognize a happy Japanese or New Guinean as easily as they can recognize a happy American. In short, the language of the emotions is universal and easily understood. This further supports the conclusion that different emotions are expressing the innate response of all human beings to certain sign stimuli, which are "turning on" the organism in different ways. We will return to trying to identify these sign stimuli later.

Hormonal Patterns and Emotion

Different emotions are not only accompanied by distinctive facial expressions; there is increasing evidence that they also are associated with different hormonal profiles. Initially attention was focused on the general physiological excitement that appeared to accompany all emotions. It was argued that emotion aroused the organism, readying it for "fight or flight" (Cannon, 1915). Heart rate, blood pressure, and muscle tension all increase with emotional excitement such as fear or anger-excitement. Selye (1956) popularized the notion of a *general adaptation syndrome,* which included a number of physiological responses that appeared to occur in all types of emotionally arousing situations, or stresses.

The brain operates through three somewhat different types of effector systems: the skeletomuscular nervous system, the autonomic nervous system, and the endocrine system. Some of the more obvious general characteristics of all

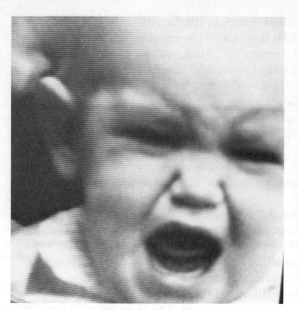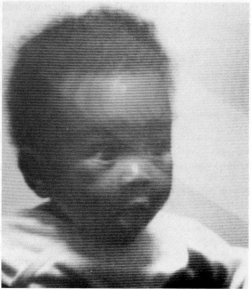

Figure 4.4.

Two Readily Recognizable Facial Expressions of Emotions in Infants. (*Left*) The expression of anger-excitement is shown on the face of a fourteen-month-old girl. (*Right*) The expression of interest-surprise can be seen on the face of a four-month-old girl (Izard, 1979).

emotions are mediated through the first two of these systems. Thus, any type of emotion-arousing stimulus—whether an electric shock or a possible sexual partner—produces at first some startle reactions, mediated through the skeletomuscular system, and some physiological change, such as increased heart rate or sweating of the palms, initiated by the autonomic nervous system.

It has not proved possible to differentiate clearly what emotion—and therefore what natural incentive—is involved on the basis of these reactions alone (Lacey, 1967). However, careful work by Mason (1975) and his collaborators has suggested that it may be possible to detect different emotional states from their profiles of endocrine response, just as it is possible to do so from differences in facial expressions. Most of the work has been done on fear and anger-excitement, because they are relatively easy to arouse and study in the laboratory. Whereas both fear and anger-excitement are accompanied by the release of cortisol from the cortex of the adrenal gland and adrenaline (or epinephrine) from the medulla of the adrenal gland, Mason has found some evidence that anger-excitement also is associated with an increase, and fear with a decrease, in sex hormone release. In his words, there are "preliminary and limited indications that different, relatively specific emotional states may be correlated with different, specific patterns of multiple hormonal responses" (Mason, 1975). If this is true, there is a physiological basis for the qualitative differences in feelings and facial expressions associated with different types of emotional arousal, for hormones are closely associated with feeling states. Thus, in thinking about how natural incentives might affect the body, we need not be limited to conceptions of general arousal but may conceive of natural incentives leading to qualitatively different emotions mediated by different hormonal patterns.

Brain Reward Systems and Emotions

A quite different line of investigation also suggests that there may be different types of affective arousal, or emotion, mediated by the brain. Olds and Milner (1954) first demonstrated that rats would press a bar to get electrical stimulation in some parts of the brain but not in others. Ever since, investigators have been pinning down more and more precisely just where in the brain electrical stimulation is rewarding and where it is not (Olds, 1977). Attention first focused on the neurons for which the catecholamines serve as neurotransmitters across the synapse from one neuron to the next. It is known that the nerve impulse travels in the nervous system via the release of tiny biochemical packets released from one neuron and picked up by receptors on the next, as well as that the biochemicals involved in different neuronal systems are different. It was first thought that the neurons served by a catecholamine transmitter, noradrenaline (a precursor of adrenaline), were the ones that, when electrically stimulated, would lead to the most active self-stimulation by rats (see Stein, 1975).

Later evidence strongly suggests that this effect, if it occurs, is indirect, and that electrical stimulation of another set of neurons is much more closely associated with self-stimulation, for which the neurotransmitter is dopamine, another catecholamine (Wise, 1980). Some investigators believe the dopamine circuits may mediate the reward system for the brain, but there is considerable evidence for independent sources of self-stimulation. The strongest such evidence comes from studies showing that opiates like morphine enhance self-stimulation (Adams, Lorens, & Mitchell, 1972). The brain also produces its own endogenous opiates, the enkephalins and endorphins, which could serve as rewards if released by emotional arousal of various types. Furthermore, there is some evidence that self-stimulation occurs in the vicinity of neurons where the neurotransmitter is serotonin (Phillips, Carter, & Fibiger, 1976), as well as in the prefrontal area, where the neural substrate has not yet been identified (Corbett, La Ferriere, & Miliver, 1982).

The assumption underlying these results is that the artificial introduction of electrical stimulation in different parts of the brain mimics the natural electrical stimulation that would occur from various types of psychological arousal, as in various emotional states. It would be useful to know whether various types of what we have been calling *natural incentives* give rise to different biochemical neurotransmitters that have been found to be rewarding. But the most that can be said at this point is that the existence of different types of reward systems in the brain provides a biological basis for a variety of types of incentives that might release the neurohormones found to be rewarding.

• POSITIVE NATURAL INCENTIVES IN INFANTS

There is much evidence that natural incentives guide human behavior, that they involve affective arousal, and that a limited number of different types of affective arousal (or emotions) may be elicited by specific natural incentives or sign stimuli. Affective arousal may be thought of as positive or negative in the sense that it either facilitates or inhibits activity intrinsically. What is needed now is more information, particularly on the positive natural incentives, since the negative ones have been more fully studied in the behaviorist tradition. Unfortunately, such information is hard to come by, particularly because it is difficult to distinguish what is natural from what is learned, since humans begin learning even before birth, in the womb.

Let us observe a one-year-old boy, Peter. One evening he was left free to crawl about on the floor among a group of adults who were seated on the floor and singing. Peter was very happy and active. He crawled everywhere, exploring new areas, pushing objects over, grasping other objects, poking a candle, sounding an unused musical instrument. In fact, the adults were understandably nervous from time to time that he would break something, push over a lighted candle and start a fire, or hurt himself as he pushed his way around the environment. To generalize about what all this activity had in common, it might be said Peter was seeking *to have impacts* on the environment.

At one point in Peter's exploration, he came across a threshold into the next room that was raised about two or three inches off the floor. He struggled to get over it and managed to do so with some difficulty. As soon as he had successfully negotiated the barrier to the other side he turned back and smiled, reversed his direction, and proceeded to climb back over the obstacles. He repeated this process six or seven times, smiling after each success. In this case, he seemed to be attracted by some kind of challenge. At the simplest level he seemed to be intrigued by doing something slightly different from what he had been doing all along, namely, crawling unimpeded in all directions. We shall call this the *variety incentive,* although much of the work on it has focused on a search for variety and new sensations rather than on new types of actions, as in this example. Also, from time to time Peter would crawl to his mother and cuddle up against her, snuggling into a pillow at his mother's side. We can think of such behavior as released by *contact incentives.*

At a somewhat more systematic level, Cicchetti and Sroufe (1976) investigated the effectiveness of thirty different types of stimulation in producing smiling in young infants. The smiling response represents a sign of positive affect that was not differentiated further into the distinctions among different types of positive affect made by students of facial expressions in infants. Among the most effective situations for producing a smile in the last five months of the first year of life were the following:

Situation	Percentage of Babies Smiling
Allow the baby to grasp yarn, then tug it three times, trying not to pull it away from the infant. Pause and repeat.	43% at 9 months
Put a cloth in your mouth, and lean close enough for the baby to grasp it. Allow the baby to pull the cloth out and replace it if this is his or her tendency.	50% at 8 months

These would seem to be examples of the *impact incentive:* the baby is getting pleasure from grasping or pulling.

Next, consider these examples:

Situation	Percentage of Babies Smiling
Say *aah,* starting low, then crescendo-ing to a loud voice, with an abrupt cutoff, then a six-second pause.	55% at 11 months
Lift the baby slowly to a position overhead, with the baby looking down back.	50% at 10 months
Place the baby in a high chair or infant seat. Crawl *across* the baby's field of vision, not toward the baby. Stand, return to starting point.	60% at 12 months
Obtain the baby's attention. Hold a human mask up so the baby can see it. Place the mask in front of your face, lean slowly to within one foot of the baby's face, and pause two seconds. Lean back slowly and remove the mask slowly.	80% at 10 months

What these situations have in common is a change in what the baby expects. In the case of the sound, an expectation is built up from the crescendo, which is abruptly changed by the cutoff. Similarly, when the baby sees the adult crawling rather than standing, or with a slightly different face than what the baby is used to, the changes in what is expected produce smiling. These seem to be clear examples of the *variety incentive.*

Finally, consider these examples:

Situation	Percentage of Babies Smiling
Give four quick pecks on the baby's bare stomach.	50% at 8 months
Say lyrically, "I'm gonna get you" ("I'm" quite protracted), while leaning toward the baby with your hands posed to grab. Then grab the baby around the stomach.	75% at 8 months
Focus the baby's attention on your fingers. Walk your fingers toward the baby; then give the baby a poke in the ribs.	60% at 10 months

These would seem to be clear examples of contact incentives that involve tactile and kinesthetic stimulation. The "I'm gonna get you" procedure also involves the variety incentive, since some surprise is involved. In contrast, a number of procedures used by Cicchetti and Sroufe (1976) evoked smiling only rarely if at all from the babies, including blowing gently at the babies' hair for three seconds, whispering "Hi, baby, how are you?" in the babies' ear, or letting the babies observe themselves in a mirror. These procedures do not involve any of the three major incentives just identifed. Cicchetti and Sroufe did not attempt to generalize about what kinds of procedures are most effective in eliciting smiling, since their interest was primarily in the effectiveness of various stimuli in producing smiles as a function of the infants' cognitive development. Chapter 5 will discuss this further, but in general the observations of Cicchetti and Sroufe support the inference that there are at least three general types of stimulation that may serve as positive incentives for human infants.

• CLASSIFICATION OF NATURAL INCENTIVES IN TERMS OF THE PRIMARY EMOTIONS

Several clues about the nature of some of the primary natural incentives have been scattered throughout the chapter. The work on emotions suggested that there might be a limited number of incentives, each primarily associated with one of the six different emotions that have been reliably differentiated in facial expressions. Observations of children either learning a language or responding to stimulation have suggested what some of the natural incentives might be. Table 4.2 attempts a preliminary classification that fits these bits of information together. The six primary emotions, as identified from facial expressions, are listed on the left side of the table and classified as positive or negative. Opposite each emotion are listed the subjective feeling states that accompany it and a possible natural incentive that gives rise to it. In some cases the fit seems quite good. For example, the evidence for the existence of a positive natural incentive for moderate variety in stimulation is excellent, as Chapter 5 will show, and the facial expression of interest-surprise is equally well documented and associated with changes in the variety incentive.

The nature of the incentive or sign stimulus for anger-excitement is less clearly defined, but Chapter 5 will review evidence pointing to the importance of an impact incentive—a pleasure that derives from having impact on the world at first physically and later psychologically. This incentive is accentuated not by interference with any goal-directed sequence, as Klinger (1977) has suggested, but by interference only with an impact or manipulation attempt. This leads automatically to an intensification of effort, which becomes recognizable as the emotion of anger-excitement. This emotion in time may develop into aggression; however, aggression is not itself a primary emotion, but a behavioral trait strongly influenced by learning and all sorts of cognitive variables (for example, thoughts about injuring or the intent to injure). Anger-excitement is considered a positive emotion because it is associated with approach, although its social effects often are regarded negatively.

Table 4.2.

CLASSIFICATION OF PRIMARY EMOTIONS AND NATURAL INCENTIVES THAT RELEASE THEM (after Ekman, 1971)

Primary Emotion (Facial Expression)	*Subjective States or Moods*	*Associated Natural Incentive Characteristics*
Positive emotions		
Interest-surprise	Feeling curious or exploratory	Variety
Anger-excitement	Feeling strong, excited, self as causal agent	Having impact
Joy-happiness-pleasure	Feeling loved, loving, peaceful, happy	Contact
Negative emotions		
Fear	Feeling fearful or anxious	Pain
Disgust	Feeling repelled or rejecting	Naturally unpleasant sensations (e.g., bitter tastes and bad smells)
Sadness-distress	Feeling unhappy or grieving over loss	Major lack of consistency with expectation

In Table 4.2, the emotion of joy-happiness-pleasure has been linked primarily to the contact sensations, which relate to sexuality, although obviously some kind of pleasure can derive from any of the positive incentives, as the research on infant smiling demonstrates. The basis for associating joy-happiness-pleasure primarily with the contact incentive lies not only in the desire to have a neat classification, but also in research that suggests this connection may exist as postulated. Underwood, Moore, and Rosenhan (1972) asked some children to think of things that made them happy and other children to think of things that made them sad. Afterward the children, who were tested individually, were told they could help themselves to some pennies available in a container nearby, but that they could also leave some if they desired for other children who could not participate in the experiment. The children who had been thinking happy thoughts left more pennies for the other children than the children who had been thinking sad thoughts or who had done no special emotional thinking. In other words, the emotion of joy-happiness-pleasure was directly connected with a concern for others, which we are supposing develops out of the contact incentives. To further test whether this is so would require seeing if children who were made happy by introducing mild variety also would be more altruistic, or whether those who had been thinking happy thoughts would do other things more, such as hit a ball harder, which Table 4.2 would associate with the impact incentive.

The negative emotions fit less well with associated natural incentives, although the connection of fear to the negative incentive from pain sensations is clear enough. The sensations giving rise to disgust are so specific it is hard to see how they can play much of a role in developing more complex motivational patterns. Naturally, pleasant and unpleasant sensations provide a basis for preferences in taste and smell, but at present no one has argued that they enter into the development of important social motives.

The poorest fit is between the emotion of sadness-distress and what Chapter 5 will call the *consistency incentive*. The problem derives in part from the fact that the emotion occurs in the absence of consistency rather than in its presence. The variety incentive places a premium on moderate degrees of novelty, but it is equally clear that there is a very powerful incentive for things to match up to expectation. The consistency incentive underlies language learning when children repeat *the dog* rather than just *dog* because they have heard *the dog* all the time. That is, when children say *dog,* they realize the inconsistency with what they have heard, which arouses distress; this, in turn, leads children to correct the mistake and say *the dog.*

The inconsistency incentive underlies the search for reduction of uncertainty and confusion—the need to produce order and predictability in a constantly changing world. The drive-reduction theorists were right in arguing that there is an incentive to reduce tension, conflict, and uncertainty. However, they were wrong in arguing it was the only incentive. The emotional sign that consistency with expectation has not occurred is sadness-distress, as reflected in facial expression, according to this line of reasoning. It is also possible to think of Solomon's negative opponent process as a major source of the inconsistency incentive, in which a strong positive affect no longer occurs after a person has become accustomed to it. This type of inconsistency is particularly likely to give rise to distress.

The classification in Table 4.2 must be regarded as a very preliminary attempt to suggest how some order might be introduced into a field characterized by considerable confusion. It can be questioned on many grounds. For example, not everyone agrees perfectly on which emotions are primary. Plutchik (1980) extends the list to eight primary emotions by separating *interest* from *surprise* and adding *acceptance,* which in his theory is associated with affiliating, whereas joy-happiness-pleasure is associated with cooperating and sexuality. Plutchik may turn out to be right, but we have followed the simpler classification primarily because *acceptance* does not lead to an identifiable facial expression and because interest and surprise appear to be on a continuum so far as facial expressions are conceived. Our analysis places greater weight on infant facial expressions than Plutchik's does, because we are searching for natural—that is, universal and innate—incentive characteristics. Thus, the fact that certain facial expressions are universal in infants and readily recognizable leads us to believe that they may be cued off by sign stimuli or incentives the observer can readily identify. Thus, we have not included additional emotions mentioned by Plutchik (1980) or Izard (1979) because of doubts about the universal recognizability of the facial expressions of these emotions in infants. There obviously are many more emotions than those listed that result from blends of natural incentives or are the product of later learning.

What is more, a very respected tradition in psychology is based on an influential experiment by Schachter and Singer (1962), which argues that there are no primary, unlearned emotions. Rather, there is only an unlearned state of affective physiological arousal, which is converted into various emotions by the subject's cognitive understanding of the situation. Chapter 12 examines this work at length and finds it does not support the conclusion that there are no fundamentally different affective states.

Chapter 5 will attempt to describe and define more carefully some of the natural incentives listed in Table 4.2. One general point about them needs to be made now. This chapter has used the term *sign stimuli* throughout, which is adopted from the ethologists to describe the external events that release innate affective responses or emotions. This describes fairly well what elicits the variety incentive: moderate environmental changes in what is expected elicits interest-surprise. In describing the baby Peter's behavior, however, we noted that some of this variation was *response produced:* It was his climbing over the threshold and the perceived novelty of what he had done that surprised and pleased him. He was not a passive responder to stimulus change; he produced it.

This is even truer of the impact incentive, for which it is hard to identify a sign stimulus that is not response produced. Peter enjoyed the sensations he experienced when he banged, grasped, or pushed something. Perhaps, as has been noted, interference with grasping or pushing serves as an additional sign stimulus to evoke more attempts to have impact, but it is the sensations from having impact that are sought as the primary source of pleasure.

• RELATION OF EMOTION TO MOTIVATION

Some theorists (Izard, 1979; Tomkins, 1962) consider emotions to be motivations in the sense that they influence behavior. As we pointed out in Chapter 3, however, the term *motivation* is used by many people as being equivalent to *determination*. That is, emotions—like habits, expectations, and so on—can be shown to *determine* or influence behavior. But in the restricted sense in which the term is used in this book, emotions do not *motivate* behavior: only motives motivate behavior. Emotions are not motives, but they are an important part of motivational systems: they indicate the presence of natural incentives. Furthermore, motives presumably are built on natural incentives, as the next chapter will attempt to make clear. Emotions also accompany motives and amplify their effects on behavior. For example, they intensify the reactions to success or failure in satisfying a motive. They provide the affective "charge" that makes motivational systems so powerful and persistent in shaping behavior. They involve a more primitive level of brain functioning that continues to influence what people say and do often without their knowing what is going on, that is, without adequate cognitive representation in the later developing cortical association areas of the brain.

NOTES AND QUERIES

1. Sign stimuli in animals tend to be quite specific and differ from one species to another. For example, whereas it is the sight of the red belly of another stickleback that releases an attack response in the male stickleback, it is the smell of urine of strange males that releases intermale aggression in mice (MacKintosh & Grant, 1966). Several species of animals attack intruders in their territory (Lorenz, 1966). It has often been inferred that humans, like other animals, have an "aggressive instinct," but the question always has been, Like which other animals? Are we most like lions, mice, or deer? What are the sign stimuli that "turn on" the aggressive response in humans? What kinds of sensations, perceptions, or situations are most likely to elicit anger-excitement in you? How would you determine if such "turn ons" were natural (part of the biological inheritance) rather than learned?

2. Solomon's opponent process theory explains why many people undergo painful experiences, like a sauna bath, to get the pleasure it automatically induces. Can you think of any painful experiences in your own life that have not been followed by pleasure? What are the implications of such instances for the theory?

3. It often has been observed that people learn languages more easily when they are young. Can you think of an explanation for this fact that would involve the operation of a natural incentive? Why might it be easier for people to get pleasure from producing the sounds they hear in childhood than to do so later on?

4.   How would you define the natural incentive involved in chewing gum? How could you determine whether it is "natural" or acquired? If you consider it a subtype of a more general natural incentive, can you think of other things gum chewers also would be likely to do or enjoy?

5.   Why does the discovery of "pleasure centers" in the brain suggest the presence of natural incentives? Would you expect to find the same pleasure centers in humans that have been found in rats? Why or why not?

6.   If the procedures initiated by Cicchetti and Sroufe represent sign stimuli that release pleasure in human infants, how would you explain the fact that in no instance did *all* the infants respond with a smile to a particular procedure?

7.   Can you think of any natural incentives that have been left out in Table 4.2? What about sensation pleasures—for example, from sights, sounds, or tastes? Can you think how possible natural incentives involved might lead to the development of motives that shape the lives of musicians, artists, or gourmets?

8.   Izard (1979) has pointed out that a greater number of different emotions can be distinguished in higher than in lower forms of life (that is, say, in human beings in comparison with salamanders or even dogs and cats). It is the face in particular in humans that reflects many different emotions. Izard argues that this is adaptive, because emotions help the organism adapt and survive, and the more differentiated the emotions are, the more flexibly the organism can adapt. If the motives are built on the natural incentives that elicit different emotions, as this chapter suggests, does this mean there will be a greater number of different types of motives in humans than lower animals? Does the fact that lower animals have more built-in responses to specific sign stimuli than humans do suggest that, among human beings, motives may be a more flexible way of incorporating natural sign stimuli into means of adapting successfully?

5

Natural Incentives and Their Derivatives

• HOW NATURAL INCENTIVES INFLUENCE THE DEVELOPMENT OF THE HUNGER MOTIVE

Much has been learned about the factors that affect eating in animals and humans. The purpose of this chapter is not to review all this knowledge, but to learn from it as much as we can about the way motives develop out of sign stimuli and the behavior they release, or what we have called *natural incentives*. The advantage of using hunger as the model for this purpose is that everyone agrees that some of the sign stimuli involved produce innate affects and that enough research has been done on eating in animals and humans to show how motives might develop out of these innate affects through learning.

To oversimplify somewhat, three types of sign stimuli influence eating: (1) sign stimuli arising from nutritional deficiency, particularly low levels of available blood sugar (Mayer, 1955; Mayer & Marshall, 1956), which increase eating; (2) sign stimuli arising from the palatability or tastiness of food; and (3) sign stimuli arising from satiety, such as a full stomach or high blood sugar level, which decrease eating. Ordinarily the mechanisms involved operate automatically to make sure the body has enough energy (represented as available blood sugar) to do its work. A person's going without food lowers blood sugar, which among other effects stimulates a portion of the midbrain that mediates affect (that is, the lateral hypothalamus), which elicits eating if food is present (Grossman, 1960). This was discovered by injecting insulin, which lowers blood sugar level and leads to increased eating. If food is tasty, it also stimulates the lateral hypothalamus (Burton, Mora, & Rolls, 1975), leading to an increased release of insulin; this lowers the blood sugar level, which stimulates the lateral hypothalamus and thus leads to more eating. Eventually a full stomach, higher blood sugar levels, and several other factors stimulate another portion of the hypothalamus and the liver to inhibit eating. Many physiological mechanisms are involved in the control of food intake (see Carlson, 1977), and their exact influence is still not fully understood. All that need concern us here is that sign stimuli built into the organism automatically and in various ways produce the responses (eating or not eating) that regulate food intake and maintain the organism.

But food is not always present, the way oxygen nearly always is, when a person or animal needs more of it. Furthermore, some objects that are eaten and swallowed are good for the organism (that is, increase the blood sugar level) and some are not; some may even be harmful or poisonous. So an individual must learn how to get the right kind of food. And learning associated with eating begins the moment the human infant is born and can no longer get nutrition directly from the mother (Marquis, 1941). Furthermore, learning about what to eat occurs easily and rapidly. For example, many studies have shown that animals very readily learn to avoid the taste of a substance that has produced illness (Garcia & Koelling, 1966), but not to avoid a taste paired with electric shock. That is, the animal seems to be preset to learn an association more easily that would keep it from eating poisonous foods than an association involving the pain of electric shock. Furthermore, animals quickly learn to prefer a diet containing a substance they need (such as salt), presumably because they are avoiding the old distress-producing salt-free diet and have found a new one that reduces the distress (Garcia, Hankins, & Rusiniak, 1974).

At what point do we begin to think in terms of motivation and motives? So long as a system works automatically without important learning having taken place, there seems little reason to speak of a motive being present. A lack of oxygen stimulates breathing; low available blood sugar stimulates the human infant to suck from the mother's breast. These mechanisms are often referred to as *homeostatic* in the sense that when a disturbance occurs, it sets in motion the response that removes the disturbance. The term *motive* is not ordinarily applied to such sequences but is reserved for instances in which important learning has taken place in connection with the affect associated with natural incentives.

At what point do we conclude learning has produced a hunger motive? A conditioned taste aversion might be described as an "avoidance motive," but it seems preferable to reserve the term *motive* for a more general type of goal. Human infants at birth must above all learn what they want—what goals or end states are associated with proper eating. Assume that the absence of food in the presence of low blood sugar levels arouses the emotion of sadness-distress (since eating is impossible) and that eating tasty food arouses the emotion of joy or pleasure. These emotions provide much of the energy behind what becomes a learned motive either (1) to relieve the distress by finding a way to eat or (2) to feel pleasure from eating. In both cases the goal defining the motive is the same—to eat—although in the first instance eating has been associated with relief of distress and in the second, with pleasure from eating. The way the two types of natural incentives may develop into motives is diagramed in Figure 5.1.

The connection between low available blood sugar and readiness to eat via stimulation of the lateral hypothalamus is what can be called a *natural incentive*—an innate connection between a sign stimulus and an affective response in the midbrain, which releases an impulse to act in a certain way if certain other conditions occur (chiefly the presence of food). Since food is not always instantly available to human infants, they experience the negative affect that automatically arises when the impulse to eat is activated and they cannot eat. In time this builds an association between the low available blood sugar cue and a threefold complex of events—namely, the absence of food, the accompanying distress, and eating to relieve the distress. This complex may be described as an affectively charged anticipatory goal response (eating to reduce the negative affect) or a goal state (since in some cases what response produces the relief of distress is not as clear as in the case of eating).

Thus, a motive may be defined briefly as *a learned, affectively charged anticipatory goal state* aroused by various cues—initially by the natural sign stimulus of low available blood sugar in the case of eating, but later by other cues such as the time of day. A motive activates the organism to learn the instrumental responses necessary to bring about the goal state.

The strength of this type of hunger motive presumably is largely determined by the frequency, intensity, and variability of the condition of "no food" being present when the organism is ready to eat. That is, the more the low available

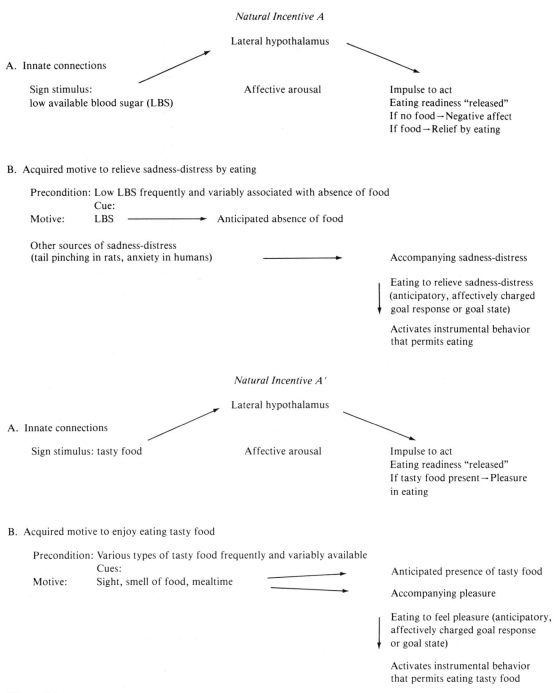

Figure 5.1.

How Two Types of Eating Motives Develop from Natural Incentives.

blood sugar cue is associated with intense negative affect under a variety of conditions, the stronger this type of hunger motive will be. Such a conclusion is supported by a number of studies showing that variable deprivation of food in infant rats is associated with unusually strong tendencies to get and eat food in adult rats (see, for example, J. M. Mandler, 1958). The hoarding is explained on the grounds that early deprivation of food increases the frequency and intensity of the negative affective arousal that occurs when the animal is ready to eat but no food is present. Thus, the natural cue, low blood sugar, as well as other associated cues, gives rise to a much stronger hunger motive to relieve distress by eating. The anticipatory goal state (the reduction in distress by eating) is much more affectively charged than it would be without the experience of variable food deprivation. Therefore food, when it appears and permits eating, is associated with a much greater relief of distress. It has acquired a much greater reward or incentive value because of the experience of deprivation, and it continues to maintain this extra value even in adulthood when plenty of food is present. Thus, the animal hoards food because it was associated early in life with relief of distress. In much the same way some people are presumed to have developed an intense interest in food and eating as a means of relieving the distress they experienced early in life in connection with eating.

Furthermore, the distress need not derive completely from lack of food to produce this effect. As Figure 5.1 points out, other sources of distress that occur during eating also can increase the motive to eat to relieve distress. If rats' tails are mildly pinched while they are eating, they eat more (Rowland & Antelman, 1976). This is surprising, because fear normally inhibits eating. The presumption is that the tail pinching creates some negative affect that eating reduces. This source of distress, like the distress from food deprivation, acts to increase the strength of the goal response of eating to relieve distress.

A similar finding has been reported for certain kinds of overweight human subjects (Schachter, Goldman, & Gordon, 1968). Subjects who were overweight and of normal weight were given various foods to eat—for example, chocolate chip cookies (McKenna, 1972)—when they were in a state of high or low anxiety. The subjects of normal weight ate fewer cookies when the anxiety was strong than when it was weak. Fear inhibited their eating. The obese subjects, however, ate equal numbers of cookies whether the anxiety was strong or weak, despite independent evidence that they are more emotional and respond more nervously to threats of various kinds. A reasonable explanation for their behavior is that anxiety has been associated with eating in the past for them, so they have a stronger motive than do subjects of normal weight to relieve distress by eating. Certainly eating can be used to relieve distress (M. C. Jones, 1924), as every mother knows who nurses or gives a bottle to calm an upset baby who is not even hungry. Perhaps obese people have developed a stronger motive to eat to relieve distress because of various experiences of negative affect associated with eating in the past. This would also explain why they eat more than is necessary to supply their bodies with the energy needed as signaled by low blood sugar levels.

The second type of natural incentive illustrated in Figure 5.1 involves tasty food as a sign stimulus. More palatable food activates the lateral hypothalamus more (Burton, Mora, & Rolls, 1975), which produces insulin release and more eating. An animal will eat much more of the same food if its taste is changed several times (Le Magnen, 1956). It is assumed that eating tasty food produces strong pleasure, so if people have this type of experience frequently, they may acquire a motive characterized by the anticipation of eating tasty food and the pleasure associated with doing so. In this case the releasing sign stimuli or cues that arouse the motive are external—involving, for example, the sight, smell, and taste of more palatable food—rather than internal, as was the previous motive complex built on the internal sign of lowered blood sugar, plus the distress caused by its absence.

Schachter (1971a) and his associates have collected a large amount of evidence demonstrating that certain overweight people are strongly influenced in how much they eat by such external cues. Compared with people of normal weight, the obese people consumed more of a good-tasting milk shake and less of a bad-tasting one (Decke, 1971). They ate more than people of normal weight when they were led to believe it was dinnertime by a clock that had been set ahead in the laboratory (Schachter, 1971a). They ate more when food cues were obvious and less when they were not obvious. For example, if nuts were in their shells they ate them less often; if they were unshelled they ate them more often than people of normal weight, who ate them equally often under both conditions.

One way to explain these results is to assume that the approach eating motive outlined in the lower half of Figure 5.1 is stronger in some overweight people as compared with people of normal weight. It might be inferred that more attention was given to providing them tasty food when they were young, so the external cues of sight, time of day, and so on, were more strongly associated with the joys of eating. Since we have concluded that these overweight people also might have a stronger motive to eat to reduce distress, obviously the eating modality should have much more importance for them than for other people, which is certainly the case. The presumption is strong that their concern with eating derives from affective experiences associated with eating, particularly early in life. This is precisely the line of reasoning advanced by Freud and his followers, who believed on the basis of clinical case studies that early affective experiences associated with eating—or the oral intake modality—lead people to fixate on or be oriented toward that modality throughout life.

Unfortunately, no studies of humans have been reported that correlate affective feeding experiences in infancy with the strength of hunger motives in adulthood or with obesity, so the hypothesis cannot be directly checked. For that matter, there is no direct evidence that obese people have stronger hunger motives, using the methods for assessing the strength of human motives described in subsequent chapters. Nevertheless, the behavior of the types of overweight people studied by Schachter and his associates is consistent with the theoretical model of the way two types of hunger motives develop as outlined in Figure 5.1.

• NATURAL INCENTIVES, EMOTIONS, AND MOTIVES

A natural incentive in humans has three components, as Figure 5.1 makes clear—namely, (1) a sign stimulus, (2) a state of central affective arousal, and (3) what is usually called a *consummatory act*—a type of response that, like eating, is released by the sign stimulus and the state of central arousal (see Cofer, 1972). It is called *consummatory* because it is aimed at satisfying whatever gave rise to it. The red belly of a male stickleback elicits aggressive behavior in another male stickleback that is aimed at the red belly. This is confusing, because the sight of the red belly, which initiates the behavior, is not identical with the consummatory experience, which comes from attacking the red belly. Nor is the sight of tasty food, which produces lateral hypothalamic stimulation and eating, exactly the same as the experience of eating tasty food, which is the *consummatory affective experience* sought. Sometimes what starts an incentive sequence is similar to the experience that consummates it, and sometimes the two are different.

Table 5.1 summarizes the relationships involved in a natural incentive sequence and shows how the motives treated in subsequent chapters develop from the natural incentives to be discussed in this chapter. The table outlines what is to come. Each of the incentives mentioned will be discussed in detail later in this chapter and the motives based on them, in later chapters. Notice that in the case of the avoidance motives, the sign stimulus differs from the consummatory experience sought. Inconsistency, conflict, and pain are sign stimuli that produce negative emotions and release acts designed to produce the consummatory experience of consistency, relief, or fear reduction. Pain and the inconsistency sign stimuli also may be referred to as *negative incentives,* although their positive aspect (consistency or relief) is used here to label them.

In the case of approach motives, the sign stimulus that sets up the natural incentive sequence initially may be the consummatory experience itself. Eating tasty food produces central affective excitement, which leads to eating more of the food and endows the sight and smell of tasty food with the power through learning to evoke an anticipatory affective goal state, thus forming the positive hunger motive. In what follows, we will use the term *natural incentive* to refer primarily to the consummatory experience and will label the incentive in terms of that experience.

Table 5.1 also shows the type of emotion as shown in facial expressions, which indicates the presence of a particular consummatory experience and the motive that is presumably acquired in connection with each type of consummatory experience. Consider the variety incentive first. As this chapter will show, there is considerable evidence that mild variation in stimulation is pleasant and sought and produces an emotion characterized by the facial expression of interest-surprise (see Chapter 4). The consummatory experience of pleasure from variety may occur by chance from changes in the environment, without the organism having done anything to bring it about. However, by the very nature of the stimulation, if the organism does nothing but passively experience it, the stimulation will become expected or boring and will lose its appeal. The con-

Table 5.1.
OUTLINE OF RELATIONS BETWEEN NATURAL INCENTIVES, ASSOCIATED EMOTIONS, AND MOTIVES

Sign Stimulus →	Consummatory Experience of	Natural Incentives — Emotion as Shown in Facial Expression →	Consummatory Acts →	Motive Acquired in Connection With
		Approach motives		
Sight or smell of tasty food	Tasty food	Pleasure	Eating	Hunger motive
Small variations from expectancy	Mild variety	Interest-surprise	Exploratory behavior	Achievement motive (Chapter 7)
Having impact, threats, interference with having impact	Having impact	Anger-excitement	Asserting, banging, and so on	Power motive (Chapter 8)
Touching, hearing, or seeing another person	Contact, rubbing, snuggling, rocking	Sexual excitement, feeling loved, loving, joy	Seeking and exchanging contact with others	Affiliative motives (Chapter 9)
		Avoidance motives		
Inconsistency, conflict	Consistency, conflict reduction	Sadness-distress	Seeking to relieve distress and increase consistency	
Large variations from expectancy				
Pain	Relief	Fear	Seeking to avoid fear	Avoidance motives (Chapter 10)
Unpleasant taste		Disgust	Spitting out	

summatory act of exploring the environment is the way in which the organism normally produces the consummatory experience from mild variation in stimulation. As the experience of variety diminishes, the organism does something to increase it. Here what started the sequence (the experience of mild variety) is also the experience sought by the consummatory act of exploratory behavior. And out of these experiences the achievement motive that will be discussed in Chapter 7 presumably develops.

In the case of the impact incentive, a baby cannot have the consummatory experience without doing something. The baby is naturally active, and in the course of pushing things around and grasping and dropping things, the baby feels the pleasurable excitement that is a built-in response to the experience of having impact. Having an impact experience is the sign stimulus for having more such experiences in an ever increasing cycle that eventually results in the facial emotion called *anger-excitement* (although, as we shall see, the term *anger* has a negative connotation that it does not deserve in its most primitive, unlearned form).

Note that here the consummatory experience or natural incentive is *response produced*. The child produces a stimulus—for example, a bang—that releases more of the same type of behavior. Out of these impact experiences develops the power motive, discussed in Chapter 8. The role of external sign stimuli in releasing the impulse to have impact is not altogether clear. There is some evidence that in humans, threats (as from strange or threatening gestures) and interference with having impact innately release anger-excitement (see Morris, 1967). These actual or potential interferences with having impact produce a negative emotional state somewhat different from pleasurable anger-excitement. In time the person seeks to release this distress through having more impact in much the same way as the absence of food develops a motive to eat to relieve distress, as outlined in Figure 5.1.

Contact experiences, such as those from snuggling, rocking, and cuddling, lead to sexual excitement or, more simply, to joy-happiness-pleasure as reflected in facial expressions. Such experiences are obtained normally by mutual exchange with another person, usually the mother or primary caretaker in the case of human infants. Eventually they endow cues from seeing or hearing such a person with the capacity to evoke anticipations of joy-happiness-pleasure from contact with such people; these develop into the affiliative motives characterized by being loved and loving, as will be discussed in Chapter 9.

Finally, mismatches between expectation and reality generate negative affect —reflected in the facial expressions of sadness-distress and fear—which generate consummatory acts designed to reduce the sadness-distress or maintain consistency. As noted already, in this instance there is a lack of fit between the experience that starts the natural incentive sequence (for example, inconsistency or pain) and the consummatory experience that satisfies or ends it (relief from the removal of inconsistency or fear). In general, experiences of negative affect from inconsistency or fear lead to the avoidance motives, which will be discussed in Chapter 10.

The outline in Table 5.1 leaves out motives associated with certain emotions represented in facial expressions—disgust, for example—which may develop into important human motives but on which no empirical work has been done. This only emphasizes the fact that the classification in Table 5.1 is preliminary and tentative. Its primary function is to suggest possible connections among natural incentives, emotions, and motives that deserve further study and to provide a framework in terms of which to organize the presentation of a large body of knowledge.

• THE VARIETY INCENTIVE

It has long been known that animals seek at least moderate amounts of novelty. White rats typically will explore a new environment unless the novelty is too strong, in which case they will freeze or even make vigorous attempts to escape (Fiske & Maddi, 1961). According to Berlyne (1967), "higher animals often find access to stimulation gratifying and properties known to raise arousal—such as novelty, surprisingness, complexity—may enhance the reward value of exteroceptive stimuli. Even pain can apparently be rewarding in small doses." Dember, Earl, and Paradise (1957) painted the walls of the two loops in a figure eight maze with two patterns of stripes. In one loop the stripes were vertical; in the other, stripes of the same width were painted horizontally. On the second day of exposure to this situation, sixteen of seventeen rats spent most of their time in the loop with vertical stripes, presumably because it provided more variety and stimulation when they ran past the stripes.

E. L. Walker (1964, 1973) extended this study by dividing a maze into four quadrants, each of which varied progressively in degree of complexity. Typically the animals started out by spending most of their time at a low level of complexity, but as they grew more and more familiar with it they moved to a higher level of complexity. This is reminiscent of the way humans with a strong achievement motive seek out more and more difficult (complex) tasks (see Chapter 7). Rats also have been shown to alternate the pathways they take to food if the pathways are comparable (Heathers, 1940) or to prefer a path to food with a barrier in it over an unobstructed path (Festinger, 1943).

McClelland, Atkinson, Clark, and Lowell (1953) attempted to systematize such observations under the general principle that moderate discrepancies from adaptation level would be found to be pleasing or rewarding, whereas large discrepancies would be unpleasant and be avoided. A completely familiar stimulus would be hedonically neutral or boring in this formulation, whereas slight variations along any of a number of dimensions would attract attention and be pleasant. Sudden large shifts from what the organism was adapted to would evoke startle, discomfort, and avoidance.

A simple experiment by Haber (1958) illustrates how the principle works. He had subjects place their hands in a bucket of water until the hands were well adapted to its temperature. Then, at the same moment, the subjects removed both hands from the bucket and immersed each in separate buckets of different temperatures, with the instructions to withdraw the hand from the bucket that was more uncomfortable. Haber found that temperatures either one degree Celsius warmer or colder than the adaptation temperature were considered more pleasant than temperatures that differed more from the adaptation temperature, producing what has been called the *butterfly curve* (see Figure 5.2). Furthermore, he found he could shift the hedonic curve upward or downward by changing the temperature of the adaptation bucket. Thus, if the hands were adapted to thirty-three degrees Celsius, a temperature of thirty-two degrees Celsius was considered pleasant, but if the adaptation level was thirty-four degrees Celsius, a temperature of thirty-two degrees Celsius was considered unpleasant. Of course, these changes take place within certain absolute limits, since all temperatures above or below certain levels are unpleasant. The phenomenon has been experienced by everyone who has tried to drink coffee and eat ice cream at the same time. If the mouth is adapted to the higher temperature of coffee, the ice cream can produce a painful reaction—a reaction much more painful than it produces without the coffee, although the temperature of the ice cream is constant.

A similar type of curve has been obtained by Maddi (1961) along the dimension of expectedness-novelty. Subjects were provided with booklets consisting of a number of pages stapled together; on some of them appeared numbers and on others, sentence stems like *In winter* or *The stranger.* The subjects were instructed to turn the pages, and when they came to a stem they were to complete it with a sentence in any way they liked. They were told that the num-

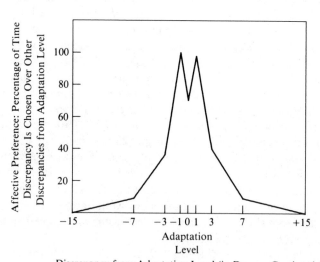

Figure 5.2.

Typical Affective Preference Curve as a Function of Temperature Discrepancies from Level to Which Hands in Water Are Adapted (after Haber, 1958).

bered pages were "included as spacers between the stems so that they might rest when not completing sentences" (Maddi, 1961). Some of the subjects were asked to predict whether a number (*N*) or a stem (*S*) was coming up next. For one group of subjects the number of pages with numbers and stems was quite regular, following an *NNS* pattern—that is, every third page contained a stem—and the subjects were asked to predict whether a number or stem was coming up next. For another group the ordering of numbers or stems had no regularity. The sentence completions produced by the subjects were objectively coded for affective tone along a scale from 1 (if they contained strongly negative affect) to 5 (if they contained strongly positive affect).

Figure 5.3 shows the results. The affective tone of the sentence completions for those experiencing regularity starts out neutral, gradually increases toward positive affect up through the third or fourth repetition of the *NNS* sequence, and then declines again. The affective reaction of these subjects to the first stem was neutral, but as they became more certain of what to expect, they reacted with positive affect when the stem occurred. However, later in the series, when they were absolutely sure a stem would occur, the occurrence of the stem no longer evoked positive affect in the sentences they wrote. For the subjects experiencing no regularity, there was no change in the affective tone of their sentence completions over time.

After the eighth repetition of the *NNS* sequence, subjects experiencing regu-

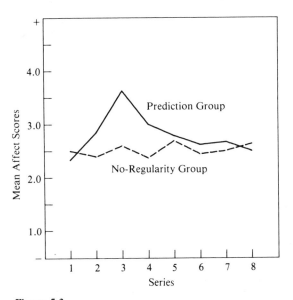

Figure 5.3.

Mean Affect Scores as a Function of Number of Series Experienced. These series constituted environmental regularity for the prediction group (Maddi, 1961).

larity were exposed to a ninth stem representing either zero discrepancy from the previous series (that is, *NNS*), a moderate discrepancy over expectation (either *NS* or *NNNS*), or a large discrepancy from expectation (either *S* or *NNNNS*). As Figure 5.4 shows, for subjects experiencing regularity, moderate discrepancies over expectation produced a more positive affect to the ninth than to the eighth stem, whereas a much larger discrepancy from expectation produced much less of a positive reaction or even a slightly negative one. Again, no marked difference in affect was displayed by those who had experienced no regularity.

The occurrence of events that are moderately different from what people expect is pleasing, whereas they react to the too familiar or the too novel either indifferently or negatively. As noted earlier, Zajonc (1980), using an entirely different technique, demonstrated that familiar items are more positively evaluated than totally new ones, although he does not explore the part of the curve in which too much familiarity breeds boredom. However, the experience is a common one in everyday life: At first you may listen to a new piece of music more or less with indifference until you become somewhat familiar with it. As the familiarity grows you confirm your partial expectations of sound sequences and rhythms and react positively. If you listen to the piece a hundred or a thousand times, however, it can become positively unpleasant.

Kagan, Kearsley, and Zelazo (1978) report a number of studies that show

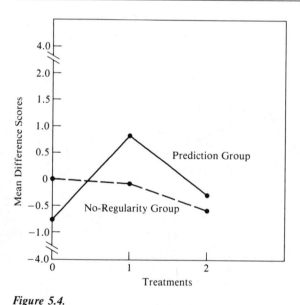

Figure 5.4.

Mean Affective Difference Scores Associated With Zero, One, and Two Degrees of Change in Order of Events (Maddi, 1961).

infants in the first year and a half of life pay more attention to and act more pleased by moderately discrepant stimuli. In their view, infants first are able to form some schema (for example, of the human face), to which they can compare a discrepant stimulus (say, a human mask without any eyes or with the features scrambled). At an early age (say, three months) the mask with scrambled features evokes considerably less attention than it does at thirteen months, because at the earlier age children have not yet formed a good enough schema of the human face to compare the discrepant stimulus with it (see also Spitz & Wolf, 1946).

A carefully designed experiment by Hopkins, Zelazo, Jacobson, and Kagan (1976) illustrates this point and also that what infants pay attention to or like depends on what they are habituated to. Infants seven and a half months old sat on their mothers' laps viewing objects exposed in a chamber in front of them. The objects were made of papier-mâché, as Figure 5.5 illustrates. The first four were red with half-inch black stripes. When the infants pressed the lever in front of them it resulted in an illumination two and a half seconds long of a stimulus object in one of the viewing compartments. During habituation they were allowed to keep illuminating the object to view it for at least three minutes or until they began to tire in doing so. They were habituated either to object A or object D in the series.

A switch then was thrown so a bar press would illuminate a comparison object in a second viewing chamber. This object also was available for viewing for a minimum of three minutes. The crucial question was which of the comparison objects the infants would be most interested in viewing, as indicated by the number of times they pressed the bar to get a look at it. As the results in Figure

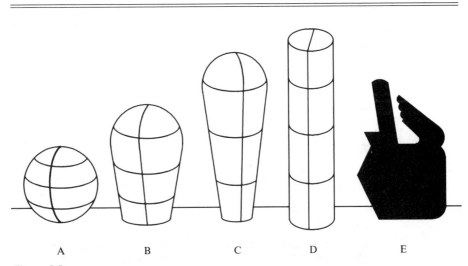

A   B   C   D   E

Figure 5.5.

Stimuli Used in Infant Habituation Study (Hopkins, Zelazo, Jacobson, & Kagan, 1976).

5.6 show, they were most interested in the object that was moderately different (second-level moderate discrepancy) from the standard object to which they had been habituated. If they had been habituated to object A they were most interested in object D, and if habituated to object D they were most interested in object A. Lesser discrepancies from the familiar object (object B after object A, or object C after object D) produced less interest, as did the most discrepant stimulus, object E. In short, the results are the same as for the Maddi experiment: moderate discrepancies from expectation are pleasurable; very small or very large discrepancies are not.

These studies define familiarity-novelty not in terms of repetition of the same event, as in the Maddi experiment, but in terms of visual/spatial dimensions. Berlyne (1967) summarized evidence that the variety incentive is appealing across a number of dimensions—familiarity-novelty, expectedness-surprisingness, clarity-ambiguity, and complexity-simplicity. (See also Berlyne & Madsen, 1973.) However the dimensions are defined, moderate variety is responded to positively, whereas extreme variety produces negative reactions and no variety produces indifference.

What is particularly noteworthy about the variety incentive is that it con-

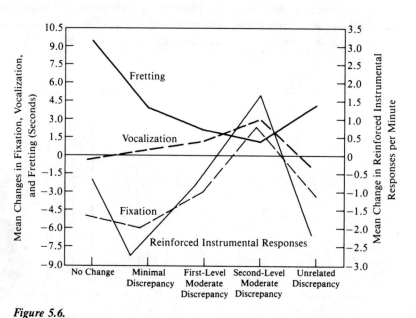

Figure 5.6.

Changes in Responsivity from the Last Two Minutes of Viewing the Standard Object to the First Two Minutes of Viewing the Discrepant Comparison Object (after Hopkins, Zelazo, Jacobson, & Kagan, 1976).

tains both unlearned and learned components. What appears innate or invariant is the degree of novelty or unexpectedness that produces the hedonic curve. Learning also plays a crucial role, because what is expected—or the situation to which the person is adapted—completely depends on experience or learning. All the natural incentives appear to operate this way: a certain type of experience innately yields the hedonic curve, but what produces that type of experience changes quickly through learning.

Individual Differences in Seeking Variety

Zuckerman (1974) has developed a sensation-seeking scale indicating that some people seek much more variety or stimulation than others. It consists of items such as *I would like to try parachute jumping; I like to have new and exciting experiences and sensations even if they are a little frightening, unconventional, or illegal; I like "wild," uninhibited parties;* and *I get bored seeing the same old faces.* In each case the subject has an opportunity to check one alternative or another one indicating the opposite preference. Obviously, many other variables besides the sensation-seeking incentive might influence the way subjects answer questions like these, but in a general way the scale does indicate real differences in the amount of stimulation people seek.

Figure 5.7 provides one of the clearest examples of this fact. Male volunteer subjects spent either eight hours of sensory deprivation or eight hours of confinement in social isolation with some pictures and music provided. The extent

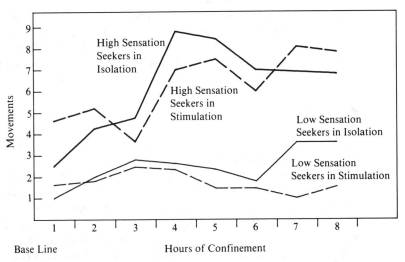

Figure 5.7.

Mean Periods of Movement per Hour of Confinement (after Zuckerman, 1974).

of bodily movements was measured "by an air mattress connected to a pressure transducer" (Zuckerman, 1974). Clearly those scoring higher on sensation seeking in fact moved much more in either condition, presumably to stimulate themselves more. In another study Zuckerman measured scalp electrical potentials evoked by different intensities of visual stimuli for subjects high and low in sensation seeking. He found the high sensation seekers (as measured by one of his scales) were augmentors. That is, the brighter the visual stimulus, the greater the electrical response in the brain measured from scalp electrodes. Those not seeking sensation did not show this effect. Apparently, sensation seekers can tolerate more such stimulation than those low in sensation seeking.

Maddi, Charlens, Maddi, and Smith (1962) also developed a measure of individual differences in seeking novelty. They compared imaginative stories written after exposure to a very monotonous tape recording with those written after exposure to a tape containing many interesting and surprising statements. The differences in the content of the two sets of stories were worked into a scoring system called "the desire for novelty." The measure is most successful in picking out those who are bored (those low on the scale) and does not correlate with other measures of curiosity or of creativity.

Beswick (1965) was more successful in deriving a measure of the extent of human curiosity. He too developed a scoring system for imaginative stories, which covered such characteristics as Wonder-Interest, Perceptual Instrumental Acts, Exploratory Role Behavior, and Intrapsychic Responses of Excitement, which were found to differentiate the stories written after exposure to curiosity-arousing experiences versus ordinary experiences. Beswick found that the test-retest reliability of the measure was high ($r = .71$ after six months); also, the measure is valid in that it correlates both with self-descriptions of orderliness and with behaviors associated with interest in novelty, as in girls' agreeing with an item like *Novelty has the greatest appeal for me.* He theorizes that being curious involves wanting to order experience on the one hand, and on the other hand being willing to experience disorder so as to bring it into order. Beswick found some support for the belief that his TAT measure tapped this characteristic in the fact that students who scored high in it took more books out of the library to read for pleasure, as well as the fact that they were more apt to spontaneously make independent inquiries of a minister about religious matters than those who scored low in the characteristic. He does not think of curiosity as a motive, but it is one in the sense that the variety incentive has more appeal for some individuals than others.

Using quite another measure, Liam Hudson (1966) has found he can distinguish between people who seek primarily novelty and those who seek primarily order. He categorized individuals according to whether they scored high or low on an intelligence test and on open-ended tests of creative fluency, such as listing as many uses of a paper clip as possible. He compared those who scored high on the intelligence tests and low on fluency tests (called *convergers*) with those who did better on the fluency tests than they did on the intelligence tests (called *divergers*). The divergers much more often were students of the arts, whereas the convergers were science concentrators. In comparison to the convergers, the divergers were more liberal and nonauthoritarian, more emotional, gave more responses involving humor or personal violence, and did much better on tests involving words rather than numbers or spatial relations. Science appeals to convergers because it involves explaining everything new in an orderly way, whereas the arts allow divergers to express their interest in novelty, change, and exciting new forms.

The Variety Incentive and the Achievement Motive

McClelland, Atkinson, Clark, and Lowell (1953) argued that the variety incentive was the basis for the achievement motive (see Chapter 7) and possibly for all motives, which it is not. For example, there is no evidence that people high in the need for Power or Affiliation are especially "turned on" by variety or moderately challenging tasks the way those high in the need to Achieve are (see Chapters 8 and 9). Since variety is a natural incentive, it can add spice to any consummatory experience; however, that is not the same as saying variety is what is primarily sought for all motive systems.

Furthermore, it is not entirely clear how the achievement motive is built on the variety incentive. The problem lies in how the transition is made from liking moderate variations in stimulus situations to liking to produce moderate degrees of variety, as in liking to *do* something better. Rats like variations in stimulation, such as traversing a maze with vertical stripes, but they soon learn to go where they can get such increases in stimulation. Does that define an achievement motive for them? The infants in the study by Kagan et al. liked to see moderately discrepant visual figures, but they also quickly learned to press a bar to get such experiences. It is well known that subjects with a strong achievement motive prefer moderately difficult tasks (see Chapter 7), just as the little boy Peter in Chapter 4 was attracted to climbing over the threshold, which involved a slight difficulty for him in getting from one place to the next. But if he were just interested in producing moderate variety, why did he not stay in the next room and explore it? Why did he turn back, climb over the threshold again, and smile at his accomplishment? One might assume that task difficulty becomes a regular form of variety, just as moderate complexity does, so moderately difficult situations become sought in themselves. Or one might assume that variety has fused with the impact incentive in mastering tasks, since obviously Peter was also pleased at producing the effect of getting over the obstacle. Research to date has not clarified this point.

• THE IMPACT INCENTIVE

Many observers have noted the great importance of exploration, manipulation, and play in lower animals and the human infant. Robert White (1960) coined the term *effectance* to describe the goal of these activities. To give a lively sense of what such behavior is like in the young child, White quotes from Gesell and Ilg (1943):

The child wants to finger the clothespin, to get the feel of it. He puts it in his mouth, pulls it out, looks at it, rotates it with the twist of the wrist, puts it back into his mouth, pulls it out, gives it another twist, brings up his free hand, transfers the clothespin from hand to hand, bangs it on the highchair tray, drops it, recovers it, retransfers it from hand to hand, drops it out of reach, leans over to retrieve it, fails, fusses a moment, then bangs the tray with his empty hand.

Even in feeding, which according to drive theory should represent the passive pleasure of tension reduction, the child becomes active. "Around one year there is likely to occur what Levy (1955) calls 'the battle of the spoon,' the moment when 'the baby grabs the spoon from the mother's hand and tries to feed itself. . . . We can be sure that the child is not motivated at this point by increased oral gratification. He gets more food by letting mother do it, but by doing it himself he gets more of another kind of satisfaction—a feeling of efficacy" (White, 1960).

Later, when the child can walk, "one observes a constant activity of carrying objects about, filling and emptying containers, tearing things apart and fitting them together, lining up blocks and eventually building with them, digging and constructing in the sandbox" (White, 1960). White feels there is "one general motivational principle" lying behind all these activities: "The word I have suggested for this motive is *effectance* because its most characteristic feature is seen in the production of effects upon the environment." In our terms, the production of effects upon the environment is a natural incentive that guides and directs much of the child's behavior. However, we will refer to it as the *impact incentive,* because the term *effectance* as described by White and understood by others includes the notions of mastery, competence, and self-determination (see Deci, 1975), which are probably later derivations of the simple impact incentive.

A noteworthy feature of the impact incentive is that children soon develop an interest in having big impacts on the environment. They seem to get satisfaction from making louder and louder noises, from knocking things about or pulling them off tables, and from assertive activities of all types. Assertiveness is particularly likely to occur if the children's ongoing manipulative activity is blocked or challenged. They react by increased intensity of effort, which quickly arouses anger-excitement. Such behavior occurs more often in boys than in girls (see Maccoby & Jacklin, 1974), but it is universally present in all children.

Having big impacts is innately satisfying; it is associated with the positive emotions in Table 4.2. However, such activities obviously are so dangerous to children and the environment that caretakers move in very quickly to suppress them. Thus, so much inhibition develops around being assertive that the satisfaction in it appears in adults only under very unusual circumstances. Zimbardo (1970) cites a number of instances in which people seem to enjoy being violent when normal inhibitions are removed. He notes that students were sometimes senselessly beaten when they were caught up in "police riots":

The ones who actually got arrested seemed to have gotten caught up among the police, like a kind of human medicine ball, being shoved and knocked back and forth from one cop to the next with what was obviously *mounting* fury. And this was a phenomenon somewhat unexpected, which we were to observe consistently throughout the days of violence—that rage seemed to engender rage; the bloodier and more brutal the cops were, the more their fury increased. (Zimbardo, 1970)

He quotes from an army sergeant who was part of an army intelligence unit that interrogated (and tortured) Vietcong prisoners: "First you strike to get mad, then you strike because you are mad, and in the end you strike because of the sheer pleasure of it" (Zimbardo, 1970). He also mentions a quarrel in which a man stabbed his girlfriend twenty-five or thirty times—far more than was necessary to kill her: he was carried away by violence, unable to stop. Zimbardo argues that this kind of pleasure in violence occurs only when natural controls are somehow removed. For instance, he found that when he "deindividuated" victims by putting them in bulky hoods, subjects were willing and able to give them much heavier electric shocks than they were when they could see the victims' faces. He conducted a field experiment to demonstrate the point more fully. Zimbardo and some graduate students began attacking an old car with a sledgehammer to see if others would follow suit. He writes the following:

> Several observations are noteworthy. First of all, there is considerable reluctance to take that first blow, to smash through the windshields and initiate the destruction of a form. But it feels so good after the first smack that the next one comes more easily, with more force, and feels even better. Although everyone knew the sequence was being filmed, the students got carried away temporarily. Once one person had begun to wield the sledgehammer, it was difficult to get him to stop and pass it to the next pair of eager hands. Finally they all attacked simultaneously. One student jumped on the roof and began stomping it in, two were pulling the door from its hinges, another hammered away at the hood and motor, while the last one broke all the glass he could find. They later reported that feeling the metal or glass give way under the force of their blows was stimulating and pleasurable. (Zimbardo, 1970)

It should be clear from these examples that the impact-anger incentive in its most primitive form does not involve the heavy overlay of learning that normally accompanies it, inhibits it, and directs it into acceptable channels. It does not even imply the intent to hurt another person, which is the way most social psychologists define *aggression*.

Distinction Between Impact-Anger and Aggression

What starts up the anger-aggression sequence? First, there is simple satisfaction from manipulation—from having impact. Then, at least as psychologists since McDougall (1908) have argued, threats and interference with manipulation satisfaction increase the intensity of the response, leading at first to excitement and then to anger and violence. Violence is not aggression, however, because it does not necessarily imply intended injury to another person. McClelland and Apicella (1945) carried out a simple experiment in which students were repeatedly criticized (insulted or threatened) by an experimenter as they were trying to sort some cards as fast as possible. The earliest response to criticism was an increased intensity of responding: the subjects began slamming the cards on the table. Later this simple assertive reaction differentiated into more instrumental responses, such as being aggressive toward the experimenter, trying to find satisfaction in what they had accomplished so far, or giving up. The most primitive response to threat, however, was undirected assertiveness, excitement, or anger.

Dollard, Doob, Miller, Mowrer, and Sears (1939), the authors of *Frustration and Aggression,* attempted to define what elicits the aggressive response by stating that any interference with a goal-directed activity would create the instigation to aggression, defined as "injury to an organism or organism surrogate." This formulation turned out to be misleading in several ways. In the first place, children dropping things or students destroying a car or slamming cards on the table all seem to be enjoying the activity for its own sake; the effect of the activity in terms of its injury to something is a secondary interpretation of what is going on. Second, their definition suggests that aggression occurs only in response to frustration when in fact, as the examples make clear, pleasure in aggression can occur without prior frustration. It is hard to imagine what frustration the students were responding to in breaking up the car. Finally, their definition directed attention away from other reactions to frustration, such as giving up or trying to find an alternative means of reaching the goal. Often interference with goal-directed activity does not lead to aggression but to other types of response.

Thus, it seems inaccurate to tie anger too tightly to frustration of just any goal. On the other hand, a challenge to an impact goal, as in threatening or criticizing someone, does seem more likely to elicit first excitement and then an increase in the intensity of response and the emotion of anger. This is not the same as blocking any goal sequence. A boy blocked in his desire to get some candy may simply decide to eat something else. No excitement need be involved. However, if he is blocked in his desire to produce an effect—to topple over a chair, for example—he pushes harder and may get quite excited. It is as if the salience of the incentive to have an impact has been increased.

Brain Reward and the Impact Incentive

There is a fair amount of circumstantial evidence that the impact incentive is served by a specific reward system in the brain, if we are correct in assuming that impact is a milder form of anger-excitement-aggression. This is certainly true in lower animals. For example, electrical stimulation in different parts of a cat's hypothalamus will produce either affective attack (hair on end, arched back, spitting) or "quiet-biting" attack (for example, pouncing on a mouse and biting it). Furthermore, the cat will press a lever to obtain the brain stimulation that produces the quiet-biting attack (Panksepp, 1971). In other words, it can be inferred that the central stimulation leading to a quiet-biting attack is pleasurable to the cat, in the sense that it will work to get the stimulation.

The hypothalamus in humans, as well as in cats, is a key portion of the brain involved in regulating the autonomic nervous system and the hormone release system, both of which play a central role in affective arousal, particularly as it involves anger and aggression. The hypothalamus regulates the "fight-or-flight" response, identified long ago by Cannon (1915) as an organism's way of mobilizing its resources when frustrated or threatened. The sympathetic nervous system is aroused, which has far-reaching effects, including increased heart rate, increased blood pressure, vasodilation in the periphery so more blood can get to the muscles, and so on. Certain neurohormones, called *catecholamines,* are the chemical messengers responsible for neurotransmission in the sympathetic branch of the autonomic nervous system. Thus, catecholamine release also is tied to the anger-aggression response regulated by the hypothalamus. The best known catecholamine is adrenaline, which accompanies anger and aggression, but its precursors noradrenaline and dopamine also play an important role in sympathetic activation. As Hamburg, Hamburg, and Barchas (1975) sum it up: "Studies in animals utilizing a variety of test situations have suggested a very powerful role of catecholamines in aggressive behavior. Catecholamines are essential for many forms of aggressive behavior, and catecholamine mechanisms are markedly altered by aggressive behavior."

Of particular interest, therefore, is the fact that electrical brain stimulation in the areas related to catecholamine release have been found to be rewarding, in the sense that animals will work to get such stimulation. It is also known that there are catecholamine pathways in the hypothalamus (Sawchenko & Swanson, 1981; Wise, 1980). This suggests that the release of catecholamines by electrical stimulation may be rewarding. The evidence for such a conclusion comes not only from the fact that hypothalamic stimulation leads to rewarding quiet-biting attack in cats, but more directly from evidence that electrical stimulation in the neighborhood of dopamine fibers, and perhaps noradrenergic fibers, is rewarding in rats (Wise, 1980) in the sense that they will press a bar to get the stimulation. It may be inferred that the rats are pressing a bar to get the electrical stimulation that releases dopamine, a catecholamine neurotransmitter, which then might be conceived of as the physiological system subserving the impact incentive.

Furthermore, drugs that increase catecholamines at the synapse between two neurons—such as the amphetamines (Axelrod, 1974) or alcohol (Borg, Kvande, & Sedvall, 1981)—increase both anger-excitement and aggression, as well as feelings of pleasure, in humans (Berlyne, 1967), once again establishing a link between the catecholamines, anger-excitement, and pleasure. What is more, the sex difference in assertiveness also is tied to a difference in catecholamine functioning. Males are notoriously more aggressive than females, even as small children (Maccoby & Jacklin, 1974), and the catecholamine system is more responsive to emotional stimuli in males than in females. For example, males respond to injections or the threat of an examination by releasing more noradrenaline and adrenaline in urine than females do (Frankenhaeuser, Dunne, & Lundberg, 1976).

Finally, physiological arousal, as from exercise or loud sounds, increases aggressiveness (Konečni, 1975). This can be understood as resulting from the fact that physiological arousal involves activation of the sympathetic nervous system, which in turn increases catecholamine release—which, according to our argument, is strongly linked to the anger-excitement-aggression response. This evidence strongly suggests that the natural incentive of having impact is served by the release of catecholamine neurotransmitters in the brain. Stein (1975) argued that a particular catecholamine transmitter, norepinephrine, provided the sole reward mechanism in the brain for all motives. He was on the right track in general, but his view needs correcting in its details.

Researchers now agree that another catecholamine transmitter, dopamine, is more important than norepinephrine. They also agree there is no good reason to assume there is only one reward mechanism. Instead, it seems more likely that there would be several neurotransmitter reward substances, perhaps one for each of the primary human incentives and the major motive systems built upon them. Certainly the evidence, so far as it goes, links the impact incentive specifically to catecholamine neurotransmitters. Conclusive proof for such a connection does not yet exist, but it certainly would not be surprising to discover that a natural incentive is hooked up with a particular type of reward system in the brain.

Impact Incentive Derivatives

Many authors have been so impressed by the importance of effectance that, like White, they treat it as a kind of master motive. As children grow they develop a sense of competence, defined often as the ability to control events. deCharms (1968) popularized the notion of personal causation and developed a measure of individual differences around whether people felt they caused events (that is, felt like an Origin) or felt they were a victim of circumstances beyond their control (that is, felt like a Pawn). *Origins* are characterized as seeing a goal as a challenge rather than a threat, setting realistic goals based on their own probability of success, and understanding the difference between controllable and uncontrollable outcomes (see deCharms & Muir, 1978). Schoolchildren in the inner city taught to think and act like Origins performed better academically and were more likely to graduate from high school (deCharms, 1976), as Chapter 14 will discuss. Feeling like an Origin can be conceived as originating from the cognitive elaboration through training of the natural impact or effectance incentive until it guides new behaviors in much the same way a motive does. For example, it has been shown that people prefer activities they have freely chosen over those they have been assigned (Perlmuter, Scharff, Karsh, & Monty, 1980), presumably because they have developed a value around being in control and have discovered they can satisfy the impact incentive more when they are in control. This chapter will return to the problem of values, or derived incentives, later.

Much research also has centered on the importance of people's feeling they can or cannot have an impact on events. Seligman (1975) popularized the notion of "learned helplessness," which results when an animal or a human being is presented over and over with a threatening situation about which nothing can be done. Thus, dogs who were shocked repeatedly in an enclosure from which they could not escape eventually became so passive that they failed to escape when shocked, even when given the opportunity to do so. This would seem to be an extreme case of extinguishing the natural incentive to have impact through learning to be helpless. On the other hand, Wortman and Brehm (1975) point out that the immediate response to a painful situation is *reactance,* the attempt to do something about it, much as we pointed out earlier that blocking the impact incentive seems to increase assertiveness. Only after repeated discovery that events are uncontrollable does a person or animal learn to be helpless.

The most important motivational derivative of the impact incentive is the power motive, which will be discussed in Chapter 8. The definition of the power motive is a "concern for having impact," a concern that presumably develops out of the many early and late learnings associated with the impact incentive.

• THE CONTACT OR SEXUAL INCENTIVES

In his paper on infantile sexuality, Freud (1905/1938) first called attention dramatically to the pleasure infants get from rhythmic tactile sensations:

> As is shown by the example of thumbsucking, there are predestined erogenous zones. But the same example also shows that any other region of skin or mucous membrane may assume the function of an erogenous zone. . . . The thumbsucking child looks around on his body and selects any portion of it for pleasure-sucking, and becoming accustomed to this particular part, he then prefers it. If he accidentally strikes upon a predestined region, such as a breast, nipple or genitals, it naturally gets the preference. . . . The rhythmic characters must play some part and this strongly suggests an analogy to tickling. . . . Pleasure-sucking is often combined with a rubbing contact with certain sensitive parts of the body, such as the breasts and external genitals. It is by this path that many children go from thumbsucking to masturbation.

Freud (1905/1938) called attention to the similarity of this type of pleasure seeking and sexual gratification: "The pleasure-sucking is connected with a full absorption of attention and leads to sleep or even to a motor reaction in the form of an orgasm. . . . He who sees a satiated child sink back from the mother's breast and fall asleep with reddened cheeks and blissful smile, will have to admit that this picture remains as typical of the expression of sexual gratification in later life."

Freud's observations were later confirmed by Kinsey, Pomeroy, and Martin (1948), who observed orgasm in boys and girls as young as four months old. They reported that orgasm in the infant involves "the development of rhythmic body movements with distinct penis throbs and pelvic thrusts, and obvious change in sensory capacities, a final tension of muscles, especially of abdomen, hips and back, a sudden release with contractions—followed by the disappearance of all symptoms" (Kinsey et al., 1948). Freud, with his usual care, also observed that infants obtained pleasure not only from the mouth and the genitals, but also from the anal region and from playing with feces. He and others (see

Spitz & Wolf, 1949) also noted the pleasure some infants get from "rocking," that is, from getting on their hands and knees and rocking vigorously back and forth. This too they classed as an expression of sexuality. The key defining characteristic of the sexual incentive for them is rhythmic tactile self-stimulation, particularly in certain body regions, which rises to a climax and then declines.

More recent studies have confirmed the innate pleasure infants get from this type of stimulation when it is provided by others, particularly the mother. Harlow (1971) and his associates demonstrated this in an ingenious series of experiments in which infant rhesus monkeys were reared with "mother" surrogates. The infant could obtain nourishment from all of the surrogates, but they were constructed to have a variety of other characteristics. The bodies of the surrogates were made of wire mesh, and some were covered with terry cloth. The rhesus monkey infants spent much more time clinging to the terry cloth mother than the wire mesh mother. Furthermore, they reacted less emotionally to a strange environment when a cloth mother with which they had been reared was present (Harlow, 1959). The presence of the wire mother, however, even though it had been the only source of food, did not reduce the infant's fear in a strange environment. In fact, the infants reared by the wire mother showed a much greater emotional response to a strange environment than monkeys reared either normally or by the terry cloth mother. Other coverings for the wire mother, such as rayon, vinyl, or sandpaper, did not increase the attractiveness of the surrogate mother for the infant monkeys.

The monkeys' behavior strongly indicates there is some innate affective response—joy-happiness-pleasure—released by the soft tactile stimulation produced by the terry cloth. Further research showed what other sign stimuli were part of the natural contact incentive: The rhesus monkey infants showed a greater preference for terry cloth mothers that were warm (rather than cold) and that rocked rather than remained stationary. In other words, they preferred the kind of rhythmic tactile stimulation Freud described. They maintained their attachment even though some of the mothers were "abusive"; that is, they blasted them in the face with air or threw them off.

Human infants also show similar attachments to being with their mothers, as the next section will describe. They enjoy being tickled—a clear example of rhythmic tactile stimulation—particularly in the stomach region, according to Cicchetti and Sroufe (1976), which is as close as they got to the genital area. The fact that people cannot tickle themselves successfully supports the idea that some such stimulation must come from another. The importance of Harlow's work with other primates is the fact that it permits a clearer definition of the innate natural incentives than is possible with humans, where mothers' attitudes and cultural expectations might be expected to teach the infant such responses.

In what sense was Freud correct in describing such a natural incentive as sexual? He did so to base his sexual theory of neurosis on what appeared to be solid biological observation, but he also used the term *sexual* so broadly that it is almost synonymous with the word *love*. In that sense, many would agree that the kind of contact gratifications he and Harlow observed are the innate bases for acquired affectional or affiliative motives. However, the sexual motive system also seems to be involved. Harlow (1971) also found that the contact gratifications in infancy, either between the mother and infant or between the infant and peers, were essential to developing normal heterosexual attraction and behavior later on. Monkeys reared on wire mesh mothers were isolated, could not relate to other monkeys, and did not form heterosexual attachments.

What still is not clear is how these contact incentives get integrated into the adult sexual motive, as well as the extent to which they are still part of such motivation in adults. Harlow's work shows that the physical contact from playing with peers soon replaces the contact gratifications received from the mother. Eventually, because of the hormonal changes that occur at puberty (see Chapter 9), the contact gratifications sought become more explicitly sexual in nature. There is also substantial evidence that children and adults continue to get pleasure from rhythmic tactual and kinesthetic sensations, since they spend so much time in amusement parks riding roller coasters and being jostled around in various machines. Some of the pleasure may derive from Solomon's opponent process mechanism described in Chapter 4 (see Solomon, 1980). That is, pleasure may be an innate consequence of the fear aroused in such situations. On the other hand, much of the jostling and rhythmic movement—swinging on swings, for example—seems quite pleasurable even when no fear is involved.

Dutton and Aron (1974) carried out an investigation that suggests that this type of stimulation may continue to be related to sexual arousal. They stationed a female experimenter near the exits from two bridges in a public park. She stopped men after they had crossed the bridges and asked them if they were willing to participate in a psychological experiment, which consisted among other things of telling a brief story about a picture. She then said that if they wanted to know how the experiment turned out they could call her telephone number, which she gave them. One bridge was a long suspension bridge over a chasm; the bridge tilted, wobbled, and swayed as people walked across it. The other bridge was quite stable. The experimenter found that the men who had crossed the suspension bridge told stories containing more sexual imagery than the men who had crossed the stable bridge. The men who had been jiggling up and down also were much more likely to telephone the girl later. In short, they appeared more sexually aroused by the experience.

Dutton and Aron (1974) and Dienstbier (1979), who conducted other similar experiments in the laboratory, explain this result as being due to the fear aroused in crossing the suspension bridge. That bridge did evoke more fear than the stable bridge, as determined by actual ratings by other subjects. Thus, it could be argued that the fear produced physiological arousal, which the men in the presence of an attractive female attributed to sexuality; when male interviewers were used, there was no difference in the sexual content of the stories written by men who had crossed either of the two bridges. According to the theory advanced by Schachter and Singer (1962), all types of physiological arousal are nearly the same, and whether they will be labeled *sexual* or *fearful* depends on cognitive factors—namely, the understanding of the situation. According to the theory, the presence of the female interviewer suggested to the men that the greater physiological arousal caused by the suspension bridge really might be sexual in nature.

As we shall see in Chapter 12, there are difficulties with this theory, and there are other possible explanations of the result. One is provided by Solomon's opponent process theory, which states that the fear from crossing the suspension bridge, much like that involved in sport parachute jumping, leads to the arousal of an opposing, or pleasurable, emotion. This theory has the advantage of explaining why the men crossed the suspension bridge in the first place—namely, to get to the pleasure that would follow the fear. Emotion attribution theory really does not explain why people would choose to cross a fearful suspension bridge if they could cross a stable one. However, Solomon's theory does not explain why specifically sexual feelings are aroused to oppose the suspension bridge fear rather than, say, the exhilaration felt after parachute jumping. A much simpler explanation is that the jiggling, joggling, and swaying is part of the sexual incentive in adults, just as it is in infants. This accounts for the interest in the suspension bridge, as well as for the increased likelihood of sexual thoughts in the presence of a woman experimenter. Despite some of Dienstbier's (1979) later experiments, it seems unlikely that inducing fear without jiggling always will increase the sexual arousal of men in the presence of women, although evidence on this point is not conclusive.

Imprinting and Attachment

Just how the contact incentives evolve into social attachments is not known, but certainly there is a shift from physical to social sources of stimulation. One explanation starts with the observation of attachments in lower animals—for example, Harlow's study of the way infant rhesus monkeys get attached to their mothers or terry cloth mother surrogates and cry when they are left alone. At an even lower level, ducklings will follow a mother duck or any moving mother surrogate to which they are exposed shortly after birth. This process is called *imprinting:* the mother normally becomes a natural incentive that is imprinted on the duckling during a certain critical period in its development.

Some psychologists, particularly Bowlby (1969), have concluded that human infants appear to be imprinted in a very similar way on their primary caretakers —usually, but not always, the mother. The infant shows the attachment through clinging, smiling, following, sucking, crying, and perhaps seeking eye contact. Which of these behaviors is displayed depends on the context, but the purpose of all of them is increasing mother proximity. According to attachment theorists, there is nothing particularly primary about clinging and its attendant incentive of contact (Ainsworth, 1973; Bowlby, 1969; Sroufe & Waters, 1977). Therefore, it is probably an oversimplification to derive all the attachment incentives from primary contact pleasures, in the manner suggested by Freud. That is, in addition to the contact incentive there may be a natural incentive (or one acquired very early and easily) based on the positive affect associated with being with others or exchanging responses harmoniously with them. (See Condon's work discussed in Chapter 9.)

On the other hand, Kagan, Kearsley, and Zelazo (1978) have provided a somewhat different explanation for the attachment phenomenon, in particular for the separation distress infants typically begin to show at around eight months of age when the primary caretaker leaves. This distress can be taken as a sign of the baby's attachment to the mother, which parallels the duckling's distress calling or the infant monkey's crying when the mother leaves. However, there are difficulties in assuming that crying indicates attachment (Kagan et al., 1978). Children sometimes cry when a comparative stranger to whom they are not attached leaves the room. On the other hand, they sometimes cry when their mother comes into the room, or they do not cry when she leaves in familiar surroundings to carry out her work around the house. "The major problem with the attachment explanation of the growth function for separation anxiety is the difficulty it has accounting for behavioral differences among children whose mothers differ in availability" (Kagan et al., 1978). That is, attachment should be stronger in infants whose mothers are readily accessible, yet children who are frequently separated from their mothers, as in day care centers, show a normal development of separation distress. They are just as likely to be distressed as children who are with their mothers all the time.

Kagan et al. (1978) believe separation anxiety is not an attachment phenomenon, but one that can be explained in terms of the variety incentive discussed earlier in this chapter. They believe that around the age of seven months a child is able to understand for the first time what it means for someone to leave the room: "During or after maternal departure the child tries to generate a cognitive structure to explain the mother's absence or a behavior to alter the situation. If he cannot do either he is vulnerable to uncertainty" (Kagan et al., 1978). If the child is uncertain, he or she is likely to be unhappy, as was noted in Table 4.2. Before the child is seven months old, the mother's leaving the room is not part of the child's cognitive schemata for understanding events, so it does not represent a major discrepancy from what is expected. Later, after about fifteen months of age, the departure is understood perfectly well, but it no longer represents a major discrepancy from the child's understanding and therefore no longer produces crying in the normal child. In other words, separation distress can be understood as an aspect of cognitive development. Such an inference also explains why the departure of a comparative stranger can produce distress at this age: children are not upset at the loss of someone to whom they are not attached, but they are upset by the realization of what someone leaving the room means, since it is disruption of expectations that is unpleasant rather than disruption of an attachment.

Whereas such theorizing can account for separation distress, it does not deal directly with the positive attachment children show for their primary caretakers or others in their environment. Little Peter in Chapter 4 spent a good deal of time going up to his mother and snuggling and rubbing himself against her, just as Harlow's infant monkeys did. The problem is how children get from this behavior to more developed social attachments. As Michael Lewis (cited in Henley, 1974) has put it so well, "a major socialization process in terms of attachment or social behavior, is to move the infant from a proximal mode of interaction (e.g., touching, rocking, holding) to a distal mode (e.g., smiling and vocalizing)."

Sexual Arousal from a Distance

Whereas rhythmic contact remains the primary mode of sexual arousal in adults, there is also some evidence that other kinds of stimulation are effective. Several observers have noted that the face and eyes are particularly potent in arousing the human infant to pleasurable smiling. Sroufe and Waters (1976) feel that eye-to-eye contact is especially important. As Rubin (1975) reports, people who are in love spend much more time looking into each other's eyes than do other people.

In most animal species, nature must arrange for the two sexes to get together and copulate in order to reproduce the species. In lower animals very specific sights, sounds, smells, or tactile stimuli elicit sexual behavior. A male moth is attracted by a smell given off by the female moth. The peahen is sexually aroused by the courtship dance of the peacock.

What about humans? Havelock Ellis (1954) has suggested that a human male can tell that a human female has reached sexual maturity by using his eyes: he can see that her body contours have changed. On the other hand, a human female can tell whether a male is sexually mature by using her ears, for a male's voice changes at puberty. The implication is that the sight of the mature female figure may have sexually arousing properties for the male, and considerable research evidence supports this assertion. When males are asked what arouses them sexually, they list primarily visual cues centering on the female body (Kinsey et al., 1948). Clark (1952) has shown that exposure to pictures of nude females will arouse sexual fantasies in men if their inhibitions are removed by alcohol. Wilson and Lawson (1976a) showed that pornographic films had the same effects on penile tumescence, again if inhibitions were removed either by the subjects' drinking or thinking they were drinking.

Kalin (1972) reported that even the presence of a fully clothed but attractive female folk singer in a small social gathering could arouse sexual fantasies in males as shown in written stories, providing the circumstances were not inhibiting. Table 5.2 summarizes some of the results of this study. Kalin counted the frequency with which stories contained references to physical sex (that is, kissing and sexual intercourse) when the singer was either present or not present, and the experiment was carried out either in an apartment setting or in a classroom, with or without alcoholic drinks being served. Under inhibiting conditions (that is, either apartment-dry or classroom-wet), the singer did not produce an increase in sexual imagery in male fantasies. However, under conditions of disinhibition (when the subjects were drinking in a relaxed social setting in an apartment), there was a large and significant increase in their sexual fantasies. Certainly the preference of males for pictures of nude females and for buying magazines that contain such pictures suggests that such stimuli have a natural incentive value for them.

Table 5.2.

MEAN FREQUENCIES OF THEMATIC PHYSICAL SEX IN STORIES WRITTEN IN SIX CONDITIONS (after Kalin, 1972)

	No Singer	*Singer*	*S − NS*[a]
1. Apartment-dry	1.18 (17)	0.70 (27)	−0.48
2. Apartment-wet	2.48 (27)	4.39 (26)	1.91[b]
3. Classroom-wet	1.80 (20)	1.31 (32)	−0.49
Drinking effect (2 − 1)	1.30[c]	3.69[c]	
Setting effect (3 − 2)	−0.68[d]	−3.08[d]	

Note: Numbers in parentheses equal number of subjects per condition.

[a]Singer − no singer conditions.

[b]In apartment-wet conditions, no singer − singer $t = 1.96$, $p < .05$ (in the predicted direction).

[c]In alcohol experiment (main effect, alcohol), $F = 11.69$, $p < .01$.

[d]In setting experiment (main effect, setting), $F = 7.57$, $p < .01$.

The evidence for the arousing value of the male voice for women is less clear, although the sexual excitement among women produced by male singers is a well-known natural phenomenon. It seems to exceed considerably the sexual arousal potential of the female voice for males, although a systematic study of this phenomenon has not yet been carried out. One attempt was made by Beardslee and Fogelson (1958) to see if rhythmic musical stimulation had more sexual arousal potential for women than for men. They found no sex differences in sexual imagery in stories written to control pictures, but when the subjects wrote stories to musical selections the results were quite different. The males responded with more overt sexual imagery, probably because at least at this historical period women were more inhibited about writing directly about sexual matters. So a symbolic sex activity score was developed that was patterned after the criteria for sexual activity described by Freud in his paper on infantile sexuality. That is, the stories written by the subjects were scored for any references to motion, rhythm, peak, and penetration—the last category being added as a metaphorical reference to sexual intercourse. If any two of these scoring categories appeared, symbolic sexual activity was scored for the story.

As Table 5.3 shows, women provided almost significantly more instances of symbolic sex activity than men did, even when writing stories to the four neutral musical selections, and the difference was much more marked for the arousing musical selections. The arousing selections contained "a pronounced emphasis on rhythm, themes with comparatively large tonal ranges, and a gradual buildup to a climax. In contradistinction, the neutral music could be characterized as having very little rhythmic emphasis and a general evenness in melody in overall construction" (Beardslee & Fogelson, 1958). Both the men and

Table 5.3.

AVERAGE SYMBOLIC SEX ACTIVITY AFTER TWO TYPES OF MUSICAL SELECTIONS (after Beardslee & Fogelson, 1958)

	Males	*Females*	*p*
Four neutral musical selections	.61	.93	< .10
Four arousing musical selections	1.20	1.93	< .01
Difference, neutral − arousing	+.59	+1.00	
Difference between differences		+.41	< .05

women were more sexually aroused by the rhythmic musical selections, but the women significantly more so. These findings need extension and confirmation, but so far as they go they suggest women may be more sexually sensitive to certain types of sound than men are.

Derivatives of the Contact Incentives: Succorance and Nurturance

Besides sexual motivation, what other motives are likely to develop out of contact gratifications? Two possibilities that readily present themselves are what H. A. Murray (1938) refers to as the needs for succorance and for nurturance, succorance being based on receiving contact gratifications and nurturance, on giving them. That is, children may get so much pleasure out of contacts with the primary caretaker that they develop a strong need for such contact, which should show up as dependence on the primary caretaker.

Sears, Rau, and Alpert (1965) and Whiting and Whiting (1975) have observed acts of dependency in children in great detail, but they have failed to make a case for the fact that there is a strong dependency *motive*. The reason may be that they defined and measured a wide variety of dependency behaviors (for example, asking for help, crying when the caretaker leaves, seeking attention and approval, and so on) and then tried to discover whether dependency was a behavioral trait by intercorrelating the extent to which children showed these behaviors. That is, would those who performed dependency act A also perform dependency acts B and C, and would children who acted dependently toward parents also act dependently toward peers? In general, they found little consistency of this type. Even children who were high in the total number of acts of dependency observed at one time period were not particularly likely to show more such acts at another time period: the average correlation for dependency scores across time periods was only .36 (Sears et al., 1965).

Whether a child acts dependently or not is more a function of the situation (the status of the two actors, the age, and the setting) than of a general tendency to act dependently. But this conclusion permits no inference about the presence of a *dependency motive*—defined as an anticipatory goal state involving being cared for—since such a goal state might be achieved by nondependent acts (for example, being a "brave" child when hurt) and since dependent acts can be instrumental in achieving other goal states. For example, a child may ask for help to solve a problem while in pursuit of an achievement goal. Furthermore, much dependent behavior, such as seeking to be with a caretaker, is clearly guided by the affiliation or attachment incentive. Thus, whether the existence of another incentive, the need for nurturance, should be postulated can be questioned. At present there is no adequate measure of the need for nurturance or any strong empirical evidence that such a need exists.

On the other side of parent-child interaction, many authors have written about the mother's or father's parental instinct—that is, their desire to care for, look after, and protect a child. Since the human infant is so helpless for so long, there obviously would be an evolutionary advantage for survival if parents were endowed with an innate responsiveness to infant helplessness that would lead to nurturance. Harlow's (1971) work on rhesus monkeys has demonstrated that clinging by the baby is a sign stimulus that evokes cuddling and caressing behavior from the mother. If a kitten is substituted for her baby, the mother monkey will try to caress it for a time; since it cannot cling, however, the mother soon stops. If another baby that does cling is substituted, the mother continues caressing. Clinging can even evoke a normal affiliative response in a "sick" monkey who had become an isolate due to prolonged separation from others (Harlow, Harlow, & Suomi, 1971).

Among humans there is also widespread evidence that mothers and some fathers (Spelke, Zelazo, Kagan, & Kotelchuck, 1973) naturally like to play with and look after their infants. Social psychologists have studied in depth the conditions under which people will stop to give assistance to a helpless person or one who cries out for help. Does a helpless person in obvious need act as a kind of sign stimulus that elicits affect and the impulse to help in a way analogous to the presumed effect of a crying baby on a parent? The evidence does not permit a clear answer. Certainly some people are Good Samaritans and stop to help needy people; however, Darley and Batson (1973) showed that even some seminary students on their way to give a talk on the Good Samaritan incident in the Bible failed to stop to help an obvious victim if they thought they were late and thus were in a hurry.

Unfortunately, neither this experiment nor the many others on the same topic shed much light on the incentives or motives involved; they focused on predicting the *action* of helping, which is a joint product of motives, incentives, skills, values, and opportunities (see Chapter 6). Thus, it is entirely possible that a victim arouses an impulse to help or nurture that could be discovered if it were measured directly, but that other factors inhibit the helping act. On the other hand, a natural incentive to nurture may not exist. It is impossible to know on the basis of present evidence, despite the large number of studies of helping behavior.

Little work has been done on measuring a motive like the need for nurturance, which might arise out of such a natural incentive as the joy-happiness-pleasure that comes from holding and helping babies. A preliminary approach has been made by Sara Winter (1969), who studied the fantasies of a mother while she was nursing her baby compared with her fantasies while her baby was in the room but not actually being nursed. The stories told after nursing contained more references to positive feelings and orientation to the present time, as well as fewer instances of instrumental or means-end thinking, than the stories written when the baby was simply present. Winter concluded that nursing mothers were characterized by a "being" rather than a "doing" orientation. In other words, mothers and other primary caretakers get contact and other gratifications out of nursing, touching, and otherwise playing with babies that may in time develop into a social motive that could be described as the need for nurturance. What is needed to demonstrate this fact is further research of the sort S. Winter began.

Finally, it is presumed that the affiliative motives—the need for affiliation and the intimacy motive—develop primarily out of the contact incentives. These motives will be fully discussed in Chapter 9.

• THE CONSISTENCY INCENTIVE

Drive-reduction theorists (see Chapter 3) readily adopted the notion that conflict could produce tension, which the organism would seek to reduce (see J. S. Brown, 1961). They reasoned further that variety was a source of conflict or confusion in the sense that the organism would not know how to behave in a new situation. Therefore, if people or animals appear to seek variety, they are doing so only to reduce tension. The rat's exploratory behavior in a new maze really is designed to reduce the tension and conflict from uncertainty (Montgomery & Segall, 1955). Thus, some psychologists always have thought organisms seek consistency in the sense that they wish to avoid conflict. The weakness of this kind of theorizing, as already noted, is that it does not adequately account for the positive enjoyment of variety.

McClelland, Atkinson, Clark, and Lowell (1953) dealt with this problem by postulating that small discrepancies from the adaptation level (or expectancy) produced positive affect, and large ones produced negative affect. They reported several studies that showed this to be the case. (See, for example, Figures 5.2, 5.3, and 5.4.) It was a short step from such a result to the inference that people would seek to avoid the negative affect resulting from major inconsistencies in what happened over what was expected. In more general terms, people would seek consistency in confirming expectations. The chief difficulty with the theory is that it proved very difficult to define in advance or generalize about what constituted a small or large discrepancy. Does a person who just misses a plane experience a large or a small discrepancy? It is small in terms of time, but large in terms of his or her expectancy of getting somewhere. Often multiple expectations are involved in real life, so it has been hard to pin down the concept of consistency in practice, when it is defined as avoiding major discrepancies from expectation.

Nevertheless, a number of independent sources of evidence suggest there is a consistency, as well as a variety, incentive. It is obviously of great adaptive significance to the organism to be able to live in a reasonably stable, coherent environment. The perceptual constancies are an example of this phenomenon. Shapes and colors are perceived as relatively the same even as they undergo significant transformations. People seen at a considerable distance are perceived as being about the same height as they would be close at hand, even though as a physical stimulus they present a much smaller image to the eye. George Kelly (1955) has theorized that people's main goal in life is to form constructs that will give coherence and order to their conception of the world, in order to enable them to understand what is going on: "Each person evolves for his convenience in anticipating events a construction system." Thus, people are able to maintain order by fitting whatever happens into their personal constructs. This is a consistency theory in the sense that people try to match up events with expectations and avoid confusion. The behavior of young children in learning a language fits here. They seek to match what they say to what they hear and avoid the discomfort of a mismatch.

At the social level the consistency incentive appears as *conformity* to social norms. Automobile drivers learn they are supposed to stop at red lights, so they stop at red lights. A man knows that he is a Mormon and that Mormons do not drink, so he does not drink. We drive on the right-hand side of the road, eat three meals a day, go to school, brush our teeth, and do thousands of things simply to be consistent—to live in a stable, predictable environment. We develop many expectations about the way things are and the way we are, and we act in conformity with these expectations. When we do not know what to expect, we conform to the expectations created by others. In a well-known experiment Asch (1951) demonstrated that if subjects hear three or four others say a shorter line is equal in length to a longer line, most will conform to the group opinion despite clear visual evidence to the contrary.

It seems unnecessary to search for underlying motives to explain why people conform to such expectations: there is tremendous economy in doing so, since conforming reduces confusion, conflict, and uncertainty. The power of the conformity incentive has been demonstrated dramatically by Milgram's (1963, 1965) well-known experiment in which subjects, when told to by an experimenter, continued to give supposed severe electrical shocks to people despite the fact that the shocks were known to be dangerous and the subjects in some instances were crying out in pain. People expect to do what they are told by authority—in this case, the experimenter. Therefore, they obeyed, despite the harm to their "victims," because not to do so would have caused even greater discomfort from disobedience to a strong expectation that they should obey authority.

Social psychologists have studied extensively the variables that affect whether a person conforms or not. Our interest here is limited to demonstrating that there is some kind of natural incentive that elicits satisfaction from matching expectations we have about ourselves, or what we perceive, to social or physical reality.

Cognitive Dissonance

Several experiments have demonstrated that inconsistency—or what has come to be called *cognitive dissonance*—motivates people to change their behavior to make it more consistent. In the original study starting this line of research (Festinger & Carlsmith, 1959), subjects first spent a long time doing dull and boring tasks. They were then paid either one dollar or twenty dollars to tell other subjects that the experiment was really very interesting. In other words, they were paid either a lot or a little for lying about the nature of their experience. Later they were all asked by another experimenter to rate how much they actually had enjoyed doing the experimental tasks. Those who were paid twenty dollars rated the tasks as slightly more enjoyable than those who had been paid nothing, who rated them as very unpleasant; those who had been paid only one dollar, however, rated the tasks as most enjoyable. Why? According to the theory, lying about the nature of the tasks created cognitive dissonance—a dissonance between what the subject is doing (lying) and his or her self-image. Being paid twenty dollars to lie seemed sufficient justification to explain to the subjects why they were doing something so unusual. Therefore, they did not change their evaluations of how pleasant the tasks were. However, subjects who were paid only one dollar to lie found they were doing something that did not fit their image of themselves as honest. They were in a state of dissonance or confusion, so they reduced the inconsistency by concluding that the tasks actually had been fairly interesting. Thus, they were no longer lying very much. This has led to a whole series of research projects demonstrating that various types of justification regularly are used by subjects to make their behavior consistent with their self-image.

Furthermore, Rokeach (1973) carried out an experiment in which he showed that demonstrating to subjects an inconsistency in their attitudes would lead to behavioral change that would reduce the inconsistency. He found that most Michigan State undergraduates ranked the value of *freedom* highest, whereas the value they placed on *equality* was somewhat lower. Rokeach pointed out the inconsistency by observing that they believed highly in *freedom* for themselves but not for others, like blacks and women, since they had rated *equality* somewhat lower. Just pointing out this inconsistency carefully in a lecture was sufficient to motivate the subjects to change their value ranking for *equality*, to increase their belief in equal rights for blacks, and to respond positively more often to a recruiting letter from the local branch of the National Association for the Advancement of Colored People.

Motives Related to the Consistency Incentive

Some people clearly are more eager to reduce cognitive dissonance than others, and some try harder to avoid "social" dissonance, or the tension that arises from not matching their behavior to social expectations. In both cases what motivates them is a desire to avoid the strong negative affect that for them accompanies inconsistency. Not much attention has been given to measuring the strength of the motive to avoid cognitive inconsistency; more attention has been given to measuring the strength of the motive to avoid social dissonance by conforming to social norms. For example, Crowne and Marlowe (1964) measured the strength of what they called the *approval motive* by asking subjects to respond to items such as *I never hesitate to go out of my way to help someone in trouble* and *I like to gossip at times*. It is socially desirable to answer *true* to the first statement and *false* to the second, although it seems highly unlikely that people would "never" fail to help someone or not like to gossip occasionally. People who give many socially desirable responses tend to behave in socially expected ways. They report to the experimenter that a boring task was really pleasant and worthwhile, and they go so far as to agree with the judgment of others that there were four knocks on a tape, for example, when there were clearly only three. In short, they distort reality to avoid the discomfort of not behaving in ways that they believe are expected of them.

However, further research has suggested that the motive behind the need for approval may be fear of rejection by others (see Chapter 10). In fact, as Chapter 10 points out, the current trend is to identify the different types of motives people have to avoid the inconsistencies leading to negative affect, depending on the source of the inconsistency—whether it be failure to meet expectations about achievement, affiliation (approval of others), or power to have impact on others. Thus, the consistency incentive, in combination with other incentives, may produce several types of avoidance motives, just as we found that an avoidance motive developed out of the distress that arose when the impulse to eat could not be fulfilled because no food was present. Up to the present, therefore, research has focused more on different types of avoidance motives than on a single consistency motive.

• INTERACTION OF INCENTIVES

So far we have been treating natural incentives as if they were independent. However, they also interact. The variety incentive combines with several others. Animals fed to satiation on one type of food will start eating again if new food is presented (arousing the variety incentive) or another animal comes in and starts eating (arousing the impact incentive). Animals sexually satiated in regard to one partner will become sexually active again if a new partner is presented (see Schein & Hale, 1965). Variety also increases sexual responsiveness in humans. So, apparently, does the impact-anger incentive. Barclay and Haber (1965) and Barclay (1969) showed that insulting students and making them angry resulted in their being sexually aroused, and vice versa: subjects who were sexually aroused showed an increase in aggressive thoughts or impulses (Barclay, 1971). This cross-linkage was unique to sex and aggression. Anger arousal did not increase general drive level or other concerns, such as the concern for achievement or affiliation; other types of arousal, such as anxiety, did not increase sexual and aggressive thoughts. Clark (1955) also found a close link between sexual and aggressive thoughts in males during sexual arousal.

As mentioned earlier, the impact and variety incentives may combine to produce the peculiar fascination that leads children and some adults to work at moderately difficult tasks. They seek the variety of something new but also get pleasure from producing the new experience themselves.

From the very beginning, natural incentives become embedded through learning in a complex network of cognitions and expectations. Some of these affect how motive dispositions are satisfied, as will be explained in the next section. Others are elaborated cognitively. For example, as has already been noted, impact experiences lead to people's conceiving of themselves as personally more or less competent—as an Origin, to use deCharms's terminology, rather than as a Pawn. That is, children not only have impact experiences; they also develop a concept or schema of the self as Origin by generalizing across these experiences, which may or may not be conscious. This self-schema may be thought of as a complex or symbolic incentive that is the product of experience with certain types of natural incentives.

Similarly, some people may develop a concept of themselves as dependent on others if they are punished for novelty seeking and too much assertiveness so that most of their natural gratifications come from contact with a caretaker. One can only speculate as to how these incentive experiences combine with each other and cumulate into various outcomes, since no direct research has been done on the problem. In fact, at this stage there is not even good agreement as to what the natural incentives are, let alone how they interact with each other.

• THE ROLE OF COGNITION IN THE DEVELOPMENT OF INCENTIVES

As is clear in the case of the variety incentive, what gives pleasure naturally changes continuously as a person's understanding grows. What seems complex and interesting to a child is boring to an adult. The number of dimensions in which an object or event can differ from expectation increases as understanding grows. For example, Martindale (1975) has applied the notion of the variety incentive to aesthetic appreciation. He has produced considerable evidence supporting the idea that in the art world, works that are moderately different from what people have been habituated to are most appreciated: "Whatever else it must be, a work of art must at some degree be novel, original, or at least different from preceding works of art" (Martindale, 1977). But repeated experience with what is novel for works of art in one period gradually produces an intrinsic pressure for more novelty in some dimension or another. Martindale has studied English poetry from the time of Chaucer to the present and found that as he predicted, there has been a steady increase in a composite, quantitative measure of variability, as he designed it, in the style of poetry. However, the dimension in which the novelty occurred shifted from one historical period to another. At one time the novelty was in word length; at another time, in phrase length; at another time, in the percentage of words occurring only once in a text; and at still another time, in the strikingness of the contrasts introduced in the poetry. Thus, the natural preference for moderate variety persists in poetry as a natural phenomenon, but there has been an enormous cognitive development of the dimensions in which the variety can occur.

The same process affects the impact and consistency incentives. What a per-

son can have impact on as a child often is limited to physical grasping or pushing. One day, however, children discover that if they leave the room they can
have impact in the sense that a parent may worry about what has happened to
them. They learn that they can have impact by arguing successfully, by graduating from college, and by collecting prestigious possessions. Similarly, in the beginning children develop cognitive expectations by observing consistency between their perceptions and physical reality: they see that a ball rolls off a table
and confirm that it hits the floor. If such a sequence fails to occur after it has
been built into a firm expectation, children are upset emotionally and seek to reduce their sadness-distress in some way.

Such cognitive expectations become more and more elaborate and differentiated with experience, so what causes sadness-distress also changes greatly. Very
quickly normative expectations also develop in the social sphere. Children learn
that if they throw their food on the floor, their mother will be angry. At first
they may repeat this response several times simply to confirm the fact that what
they expect to happen will indeed happen. From here they go on to develop
very complex expectations of how to behave in the social area, which they normally confirm by behaving that way, because not to do so is innately distressing.
The need for consistency is the same at various stages of maturity, but how the
consistency is defined becomes enormously elaborated through experience and
cognitive development.

• SYMBOLIC INCENTIVES, OR VALUES

Eventually people develop conscious values that guide their attitudes and
behaviors. Sometimes it is easy to see how these values could have developed
through cognitive elaboration from natural incentives, and sometimes it is not
easy. For example, most U.S. citizens rank *freedom* as their most important
value (Rokeach, 1973). It can readily be seen how belief in freedom develops out
of the impact incentive if children are allowed a fair amount of freedom in pursuing that incentive. That is, having obtained a lot of satisfaction from impact,
they might easily develop the conscious thought that it is "good to be free" so
as to be able to have impact in all sorts of ways. It also can be understood how
people could come to value *security* consciously if they had experienced much
pain and fear in growing up. But how can people derive a belief in the importance of *equality* or *salvation?* Such values appear to develop out of the general
understanding people of a particular culture develop as to how the world works.
They have no obvious source in natural incentives. In other cases, a value may
have many sources. Money is commonly believed to be an important value or
social incentive, but money means different things to different people. For some
it means security; for others, the opportunity to have impact or to be considered
important; and for still others, a measure of how well they are doing at some
job (see McClelland, 1967).

Psychologists are uncertain about just what values are most important to
study. Rokeach (1973) has done a lot of interesting research on a representative

list of eighteen terminal (end-state) and eighteen instrumental values. Subjects are asked to rank order each set of eighteen values in the order of importance for their own lives. As Tables 5.4 and 5.5 show, considerable variation exists from one type of subject to another in regard to what is most important to them. *Salvation* is ranked fourth in importance by U.S. women but twelfth in importance by U.S. men. On the other hand, men rank *a comfortable life* fourth in importance, whereas it is only thirteenth in importance to women. Physical scientists regard it as much more important to be *self-controlled* than do humanities majors, whereas the latter regard *forgiving* as much more important than do the former.

The importance of such values also varies across cultures. *National security* is second in importance to Israelis but only seventeenth to U.S. citizens, a not very surprising finding in view of the threats to Israel's existence from the Arab world.

Values have a strong cognitive component. They grow out of people's understanding of the world and of what their culture regards as most important. Values are conscious. Motives, on the other hand, are less cognitively elaborat-

Table 5.4.

TERMINAL VALUE MEDIANS AND COMPOSITE RANK ORDERS FOR U.S. MEN AND WOMEN (after Rokeach, 1973)

Terminal Value	Male N = 665	Female N = 744	p
A comfortable life	7.8 (4)	10.0 (13)	.001
An exciting life	14.6 (18)	15.8 (18)	.001
A sense of accomplishment	8.3 (7)	9.4 (10)	.01
A world at peace	3.8 (1)	3.0 (1)	.001
A world of beauty	13.6 (15)	13.5 (15)	—
Equality	8.9 (9)	8.3 (8)	—
Family security	3.8 (2)	3.8 (2)	—
Freedom	4.9 (3)	6.1 (3)	.01
Happiness	7.9 (5)	7.4 (5)	.05
Inner harmony	11.1 (13)	9.8 (12)	.001
Mature love	12.6 (14)	12.3 (14)	—
National security	9.2 (10)	9.8 (11)	—
Pleasure	14.1 (17)	15.0 (16)	.01
Salvation	9.9 (12)	7.3 (4)	.001
Self-respect	8.2 (6)	7.4 (6)	.01
Social recognition	13.8 (16)	15.0 (17)	.001
True friendship	9.6 (11)	9.1 (9)	—
Wisdom	8.5 (8)	7.7 (7)	.05

Note: Figures shown are median rankings and, in parentheses, composite rank orders.

Table 5.5.

SIGNIFICANT VALUES DIFFERENTIATING HUMANITIES, SOCIAL SCIENCE, AND PHYSICAL SCIENCE MAJORS AT FLINDERS UNIVERSITY IN SOUTH AUSTRALIA (after Rokeach, 1973)

	Humanities	*Social Sciences*	*Physical Sciences*	p^a
	$N = 103$	$N = 162$	$N = 198$	
Terminal values				
A comfortable life	14.4 (17)	13.3 (14)	12.2 (13)	.001
A world of beauty	10.9 (13)	13.0 (13)	12.9 (15)	.001
Instrumental values				
Ambitious	10.8 (14)	7.8 (6)	7.8 (6)	.01
Capable	10.1 (12)	8.7 (11)	8.0 (7)	.05
Forgiving	7.8 (6)	8.2 (9)	9.7 (12)	.05
Imaginative	8.4 (7)	12.8 (16)	12.4 (16)	.001
Intellectual	9.1 (10)	11.4 (14)	11.5 (15)	.05
Self-controlled	10.2 (13)	8.1 (8)	7.7 (5)	.05

Note: Figures shown are median rankings and, in parentheses, composite rank orders.
[a]Kruskal-Wallis test.

ed, are tied more directly to natural incentives and emotions, and often are unconscious. Both motives and values shape behavior, but they should be thought of as independent determinants of behavior. (This will be discussed further in Chapters 6, 12, and 13.) Sometimes people speak of values motivating behavior in the sense that an Israeli may be "motivated" by a concern for national security. As has been repeatedly emphasized, however, it is more correct to say that national security activates or helps determine a response, and to save the term *motivation* for situations in which a motive is actually involved rather than some other determinant of behavior.

Natural incentives may be cognitively elaborated into symbolic incentives, or values, which guide and direct much of conscious behavior. On the other hand, the motives built on natural incentives also continue to influence behavior at another level. The point is dramatically illustrated by a physician's description of the behavior of a patient damaged in the frontal lobe, where cognitive elaboration takes place:

> For example, one former patient, whom I will call Mr. Jones, had his right frontal lobe destroyed by a tumor. Mr. Jones had difficulty with voluntary tasks that were verbally requested, despite the fact that he understood what was wanted of him. When asked to pick up his water glass, for example, he made no response. "Do you understand what I want you to do, Mr. Jones?" I asked. "Yes. You want me to pick up the glass." "Have you done that?" "No." "Can you?" "Yes." "Go ahead and

pick it up then," I urged him. No response. If he was thirsty, however, he would pick up the glass and drink from it spontaneously. (Cytowic, 1981)

The man's more primitive, unconscious motivational system, built on the natural incentive for drinking, was still intact and could activate the necessary response, but the cognitively elaborated conscious intent to drink no longer functioned.

NOTES AND QUERIES

1. Perry's recurrent dream from *In Cold Blood,* described in Chapter 2, ended up with a vision of an oral paradise in which there was abundant wonderful food and drink. In what way could this be taken to mean that Perry had a strong hunger motive? Which of the two types of hunger motives outlined in Figure 5.1 does the dream most probably represent? Why? What types of childhood experiences surrounding eating would be likely to produce this motive?

2. If people eat a lot, does it mean they have a strong hunger motive? List some reasons other than hunger that would lead people to eat excessively. If people do not eat much, does it mean they have a weak hunger motive? In the condition called *anorexia nervosa,* people have great difficulty eating enough to maintain their weight. Can you imagine a learning scenario in which they might have developed a strong motive that somehow is satisfied by not eating?

3. Tying the achievement motive to the variety incentive creates a difficulty over whether some discrepancies from expectation are more pleasurable than others. In the Maddi (1961) experiment, if a sentence stem occurred either a little earlier or a little later than expected, it produced positive affect. However, in the area of achievement it seems unlikely that an infant or an animal would like a slight deviation in the *less* complex direction as much as a slight deviation in the more complex direction. Would the rats, after being adapted to a complex environment for some time, spend more time in a simpler environment? It seems unlikely. In much the same way it seems unlikely that a child, having become adapted to playing with a complicated toy, would prefer working with one that was simpler. There seems to be a built-in bias toward getting pleasure from more complex or difficult tasks that is not captured by the idea that any slight deviation from expectation is pleasurable. How would you define the natural incentive, if it indeed involves more than simple variety? Could we think in terms of a complexity incentive?

4. List some ways in which you enjoy having impact. Do they involve primarily physical activities or relationships with people? How often do they involve aggression in the sense of intent to injure another person? Compare the lists prepared by men and women. If there are differences, what do they mean?

5. The eyes are said to be an important source of sign stimuli in humans. For example, a certain type of glance is supposed to elicit fear or anger and another type, love and affection. How would you describe the difference between these two types of glances? Having made the distinction, how would you determine by experiment whether you were right? Can you think of an experiment that would indicate whether the emotional responses to these glances were innate or learned?

6. In what ways could the increased production of sex hormones at puberty affect the way in which natural incentives in the sexual area function? Consider all the aspects of a natural incentive as outlined in Figure 5.1.

7. Do you agree with Freud that love is based on contact incentives, or do you think it might be based on some other type of natural incentive? Why or why not? What other type of natural incentive might be involved?

8. From the results of Sara Winter's study of nursing mothers, would you theoretically expect women to develop a stronger need for Nurturance (if it could be measured) than men? Why or why not?

9. Whereas the present trend in motivation research is toward measuring different types of avoidance motives, make a case for the fact that in addition there may be a natural incentive for cognitive consistency, which might develop into a stronger concern for this goal state in some people than others. How would you detect its presence?

10. The chapter treats values as independent cognitive derivations from natural incentives. Does this suggest that important values might be named for the same natural incentives for which the motives are named? How can you decide what the important values are?

11. Freud (1927/1957) remarks in *The Future of an Illusion* that "there are two widely diffused human characteristics which are responsible for the fact that the organization of culture can be maintained only by a certain measure of coercion: that is to say, men are not naturally fond of work, and arguments are to no avail against their passions." After reviewing the evidence in this chapter, do you agree with Freud's conclusions? How would you specifically answer his contention that people are not naturally fond of work?

6

Measures of Human Motive Dispositions

• THE MOTIVATIONAL SEQUENCE

What is needed now is a general model of motivated behavior. Experimentalists deal with *motivation*—with short-term situational influences like food, variety, requests for obedience, or electric shock that arouse approach or avoidance behavior immediately. Personality theorists or clinicians typically think in terms of *motives,* that is, stable dispositions that organize or explain much of what a person says and does. How do these two approaches fit together? What exactly is a motive disposition, and how should individual differences in its strength be measured? According to clinicians, some people, like Freud, have a strong need for fame, recognition, or power. How do we determine how weak or how strong the power motive is in different individuals? How is a disposition like the power motive aroused by a situation, and when aroused, how does it influence what the person does? These are the questions to which this chapter is addressed.

Motives are based on emotionally arousing incentives, which were discussed in the previous chapters. The incentives start out by being natural in the sense that they innately give rise to different types of positive or negative emotions. As we have seen, however, their nature changes rapidly with learning. The moderate degree of variety that produces positive emotional arousal at one time produces only boredom after exposure to new material. The pleasure children derive from the impact of dropping a spoon wanes as they move on to seeking bigger impacts.

Eventually a cognitive schema develops that organizes for children the category of situations that evokes different types of positive or negative emotional arousal. From the subjective point of view, these cognitive schemata may be called *goals* in the sense that the person learns to seek out (or avoid) the situations involved. Looked at from the point of view of the observer, they are referred to as either *positive* or *negative incentives,* since the person is seen to approach or avoid the situations involved.

In growing up, some people may develop more elaborate schemata associated with a given incentive than other people do. While all children start out enjoying having impact, some parents may strongly discourage this activity, so their child does not develop much pleasure from it or develop a good concept of how to attain pleasure in this way. Other parents may allow or even encourage the activity, so their child develops a more elaborate schematic representation of the many different ways in which he or she can get pleasure from having impact. Some parents may begin to verbalize the desirability of pursuing power goals by admiring their child for acting assertively or by encouraging him or her to fight back. In time, as the previous chapter showed, the child may develop a conscious value for being assertive or influential, although he or she may also pursue power goals without placing a conscious value on them.

In either case, many more situations get connected through learning with power goals or incentives. At home, a simple request to turn off the television may produce a defiant, assertive refusal. At school, playing basketball may evoke a strong competitive response. Even in a social situation among friends, children may find ways of calling attention to their importance. When a variety of cues consistently arouses a class of incentives or goals, we may speak of a motive having been formed. Obviously, there will be differences in the strength of such a motive, depending on the experiences of the person. So it will be important to find a way to measure these differences in strength. The cues or stimulus situations that give rise to these motives may be referred to as *demands*, since they regularly give rise to a motive state.

The way these facets of motivation fit together into a motivational sequence is illustrated in Figure 6.1. *Demands* (A), or arousal cues, made in terms of *incentives* (B), will—if they contact an existing *motive disposition* (C)—lead to *aroused motivation* (D), which combines with cognitions, habits or skills to produce the impulse to act, which combines with opportunities to produce action. As Chapter 3 noted, some writers (Atkinson & Birch, 1978; Weiner, 1980a) use the term *motivation* to refer to the end product of *all* the personal determinants of action (including habits and cognitions), but we will restrict the use of the term here to mean an aroused motive.

Figure 6.1 gives three examples to illustrate how the motivational sequence operates. Hunger is described in the behaviorist tradition as a primary drive. It is primary only in the sense that recurrent physiological demands (for example, low blood sugar) get associated very early and very strongly with the incentive of eating, which involves taste sensations. (See Figure 5.1.) In time, through learning, even a simple cue like noticing that it is time for supper is enough to contact or arouse the eating motive complex, which then arouses the intent to eat. Ordinarily we do not think much about individual differences in the strength of the eating motive, although the overweight people described in Chapter 5 spent much more time thinking about eating, preparing to eat, trying out different kinds of foods, and so forth. Whether the aroused motive to eat leads to actual eating obviously depends on opportunities (whether food is available), cognitions (whether the person eats the available food), and habits (whether the person usually eats at this time).

The second example in Figure 6.1 concerns the power motive. Suppose a girl is about to play a tennis match. Just being in a competitive situation is probably enough of a demand to contact the incentive of having impact or acting powerfully, or her coach may actually verbalize the demand by telling her to "get in there and fight." The coach's mentioning the incentive does not automatically arouse the intent or desire to win. It depends on whether the incentive used is part of the power motive system the girl has developed. If she has a greater need for power, then the incentive will contact it and lead to the intent to win. Whether her aroused power motivation leads to aggressive acts will depend on the situation, or opportunities (whether she is winning or not); her values (whether she thinks it is wrong to display temper on the court); and her habits (whether she is accustomed to throwing her racket away when she misses).

The third example is drawn from the type of material analyzed by Freud and other clinicians in order to demonstrate that the model works equally well

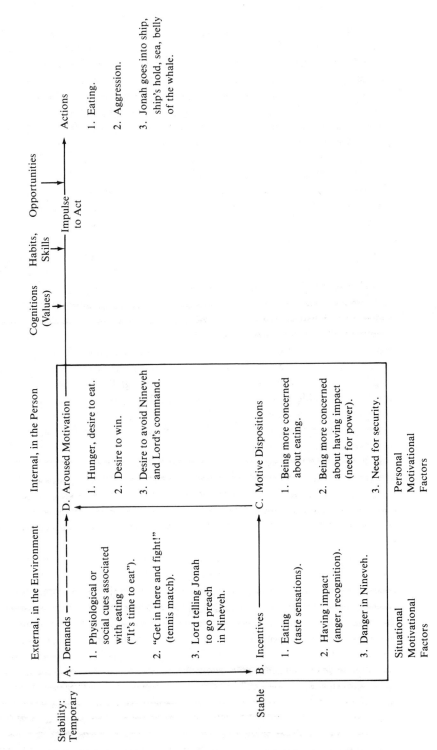

Figure 6.1.

Elements in the Motivational Sequence Leading to Action.

for such analyses. In the Bible there is a story about Jonah being swallowed by a whale in a kind of dream sequence. The Lord calls Jonah to preach against wickedness in the city of Nineveh. Jonah refuses and runs away in a ship, which gets caught in a storm. He falls asleep in the hold, eventually gets thrown into the sea to appease the gods, is swallowed by a whale, asks the Lord for forgiveness, and is vomited up on the dry land, safe and sound, after three days in the whale's stomach. Jonah's motive is not hard to identify: he is running away and going from one hiding place to another—first in the ship, then in its hold, then in sleep, then in the ocean, and finally in the whale's belly.

The motivational sequence leading to his actions can be conceptualized in the usual way, as Figure 6.1 illustrates. The demand is that he go preach in Nineveh, but Nineveh apparently is a negative incentive for him: it represents danger. This negative incentive contacts his need for security, which arouses the intent to avoid Nineveh and the Lord's command to go there. The actions Jonah takes all seem designed to satisfy his need for security. The only thing unusual about the story is that in real life a whale's stomach would not provide an opportunity for hiding.

As we shall see, thoughts are good places to look for motivational effects, because they are not as dependent as actions are on values, skills, and opportunities in order to be expressed. In real life, Jonah's need for security may have led only to the action of not going to Nineveh; we would have been left trying to determine why he did not go, when there might have been many reasons. He might like it where he is; he might have had a girlfriend somewhere else; he might not be able to get work in Nineveh. It is only as we get more of his thoughts represented here by such dream acts as sleeping in the middle of a storm or being swallowed by a whale that we have an easy time inferring what his primary motive was.

The Jonah story also illustrates that fear or avoidance motives built on negative incentives operate in the same way as approach motives. They are triggered by cues, which evoke a negative incentive (the threat of pain or discomfort), which contacts a stronger or weaker need to avoid that situation, which arouses in turn a stronger or weaker immediate impulse to avoid the danger.

Figure 6.1 also illustrates how two facets of the motivational sequence can be thought of as external to the person in the environment, namely, the demands and the incentives. In an experiment, investigators usually manipulate these two variables: they ask subjects to do something (a demand) for a variety of possible incentives (to please the experimenter, to earn some money, to show how good they are, and so on). Presented incentives become goals inside a person only when they contact a relevant motive disposition. Thus, the motive disposition and the aroused motive are the two variables that can be thought of as inside the person. The facets of the motivational sequence may also be classified in terms of whether they are temporary or stable. Demands and aroused motives are specific to a particular situation and therefore are temporary. Incentives like money, food, or the challenge of moderate risk are relatively stable aspects of the sequence, as is the motive disposition the subject brings to the experiment.

Each of these four aspects of the motivational sequence will now be discussed in more detail.

Demands

Demands may be classified as biological or social. For a long time psychologists concentrated on studying biological demands, such as hunger, thirst, and pain from electric shock, because they appear to be simpler and easier to define and manipulate systematically. Strictly speaking, these demands are not motives when they first occur. They may produce restless behavior, as when a baby first experiences arousal from low blood sugar levels, but the behavior does not satisfy the criteria of being motivated—that is, of being organized or directed toward an anticipated goal state—until the baby has formed a learned connection between a demand and what will satisfy it, namely, eating food. A biological need caused by a lack of food will, through learning, very quickly and dependably cue off a desire to get food. So it is proper to speak of a hunger motive having developed out of this regular biological demand, but it is nevertheless important to realize that the demand and the motive are separate. In exactly the same way a social demand, such as a father's command to a little boy to drink his milk, does not at the outset automatically lead to the *impulse* to drink the milk, or to behavior that could be classified as motivated. The boy must learn that the command ties in with some incentive-motive system before he will obey it. Many demands acquire motivating characteristics quite rapidly, but they do not have them initially.

Social demands can be just as powerful as biological demands. The basic tool of psychologists, the experiment, would not work unless the force of social demands was very great. Think of the tens of thousands of undergraduates who faithfully do even the most bizarre things at the request of psychological experimenters year after year! It would be a rare biological demand that could produce such consistent behavior from human subjects. The ready compliance of the hypnotized subject to the experimenter's command is well known, but as Martin Orne (1962) has pointed out, the average subject, even in a nonhypnotized condition, also will do almost anything the experimenter asks him to do. The experimenter has only to say, "This is an experiment. Go and lie down on the table." Almost every subject will do so without hesitation.

Remember that none of these demands is effective unless it contacts some incentive-motive complex. Just because an experimenter asks some college students to try to do as well as they can on some tasks given to them does not mean that all the students will accept the goal of doing well. Whether they accept it or not depends on the strength of their need for Achievement (see Chapter 7). The reason social demands often are so effective is that they call on the natural consistency incentive discussed in Chapter 5. People do what they are asked to do because it is satisfying to do what is expected or what they and others have often done before in the situation. In any case, the effectiveness of demands or instructions for arousing intents must always be evaluated in terms of the incentives and motive dispositions present in the situation.

Effect of Increasing Demands on Performance.   In general, stepping up demands increases performance. This is why parents urge their children to do well in school or to "hitch their wagon to a star," and why coaches spend time urging their players to try harder. Psychologists demonstrated long ago that the more demanding the task, the more effort the subject puts out (Ach, 1910). More recently, Locke, Shaw, Saari, and Latham (1980) reviewed data showing that setting higher goals leads to better performance than setting easy goals in all sorts of tasks from logging to typing to simple clerical tasks like adding and card sorting. In other words, people normally do better when greater demands are made on them to perform.

Does this justify setting impossibly difficult goals for people to get them to put out more effort? Not really, because the relationship between demand and performance is more complicated than such a conclusion implies. In 1908 Yerkes and Dodson concluded that increasing demands lead first to an increase and then to a decrease in the efficiency of performance. Animals' problem solving seems to be best when their drive strength is moderate rather than extreme. So if demands increase drive strength or aroused motivation, they could have a negative influence at very high levels.

In a typical study, Birch (1945) observed how chimpanzees solved problems to get food when their demand for food was increased by depriving them of it for up to forty-eight hours. For instance, in one task the caged chimpanzees had to use a short stick to bring in a string attached to a longer stick that could be used to reach the food. After going without food for only two hours, the chimpanzees were desultory in their approach to problems like this; most of the time they failed altogether to solve them in the maximum allotted time of one hour. The average time taken for all tasks (counting one hour for failure to solve the task) was about thirty-four minutes. As the chimpanzees got hungrier and hungrier, failures became fewer, and the average time taken to solve the problems dropped after twenty-four hours of food deprivation to around eleven minutes. However, if they were deprived of food for forty-eight hours, their efficiency fell off, and the average time taken to solve the problems rose to about twenty-one minutes.

Inefficiency at low and very high demand was qualitatively different, however. When the animals were not very hungry, they simply did not try very hard to solve the problems, because they were not very interested in the food. When they were extremely hungry, on the other hand, they were overexcited and focused so directly on the goal that they could not take the time to figure out how to solve the problem. After forty-eight hours of going without food, the chimpanzee Art persistently reached directly for the food with the short stick, in one instance making as many as twenty-six consecutive unsuccessful sweeps. The intensity of the demand prevented him from taking the time to "think out" the problem. It lowered his efficiency by narrowing the focus of his attention.

People put under great pressure to solve difficult problems make more errors, and their efficiency decreases (see Heckhausen, 1980; Schneider & Kreuz, 1979). This type of observation led Thurstone (1937) to suggest that there may be an optimal level of demand to get the highest quality of performance for tasks of different difficulty. Increasing demand at first facilitates the utilization of cues relevant to performing the task (Bruner, Matter, & Papanek, 1955), but very intense demand may distract people, cause them to become anxious and not see relevant cues, lead them to make errors (Patrick, 1934), and perhaps even quit trying altogether. In short, the relationship between increasing demand and efficiency is curvilinear, assuming an inverted *U* shape; also, the more complex the task, the lower the optimal level of demand.

Stennett (1957) reported a representative study showing this effect. Subjects were asked to try to keep noise at a minimum by turning a knob to a "null point" whenever noise occurred in an auditory tracking task. Their performance score was the number of seconds in a one-minute trial in which they managed to keep "on target" (no noise). Muscle tension and skin resistance (to measure palmar sweating) were recorded from the unused left arm to get estimates of physiological activation. Subjects were tested under three types of demand for good performance. In the low demand condition, subjects were told from time to time that they should track as usual, but that the experimenter was simply calibrating the apparatus and could not record their score. In the optimal demand trials, the experimenter encouraged the subjects to perform better and offered them small sums of money (twenty-five cents) to improve their scores. In the high demand trials, they were told the best score that had ever been made with the apparatus and urged to break the record. They were offered five dollars for each trial in which they equaled or bettered the record, or two dollars plus avoidance of electric shock to their leg. As Figure 6.2 makes clear, the activation level as measured by muscle tension increased regularly as the level of demand for better performance increased, but performance was best under moderate levels of demand and activation. Other investigators (for example, Duffy, 1962) have shown that a variety of factors enter in to complicate the simple relationship shown here and assumed by the Yerkes-Dodson law. In fact, surprisingly few studies confirm its existence, partly because the investigators have not conceived of demand as only one aspect of the motivational sequence to be considered and kept under control.

The distracting effect of too much demand is also illustrated by research on the effects of induced muscular tension on learning. In these experiments subjects see three-letter nonsense syllables like *BMT* exposed briefly in a small window. They are to learn to anticipate and say out loud what letters will be exposed next when they see a given nonsense syllable. They perform this task under normal conditions and also when squeezing a hand dynamometer at various fractions of the maximum squeeze they can make on the instrument. As Figure 6.3 shows, a mild squeeze on the dynamometer, at about one quarter of the maximum grip, facilitated learning; however, when the subjects were forced to squeeze at about three quarters of their maximum grip, learning actually fell below what it was when no squeezing was required (Courts, 1939). The induced muscular tension can be thought of as equivalent to increasing demand such as would be mobilized by stronger, external incentives; if this is so, the expected relationship is obtained; increased demand first increases performance and then decreases it. Very probably it decreases it, because, as in the case of the chimpanzee Art, the increased pressure distracts the subject from concentrating on the performance itself.

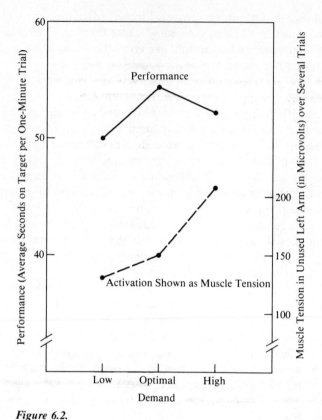

Figure 6.2.

Relationship Between Increasing Demand, Activation Level, and Performance. Two values for the optimal condition have been averaged for simplicity in presentation (after Stennett, 1957).

It is important to remember, however, that demands have an effect on performance only if they contact motives in the individual, as Figure 6.1 makes clear. Laboratory studies such as those just reviewed, or the field studies summarized by Locke (1968, 1975) show the effects of demands on performance only because subjects are willing to commit themselves to trying to do what the experimenter asks them to do (that is, learn to anticipate nonsense syllables and squeeze a dynamometer). In real life, if demands are set too high, people may give up trying altogether or become so anxious that they perform very badly.

Incentives

Incentives are emotionally arousing stable characteristics of the environment or person-environment interactions that people seek out (positive incentives) or

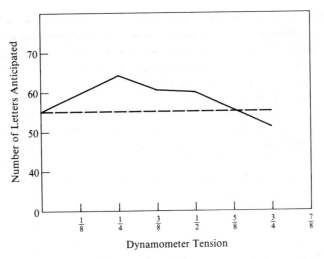

Figure 6.3.

Relationship Between Number of Letters Correctly Anticipated and Dynamometer Tension (after Young, 1961, after Courts, 1939).

avoid (negative incentives). Chapters 4 and 5 discussed at length the various forms incentives take. They differ from demands in that they are less specific to a particular time and place. Suppose an experimenter says to a group of subjects, "You are to work on these arithmetic problems, and I will give a prize of $2.50 to the one of you who solves the most problems in twenty minutes." The experimenter is making a demand at a particular time and place for performance from some particular individuals but is using a generalized incentive— money.

Atkinson (1958) carried out such an experiment in which money and another incentive were introduced. Ten to twenty undergraduates were assembled in groups and told they were going to compete for monetary rewards by seeing who could solve the largest number of arithmetic problems in the time allotted. Along with a test booklet, students were given an instruction sheet telling them how large a money prize they might win and what their chances of winning it might be in terms of how many others they were competing with for it. The money prize offered was either $2.50 or $1.25 for the best performance, and the chances of winning it were for some students one out of twenty, for others one out of three, for others one out of two, and for others three out of four. That is, in the last instance the three best performers out of the four competing all would get the prize.

As Table 6.1 shows, those who were competing for $2.50 performed significantly better than those who were working for a possible $1.25, regardless of the odds under which they were working. Notice also that a higher money reward maintains higher performance, particularly when the expectancy of winning is very low (odds, one in twenty) or very high (odds, three in four). In other words, money seems to work best when other incentives are not operating—in this case, the achievement incentive, which is optimal when there is a moderate chance of winning. As the means at the bottom of Table 6.1 show, performance is best when the achievement incentive is optimal—when the person has a fifty-fifty chance of getting the prize (see Chapter 7). If the odds are very long (one in twenty), the achievement incentive has less attraction, because the person is unlikely to win. If the odds are short (three in four), it also has less attraction, because nearly everyone will win. In these two situations where the achievement incentive was less important, the larger money reward had the most effect. When the achievement challenge was greater at moderate odds, the larger money reward had less influence. The reverse also was true: when the money incentive was less important ($1.25), the achievement incentive—as represented by the difference in performance at one-in-twenty versus one-in-two odds—had a stronger effect than when the money incentive was more important ($2.50).

Money as an incentive is misleadingly concrete. Psychologists use it in experiments because it is easier to manipulate than other incentives. However, it always takes on the meaning of the particular motivational situation in which it is employed as an incentive. For example, even in the experimental situation reported in Table 6.1, it is doubtful that the students were working harder just because they were offered a somewhat larger money prize. Is it reasonable to believe that $1.25, even in noninflated money, would mean that much to a college undergraduate? Instead, the larger prize offered by the experimenter simply may have meant to the students that a prestige figure placed a higher value on their performing faster, and their desire to please the experimenter was proportion-

Table 6.1.

EFFECT ON PERFORMANCE OF MONETARY INCENTIVE AND EXPECTANCY OF WINNING (after Atkinson, 1958)

Incentive		Expectancy of Winning (Difficulty)[a]				Incentive Means
		1/20	1/3	1/2	3/4	
$2.50	N =	18	18	18	18	
Mean score		50.3	51.8	54.1	51.7	52.0
$1.25	N =	13	13	13	13	
Mean score		45.0	50.8	52.0	45.7	48.4
Difference		5.3	1.0	2.1	6.0	4.6
Expectancy means		48.0	51.4	53.2	49.2	

[a]Fifty is an average score for the group on two tasks—arithmetic and drawing X's in circles. Incentive difference is significant at $p < .01$, difficulty differences at $p < .05$.

ately increased. In fact, in another experiment Atkinson and Reitman (1956) reported that girls with high affiliative needs were particularly likely to work harder when a monetary incentive was offered—presumably because they were precisely the ones who would be more interested in pleasing the experimenter.

Motive Dispositions

Demands are couched in terms of incentives that must contact motive dispositions if motives that ultimately influence action are to be aroused. What exactly are motive dispositions? We have described them as representing individual differences in the strength of anticipatory goal states or the networks of associations built up around natural incentives. If a boy—through encouragement or on his own—gets a good deal of pleasure from doing well at moderately challenging tasks, he will tend to develop a stronger achievement motive in the sense that more situations will cue off for him, and more frequently, the anticipation of getting satisfaction from doing such things.

The possibility of satisfaction from such an incentive situation is seen internally as a goal. The goal may not be conscious. The boy may not know why he is attracted to working on challenging tasks. He—or we as observers—may be aware that he works more energetically at such tasks, is more aware of the possibilities for satisfaction from this type of performance, and learns more quickly to do whatever is necessary to get this type of satisfaction. That is, as in the behaviorist tradition, we infer the presence of a central motive state when a person is more active or energetic in pursuing a goal, more sensitive to cues relating to the goal, and quicker to learn what is needed to get to the goal. In other words, motives drive, orient, and select behavior. So we may define a motive disposition as a *recurrent concern about a goal state that drives, orients, and selects behavior.* The word *concern* in the definition gives away the fact that we are primarily interested here in human beings; as we shall see, concerns can be directly measured in the thought processes of humans, but they must be inferred from the actions of animals. Concerns can be inferred from actions, but it is much more difficult and hazardous to do so than to measure the concerns directly.

The goal state that defines a motive can be the same as or different from the incentive present in the demand that is supposed to motivate behavior. Thus, in Table 6.1, the achievement incentive (defined as moderate challenge) will activate individuals who have a stronger concern about this incentive—namely, those we say have a stronger achievement motive—more than those who do not have such a recurrent concern (see Chapter 7). For the latter the incentive does not contact the achievement motive disposition, so if the person performs at all, it must be out of some other motive, such as the desire for social approval or the motive built on the consistency-conformity incentive. The problem in all of this is to measure recurrent concerns or motive dispositions, since now we have moved from the external world to inside the person, and it is harder to know just what is going on inside a person than what is going on in the environment. This is the main problem to which we soon will turn our attention.

Aroused Motivation

The final outcome of a motivational sequence is an aroused motive to act in such a way as to satisfy the motive disposition that has been engaged by demands or arousal cues referring to some incentives relevant to the motive. This motivation to act combines with cognitions (values), skills, and opportunities to produce the particular acts that occur.

Often in real life, all these determinants of action are implicit in the form of a very specific behavioral intent, such as when a man says he cannot find a shirt and "I want to go to the store to buy a shirt." From such a stated intent, it is often safe to predict that he will walk out of the house, get into a car, drive to the center of town, park, put a dime in the parking meter, walk into the store, pick out a shirt, pay for it, bring it home, and put it on. Notice that we can predict action in this case from the motivational intent because we know there is a store where he can buy a shirt, that he can drive a car, that he has the money to buy the shirt, that he has the time to do it now, that he values wearing a shirt, and so on.

On the other hand, statements of general intent, such as "I want to do well in school," are of little value in predicting action—in this case how well the person will do—because the other determinants of action are not so well known, such as the person's academic skills, the opportunities provided for studying versus enjoying life, and so on. Furthermore, even the expression of such an intent is influenced by factors other than motive dispositions, such as the positive value people place on academic success, the social desirability of saying one wants to do well in school, and so on. In short, statements of conscious intent are generally not good indicators of an aroused motive, because they are the product of many factors other than motive strength.

Psychologists interested in understanding intents usually have relied on simple statements of wishes or choices and concentrated on the situational factors that influence them. For example, Atkinson (1957) worked out a system showing that the intent or desire to choose an alternative is a joint function of motive strength multiplied by attractiveness multiplied by the difficulty of attaining the alternative. In commonsense terms, children's desire for a piece of candy is a joint function of their hunger, how big and delicious the candy is, and how much they must pay for it. Atkinson's model will be explained in Chapter 7. The point to keep clearly in mind here is that this kind of intent or impulse to act is not identical with the concept of an aroused motive, as shown in Figure 6.1. It may, under certain very specific conditions, indicate the presence of an aroused motive, but ordinarily such an intent is more complexly determined.

Demands can easily influence aroused motives. In fact, most of the time we act as if all we have to do to get somebody to do something is ask them to do it. And so far as many normative situations are concerned, we can indeed rely on demands' arousing an impulse to act, without worrying about what incentives and motive dispositions are involved. A father tells his daughter to drink her milk, and she does. A boss asks a worker to get back to work, and he does.

Actually, behind the success of such demands lie various incentives and motives, but for practical purposes they can be ignored until something goes wrong and a demand does not produce the expected intent or aroused motive.

Over forty years ago psychologist Kurt Lewin (1935) and his students got interested in what appeared to be a natural impulse to complete an interrupted task. They allowed subjects to complete some tasks and stopped them in the course of performing others; they found that the subjects remembered the incompleted tasks better than completed tasks and returned to resume working on them if given the opportunity. What appears to be responsible for the effect (named the *Zeigarnik effect* after its discoverer) is the implicit demand, accepted as a norm by most adults, that people should finish a job that has been started. Shifting the demand character of the situation alters the motive aroused. If the experimenter suggests that the subjects are to show how well they have done, they tend to recall more completed tasks (Atkinson, 1955). If subjects are asked to imagine themselves failing before a large audience in a directed daydream, another implicit demand is implanted—to prove they are not failing—and they recall more completed tasks than uncompleted tasks (Russ, cited in Heckhausen, 1967).

Aroused motive states need not be conscious, as Chapter 1's review of Freud's work made clear. They can influence behavior without a person's being aware that an unconscious wish existed until later evidence reveals its presence. This fact provides still another reason why conscious motives or stated interests should not always be taken at face value as indicators of the strength of aroused motives.

• AROUSING MOTIVES TO DETECT THEIR UNIQUE EFFECTS ON BEHAVIOR

Motive dispositions are the obvious key to understanding a motivational sequence, for without knowing what motives people bring to a situation, it is impossible to know how they will react to a demand or an incentive. Laboratory experiments on motivation can be carried out, because most subjects bring motives to the situation that the experimenter can appeal to in getting them to do what he or she wants them to do. The fact that subjects sometimes do not do what they are expected to do calls attention to the fact that individuals differ even in the motive dispositions they bring to an experiment. What are some of these motives? How can individual differences in their strength be measured?

One way to detect individual differences in motive strength is to find some behavior that is the unique effect of the motive and use it as an index of the strength of the motive. Thus, if we could show that whenever people were angry their heart beat faster, and the angrier they were the faster their heart beat, we might try to use heart rate as an index of how angry a person was. However, the effect has to be unique to the state that produces it. Otherwise we make mistakes in inferring backward from effects to their cause. We can infer a person is angry from an increased heart rate if anger—and anger only—produces such an effect, which is clearly not the case. Increased heart rate can also result from fear or sexual arousal.

This is the difficulty in trying to reason from actions to the motives that produced them. As we have repeatedly emphasized in discussing Figure 6.1, many factors other than aroused motives enter into determining an action like eating or doing well in school. Yet people continuously make the mistake of inferring that because people are doing well in school, they have a strong need for achievement, or that because others eat a great deal, they are always hungry. In fact, people may do well in school because they are intelligent (have academic talent); because they have developed good study habits; or because they are motivated by a variety of goals unrelated to achievement, such as the need for social approval or the need to be considered an important person.

Such considerations led psychologists to seek unique effects of aroused motives in perception or apperception (that is, fantasy). As Chapters 1 and 2 pointed out, Freud and other clinicians repeatedly demonstrated that fantasy—particularly dreams—provided excellent opportunities for inferring the presence of different types of motives. This is because fantasies are less influenced by nonmotivational determinants like skills and opportunities than actions are. People can dream about doing all sorts of things they have neither the skill nor the opportunity to do in real life. Thus, it is safer to infer from the fact that a girl dreams about being president of her class that she has a desire to be important than it would be if she actually were president of her class: in the latter instance the behavioral result might be determined primarily by her social skills or the lack of good alternative candidates rather than by her desire to be important.

In reviewing the behaviorist tradition we found that Skinner had also concluded that operants—that is, "spontaneous" responses—reflect goal-directed striving more directly than respondents do for the same reason. Respondents, by definition, are more determined by the external stimulus situation, whereas operants are determined by whatever cues they carry inside themselves. In Skinnerian terminology, fantasies are "covert operants." They have the advantage of all operants in more sensitively reflecting motivation. Furthermore, since they are covert (that is, thoughts rather than overt acts), they have the further advantage of not depending on skills or opportunities.

Effects of Arousing the Hunger Motive

Why not arouse motives experimentally and look for their unique effects in fantasy? Atkinson and McClelland (1948) did just that in an early study that compared the content of imaginative stories written after subjects went one, four, and sixteen hours without food. The objective was to detect precisely how fantasies of hungry young men differed from their fantasies when they were not hungry. The experiment was done in such a way that the men involved did not realize that the effect of hunger on imagination was being investigated; otherwise, they might have written the kind of stories they thought hungry people should write. In other words, the experimenters tried to eliminate a nonmotivational or cognitive determinant of the fantasy responses. This was done by assigning some submariners to quarters late in the afternoon so they could sleep late and participate in some psychological research the next morning, some sixteen hours after their previous meal. Other subjects wrote stories one hour after they had finished the noon meal, and again four hours afterward (just before supper). The content of the stories was searched to identify fantasy elements that were present when the hunger motive was strong and not present when it was weak.

The results contained a surprise, as Figure 6.4 illustrates. Hungrier men did not have fantasies of eating a lot of delicious steaks and desserts, as one might have supposed. Conventional wisdom assumes that hungry people dream of food, so that if people think a good deal about eating, they must be hungry. But this does not turn out to be true. The category labeled *goal activity* in Figure 6.4, which represents thoughts about eating, declines in frequency as hunger increases. In contrast, the category labeled *instrumental activity,* which has to do with activities or objects associated with getting food, increases with hours of food deprivation. Stories dealing with food deprivation—particularly with black market activities to overcome shortages—increased. After the fact, it is easy to understand how it is more adaptive for hungry people to think about ways of getting food rather than just passively dream of eating. In another part of the experiment the subjects were shown a very dim slide, supposedly of three objects on a table. The hungrier subjects more often reported that they were knives, forks, spoons, and plates than the less hungry subjects, but they did not more often mention eatables.

So an aroused motive state—namely, hunger—has some unique and rather unexpected effects on fantasy. It is doubtful if these effects would have been obtained if the subjects had known they were purposely being deprived of food. For Sanford (1937) has shown that subjects who fast voluntarily for an experimenter do think more often about food. They do what they expect they should do. Keys (summarized in Sherif, 1948) reported that conscientious objectors in World War II *voluntarily* undergoing starvation spent a good deal of time fantasizing about things to eat. However, these fantasies also might have an adaptive significance, since if the visions of eating had become strong enough, the volunteers might have broken their fast. In other words, in this case the subjects' cognitions or expectations were quite different from those of the submariners, who did not know that hunger was the object of study.

Individual Differences in the Strength of the Hunger Motive

Atkinson and McClelland (1948) also developed an overall "need for Food" score based on giving one point for the presence of a characteristic in a story that appeared more often after sixteen hours than one hour of food deprivation and subtracting one point for a story characteristic that decreased in frequency from one to sixteen hours of food deprivation. This score averaged 0.74 for subjects who had gone one hour without food, 1.57 for subjects who had gone four hours without food, and 4.05 for subjects who had gone sixteen hours without eating. In contrast, when subjects were asked to rate how hungry they were,

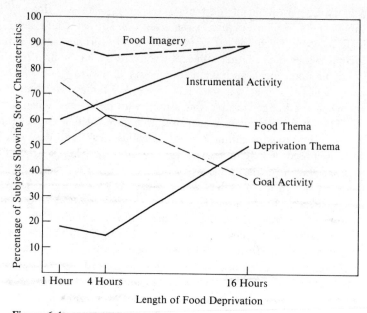

Figure 6.4.

Percentage of Subjects Showing Selected Food-Related Story Characteristics as a Function of Increasing Hunger (after Atkinson & McClelland, 1948).

they judged themselves to be significantly more hungry after four hours than after one hour of going without food, but after sixteen hours they were no hungrier than after four hours. Thus, self-ratings of the strength of the hunger motive provided a less sensitive index of hours of food deprivation than did the measure based on fantasy.

The next logical step would have been to obtain need for Food scores from subjects when the hunger motive was not aroused—say, two or three hours after a meal—and to use them as a measure of individual differences in the strength of the motive. That is, people who scored very high in the need for Food even when the motive was not aroused might be assumed to be chronically hungry, so to speak. At least, they chronically think like hungry people do—namely, about the absence of food or about getting food. Such people might be further expected to eat more or eat more often than people for whom the need for Food score is low.

Such a study has not been carried out, although Schachter and his associates have extensively investigated overeating, which might be considered a sign of a chronically aroused hunger motive. They too obtained a somewhat surprising result (Schachter, 1971b). Overweight subjects are more influenced by external cues than underweight or normal subjects are, as was noted in Chapter 5. They eat more when it is time to eat or when food cues are present than normal subjects do. But they eat less and find it easier than subjects of normal weight to skip meals and fast when external cues are not present. Table 6.2 gives a typical result. In this experiment subjects were given a break after doing some work in the laboratory and told they could eat as many sandwiches as they liked during the break. In one condition, one sandwich was put out and the subjects were told there were others in the refrigerator if they wanted more. In the other condition, instructions were the same except three sandwiches were put out. In the one-sandwich condition, the overweight subjects ate fewer sandwiches—about 1.5 on the average—than the normal subjects, presumably because when they ate up one sandwich no more food cues were present. However, when three sandwiches were offered, the overweight subjects ate significantly more than the normal subjects and more than they did under the one-sandwich condition.

There are several possible explanations for this result, but one possibility not investigated by Schachter and his associates is that overweight subjects are chronically hungrier than normal subjects. If they are, their behavior could be explained by Atkinson and McClelland's (1948) results. In that study also, hungrier subjects did not think more often about food cues when they were absent. Thus, a hungrier subject might not be expected to imagine more vividly the sandwiches in the refrigerator and thus be led to get more of them to eat. On the other hand, in another part of the Atkinson and McClelland experiment, subjects were shown some vague objects exposed on a slide, which they were told were a bowl and a cake. They were asked to judge which was larger, and the hungrier subjects said the cake was larger more often than did the less hungry subjects (McClelland & Atkinson, 1948). Thus, it would be expected that if food cues were actually present, hungrier subjects could see them more vividly and be led by the food incentive to eat more. For a comparable effect of need on perception, see Bruner & Goodman (1947).

However, without a direct measure of the strength of the hunger motive in obese and normal weight individuals (as obtained, for example, from the need for Food score developed by Atkinson and McClelland), it is impossible to

Table 6.2.

EFFECTS OF PRESENT OR ABSENT EATING CUES ON EATING BY OVERWEIGHT AND NORMAL WEIGHT SUBJECTS (after Schachter, 1971b)

	Mean Number of Sandwiches Eaten When Offered	
Subjects	*Eating Cues Absent (One Sandwich Offered)*	*Eating Cues Present (Three Sandwiches Offered)*
Normal weight (*N*)	1.96	1.88
Overweight (*O*)	1.48	2.32
Difference (*N − O*)	.48	−.44
p	< .05	< .05

know whether the obese subjects are, in fact, chronically hungrier. All that can be said is that the finding on the importance of external cues for obese subjects is consistent with other research on the effects of hunger on perception and fantasy. The Schachter research also illustrates once again the difficulty of using an action measure to determine the strength of a motive, for overeating could be caused by many factors other than a strong hunger motive. It might be the result of a defect in fat metabolism, hypothalamic malfunction such as characterizes obese rats (see Schachter, 1971a), or eating habits of long standing.

• MEASURING THE STRENGTH OF SOCIAL MOTIVE DISPOSITIONS

Coding Thought Content for the Achievement Motive

The procedure adopted in the hunger experiment (Atkinson & McClelland, 1948) has been followed in a number of other studies designed to detect the unique effects on fantasy of arousing different kinds of social motives. In the first of these, attempts were made to arouse the achievement motive by telling some young men that performance tests they were taking would give an indication of their general intelligence and leadership capacities, and then manipulating the amount of success and failure they experienced on those tests (McClelland, Atkinson, Clark, & Lowell, 1953). Shortly afterward, subjects were asked to write brief, five-minute stories to a series of four to six pictures for what was sometimes described as a test of creative imagination and sometimes as a picture-story exercise (to deemphasize the testing character of the fantasy collection technique). Some of the pictures were taken from the Murray Thematic Apperception Test (1938), and some were chosen specifically for this study, such as the one in Figure 6.5.

Characteristics of stories written after achievement motive arousal were carefully compared with characteristics of stories written when no attempt to manipulate motivation was made (called the *Neutral condition*). The chief difference was in a characteristic labeled *achievement imagery,* which was defined as being present in a story when someone was involved in doing something better. "Doing better" involved an implicit or explicit *standard of excellence*—for example, winning a contest; fixing a machine; attaining a unique accomplishment, such as inventing something; or being concerned over a long period of time with a performance goal, such as in pursuing a career to become a doctor. *Involvement* was indicated by an explicit statement of a desire or intent to do well; by affective concern over goal attainment (feeling good after success or bad after failure); or by extraordinary efforts to achieve a goal, as in "the boy is working *very carefully* on his essay."

Once a story was identified as being achievement related because of the presence of such imagery, it was searched for other characteristics that differentiated the stories written under achievement-oriented versus neutral conditions. A number of such characteristics were found and carefully defined so that two

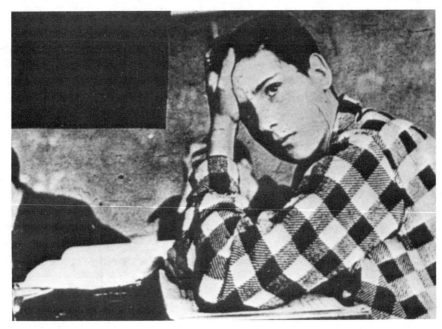

Figure 6.5.

Picture Used in the Standard Series for Eliciting Stories to Be Scored for *n* Achievement (McClelland, Atkinson, Clark, & Lowell, 1953).

trained judges could agree almost perfectly on their presence or absence in a story. They are listed in Table 6.3, which also shows the percentage of stories containing each characteristic under relaxed and achievement-oriented instruction conditions. Thus, 33 percent of the stories written under achievement-oriented conditions contained explicit statements of the need or desire to achieve, as compared with only 10 percent of the stories written under relaxed conditions.

The categories make sense when they are conceptualized as part of a problem solving sequence, as illustrated in Figure 6.6. In this sequence the person is seen as trying to achieve a certain goal, defined here in terms of the achievement imagery definition. In thinking about the goal, the person may express a specific need for it, as well as anticipate getting it or not getting it and feeling good if he or she gets it or not good if he or she does not get it. The person may be pictured as encountering obstacles on the way to getting the goal—either in himself or herself or in the environment—and as taking various actions to reach the goal or overcome the obstacle to the goal. In the course of taking these actions, the person also may get help. It is as if the arousal of the achievement motive increases the probability that the person will think about all aspects of a problem-solving sequence.

To get an overall achievement motive score for an individual, the presence in a story of any one of the categories in Table 6.3 is counted as +1. A story containing no imagery related to achievement is scored −1. Originally, working at a task in a way that is not quite strong enough to be given a +1 was scored as 0 (for task imagery), but in later use both unrelated and task imagery were scored as 0. A given characteristic was scored only one time per story, even

Table 6.3.

EFFECT OF ACHIEVEMENT AROUSAL ON CHARACTERISTICS OF IMAGINATIVE STORIES
(after McClelland, Atkinson, Clark, & Lowell, 1953)

	Percentage of Stories Showing Characteristic Under Two Conditions	
Story Characteristic and Example	*Relaxed* *(N = 156 Stories)*	*Achievement-oriented* *(N = 156 Stories)*
Achievement imagery "He is trying to run faster."	25	54
Need "He wants to do well."	10	33
Positive anticipatory goal state "He is thinking how great he will feel if he does."	4	15
Negative anticipatory goal state "He is thinking how badly he will feel if he fails."	6	14
Positive goal state "He is happy he succeeded."	2	15
Negative goal state "He is unhappy he failed."	6	9
Actions "He has been practicing every day for a week."	3	25
Obstacle in the environment "His mother thinks he is crazy to spend so much time running."	6	6
Obstacle in the person "He worries so much it slows him down."	3	13
Help "His coach has given him some good advice on how to improve."	3	10
Achievement theme[a]	18	45
Mean *n* Achievement score[b]	1.95 (SD = 4.3)	8.77 (SD = 5.3)

[a]The whole story deals with an achievement theme. No other significant theme was mentioned.

[b]The mean *n* Achievement score is obtained by adding one point for each characteristic coded per story and subtracting one point for each story totally unrelated to achievement. All differences are significant except for *obstacle in the environment* and *negative goal state*.

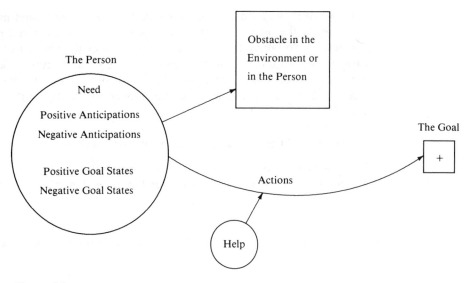

Figure 6.6.

A Problem-solving Model for Conceptualizing Motive Subcategories (Winter, 1973, after McClelland, Atkinson, Clark, & Lowell, 1953).

though it occurred several times, to avoid giving extra credit for more verbally fluent subjects. However, in recent years it has also been the regular practice to correct for verbal fluency by adjusting the motive score statistically for the total number of words in all the stories.

The sum of such characteristics present in all stories (a protocol) written by a subject is called the "*n* Achievement score," following H. A. Murray's (1938) practice of abbreviating *need for Achievement* to *n* Achievement. It is obviously jointly determined by the number of achievement cues in pictures, instructions, and individuals, as Figure 6.7 illustrates. That is, the *n* Achievement score per story increases as a function of how related the pictures are to achievement, increases as instructions get more achievement oriented, and increases as individuals differ in their overall *n* Achievement score. The three determinants combine in a simple additive fashion such that a person with a low *n* Achievement score overall, when responding to a picture containing no achievement cues under relaxed conditions, is very unlikely to put any achievement thoughts into a story written under those conditions. On the other hand, a person with a high *n* Achievement score overall, when responding to a high cue picture under achievement-oriented conditions, is most likely to tell a story saturated with achievement content. There do not seem to be any interaction effects in the sense that moderate cue pictures, for example, might differentiate better than high or low cue pictures between relaxed and achievement arousal conditions.

External events also can influence the content subjects put into their stories. Figure 6.8 shows how achievement imagery increases in stories written by students when they are to take an examination at some later point in time. The more nearly the picture represents the examination situation and the closer the students are to taking the examination, the greater the amount of achievement imagery written into the stories. Thus, a medium cue picture evokes little achievement concern a year before the examination, somewhat more three weeks before the examination, and much more on the day of the examination itself.

Coding Thought for the Power and Affiliation Motives

The same approach was adopted to develop scoring systems for the need for Affiliation (*n* Affiliation) and the need for Power (*n* Power), as will be described in

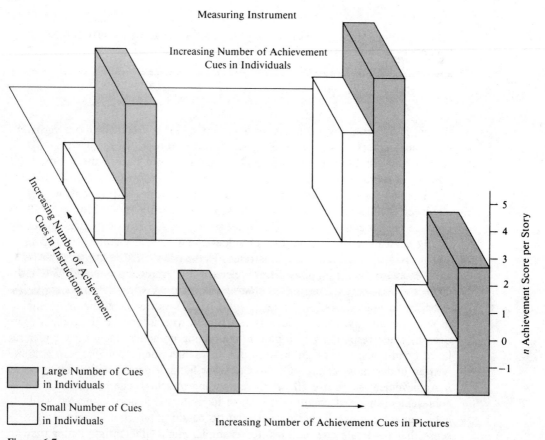

Figure 6.7.

Graphic Representation of Joint Determination of *n* Achievement Score Obtained from a Single Story by Number of Achievement Cues in (1) Pictures, (2) Instructions, and (3) Individuals (McClelland, Atkinson, Clark, & Lowell, 1953).

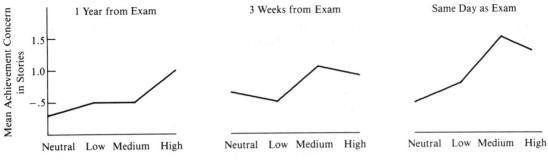

Figure 6.8.

Mean Achievement Concern in Stories Written to Pictures of Increasing Similarity to an Examination, Plotted Separately for Groups of Students for Whom the Examination Was Increasingly Near (Heckhausen, 1967, after Fisch).

subsequent chapters. Thus, any given story is normally scored for several motives.

Table 6.4 illustrates how stories written to the same picture can have quite different motivational content. The stories in Table 6.4 are artificially constructed to illustrate some of the aspects of coding systems developed from studies in which these motives were aroused to define and measure *n* Achievement, *n* Affiliation, and *n* Power. The story in the left column contains most of the elements that appeared more often in stories written by young men after the achievement motive had been aroused. The primary decision about whether to score a story as achievement oriented depends on whether there is some concern to do well or to do better expressed in the story. Here George clearly cares about producing the most practicable drawings so he can build a bridge. Other aspects of the story mention that he is thinking about how happy he would be if he achieved the goal, how he must act so as to overcome blocks in the world, and how unhappy he is when he fails to achieve the goal. It is a nonobvious finding that arousing achievement motivation just as often led subjects to think about failure as about success and joy in winning.

Affiliation concerns were aroused by exposing young men to a situation in which they were publicly judged by their peers on their popularity and personal characteristics. Under these conditions their stories reflected a greater concern for establishing, maintaining, or repairing friendly or affiliative relationships (Shipley & Veroff, 1952). In the artificial story constructed in the middle column of Table 6.4 to reflect this type of arousal, George is described as concerned about maintaining his affiliative relationship with his wife, about personal and environmental blocks that interfere with this relationship, and about his desire to maintain it and to take steps to repair it.

Power motivation has been aroused in a variety of ways (see Winter, 1973).

Table 6.4.

TYPICAL STORIES WRITTEN WHEN ACHIEVEMENT, AFFILIATION, AND POWER MOTIVES HAVE BEEN AROUSED TO A PICTURE OF A MAN AT A DRAWING BOARD

Achievement Arousal	Affiliation Arousal	Power Arousal
George is an engineer who *(need, +1) wants to win* a competition in which the man with *(achievement imagery: standard of excellence, +1) the most practicable drawing* will be awarded the contract to build a bridge. He is taking a moment to think *(goal anticipation, +1) how happy he will be* if he wins. He has been *(block, world, +1) baffled by how to make such a long span strong,* but remembers *(instrumental act, +1) to specify a new steel alloy* of great strength, submits his entry, but does not win and *(goal state, negative, +1) is very unhappy.*	George is an engineer who is working late. He is *(affiliation imagery, +1) worried that his wife will be annoyed* with him for neglecting her. *(block, world, +1)* She has been *objecting* that he cares more about his work than his wife and family. *(block, personal, +1)* He seems *unable to satisfy* both his boss and his wife, *(need, +1)* but he *loves her* very much, and *(instrumental act, +1)* will do his best to *finish up fast* and get home to her.	This is Georgiadis, a *(prestige of actor, +1) famous architect,* who *(need, +1) wants to win a competition* which will establish who is *(power imagery, +1) the best architect in the world.* His chief *rival,* Bulakovsky, *(block, world, +1) has stolen* his best ideas, and he is dreadfully afraid of the *(goal anticipation, negative, +1) disgrace of losing.* But he comes up with *(instrumental act, +1) a great new idea,* which absolutely *(powerful effect, +1) bowls the judges over,* and he wins!
Thema +1, Total *n* Achievement score = +7.	Thema +1, Total *n* Affiliation score = +6.	Total *n* Power score = +7.

In one study, student candidates for office wrote stories while they were waiting for the election returns to be counted. In another, they wrote stories after they had been exposed to the influence of an impressive leader (a film of John F. Kennedy making his inaugural address). Gradually it appeared that the kernel of the unique effect these different arousal situations were having on thought content lay in the area of *having impact* on others or being considered strong, important, or powerful. Thus, in the right column of Table 6.4, Georgiadis is described as wanting to win a competition, just as George is in the achievement story. This time, however, it is clear that winning implies an enhanced reputation. The concern is not with doing better but with being recognized as the best architect in the world. Other aspects of this story illustrate the characteristics of a well worked out motivational sequence involving rivals, fears, and means of having impact.

Every time an aspect of either the *n* Achievement, *n* Affiliation, or *n* Power motivational sequence is mentioned in such stories, as indicated by the words in italics, it is counted as $+1$. An additional point is added for thema if the story is mostly about a particular subject, and an overall score for the story is obtained by summing the number of different elements present. Few of the characteristics of the overall coding scheme appear in any given story, but people are asked to write from four to six stories so that they have several opportunities to include ideas that would be scored under one or the other of the motive-coding systems. A score for all stories is called a person's *n* Achievement, *n* Affiliation, or *n* Power score. Once the motivational codes have been established from the arousal experiment, individual differences in the strength of a motive are assessed by having people write stories under neutral conditions so that the observer can discover what they spontaneously think about when they are not under the pressure of any particular motivational demand. What is being measured is how often thoughts spontaneously turn to achievement, to power, or to affiliation goal states. Note that subjects do not know what they are supposed to write in stories of this kind, so conscious values and expectations have less effect on what they write; therefore, this writing is a purer measure of their motive dispositions. The method provides a means of assessing directly the *recurrent concern for a goal state,* which is the essence of the definition of a motivational disposition.

Whereas the motives most commonly studied have been the achievement, affiliation, and power motives, the technique of deriving scoring codes for motives through motivational arousal is completely generalizable, and it has been used to study other motives as well. For example, some soldiers wrote stories ten hours before, one-half hour after, and ten hours after, an atomic explosion during which they were stationed in trenches 4000 yards from the point of the detonation (Walker & Atkinson, 1958; see Chapter 10 of this book). The danger (a "demand" characteristic) elicited more fear-related motivation in stories written before the explosion than in those written when the danger had passed.

In Chapter 1 we discussed the effects of sexual arousal on fantasies, and in other places we will deal with other concerns discovered to result from motivational arousal.

Adequacy of Various Measures of Individual Differences in Motive Strength

Coding stories for various types of goal-oriented content is not the most popular means of measuring individual differences in motive strength. It derived from H. A. Murray's research reported in *Explorations in Personality* (1938), but so also did the method of assessing motive strength by asking subjects how much they agreed with various statements related to different motives. Table 6.5 lists some items Murray also used to evaluate the strength of a person's *n* Achievement, *n* Affiliation, and *n* Power. One obvious advantage of this approach is that it is so much cheaper than coding thought content; a subject's replies—say, on a scale of $+3$ to -3 for each item—can be recorded and can be read by a machine and a person's total score automatically computed without any effort on the part of the experimenter. So a number of measures of motive strength

Table 6.5.

EXAMPLES OF SELF-REPORT ITEMS USED BY MURRAY TO ESTIMATE
THE STRENGTH OF VARIOUS NEEDS (after H. A. Murray, 1938)

Need for Achievement

1. I set difficult goals for myself, which I attempt to reach.
2. I enjoy relaxation wholeheartedly only when it follows the successful completion of a
substantial piece of work.
3. I work like a slave at everything I undertake until I am satisfied with the result.
4. I enjoy work as much as play.

Need for Affiliation

1. I am in my element when I am with a group of people who enjoy life.
2. I become very attached to my friends.
3. I like to hang about with a group of congenial people and talk about anything that
comes up.
4. I go out of my way just to be with my friends.

Need for Power (Dominance)

1. I enjoy organizing or directing activities of a group—team, club, or committee.
2. I argue with zest for my point of view against others.
3. I usually influence others more than they influence me.
4. I feel that I can dominate a social situation.

Note: In Murray's questionnaire the statements for a given need are not presented consecutively, but are
interspersed with others. In later versions of this type of questionnaire, items are included so disagreement also
indicates strength of the need in question, and pairs of statements equated for social desirability are presented so
the choice is not dictated by the tendency to give desirable responses.

based on such self-reports have been carefully developed over the years, including the Edwards Personal Preference Scale (1957), the Jackson Personality Research Form (1966), and the Mehrabian Scales for Achievement and Affiliation Orientation (1969, 1970). How do these measures of motive strength stack up against those obtained from coding thought content? Which is the better method of assessing motive strength?

Murray believed the best method of measuring motive strength was to include information from both these sources, as well as from any other source, such as interviews or behavior in games or role-playing situations. In the assessment centers he designed, a relatively small group of persons was studied intensively over a period of days by a number of expert observers. Subjects were interviewed, tested in a large number of different ways, and watched as they participated in various group activities. Each observer made preliminary estimates of the strength of the subjects' various motives based on all the information available to him or her. Then the observers came together in a diagnostic council in which they discussed at length all the information obtained and estimated the strength of a person's motivation in a particular area. The final judgment by the diagnostic council of, say, the strength of a person's *n* Achievement, was considered to be the best possible way of arriving at the truth about that motive for that person. How does this method of measuring individual differences in motive strength—which we call the *clinical method*—stack up against the self-report method or the method of estimating motive strength from coding spontaneous thought content? Which is the best method?

important

• ALTERNATIVE MEASURES OF MOTIVE STRENGTH EVALUATED ACCORDING TO THE CRITERIA FOR GOOD MEASUREMENT

To answer such questions, we must review the criteria for a good measure of any characteristic. Table 6.6 lays out the major criteria and illustrates how each applies to a physical variable, such as temperature, and a psychological one, such as motivation. The *sensitivity* criterion requires that a measure fluctuate or vary systematically with the presence or absence of, or change in, a characteristic of which it is supposed to be an index. If a lighted match is brought near a column of mercury in a glass tube and the mercury does not rise, the mercury is an insensitive indicator of temperature change. If a self-report does not indicate fear when we know the person is about to make a parachute jump (Epstein, 1962), self-report is not a sensitive indicator of a motive state.

The *uniqueness* criterion requires that the indicator not be influenced by variables other than the one it is supposed to be measuring: if the mercury rises as pressure is applied, a high reading can reflect pressure rather than heat. It was on this ground that we questioned the value of using action as an index of motive strength, because actions such as doing well in school may result from intellectual factors that have nothing to do with motivation.

The *reliability* criterion really has two aspects. In the first place, two observers reading the same index at the same time should give the same report. In the second place, two observations of the same characteristic of the same person under the same conditions should agree.

The *validity-utility* criterion is the most important of all, because it is possible to get a measure that is sensitive, unique, and reliable but that is quite unimportant in that it does not tell anything else about what the person will do in a variety of situations. Psychology, like all science, is an economizing game, the goal of which is to measure the least number of variables that will give the most information about how a person will behave in a variety of situations. In practice, the validity-utility of a measure of human motive strength is judged by the network of correlations (Cronbach & Meehl, 1955) established between it and other things the person does. The network also must make theoretical sense. That is, to be sure we have a measure of motive strength and not some other variable, it must be shown that people who score high on the measure behave as if they were more motivated in this area; for example, if they are high in

Table 6.6.

CRITERIA FOR A GOOD MEASURE OF TEMPERATURE AND MOTIVATION

Criteria of a Good Measure	Meaning	Application to	
		Temperature	Motivation
Sensitivity	Index reflects underlying variable sensitively.	Column of mercury rises regularly as heat is applied.	Behavioral index reflects induced motivational states.
Uniqueness	Index reflects changes in that variable only.	Column of mercury does not rise as pressure is applied.	Behavioral index is relatively uninfluenced by habits, values, and so on.
Reliability	Index gives same reading under same conditions.	Mercury rises to same point if same heat is applied.	Behavioral index gives same value for an individual on repeated testing.
Validity-utility	Index reflects a variable of importance.	Temperature as measured by a thermometer is theoretically and practically useful in predicting what will happen to substances under various conditions.	Motive index shows theoretical properties of a motive and is useful in predicting behavior under various conditions.

n Achievement, they must be more energetic in achievement situations, they must be more sensitive to achievement cues, and they must learn material related to reaching the achievement incentive faster.

Let us now see how each of the three methods of measuring individual differences in motive strength stacks up against the four criteria of a good measure.

Sensitivity

The thought content codes for measuring motive strength pass the sensitivity criterion for a good measure, because they were derived by comparing and contrasting differences in fantasy under unaroused and aroused conditions. The self-report measures pass it less adequately. As mentioned earlier, the thought measure of need for Food (*n* Food) increased monotonically with hours of food deprivation, but self-ratings of hunger did not increase appreciably between four and sixteen hours of food deprivation. Parachute jumpers do not report being as afraid as physiological indexes suggest they are, probably because they are suppressing their feelings of fear in order to go through with the experience. Similarly, self-reported fatigue ratings do not increase in a simple fashion with hours of going without sleep, whereas thought codes do (see, for example, E. J. Murray, 1965).

Personality theorists working with questionnaires usually distinguish between a *trait measure* (asking people what they want usually) and a *state measure* (asking people what they want right now; see Spielberger, Gorsuch, & Lushene, 1970). This corresponds to the distinction between a motive disposition and an aroused motive. To satisfy the sensitivity criterion, theorists should show that an aroused motive (for example, anxiety in response to a threat) increases the state anxiety score and that this somehow relates to the trait anxiety score the person also reports. So far little research has been carried out on whether motive self-reports are sensitive to motivational arousal; what little there is suggests that they are not likely to be sensitive, since they are strongly influenced by other variables, for example, the conscious value placed on particular motive states such as appearing not to be very anxious.

The clinical method of estimating motive strength can hardly be evaluated against the sensitivity criterion, because by definition it includes all sources of information, including the fantasy codes, which do pass the sensitivity criterion. However, since the final clinical judgment also includes self-report measures, which are relatively insensitive to motivational changes, it might be inferred that they are not as sensitive to motive changes as the fantasy measures are by definition.

The sensitivity criterion also implies that the effects of variations in motive strength on thought content will be the same for all people everywhere. Heat applied to a column of mercury will cause it to rise in Peoria and Timbuktu in exactly the same way. But is this true in psychology? Does achievement motive arousal have the same effects on fantasy in different cultures? Perhaps in some cultures it will lead to thoughts about achieving cooperatively, and in others it will lead to thinking about doing things individualistically, as Maehr and Kleiber (1981) have argued. In *The Achievement Motive* (McClelland et al., 1953) it was reported that Navaho males responded to achievement arousal in the same way other males did. That is, they wrote more stories containing achievement imagery (as defined from earlier arousal experiments on people in the United States) than did Navaho males under relaxed testing conditons. Since then, the basic achievement arousal experiment has been replicated in Germany (Heckhausen, 1963), in Brazil (Angelini, 1959) and in Japan (Hayashi & Habu, 1962). The thought characteristics associated with achievement arousal seem to be much the same across different cultures.

On the other hand, some early results obtained using women subjects raised some doubts as to the generality of this conclusion. Neither the achievement-arousing instructions nor the experiences of success and failure that worked for men served to increase the n Achievement scores of women exposed to the same conditions. For example, in one study the mean n Achievement score for college males was -1.46 under relaxed conditions and 3.46 after failure, whereas for college females the mean scores were 1.24 and 0.93, respectively (McClelland et al., 1953). Apparently either the aroused achievement motive affects women's thought processes differently than it affects men's, or the achievement-arousing instructions that were used failed to arouse the motive for women.

The first possibility raises some very serious questions about this whole approach to motive measurement, because it would mean that a whole different scoring system would have to be developed to assess achievement motive strength in women. Fortunately, this did not prove to be necessary for two reasons. In the first place, it was found that *n* Achievement scores for women (using the scoring criteria developed from the arousal experiments with men) correlated with female performance in the same way as for men. That is to say, women who scored high in *n* Achievement behaved in the same way as men who scored high in *n* Achievement, indicating that the measures were as valid for women as for men. In the second place, it was found that the achievement-oriented instructions used to arouse men simply were failing to arouse the achievement motive in some groups of women. In later arousal studies (for example, French & Lesser, 1964), references to the importance of intellectual, career-oriented achievement did increase achievement motivation in women (see Stewart & Chester, 1982). Furthermore, in Germany, Brazil, and Japan, the male achievement-orienting instructions produced the same effects on women's as on men's fantasy. In addition, it was found that judging popularity and personal attributes in public served as achievement incentives for some U.S. women in the sense that under these conditions, women's stories showed the same rise in achievement concerns as the men's stories did when their intelligence and leadership capacity were the incentives used (McClelland et al., 1953).

Thus, methods of arousing the achievement motive (demands plus incentives) may differ in various subgroups of the human population, but so far no one has reported any special fantasy effects of achievement motive arousal that are not included in the coding system originally developed for young men in the United States. Unfortunately, not enough research has been done in other cultures on arousing motives to be sure the same conclusion can be drawn about thought content related to the power and affiliation motives.

Uniqueness

How do the various methods of assessing motive strength stack up against the uniqueness criterion? The clinical method fails it signally. Suppose a number of clinicians pool their judgments of a patient's motivation for treatment, as in a Menninger Clinic study (Luborsky & Sargent, 1956). They all use a number of clues based on their knowledge of a patient's test scores, social behavior, or conduct in a therapeutic hour. Each clinician makes a numerical estimate of how motivated for treatment a particular patient is, and by and large they agree. Is this not the best possible estimate of a patient's motivation? But note in the diagram in Figure 6.9 that the judges' ratings of the level of psychosexual development and ego strength correlate highly with their ratings of motivation for treatment. Furthermore, levels of psychosexual development and ego strength are themselves highly correlated. In other words, the clinicians could not really distinguish very well among these three variables. Because of their common training in the psychoanalytic tradition, they found it difficult to imagine a person at a low level of psychosexual or ego development also being highly motivated for treatment. So it is not clear what clues the judges were actually using in rating the patient's motivation. They may have been responding primarily to his or her level of psychosexual or ego development. If so, the estimate of motivation is really not a measure of motivation at all, but of other things that, in the judges' minds, imply that the patient is motivated to a greater or lesser degree. In short, if the judges are allowed to use many clues in arriving at their assessment of motive strength, the measure is "impure," a hodgepodge of assessments of many different response tendencies the judges believe are related to motive strength.

Self-reports also do not pass the uniqueness criterion very well, in part because they are subject to various types of response biases. For example, some subjects are "yea sayers"; others are "nay sayers" (Couch & Keniston, 1960). The yea sayers tend to agree more with all sorts of statements and the nay sayers to disagree more. A high score on the first four items in Table 6.5 may indicate not only a higher *n* Achievement, but also a greater tendency to agree with any and all statements. Schedules can be corrected for this bias by equalizing the number of statements that have to be agreed or disagreed with in order to get a high score.

Another type of bias comes from the fact that most people tend to agree more with socially desirable items. This bias can be corrected by equating items for their social desirability and forcing the subject to choose between them (Edwards, 1957; Jackson, 1966).

However, the main difficulty with self-ratings so far as the uniqueness criterion is concerned is that they reflect the person's self-image and values. Thus, most U.S. citizens feel they should have a high achievement motive and will agree with statements indicating that they do. On the other hand, most U.S. citizens feel they should not be high in the power motive and will disagree with items indicating that they have such a need. Once in a discussion section for a class in motivation, a student vehemently argued for nearly the whole hour that his *n* Power score obtained from the picture-story method was too high. By the end of the time, everyone in the class was convinced that the student's score was exactly right.

The main contribution of the Freudian revolution to personality theory was

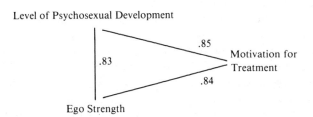

Figure 6.9.

Intercorrelations of Personality Variables as Rated by Judges at the Menninger Clinic (Luborsky & Sargent, 1956).

the demonstration that people's conscious values and unconscious motives are not necessarily the same. This book will adopt the convention of referring to self-report measures of motive strength as *values* (abbreviated to *v*) to avoid confusion on this point.

People's values as reflected in self-ratings have a number of determinants that are not motivational in character. For example, Lynn (1969) developed a self-report measure of *v* Achievement in which entrepreneurs scored higher than students. He inferred from this fact that he had a good measure of achievement motive strength, since entrepreneurs should score higher than students. What he failed to take into account, however, was that entrepreneurs know they have been more successful; if asked, they will say they set difficult goals, prefer work to play, and so forth, because that readily explains to them why they have been more successful. What is taken as an indication of their achievement motive strength is really simply a part of their overall self-image.

Do the thought measures pass the uniqueness criterion? To begin with, in general they are uninfluenced by values or response sets. People who respond to questionnaires showing that they highly value achievement, affiliation, or power do not usually score significantly higher on the corresponding motives as scored in fantasy (see Child, Frank, & Storm, 1956; deCharms, Morrison, Reitman, & McClelland, 1955). Those who value social approval, as measured by the Crowne-Marlowe measure (1964), also do not score higher on any of the three social motives, as checked in a sample of seventy-six adults studied by McClelland, Constantian, Pilon, and Stone (1982).

Can a person fake a high motive score by writing stories with the necessary characteristics? If so, a high score might be obtained even though the motive level was low. Asking subjects to fake a high *n* Achievement score did not produce a significant increase in the mean *n* Achievement score (McClelland et al., 1953), but obviously anyone who has learned the scoring systems as outlined in Table 6.4 can fake a high score. Curiously enough, however, if after learning to fake a high score people tend to think that way much of the time, the motive in fact would appear to have greater salience for them. As we shall see in Chapter 14, one of the ways of increasing motive strength is to teach people to write stories saturated with the thoughts characteristic of people with a strong motive.

The Effect of Conditions of Test Administration on Imaginative Stories.   A more serious problem arises from the fact that story content is very easily influenced by the conditions of test administration, as the arousal experiments demonstrate. This means that the score in an individual's stories may not be the result of the person's own motivation so much as the result of other factors in the testing conditions (see Figure 6.7). Ever since Murray's time it has been stressed that if stories are to reflect personal characteristics, they must be obtained under relaxed conditions in which the subject feels natural and spontaneous. McClelland et al. (1953) reported that ego involvement tended to inhibit the ability of the subjects to fantasize, making their stories unable to be scored.

Lundy (1981a) has systematically investigated the problem by comparing the results obtained when stories were written under the usual relaxed or informal conditions with those written after the introduction of three forms of "pressure" that he thought would evoke stereotyped stories not based on personal motives. He told one group of subjects that the story writing was a test that would reveal "hidden personality tendencies" including "imperfections or minor defects in the personality" (Lundy, 1981a). He stressed to another group of subjects that they should be very careful in writing their stories because he wanted to get them under conditions "which are standardized and carefully controlled" (Lundy, 1981a) so that he could compare the results for normal subjects with those written by people who were psychotic or brain damaged. Before asking a third group to write stories, Lundy simply administered a personality test dealing with affiliative matters, which was supposed to tell them whether they were the kind of person who was always at ease or quite insecure in groups. He felt that all the special instructions would make the subjects more cautious and more likely to write stereotyped stories rather than ones reflecting their personal motives. He developed a special coding device, called the *ego control score,* to see if in fact this occurred. The score measured the amount of incoherence in a story—that is, as shown by jumping from one thought to another—and the amount of transcendence as shown by the subjects' bringing in characters and objects not in the picture.

All three types of special instructions designed to increase pressure decreased transcendence and incoherence; this significantly increased the ego control score, showing that the stories were more stereotyped. What is even more important is that the motive scores obtained when stories were written under special instructions lost their validity. That is, they no longer correlated with behaviors characteristic of the motives in question, as they had when obtained under relaxed conditions.

Lundy also had obtained a number of other measures of the usual correlates of *n* Achievement, *n* Affiliation, and *n* Power, such as the kinds of television shows the students typically watched. He found, as expected, that the subjects higher in *n* Achievement were more likely to watch information shows on television, those high in *n* Affiliation were more likely to watch soap operas and comedies, and those high in *n* Power were more likely to watch sports on television than students low in any of these motives. This was true, however, only when the motive scores were obtained under relaxed conditions. When the students felt threatened in any way because of the instructions, the validity coefficients —that is, the correlations with activities associated with the motives—were reduced significantly and, for all practical purposes, they disappeared. Figure 6.10 summarizes the results in a very striking way. It shows that the classes that took the test under relaxed conditions—referred to as the *personal schemata group*—all scored low in ego control and high in the validity estimates of the motive scores obtained. The reverse was true for the three types of special instruction groups: they scored higher in ego control and lower in the validity of the motive measures obtained.

In another study, Lundy (1980) reviewed all reports between 1966 and 1980 that included a measure of *n* Achievement, *n* Affiliation, or *n* Power. He found, for example, that of the 195 reports that employed a measure of *n* Achievement,

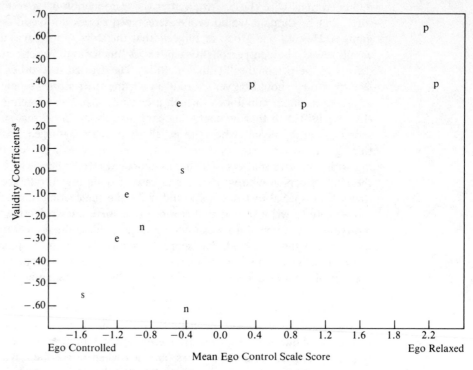

^aFisher *z*-transformations to normalize the distribution of coefficients.

Figure 6.10.

Scatterplot of Validity Coefficients and Mean Ego Control Scale Scores for All Classes (Units of Analysis) in the Study. p = personal schemata group; n = normative group; s = structured group; e = ego-threatened group (after Lundy, 1981a).

124 found significant differences using this measure, and fifty-one reported insignificant differences. He then went on to look for factors that might be responsible for the fact that some investigators found the measure to be valid and others, invalid. Among the factors that were important was the status of the test administrator. When the administrator was an authority figure—which could be interpreted as introducing some kind of pressure on the subjects—the validity coefficients of the motive measures were very much less than when the administrator was a fellow student or behaved in a casual manner. Lundy also found that manipulations of instructions strongly affected the validity of the scores obtained by the test. Even simply calling the story-writing procedure a *personality test* rather than a picture-story exercise adversely affected the validity of the scores obtained from the stories.

In short, motive scores obtained from imaginative stories do not uniquely reflect motive differences under all conditions of test administration. It is extremely important that the conditions of administration be relaxing for the results to satisfy the uniqueness criterion. What is particularly valuable about Lundy's research is that he has developed a measure of ego control that can serve as a check for experimenters as to whether or not they have succeeded in relaxing the subjects taking the test. If the average ego control score is too high, there is evidence that other factors will influence the motive scores and that they will no longer be good indicators of motive strength.

Reliability

Fantasy measures of human motives pass the sensitivity and the uniqueness criteria for a good measure, but they have difficulty satisfying the reliability criterion. In fact, fantasy makes many psychologists nervous, because it has a "now you see it, now you don't" quality that is the very antithesis of good scientific measurement. One analyst sees one motive pattern in a dream, while another sees something else. The problem of getting high observer agreement has been solved for measures of the sort illustrated in Table 6.4. The criteria for the presence or absence of achievement, power, or affiliation imagery and their subcategories are so objective that it is possible to train observers to agree almost perfectly on the scores they obtain for a given set of stories.

Coding Reliability.   Two methods of testing coding reliability have been used. The first involves the percentage of agreement on the presence of a category. Suppose two judges, A and B, score six stories for the presence or absence of achievement imagery. Suppose Judge A scores achievement imagery in Stories 1, 3, and 5, and Judge B scores it in Stories 1, 3, 5, and 6. The percentage of agreement is computed by multiplying the number of stories in which they agreed the category was present (namely, three) by two ($3 \times 2 = 6$) and dividing by the sum of the number of times each judge scored for the presence of the category ($3 + 4 = 7$). This gives a ratio of 6/7, or 86 percent, which is a representative figure for the amount of agreement usually found for different categories in the various motive scoring systems.

Note that in this ratio it is necessary to have a denominator that covers how frequently a judge scores a given category, since this tends to vary somewhat; if we only looked at the percentage of agreement, without taking the level of scoring into account, it would be technically possible to get fairly high agreement if one judge scored every story as containing the category.

The percentage of agreement is a conservative reliability estimate, because it does not include agreement on the absence of a category. The reason it does not is that some of the categories are quite infrequent, so including agreement on absence could overestimate the reliability of coding. For example, suppose Judge A scores "help" in the *n* Achievement scoring system in Story 1 and Judge B, in Story 3. There is perfect disagreement on presence; however, they do agree that the category is absent in four of the stories, which would yield a percentage of agreement score of $(2 \times 4)/12$, or 75 percent, which seems like an overestimate.

Another way of checking coding reliability is to correlate the total scores for an individual obtained by two different coders. These correlations between well-trained scorers run between .85 and .95, indicating that two different judges arrive at about the same score for the same person (see McClelland et al., 1953; Winter, 1973). The only difficulty with this measure is that it is still technically possible to get high correlations between two sets of scores while one judge is scoring more than the other judge overall, so the mean scores for a group of subjects could be higher for Judge A than for Judge B even though their agreement on the rank order of the two sets of subjects was nearly perfect. Thus, the same judge must be used in scoring all subjects to be compared, or the two judges must be calibrated very carefully so as to arrive at the same level of scoring.

Test-Retest Reliability.   The second meaning of *reliability* involves whether testing individuals on repeated occasions yields the same motive score. One traditional way of checking for this kind of reliability is to divide the test into two equal halves and see if the person scores the same on both halves. This is sometimes referred to as the *split-half method* of estimating reliability. For example, if a student gets an *n* Achievement score of 4 on Pictures A, C, and E, he or she should get a score of 3 to 5 on Pictures B, D, and F rather than, say, a score of -1, which would indicate great inconsistency in the two halves of the test. The correlation from sets of *n* Achievement scores obtained from two groups of three pictures each was reported to be as high as .64 in *The Achievement Motive* (McClelland et al., 1953), but a later review of research suggested that these internal consistency correlations generally run from .30 to .40, indicating unsatisfactory reliability by traditional psychometric standards (Entwisle, 1972). In contrast, internal reliability correlations for self-report measures are much higher, from .70 to .90 (Entwisle, 1972; McClelland, 1980).

However, Atkinson, Bongort, and Price (1977) have argued that traditional psychometric theory is wrong in assuming that the response to any test item (here, a story written to any picture) is an isolated and completely independent test of the strength of some underlying characteristic such as *n* Achievement. Instead, they have developed a theory that stresses the continuity of the thought stream. In their view, response tendencies having to do with achievement, affiliation, or power are continuously competing for expression in thought. If the achievement tendency is expressed in connection with the first picture, its expression "uses up" the tendency and reduces it in strength so that the next strongest tendency—say, for affiliation—will appear in the next story. Thus, there is no reason to expect consistency in response tendencies from one item to the next. In fact, a well-known phenomenon in psychology, called *associative refractory phase* (see Telford, 1931), states that subjects are unlikely to repeat an association they have just given.

Atkinson and Birch (1978) took their analysis further and developed a computer program that, with certain built-in assumptions, generated curves like those shown in Figure 6.11. In this simulation there are three tendencies competing for expression. It is further assumed that the subject is telling four stories, which divide the time line into equal quarters. Tendency X is for achievement. If we sum the time spent expressing X in the four stories (when the tendency to write about X was stronger than the tendencies to write about Y and Z), we obtain the values of 7, 3, 4, and 5. If we compare the achievement tendencies expressed for Stories 1 and 4 with those for Stories 2 and 3 on two alternative halves of the test, we get values of 12 and 7, indicating a major discrepancy, or low internal inconsistency.

Using their program, Atkinson, Bongort, and Price (1977) generated twenty-five computer simulations; in each, subjects were arbitrarily classified as high, middle, or low in *n* Achievement. They then measured the percentage of time that each subject would spend thinking about achievement, according to their computer simulation with different assumptions about the internal consistency measures from one time period to the next. Their measure of the validity of the *total time spent thinking about X measure* was the extent to which it agreed with the *n* Achievement level assigned to an individual in advance in the computer program. That is, if a person was assigned to the top third of the *n* Achievement scoring distribution in advance, he or she should be in the top third of those spending time thinking about achievement in the computer simulation.

In Figure 6.12 they plotted construct validity (the percentage of subjects

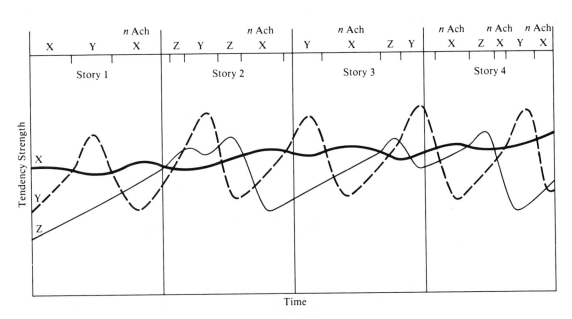

Figure 6.11.

Response Tendencies Competing for Expression During the Telling of Four Stories (after Atkinson, 1980).

correctly placed in various thirds of the *n* Achievement distribution by the time-spent measure) against a measure of internal consistency (here, Cronbach's alpha, a more generalized measure of internal consistency than the usual split-half correlations). Notice that the overall time spent thinking about achievement is an excellent index of "true" *n* Achievement scores, even when the internal consistency measure is very low or even, in one case, negative. Their conclusion is that "the construct validity of thematic apperceptive measures does not require internal consistency reliability as supposed by traditional test theory" (Atkinson et al., 1977).

Not everyone accepts all the assumptions involved in the computer model generated by Atkinson and Birch. Others will remain perplexed by the practical problem of deciding which score to use if, in fact, they are different on different halves of the test. But at the least this approach suggests that the need for internal consistency in measures of this sort must be carefully thought through.

Another way to look at the fantasy measures of motive strength is in terms of a multiple regression model in which the pictures represent independent estimates of the true score. In multiple regression it is advantageous for several de-

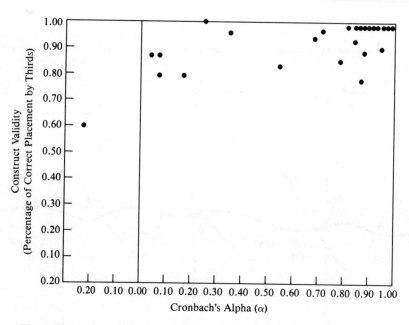

Figure 6.12.

Relationship of Construct Validity and Internal Consistency (α) in Twenty-five Simulations of TATs Varying Design and Parameter Values. *Construct validity* refers to the percentage of subjects correctly placed by total time in achievement activity into rank-ordered thirds of true motive strength defined by computer input (after Atkinson & Birch, 1978, after Atkinson, Bongort, & Price, 1977).

terminants of an overall score to be uncorrelated with each other, because their contribution to the total score will be greater if each is not influenced by its association with another determinant. McClelland (1980) puts it this way: Motives in psychology are used to explain *"inconsistencies* in behavior just as habits explain consistencies. When a hungry dog is trying to get out of a cage to get to food, it will try a wide variety of *different* responses. Why should we expect it to provide internally consistent responses? If it is whining, it may not be scratching; if it is trying to push through the slats, it is not pawing at the latch. One would not expect high correlations among these responses any more than one would expect signs of achievement motivation in different stories to be highly correlated." It is the total sum of all these different responses that should be the best indicator of motive strength.

The Influence of the Set to Be Creative or Consistent.   But here again a problem arises. The correlation of the total *n* Achievement or *n* Power score from a set of four to six stories obtained on one occasion is not very close to the same scores obtained from the same individual on a second occasion. The correlations typically run from .20 to .40 (Entwisle, 1972; McClelland et al., 1953; Winter, 1973), again suggesting a reliability that is too low for the measures to be taken very seriously. Part of the reason for this variability lies in the fact that the chief requirement for a true reliability test is not met, for the subjects are not in the same situation the second time they take the test. They are set to respond differently the second time. They have seen the pictures before and wonder why they are being asked to take the test again. The instructions tell them to "be creative," which they interpret to mean that they should tell "another story" to the same picture. They are set to be creative. If they tell different stories to the same pictures, they are unlikely to get similar motive scores. If different pictures are used, the test-retest correlations are scarcely any higher, perhaps because the subjects are still under the impression that they should be creative and tell different stories, but more probably because the subjects find the experience strange and wonder what is going on.

As Lundy's results discussed in the previous section show, if subjects feel in any way threatened by the procedure and not completely relaxed, the scores obtained seem to be the product of normative or stereotyped, rather than personal, schemata. There is still the problem of which score to use for a given individual, and in general, research has shown that the scores obtained from the first testing are more valid than those obtained on second testings, probably because the second testing is not understood by the subjects (see Atkinson, 1980).

Winter and Stewart tested the possiblity that it was the "be creative" set that lowered test-retest correlations. They instructed the subjects as follows: "Do not worry about whether your stories are similar or different from the stories you wrote before. Write whatever stories you wish" (Winter & Stewart, 1977). Under these instructions the test-retest correlation for the *n* Power score rose to .58, as contrasted to correlations in the .20s when the second test was administered with the usual "be creative" instruction. In testing some high-school students a year later, Lundy (1981b) also told them they were free to tell stories that were the same as or different from those they told last time. He obtained a test-retest correlation of .56, which compares favorably with the stability of measures obtained from questionnaires after one year.

In a sense, the reliability issue is the obverse of the sensitivity criterion. Motive measures based on coding spontaneous thought patterns are unusually sensitive to situational disturbances, so replicating experiments and getting the same scores for individuals on two different occasions represent more difficulties than are common in psychological research. Nevertheless, they do yield reliable results if care is taken to keep the subjects relaxed and unusual response sets are removed.

Klinger (1968) understood this problem but attempted to solve it in the wrong way. He tested subjects alone in a seven-by-seven-foot soundproofed room, eliminating all personal contact with the experimenter. Instructions were given to the subject by means of signs, audio tapes, slides, and films. They were asked to sit quietly for twenty-five minutes in order to reduce such things as associative variability. This did not increase the reliability of the measures obtained, but as Winter (1973) points out, the situation for the subject was a very peculiar one; it was not at all patterned after H. A. Murray's early insistence that subjects must be kept relaxed and spontaneous, the conditions which have been shown ever since to yield the most valid and relaible motive scores.

Test-retest and internal reliability correlations for self-report and clinical estimates of motive strength are much higher—in the range of .70 to .90. So far as the clinical judgments are concerned, the high correlations do not mean much, because—as the last section pointed out—the judges are responding to some overall picture of the subjects rated, which remains stable, rather than to the specific motivational aspects of the subject's personality.

The reported consistency of self-reports represents an exaggerated estimate of "true" consistency for several reasons. The most important is that subjects answering a questionnaire are set by the instructions to respond consistently, since they are told to be honest and frank. If they answer a question differently on a second occasion, they might easily feel either dishonest on one occasion or the other, or at the very least, foolish in not knowing themselves very well. The tendency toward consistency is abetted also by response sets like the tendency to admit or deny unfavorable characteristics or to agree or disagree with most items.

Furthermore, the subjects are typically asked more or less the same question in a dozen different ways (see Table 6.5). If people say in one part of the questionnaire that they are very attached to their friends, it might seem like a reflection on their honesty or intelligence to say in another part of the questionnaire that they do not go out of their way to be with their friends. If they had said that they set difficult goals for themselves, it just seems reasonable that they should also agree that they work like a slave.

Worst of all, many motivational inventories contain items referring to the past, which ought to evoke the same response every time the subject answers the question. If subjects say they can remember "playing sick" to get out of something, they should say that every time they are confronted with the item. A difficulty with items like these is that they have to continue to be scored as indicating the presence of a particular need even though a person might have changed. In this case, sensitivity is sacrificed to reliability. Despite these difficulties, most self-report motive inventories have satisfactory, though somewhat inflated, reliability.

Validity-Utility

From the behaviorist tradition covered in Chapter 3, we learned that motives drive or energize, orient, and select behavior. A more motivated animal is more energetic, it directs its attention toward cues relevant to the motive more readily, and it learns more quickly to take the acts that lead it to the goal it is seeking. So presumed measure of motive strength in people should satisfy these criteria in order for the measures to be considered valid indicators of differences in motive strength. That is, people high in *n* Achievement, as compared with people low in *n* Achievement, should be more energetic in producing achievement-related acts, should be more sensitive to achievement-related cues, and should learn material related to *n* Achievement incentive more quickly. The motive measures based on operant thought content have been tested against these criteria, whereas self-report and clinical judgments for the most part have not. Scattered throughout the chapters on the different motive dispositions are many studies indicating the validity-utility of the measures, so it is only necessary here to give a brief summary of the type of study that demonstrates validity according to these criteria. So far as the *energizing* criterion is concerned, studies have shown that the *n* Achievement score is associated with more frequent entrepreneurial acts (Andrews, 1967), the *n* Power score with more frequently getting into arguments (McClelland, 1975), and the *n* Affiliation score with more frequent affiliative acts (Constantian, 1981; see Chapter 13 of this book).

So far as the orienting or sensitizing function of motives is concerned, an early study (McClelland & Liberman, 1949) demonstrated that subjects high in *n* Achievement showed faster recognition of achievement-related words rapidly presented in a tachistoscope if the words were positive (like *success*) rather than negative (like *failure*). It was as if they were "preset" to see such words so that they recognized them sooner than other subjects. The same effect has been demonstrated even more dramatically for subjects high in *n* Power as they are exposed to pictures representing power or neutral cues.

Through electrodes attached to their scalps over the occipital area of the brain, which receives visual sensations, it has been shown that subjects high in *n* Power respond with a greater electrical potential change to pictures representing power than to neutral pictures as early as 0.1 to 0.2 second after the picture has been exposed. Those low in *n* Power show no difference in visual responsiveness to power and neutral pictures (McClelland, Davidson, & Saron, 1979; see Chapter 8 of this book). What is particularly important about this finding is that it demonstrates that compared with subjects low in *n* Power, the brains of subjects high in *n* Power are preset to respond more strongly to power cues in the occipital area, where visual information is first projected. The difference is in the receiving system, and not just in the verbal or motor response to motive-related cues.

So far as the criterion of facilitating learning is concerned, high *n* Achievement was early shown to lead to improvement in performance where the task was difficult enough for improvements to occur. Figure 6.13 shows the relevant findings. Subjects were asked to unscramble letters like *WTSE* to make a word and continue doing so for twenty minutes (McClelland et al., 1953). Subjects high and low in *n* Achivement started out at about the same level of performance in the first four minutes. By the last four minutes, however, the subjects high in *n* Achievement were unscrambling somewhat more than five words more in the four-minute period than they had at the beginning, whereas those low in *n* Achievement were performing pretty much the same at the end as they had been at the beginning.

The difference in gains is highly significant. Similar studies have been carried out for the other motives. Subjects high in *n* Power learned associations faster between pictures and words if they are power related than did subjects low in *n* Power, whereas there was no difference in learning speed if the picture-word pairs were unrelated to power (McClelland, Davidson, Saron, & Floor, 1980). Subjects high in *n* Affiliation learned complex networks of social relationships more quickly than did subjects low in *n* Affiliation (see Chapter 9).

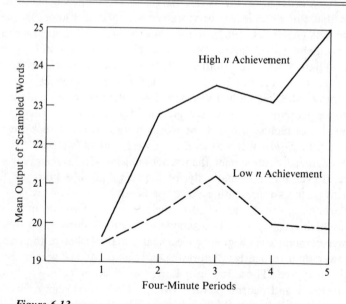

Figure 6.13.

Mean Output of Scrambled Words per Four-Minute Period for Subjects with High and Low *n* Achievement Scores (McClelland, Atkinson, Clark, & Lowell, 1953).

A Comparison of the Validity-Utility of Self-report and Fantasy Measures of the Need for Achievement. In one study, the ability of a motive score based either on fantasy coding or on self-report to satisfy the validity-utility criterion for a measure of motive strength was directly compared. The results are shown in Table 6.7. Here the orienting function of a motive is assessed by the proportion of subjects taking moderate risks in a ringtoss game. The expectation is that subjects high in *n* Achievement should focus their attention more on what has been defined as the achievement incentive—that is, a moderately challenging task. Subjects classified as high in *n* Achievement by the fantasy measure do significantly more often focus attention on the moderately challenging task, as expected according to theory.

But if subjects are classified as high in *n* Achievement by the self-report measure—here obtained from the Edwards Personal Preference Schedule (1957)—they do not behave according to expectation but even focus on the achievement incentive less often than those low in *n* Achievement according to the self-report measure. The energizing function of motivation was measured in this study by the percentage of subjects persisting longer than average when they were taking a final examination. Once again the fantasy measure correctly predicts who will persist longer, and the self-report measure does not.

Table 6.7.

VALIDITY-UTILITY OF FANTASY AND SELF-REPORT MEASURES OF *n* ACHIEVEMENT IN PREDICTING BEHAVIOR (after Atkinson & Litwin, 1960)

Motive Function	*Fantasy Measure*	*Self-report Measure*
A. Orienting	Percentage taking moderate risks in a ringtoss game	
High *n* Achievement	61	36
Low *n* Achievement	36	62
	$p = .04$	$p = .02$
B. Driving	Percentage persisting longer than average in a final examination	
High *n* Achievement	60	42
Low *n* Achievement	32	55
	$p = .03$	n.s.
C. Selecting	Percentage above average in final examination grade	
High *n* Achievement	64	58
Low *n* Achievement	32	46
	$p = .02$	n.s.

So far as the selecting function of motivation is concerned, subjects classified as high in *n* Achievement by the fantasy measure performed better on the final examination, suggesting either that the motive had led them throughout the course to learn the material better or that they dealt with the questions more efficiently at the time of the test itself. And once again, the self-report method of classifying subjects as high or low in *n* Achievement did not successfully predict which ones would perform better on the final examination. This last result is somewhat atypical for reasons that will be discussed later, since subjects high in *n* Achievement do not usually get higher grades. However, the results are included here because they compare the validity of the two ways of measuring motive strength against the three validity criteria for a motive in the compass of a single study.

The fact is that those who use self-report or clinical assessment methods of measuring motive strength have relied heavily on the "face validity" of their measures. It is enough to observe that items like those in Table 6.5 obviously deal with the content of various motive systems. Why worry if people classified as high or low by this method actually behave as they ought to behave if they were more or less motivated on the dimension in question? Yet as we have seen, the self-reports may reflect other variables, like values, that are not motives, and it is only by using the functional criteria for the presence of a motive that we can distinguish between motives and values.

Values do influence behavior. For example, deCharms et al. (1955) report that students with high self-reported achievement drives were more likely to be influenced by a professor's opinions on the quality of a painting than students low on this measure. So those who say that they work hard and strive for achievement clearly *value* achievement in that they tend to look for standards of excellence in judging the worthwhileness of something. Conscious values can clearly affect judgments without leading to behavior that can be regarded as motivated.

A number of self-report measures of differences in motive strength have been developed, because they are cheaper and easier to use (Atkinson & O'Connor, 1966; Edwards, 1957; Hurley, 1955; Jackson, 1966), but they either have not been tested against the validity criteria or have not shown good validity-utility. The one exception is a carefully designed achievement orientation test developed by Mehrabian (1969). The items on the test were taken from achievement motivation theory and do not deal as openly with achievement values as those in the early Murray schedule and its later derivatives. For example, Mehrabian included items such as "I think more of the future than the present or the past" or "I would rather work on a task where I alone am responsible for the final product than one in which many people contribute to the final product." He found that a thirty-four-item scale of this type correlated significantly with the *n* Achievement score obtained from fantasy and also had some validity in the sense that people who scored high on it correctly solved more problems than those who scored low on it. However, the correlation with the fantasy *n* Achievement score is not high, and the Mehrabian measure has the disadvantage of correlating significantly with measures of social desirability, indicating that it is not a pure measure of motive strength. Thus, there is little justification for using it as a substitute for the fantasy *n* Achievement score, which has been extensively validated.

In summary, it is clear that the measures of motive strength based on coding thought content are better than the measures obtained from self-reports or clinical judgments for a variety of reasons. The fantasy measures were more carefully derived by actual comparison of how people think when a motive is aroused as compared with how they think when it is not aroused. The fantasy measures provide a more unique index of motive strength, since they are relatively uninfluenced by values, response biases, and other determinants of behavior. They are probably as reliable as the self-report measures when the concept of reliability is properly understood, and they certainly have more proved validity by the criteria generally established in behavior theory for determining whether behavior is motivated or not. The major difficulty with the fantasy measures is that they are very sensitive to situational influences, and great care must be taken when stories are obtained to be sure subjects are relaxed and spontaneous. Self-report measures of motive strength are reliable and inexpensive to obtain, and they provide a good index of a person's value orientations. As measures of motive strength, however, they have shown little validity-utility. Whereas clinical judgments of motive strength may seem to have more face validity, since they take everything into account, they are practically worthless as independent measures of motive strength alone, precisely because they take so much into account. That is, it is difficult to know how much a rating reflects motive strength or any number of other variables.

For these reasons, the emphasis in this book is on research done using the fantasy measures of motive strength, because they deal more narrowly with problems of motivation per se. However, the influence of information obtained in self-reports will be discussed again in Chapter 12, on cognitive influences on motivation, and in Chapters 13 and 14, which deal with the interaction of motives and values in determining response strength and in changing behavior.

NOTES AND QUERIES

1. In the muscle tension experiment, it is usually assumed that increased tension somehow directly affects the learning. But the result obtained might also be explained in motivational terms. Try to make such an analysis. Remember that the subject is trying to please the experimenter by doing two things at once—squeeze a dynamometer and learn some nonsense syllables. How could increasing emphasis on the first task at first facilitate and then inhibit performing the second? Would such an analysis suggest that the inverted *U* effect might be obtained by requiring the subject to perform *any* two tasks, even if one did not involve direct physiological arousal?

2. The text suggests several reasons why very heavy demands may make performance less efficient. What are they? Has your performance ever suffered when either you yourself or others expected too much of you? Why?

3. The text states that the money incentive means different things, depending on the motives of the people involved. Give some examples. For instance, what might the money incentive mean for poor people, for people with a strong achievement drive, or for people concerned about fair pay?

4. Under what conditions is an intent or desire for something most likely to indicate the presence of an aroused motive? According to Figure 6.1, such a situation shold occur when the other determinants of an intent are minimized or held constant. Describe some situations in which this happens.

5. If different incentives arouse the achievement motive for different groups of people, does that mean we have to think in terms of different kinds of achievement motivation? For example, some women's achievement motive is not aroused by references to their leadership capacity but by references to their social skill; offering money rewards increases *n* Achievement more in working-class than in middle-class people (see Douvan, 1956). What exactly does this mean? Is the motive itself different in different groups, or is the way it is expressed likely to be different?

6. Several organizations have been trying to teach people "success" motivation. Is there such a thing as success motivation? How does it relate to *n* Achievement or other motives psychologists measure?

7. Why do you think arousal instructions that increased *n* Achievement in men in the United States also tended to arouse the achievement motive in women in other countries more consistently than in the United States?

8. Blood pressure varies greatly depending on what a person is doing, yet physicians believe their measures of blood pressure are reliable enough to be depended on. What precautions do they take to insure greater reliability of their measures? Is what they do analogous to what should be done to insure the reliability of measures of motive strength obtained from fantasy?

9. Validity-utility is sometimes defined in terms of whether something is measuring what it is supposed to be measuring—that is, is it giving a *true* estimate of the characteristic in question? But how do you know what provides a *true* measure of a motive? If a person says "I have a strong need to achieve" over and over again, is that not valid evidence that he or she truly has a strong need for achievement? Why or why not?

10. Suppose an experimenter (a faculty member) says to a student, "I want you to perform as well as you can on this experiment, in which you will get a mild shock for mistakes." Make as complete a descrition as you can of all the incentives and motives that might be involved for the student. If your picture of the motivational situation turns out to be complex, might this explain why the results of such experiments are often confusing?

11. If measures of anxiety state go up under the threat of electric shock, do you think that means self-reported anxiety would provide a good estimate of the

anxiety avoidance motive? For example, suppose people exposed to the threat of shock say they are "nervous" more often. Does that mean people who say they are nervous in general, even when they are not threatened by shock, are more likely to have a stronger anxiety avoidance motive? Why or why not? In other words, might the response pass the sensitivity, but not the uniqueness, criterion of a good measure?

12. The fantasy measure of motives employs written daydreams, but Freud based his analyses on night dreams. What would be the advantages and disadvantages of asking subjects for dreams they had had and scoring them? (For a reference, see LeVine, 1966.)

Part 3

*Important
Motive Systems*

7

The Achievement Motive

In Chapter 6 we examined in detail how individual differences in motive strength can best be measured, because in science, measurement is of central importance. Without it we would still be in the position of McDougall, speculating about what motives there are and how they affect behavior. This chapter and the next chapters in Part 3 attempt to summarize what has been found out about several social motives that have been measured by the method recommended in Chapter 6—by coding fantasy or spontaneous thought patterns. For each motive we will start by explaining how the method of measuring it in fantasy was developed, then turn to the evidence indicating it really is a measure of a motive using the validity criteria established in Chapter 6, and finally summarize what is known about how people behave who score high in the motive measured in this way. Naturally, there has been curiosity about how people develop a strong motive of one type or another, so at the end of each chapter is a section summarizing what is known about how people acquire such a motive.

The emphasis on measurement may seem boring or unnecessary, but the fact is that progress has been made in the field of motivation only as some standardization in measurement occurred. Before that, investigators kept coming up with different or contradictory results or insisting that what was really meant by some motive, such as the need to achieve, was quite different from what somebody else had claimed. For example, do you think Jesus had a strong need to achieve? He certainly was ambitious in his efforts to save the world. In fact, he was so ambitious that he gave up his life for the cause. The whole point of this chapter is that once the method it describes of measuring the need to achieve has been established and accepted, the question about Jesus can be empirically answered. His sayings can be scored for achievement imagery, and the frequency of this imagery can be compared with its frequency in the sayings of others. If Jesus scores high, then *by definition* he has a high *n* Achievement. Otherwise, he does not. There can be no further argument on the point.

Thus, it is obviously of primary importance to establish how the motive is measured in the first place. The scientific meaning of a concept like the need to achieve is defined by how it is measured once that has been established. Of course, the method of measurement can be questioned, or another method proposed, but whatever the method, it must pass the criteria for a good measure discussed in Chapter 6. The measures described in this and subsequent chapters for the most part do pass those criteria and have led to the accumulation of some very new and exciting information about the way certain key social motives govern our behavior both individually and socially.

• MEASURING THE NEED FOR ACHIEVEMENT

The strength of the achievement motive in individuals is best measured by the *n* Achievement score derived from coding the thought content of imaginative stories, as explained in Chapter 6. The *n* Achievement score is usually obtained from stories written to pictures, but it also can be validly obtained from stories written to sentence stems such as "A father and his son looking out at a field" (McClelland, 1977a) or from the French (1958a) Test of Insight, in which the subject is asked to explain why a man behaves as he does in a brief written description, such as "Joe is always willing to listen" or "Ray works much harder than most people." Heckhausen (1963) used the picture-story format but developed a slightly different coding system for n Achievement that yielded four separate measures: Hope of Success (HS), Fear of Failure (FF), the difference between the two (HS − FF, or the Net Hope score), and the sum of HS + FF.

Atkinson (1958) and his students also were interested in the negative aspect of achievement motivation, or fear of failure, and developed a Resultant Achievement Motivation (RAM) score, which was obtained by cross-classifying n Achievement scores with scores on a Test Anxiety questionnaire developed by Mandler and Sarason (1952). Subjects above the median in n Achievement and below the median in Test Anxiety are considered to be most clearly oriented toward approaching achievement, whereas those below the median in n Achievement and above the median in Test Anxiety are considered to be most oriented toward avoiding achievement (or fearing failure; see Atkinson & Litwin, 1960). Most of the results Atkinson and his students report are obtained by contrasting the performance of these two groups.

However, it is not entirely clear—either on theoretical or empirical grounds—that the fear of failure is the direct opposite of the need to achieve (as assumed by this procedure). Therefore, in this chapter we will consider so far as possible only the effects of the achievement motive by itself on behavior, leaving the treatment of the fear of failure and other avoidance motives to Chapter 10.

One other method of measuring n Achievement levels has been used with some success. It is based on Aronson's (1958) finding that individuals high in n Achievement in fantasy spontaneously draw different shapes—that is, doodle differently—as compared with individuals low in n Achievement. The former draw more discrete S shapes and diagonals, whereas the latter produce more "fuzzy" multiple waves: in short, people low in n Achievement "scribble" more, make less effort to introduce variety, and are satisfied with simple repetitive motions. A simple test of this difference can be obtained by flashing very briefly a couple of slides with some barely visible markings on them and asking the subject to reproduce them. Since nothing much can be seen, what the subjects produce represents their spontaneous drawing tendencies, which can be coded to yield an n Achievement index, scoring +1 for diagonals and S shapes, and −1 for multiple waves and a few other such characteristics.

This index has the advantage that it is apparently even less influenced than the picture-story exercise by the subject's sets introduced by test administration conditions, as reviewed by Lundy (1981a). McClelland (1961) found it to correlate better than the verbal measure with theoretical behavioral correlates of n Achievement in a cross-national study involving different test administrators in different countries. It has also been used to estimate n Achievement levels in ancient civilizations—particularly those with no written records—since it can be applied with minor changes to pottery designs (see Chapter 11). However, since it lacks "face validity"—that is, it does not have obvious meaning in itself—it has not been widely used.

As Chapter 6 mentioned, there have been many attempts to develop "objective" measures of the strength of the achievement motive by employing various questionnaires. None of these measures has proved to be a consistently valid indicator of the strength of the achievement motive in the sense that it passes the criteria for a good measure described in Chapter 6 as well as the *n* Achievement score does.

Typical of such attempts is Schmalt's Achievement Motivation Grid (1976). Following a procedure adopted some years earlier in the Iowa Picture Interpretation Test (Johnston, 1957), Schmalt asks subjects to look at pictures and pick statements that describe what the characters in the pictures are thinking. The various statements written below the pictures represent aspects of the *n* Achievement scoring system. Achievement motive scores obtained in this way do have some predictive value for goal-setting behavior, but not for other well-known characteristics of achievement motivation measured by coding fantasy. The result is typical of such research, because a conscious cognitive, evaluative component is much more strongly present in picking choices among alternatives in a questionnaire than in generating spontaneous responses to a picture or a sentence stem. This cognitive, evaluative component is not part of the motive system per se, although it influences it in many ways (see Chapter 12). In everyday language it represents values (that is, the extent to which a person values achievement) rather than motives (that is, the extent to which a person gets satisfaction from thinking about or doing things better; see also Chapter 5).

• EVIDENCE THAT THE NEED FOR ACHIEVEMENT SCORE MEASURES A MOTIVE

As we concluded from studying the behaviorist tradition in Chapter 3, motives drive, orient, and select behavior. Chapter 6 presented some preliminary data showing that individuals who score high on various fantasy-based motive coding systems generally behave differently in these three respects from those who score low on the same motive-scoring systems. As compared with subjects low in *n* Achievement, those who score high in *n* Achievement show various signs of a higher level of physiological activation: They show more muscle tension when concentrating on a task (Mücher & Heckhausen, 1962); a stronger galvanic skin response, indicating more imperceptible sweating due to activation of the sympathetic nervous system (Raphelson, 1957; Vogel, Baker, & Lazarus, 1958); and a higher critical flicker fusion frequency (Wendt, 1955). That is, if two adjacent lights are flicked on and off in rapid succession, they will eventually fuse into perceived motion from one to the other, if the time between the two lights is short enough. A measure of alertness or vigilance can be obtained by determining how short the interval between the two lights must be before the person reports apparent fusion or apparent motion. Subjects high in *n* Achievement report fusion only after a much shorter period of time has elapsed between the two light flashes, indicating greater vigilance than subjects with low *n* Achievement.

The fact that subjects low in *n* Achievement sometimes show signs of greater physiological arousal (see Raphelson, 1957; Vogel et al., 1958) appears to be due to the fact that very often subjects low in *n* Achievement are high in another motive—namely, the fear of failure, which, since it is anxiety producing, leads to physiological arousal.

Subjects high in *n* Achievement are also more oriented toward or more sensitive to certain stimuli. As compared with those low in *n* Achievement, they perceive achievement-related words more quickly when they are exposed very rapidly in a tachistoscope (McClelland & Liberman, 1949; Moulton, Raphelson, Kristofferson, & Atkinson, 1958). That is, they pay more attention to cues related to performance improvement. Bartmann (1965) showed that they gained more in learning how to do a task from a period of programmed instruction than subjects low in *n* Achievement. They tend to recall more interrupted tasks in a context in which interruption may be interpreted as not doing very well (Atkinson, cited in McClelland et al., 1953).

This greater attention to the performance aspects of a situation also promotes better learning. As compared with subjects low in *n* Achievement, those who score high perform better at anagrams and scrambled word tasks (see Chapter 6), mental arithmetic (Wendt, 1955), and conceptual problems requiring insight (see Heckhausen, 1967). What is common to these tasks is that they are at least moderately challenging. Tasks that are too easy or routine—such as canceling *e*'s and *o*'s—do not always elicit better performance from those higher in *n* Achievement, nor do impossibly difficult tasks, as we shall see in a moment. In any case, there is ample evidence that *n* Achievement as measured in this way leads to learning or performance improvement, thus satisfying the third criterion for the existence of a motive—namely, whether it serves to select out and make more likely certain responses after they are rewarded.

Much energy has gone into trying to determine whether there is a relationship between *n* Achievement and grades in school. Usually such a relationship is not found to be significant; this has led a number of investigators (see Entwisle, 1972) to conclude that the *n* Achievement score cannot be valid because it does not predict scholastic achievement. However, there is no theoretical reason for predicting that high *n* Achievement should lead to better performance in the classroom under all conditions, any more than there is reason to believe, as explained earlier, that high *n* Achievement should always lead to better performance regardless of the incentives present (see Table 7.1 in the next section). If there is strong achievement pressure (see McKeachie, 1961; Wendt, 1955) or if extrinsic incentives of any kind are introduced, there should be no relationship between high *n* Achievement and grades. Nor should there be a relationship if the work is very easy or much too hard. In other words, the relationship should exist only when an achievement incentive or challenge exists. To expect otherwise is like contending that hunger as a drive should lead to better performance even if its incentive of food is not present (see McClelland, 1980).

• WHAT IS THE INCENTIVE FOR THE ACHIEVEMENT MOTIVE?

If food is the reward or incentive for the hunger drive, what is rewarding for the achievement motive? We have repeatedly emphasized that "doing something better" is the natural incentive for the achievement motive. It now is time to become more precise, for people can do better for all sorts of reasons—to please the teacher, to avoid criticism, to gain the approval of a loved one, or simply to get some time off from work. What should be involved in the achievement motive is doing something better for its own sake, for the intrinsic satisfaction of doing something better.

The point is nicely illustrated by an experiment conducted by French (1955). Having first obtained *n* Achievement scores from story completions for the Test of Insight under standard conditions, French varied the incentives provided for performing better at a digit-symbol substitution task on a second occasion. Her subjects were officer candidates in school at a U.S. Air Force base. Using a code that showed which digits went with which letters, the subjects were to put the appropriate digits under each of a long series of letters typed out below the code. To one group of subjects she said in a casual, friendly way, "We are just experimenting today and we appreciate your cooperation very much. We want to find out what kind of scores people make on these tests." Table 7.1 lays out the motivational sequence in the terms used to describe it in Figure 6.1. The *demand* to do the task is stated here in terms of an *incentive* to please the experimenter, which should be appropriate to a motive disposition to affiliate with others (*n* Affiliation; see Chapter 9), meaning that the *aroused motivation* to do well should be highest in subjects for whom the need for affiliation is aroused.

A second group of subjects were told in a formal and serious manner by an airman that the tests they were taking measured "a critical ability—the ability to deal quickly and accurately with unfamiliar material. It is related to general intelligence and will be related to your future career. Each man should try to perform as well as possible." In other words, the *incentive* was for individuals to show how capable they were, which should be related to the need to achieve.

Finally, a third group was told that "the five men who make the best scores in five minutes will be allowed to leave right away—the others will have more practice periods and more tests." Here the *incentive* is to leave early and get out of work, which should appeal particularly to those who dislike work or need rest.

French also measured the degree to which the affiliation and achievement motives were aroused by administering a second form of the Test of Insight just after she gave the instructions mentioning different incentives to the various groups. She found, as expected, that mentioning the achievement incentive had the greatest effect on arousing achievement motivation for those high in dispositional *n* Achievement on the first test (mean level = 6.27). The level of achievement motivation aroused for these subjects from the other incentives was lower (mean = 4.20 for the Relaxed condition and 5.40 for the Time-off condition). The level of achievement motivation aroused for those low in dispositional *n* Achievement was significantly lower across all incentive conditions, as expected. For those high in *n* Achievement, the picture is quite consistent and easily understandable: the *demand* to do the task couched in terms of achievement *in-*

centives contacted their high achievement *motive disposition* and aroused more achievement *motivation,* which expressed itself in performing better.

As Table 7.1 shows, introducing an achievement incentive for the subjects —to show how capable they were—produced the highest average number of digit-symbol substitutions, but its effect was most marked on those who had scored high in dispositional *n* Achievement on a previous occasion. Under this incentive the subjects high in *n* Achievement produced almost twice as many substitutions as those low in *n* Achievement. On the other hand, the two other incentives—involving affiliation or time off from work—did not elicit better performance from those high in *n* Achievement as compared with those low in *n* Achievement.

For Group 1, mentioning an affiliative incentive for doing the task ("to please me") meant the men for whom this instruction had aroused the affiliation motive performed significantly better. In this group the correlation between aroused affiliation motivation and subsequent performance was .48, $p < .01$, as compared with similar correlations of $-.02$ and $-.13$ in the other incentive groups. In other words, any affiliation motivation aroused in the other conditions did not lead to better performance, because better performance was not tied in these conditions to the affiliative incentive. To put it another way, aroused affiliation motivation will lead to better performance if better performance is cognitively understood to be the way to satisfy the affiliation motive (that is, to please the experimenter). This makes the point once again that better performance does not always signify more aroused achievement motivation. Better performance can be undertaken to satisfy many different motives.

What motivation was aroused in the group promised time off cannot be determined very well, because only achievement and affiliation motivation were scored. Those low in dispositional *n* Achievement had the highest level of aroused achievement motivation in this condition, but it is possible that it was avoidance motivation (which could have shown up in one of the measures of fear of failure; see Chapter 10) that led them to work harder to escape from work. It is also possible that for such people the motivation to achieve is aroused primarily by external pressures, or that some other type of motivation was aroused that was not scored.

The main point is that those high in *n* Achievement actually performed somewhat less well than those low in *n* Achievement when the incentive was time off from work. So subjects high in *n* Achievement do not always perform better than those low in *n* Achievement. They apparently perform better only when an achievement incentive is present in the situation. As these results suggest, an achievement incentive is one in which a person gets satisfaction from doing something better *for its own sake,* or to show that he or she is more capable of doing something. As Deci (1975) has shown in a number of experiments, if extrinsic incentives are provided for doing something, the intrinsic satisfaction from doing it well tends to be lost, and subjects high in *n* Achievement do not perform better under such conditions.

Evidence for the importance of intrinsic achievement satisfaction to subjects

Table 7.1.

INFLUENCE ON PERFORMANCE OF VARIOUS INCENTIVES IN COMBINATION WITH *n* ACHIEVEMENT (after French, 1955)

A. Demand ⟶	B. Incentive ⟶	C. Motive Disposition ⟶	D. Aroused Motivation	*Work Output: Average Digit-Symbol Substitutions*
Group 1 Do this task	To please me	Need for approval or affiliation	To work to get approval	16.5: High *n* Achievement = 17.7 Low *n* Achievement = 15.4
Group 2 Do this task	To show your intelligence and leadership ability (how capable you are)	Need for Achievement	To work to do better	23.5: High *n* Achievement = 29.8 Low *n* Achievement = 16.7 $p_{difference} < .01$
Group 3 Do this task	Best five can leave early and get time off from work	Need for rest, escape from work situation	To work to escape	20.3: High *n* Achievement = 18.2 Low *n* Achievement = 22.5

high in *n* Achievement comes from a number of sources. For example, Wendt (1955) found that when subjects were performing complex mental arithmetic tasks, those high in *n* Achievement did significantly better than those low in *n* Achievement so long as the experimenter left them alone. However, if the experimenter scheduled the work by constant reminders of what the subjects should be doing, the better performance of those high in *n* Achievement tended to disappear. In an entirely different situation, McKeachie (1961) studied the joint effect of teaching style and students' motive levels on grades obtained in college. He found that when external achievement cues in the classroom were judged to be high, students high in *n* Achievement tended to do less well in the course than those low in *n* Achievement. To put it the other way around, if achievement cues were low—that is, if the instructor did not make a point of encouraging competition or setting high standards of achievement—those high in *n* Achievement tended to do better than those low in *n* Achievement. That is, they readily find intrinsic satisfaction in achieving, but external promptings tend either to distract them or to encourage the students with low *n* Achievement to do better.

Moderate Task Difficulty as an Achievement Incentive

In the French experiment summarized in Table 7.1, the nature of the achievement incentive was spelled out for the subjects by the experimenter. However, in most of the work in this area, the achievement incentive is defined by the intrinsic difficulty or challenge of the task. If the incentive is to "do better," neither a very easy task nor a very difficult one provides an opportunity to do better. If the task is easy there is no question of doing it better, since anyone can do it; if it is very difficult there is also no question of doing it better, because everyone is likely to fail in attempting it.

It follows that moderately difficult tasks should provide people the best opportunity of proving they can do better. A large number of empirical studies have demonstrated that subjects high in *n* Achievement prefer working on moderately difficult tasks in which the probability of success lies somewhere between .30 and .50. The reason is that they should prefer working under conditions where the achievement incentive is maximal. Subjects low in *n* Achievement show quite a different preference curve for tasks differing in difficulty.

Some typical results are shown in Figures 7.1 and 7.2, as reported by deCharms and Carpenter (1968). The subjects were over two hundred children from the fifth and seventh grades in inner city schools. After being given the standard test for *n* Achievement, they were familiarized with a set of words to be spelled and arithmetic problems to be solved that were carefully graded into levels of difficulty: "After all children had attempted all items, the various levels of difficulty were explained to them and their own ability at each level was impressed upon them by pointing out how many they had completed correctly" (deCharms & Carpenter, 1968). It was then explained to them that they would take a test individually in which they could choose the level of difficulty of each item they would attempt. They would get more points for performing an item correctly at a more difficult level. The subjects also knew what their probability of success was at the level of difficulty they chose, because they could look back at their previous performance at that difficulty level. That is, there were ten items at each difficulty level, and if they had done two correctly at that difficulty level previously, their probability of success at that level of difficulty would be two out of ten, or .20.

Figures 7.1 and 7.2 show that subjects high in *n* Achievement regularly chose to work at difficulty levels where their probability of success was moderate (from .30 to .50), whereas subjects low in *n* Achievement showed no such preference. If anything, they biased their choices toward very difficult items where their probability of success was quite low (from 0 to .20). In the case

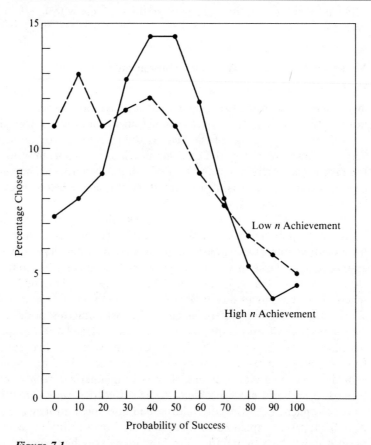

Figure 7.1.

Percentage of Tasks Chosen at Each Level of Probability of Success on the Arithmetic Risk-taking Task by Subjects Above and Below the Median *n* Achievement Score (after deCharms & Carpenter, 1968).

of spelling, there was a trend for the subjects low in *n* Achievement to choose very easy items, which has also been found in other studies (see McClelland, 1958a).

Atkinson's Model for Predicting Moderate Risk Preference

In a classic paper, Atkinson (1957) presented a formal model that explained these results. He assumed that the strength of the tendency to achieve on a task (or the strength of preference for various tasks) is a joint function of the motive to achieve, the expectancy or probability of success (P_s), and the incentive value of success (I_s), where incentive value is defined as one minus the

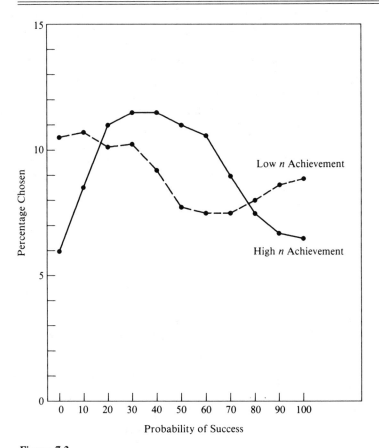

Figure 7.2.

Percentage of Tasks Chosen at Each Level of Probability of Success on the Spelling Risk-taking Task by Subjects Above and Below the Median *n* Achievement Score (after deCharms & Carpenter, 1968).

probability of success $(1 - P_s)$. In other words, it is assumed that the value of success is directly proportional to its difficulty. As Table 7.2 illustrates, if the probability of success is moderate, or fifty-fifty, the product of $P_s \times I_s$ is maximal, explaining why moderately difficult tasks have the largest incentive value. As Table 7.2 also makes clear, if the motive to achieve (M_s) is higher, as in high *n* Achievement, the preference for moderately difficult tasks over either easy or difficult tasks should be even greater (.75 to .27 versus .25 to .09).

The model also suggests that even those low in *n* Achievement should show some preference for moderately difficult tasks, which is not the case, as Figures 7.1 and 7.2 show. However, Atkinson handled this problem by assuming that subjects low in *n* Achievement are actually afraid of failure and tend to avoid moderately difficult tasks for this reason, thus canceling out this preference (see Chapter 10).

Atkinson's model introduced a confusion in terminology, as already mentioned, which must be made explicit to avoid trouble. He sometimes referred to the product of the three variables in Table 7.2 as the *aroused motivation to achieve,* which confuses the aroused achievement motivation with what we have called the *impulse to act* (or to choose one task over another)—which is a product of motivational and nonmotivational variables and which Hull called *excitatory potential* (see Chapter 3). The level of achievement motivation aroused in a situation can be determined by giving a TAT under conditions of arousal (and comparing the *n* Achievement level obtained with its level under normal testing conditions), but Atkinson did not mean (and has never shown) that the aroused achievement motivation level measured in this way is a joint function of the three determinants in Table 7.2. Rather, he meant to predict with his formula the tendency to approach or work hard at various tasks, which should be distinguished from the achievement motivation actually aroused, as shown in the motivation sequence outlined in Figure 6.1.

Table 7.2.

AROUSED TENDENCY TO ACHIEVE AS A JOINT FUNCTION OF MOTIVE TO ACHIEVE (M_s), EXPECTANCY OR PROBABILITY OF SUCCESS (P_s), AND INCENTIVE VALUE OF SUCCESS (I_s), WHERE $I_s = 1 - P_s$ (after Atkinson, 1957)

Task	*Low n Achievement:*				*High n Achievement:*			
	$M_s \times$	$P_s \times$	I_s	$= Approach$	$M_s \times$	$P_s \times$	I_s	$= Approach$
Task A (hard)	1 $\times$	0.10 $\times$	0.90 $=$	0.09	3 $\times$	0.10 $\times$	0.90 $=$	0.27
Task B	1 $\times$	0.50 $\times$	0.50 $=$	0.25	3 $\times$	0.50 $\times$	0.50 $=$	0.75
Task C (easy)	1 $\times$	0.90 $\times$	0.10 $=$	0.09	3 $\times$	0.90 $\times$	0.10 $=$	0.27

Atkinson's model explains quite well the actual distribution of choices for tasks of different difficulty, as Table 7.3 demonstrates. To test it, Litwin (1958) used a ringtoss game in which choosing to stand at different distances from the peg represented choosing tasks differing in difficulty. He had determined the incentive value of a ringer from different distances by asking a number of students how much money up to one dollar should be awarded as a prize for a ringer from each distance. The second column in Table 7.3 gives the answers he received. He also asked the subjects to estimate what the chances in one hundred were of an average person throwing a ringer from the same distances. The results are recorded as perceived success probability (P_s) in the fourth column in Table 7.3. Litwin observed that the money reward column matched closely the perceived difficulty of the task, as estimated from the reciprocal of the probability of success ($1 - P_s$). Choices or the approach tendency then should be a joint function of expectancy of success (P_s) times the value of success at that level of difficulty figured either in terms of money or difficulty ($1 - P_s$). He multiplied the two variables, $P_s \times (1 - P_s)$, and compared the predicted attractiveness of various distances with the distribution of distances from which students actually chose to throw. The curves match fairly well. The value times probability of success equations predict that most choices will fall between Lines 10 and 15, with fewer at shorter and longer distances, and this is what happened.

Other psychologists have worried about the best way to estimate the incentive value of tasks of different difficulty. Calculating it on the basis of $0.9 - P_s$

Table 7.3.

THEORETICAL AND ACTUAL ATTRACTIVENESS OF TASKS OF DIFFERENT DIFFICULTY IN A RINGTOSS GAME (after Litwin, 1958)

	Value		*Success Probability* P_s		*Incentive Value (Predicted Attractiveness, Value × Expectancy)*		*Proportion*
Lines Distant from Peg[a]	*Cents for Ringer*	*Difficulty ($1 - P_s$)*	*Perceived*	*Actual*	*Cents × P_s*	*Difficulty × P_s*	*Actual Choice Out of 400 Times*
1–3	$0.04	.01	.99		.04	.01	.00
4–6	0.14	.12	.88	.70	.12	.11	.05
7–9	0.29	.30	.70	.31	.20	.21	.09
10–12	0.50	.45	.55	.20	.27	.25	.33
13–15	0.62	.62	.38	.15	.24	.24	.34
16–18	0.81	.75	.25	.14	.20	.19	.18

[a]Lines started ten inches from peg, and subsequent lines were ten inches apart.

instead of $1 - P_s$ gives results in this instance that more closely approximate where people actually stood, for they apparently tended to underestimate in practice the real difficulty of what they were attempting. That is, as a comparison of Columns 4 and 5 in Table 7.3 illustrates, they perceived the probability of success as greater than the actual probability of success. Thus, they stood farther away more often than they should have, according to the model. This is also true of the results shown in Figures 7.1 and 7.2. That is, the actual peak preference for task difficulty is in the .30 to .40 range rather than .50 as predicted by the model (see Schneider, 1978).

Teevan, Burdick, and Stoddard (1976) have even argued that incentive value is not always inversely related to task difficulty. They found that whereas it was true that subjects tended to associate larger incentives with greater task difficulty (lower probability of success), this seemed not to be the case when subjects were asked *in advance* how important it was to them to succeed at tasks of varying difficulty. Under these conditions, subjects said it was most important to them to succeed at the easiest and not the hardest tasks, in an apparent reversal of the Atkinson assumption. However, this may only have meant that they feared looking ridiculous for failing at very easy tasks, and not that they *valued* success at the easy tasks more in the Atkinson sense.

Atkinson and Litwin (1960) also classified subjects in this experiment according to whether they were high or low in *n* Achievement. Those with high *n* Achievement tended to choose moderately difficult tasks (throwing from Lines 10 to 15) significantly more often than those with low *n* Achievement. In other words, they showed the same trend as the whole group, only more so. This is as it should be according to the model outlined in Table 7.2. A further example will make the point even clearer:

Motive Strength	$\times$	P_s	$\times$	I_s, or $1 - P_s$	=	Resultant Approach Tendency
4	$\times$	.50	$\times$	.50	=	1.00
4	$\times$	.70	$\times$	.30	=	0.84
				Difference	=	0.16
1	$\times$	.50	$\times$	.50	=	0.25
1	$\times$	.70	$\times$	.30	=	0.21
				Difference	=	0.04

That is, the difference in the attractiveness of a moderately difficult task ($P_s =$ .50) over an easy task ($P_s = .70$) is greater (.16) for those high in *n* Achievement than for those low in *n* Achievement, where it equals .04. The greater preference of subjects with high *n* Achievement for moderately difficult tasks has been confirmed in a number of different studies (see Figures 7.1 and 7.2). For example, Heckhausen (1963) found that they typically chose to work on mazes that were only slightly more difficult (not easier or much harder) than mazes they had succeeded in tracing earlier.

A Cognitive Explanation of the Preference for Moderate Risk

Weiner (1980a) has argued that the reason subjects with high *n* Achievement choose moderately difficult tasks is that such tasks are more diagnostic of how well they are doing. If the task is easy they will not know whether success was due to their efforts, because everyone can do it, and if the task is difficult they will also not be able to tell what their efforts produced, because they will fail. Thus, they seek moderately difficult tasks to get information on the impact of their efforts on performance. In other words, they prefer these tasks not because they get more pleasure out of working with them in Atkinson's sense, but because they can find out better from performing such tasks whether they can attribute their success to their own efforts—which is the way Weiner defines *n* Achievement (see Chapter 12).

Trope (1975) created a situation in which the diagnostic value of a task varied independently in relationship to its difficulty level. Diagnosticity was varied by telling the subjects that 90 percent of subjects with high ability can do the task as compared with only 60 percent of subjects with low ability. For another task the comparable figures were 52 percent success for the high ability person and 48 percent success for the low ability person. Under these conditions subjects with a presumably strong achievement motive more often chose to work on the easier task with high diagnostic value (90 percent versus 60 percent) rather than on the more moderately difficult task with low diagnostic value (52 percent versus 48 percent).

There is some evidence that subjects high in *n* Achievement prefer moderately difficult tasks because they have more feedback value. W. U. Meyer (1975) carried out the following experiment on a group of police trainees in Germany:

> Each subject was asked to imagine a situation where he had to shoot at a target with 10 rings from 9 distances. For each distance, difficulty was conveyed by social norms indicating what percentage of prospective policemen hit the "10" on the target (2, 6, 13, 32, 52, 73, 81, 85, and 98% respectively). The subjects then had to imagine that they were going to shoot from each distance once and they would maximally concentrate on one shot. Given these conditions, the subjects estimated their probability of hitting the 10 on the target from each distance. After indicating the specific probability levels, the subjects were asked: "Suppose that immediately after shooting from each distance the target disappears. You have no feedback whether you were hitting or missing the 10. Suppose further that you can get feedback about hitting or missing the 10 on the target for *one distance* (assume that there is no other feedback possible). At what distance would you like to know if you were hitting or missing the "10"?"

Figure 7.3 is from a reanalysis of Meyer's data by Heckhausen (1975). It shows that the subjects higher in *n* Achievement chose much more often to get feedback on how well they were doing at moderate levels of difficulty for them. Subjects low in *n* Achievement showed no particular trend, or if anything, preferred getting feedback for low probability of success. This suggests, but does not prove, that the subjects high in *n* Achievement were making their choices in

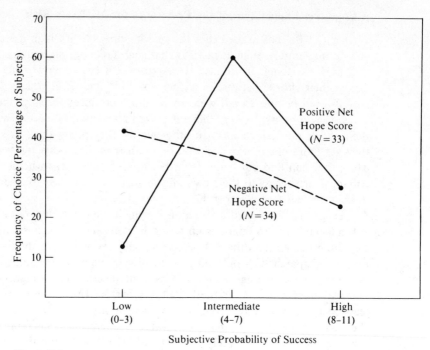

Figure 7.3.

Frequency of Information Choice Within Low, Intermediate, and High P_s Range for Subjects with Positive and Negative Net Hope *n* Achievement Scores (after Heckhausen, 1974).

order to get feedback, for it is possible that the tendency to choose moderate levels of difficulty here was simply a generalization of their tendency always to do this rather than because the instructions told them they would get feedback at this level. Unfortunately, Weiner's attempts to show that subjects high in *n* Achievement prefer more diagnostic tasks are inconclusive, because he used an objective test measure of *v* Achievement rather than the usual *n* Achievement score based on spontaneous thought content.

• HOW HIGH NEED FOR ACHIEVEMENT AFFECTS PERFORMANCE

Influence of Variations in the Challenge a Task Presents

So far, research findings indicate that subjects high in *n* Achievement prefer working at levels of moderate risk where the probability of success is somewhere in the range of .30 to .50. They are more attracted to such tasks, but do they actually perform better when the challenge is moderate? Many studies have shown that they do. A typical result is shown in Figure 7.4. In this study subjects were asked to try to solve sixty anagrams placed on a page (Raynor & Entin, 1982b). They were told that in order to be successful and move on to the next task, they had to complete either fifty-four, thirty, or six out of the sixty anagrams in the time allotted. If they did not meet the "moving-on" criterion, they had to sit quietly while others continued to work. As Figure 7.5 shows, when the moving-on criterion was of moderate difficulty (requiring half of the anagrams to be solved), those high in *n* Achievement performed significantly better than when the moving-on criterion was either very difficult or very easy. Furthermore, those low in *n* Achievement did not show this pattern at all. Karabenick and Yousseff (1968) also showed that subjects high in *n* Achieve-

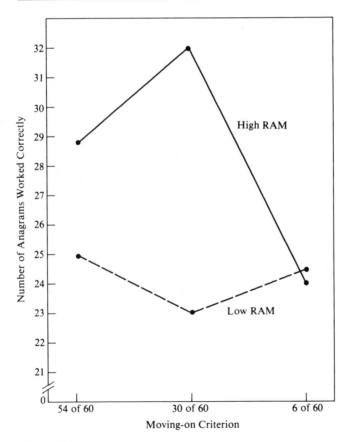

Figure 7.4.

Number of Anagrams Worked Correctly as a Function of Resultant Achievement Motivation (RAM) and Moving-on Criterion (after Raynor & Entin, 1982b).

ment performed better than subjects low in *n* Achievement only when learning moderately difficult paired associates as compared with very easy or very difficult ones.

Atkinson (1958) had reported a similar result earlier in an experiment, some of the results of which were reported in Table 6.1 in Chapter 6. In this study subjects understood that they had different probabilities of success because they were competing either with a larger or smaller number of other students. As Figure 7.5 shows, the subjects high in *n* Achievement performed significantly better at middle levels of probability of winning (one in three or one in two) as compared with a very slight chance of winning (one in twenty) or an almost certain win (the best three out of four students getting the money award). In this case, a probability of success of fifty-fifty produced better performance even for those low in *n* Achievement, as ought to be the case according to the Atkinson model presented in Table 7.2. The effect of the intrinsic challenge of tasks of different difficulties is accentuated in Figure 7.5 because the extrinsic, monetary incentive was relatively low. Even so, it may have accounted for the extra effort from those low in *n* Achievement at $P_s = .50$, as contrasted with the result in

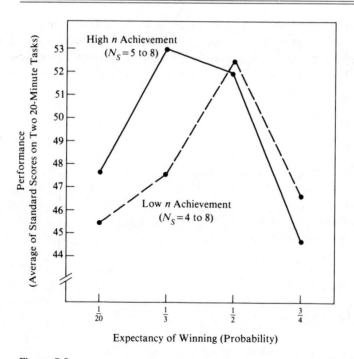

Figure 7.5.

Performance as a Function of *n* Achievement and Expectancy of Winning When the Monetary Incentive Is Low (after Atkinson, 1958).

Figure 7.4, because they thought they had a better chance of getting the money reward.

One difficulty in generalizing about the behavior of those low in *n* Achievement is that they are working in various performance situations for a variety of incentives induced by the instructions and the setting other than the achievement incentive of primary interest. Also, the definition of low *n* Achievement varies from study to study: in the Atkinson study it is simply those who are below the median in *n* Achievement, whereas Raynor and Entin (1982b) followed the later Atkinson procedure of combining the *n* Achievement score with a test anxiety score so that a person low in resultant achievement motivation (RAM) is defined as someone low in *n* Achievement and high in anxiety, indicating fear of failure. Whatever the results for those low in *n* Achievement, the findings do agree that those high in *n* Achievement perform better under conditions of moderate challenge.

At first glance the results for the easiest competition, where chances of success are three out of four, or .75, would seem to present a problem for the Atkinson model outlined in Table 7.2, for under this condition the subjects low in *n* Achievement perform, if anything, somewhat better than those high in *n* Achievement. This result cannot be predicted by a model that allows only for motive strength to combine multiplicatively with P_s, since according to the model, those high in *n* Achievement will always do better at all tasks, no matter how easy or hard they are.

What is happening here is that those with high *n* Achievement are *perceiving* the easy task as even easier for them, so it has little incentive value to combine with their high motive strength. See the following numerical example:

M_s ×	P_s ×	I_s, or $1 - P_s$ =	Approach Tendency
	Stated = .75		
3 ×	Perceived = .95 ×	.05 =	.14
1 ×	Perceived = .75 ×	.25 =	.19
	Difference in favor of low *n* Achievement	=	.05

In the example it is assumed that the stated probability of success of .75 is perceived by those high in *n* Achievement as $P_s = .95$, which then yields an approach tendency by multiplication that is actually less than that for the subjects low in *n* Achievement despite their lower motive strength. In general, people with high *n* Achievement estimate tasks to be easier for them at the outset (McClelland et al., 1953; Pottharst, 1955), so they are attracted to, and work harder at, more difficult tasks and less hard at easy tasks than people with low *n* Achievement.

Responding to Moderate Challenges in Everyday Life

Hoyos (1965) applied Atkinson's risk-taking model to driving. He predicted that individuals with high *n* Achievement should be better drivers because they would avoid extreme risks; in fact, he found they were less often involved in accidents and traffic violations. However, they took more calculated risks, such as overloading, driving without a license, or committing parking violations.

O'Connor, Atkinson, and Horner (1966) used the risk-taking model to explain the effects of ability grouping on performance in the classroom. They reasoned that in a normal classroom where children of very different abilities are present, those with high ability perceive the probability of success to be high, whereas those of low ability perceive it to be low. In such classes students with high *n* Achievement, in comparing their performance with that of other students, would not be maximally challenged, for they would see that they could easily do better than the really poor students and that they did not stand a chance of doing better than the very good students. If they were grouped with students of similar ability in homogeneous classes, however, they should be more often presented comparisons in which they would stand around a fifty-fifty chance of doing better than the other person; this corresponds to the optimal achievement incentive value according to Atkinson's model. The results of comparing the performance of students high and low in *n* Achievement when in homogeneous or heterogeneous classes are shown in Table 7.4. Clearly, at all ability levels, subjects high in *n* Achievement do much better than those low in

Table 7.4.

MOTIVATIONAL EFFECTS OF ABILITY GROUPING IN SIXTH GRADE: PERCENTAGE OF STUDENTS SHOWING ABOVE-MEDIAN GROWTH FOR THEIR INTELLIGENCE LEVEL IN READING AND ARITHMETIC ON CALIFORNIA ACHIEVEMENT TEST (after Atkinson & Birch, 1978, after O'Connor, Atkinson, & Horner, 1966)

Resultant Achievement Motivation (n Achievement–Test Anxiety)	*Homogeneous Classes*		*Heterogeneous Classes*	
	N	*Percentage Above Median*	*N*	*Percentage Above Median*
	IQ 125 and above			
		Both Areas		Both Areas
High	24	71	37	46
Low	10	50	27	37
	IQ 113 to 124			
		Both or One Area		Both or One Area
High	11	90	17	41
Low	17	65	19	58
	IQ 112 and below			
High	8	88	8	38
Low	23	52	14	36

Note: When all levels of intelligence are combined, the difference between motivation groups within the homogeneous classes and the difference between classes for the high motivation group are statistically significant.

n Achievement in homogeneous classes, whereas they do not do significantly better in heterogeneous classes. This result is a nice confirmation of the predictive value of Atkinson's model.

Persistence

The risk-taking model has also been applied to explaining the tendency to *persist* in working at tasks of different difficulty levels. At first it was thought that subjects high in *n* Achievement would persist longer in working at any task. For example, French and Thomas (1958) found that 47 percent of the subjects high in *n* Achievement persisted up to the time limit in working at an insoluble task, as compared with only 2 percent of those low in *n* Achievement.

However, Feather (1961) reasoned that persistence ought to depend on probability of success according to Atkinson's model. That is, subjects high in *n* Achievement should persist longer when they begin to fail at an easy task than when they fail at a very difficult task. He in fact found this to be the case, as Figure 7.6 illustrates. The figure also suggests why this difference should be obtained: As a subject begins to fail at an easy task that is supposed to have a .70 probability of success, the perceived probability of success begins to get less and moves into the area of maximal attraction for subjects high in *n* Achievement—namely, the area of moderate probability of success. On the other hand, a hard task with a probability of success of only .05 should have little attraction for subjects high in *n* Achievement; as they begin to fail, it should have even less attraction, and persistence should be low. Thus, whether subjects high in *n* Achievement persist when they begin to fail at a task depends very much on the perceived difficulty of the task.

Feather predicted and found the reverse result for subjects low in *n* Achievement: they persisted longer after failure at a difficult than at an easy task (see also Feather, 1963). This result is predicted from Atkinson's model, because subjects low in *n* Achievement are perceived as fearing failure and avoiding tasks of moderate difficulty (see Chapter 10). It follows that success at easy and difficult tasks would have the opposite effect. Since success at an easy task ($P_s = .70$) would increase the probability of success even more, the attraction of continuing to do the task would be less for those high in *n* Achievement, and they would tend to stop doing it. On the other hand, success at a very difficult task might move the probability of success into the region of greater attractiveness for those high in *n* Achievement.

Effects of Too Much Motivation on Performance

As noted in Chapters 3 and 6, psychologists have found evidence that too much motivation can interfere with performance. So far no one has demonstrated a curvilinear, or inverted U-shaped, relationship between *n* Achievement and performance, indicating that too high a level of *n* Achievement leads to somewhat lower performance than a moderate level of *n* Achievement. However, several studies have shown that if *n* Achievement is associated with a high *n* Affiliation,

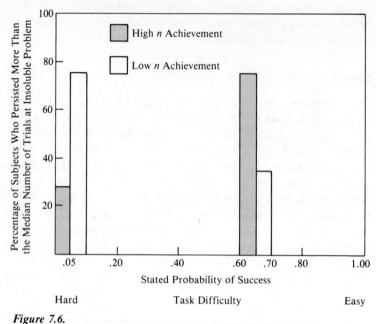

Figure 7.6.

Relationship of High and Low *n* Achievement to Persistence at Easy and Difficult Tasks After Failure (after Feather, 1961).

and incentives for both motives are present in the situation, performance can suffer. For example, Entin (1968) asked junior high school boys to solve arithmetic problems under either one of two types of feedback conditions. In one instance they were told privately how well they had done—which was assumed to be relevant to the achievement motive—and in the other condition their scores were listed publicly where all could see them—an incentive relevant to the affiliation motive, because subjects high in *n* Affiliation tend to want social approval (Chapter 9).

In a reanalysis of Entin's results, Atkinson and Birch (1978) assumed that subjects who were low in *n* Achievement and *n* Affiliation and who received private feedback would have the lowest level of motivation to perform, whereas those high in both motives and receiving public feedback would have the highest level of motivation. Subjects with other combinations of motive strength and feedback were considered to be moderately motivated. The data in Figure 7.7 from this study show the inverted U-type curve supposedly characterizing the relationship between increasing motivation and performance. Neither the subjects with the lowest or highest motivation performed as well as those with a more moderate combination of motives and incentives to perform.

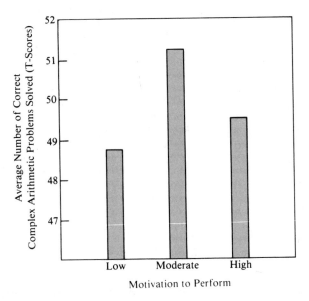

Figure 7.7.

Effect of Increasing Motivation to Perform on Efficiency (after Atkinson & Birch, 1978, after Entin, 1968).

Similar results were obtained in a study by Sorrentino (1974). Instead of using the incentive of private versus public feedback, he employed the incentive of contingent versus noncontingent paths to going on to the next task, as explained in connection with the moving-on criterion used with the experiment summarized in Figure 7.4. Under contingent conditions subjects were under pressure to achieve a certain level of performance before they could continue with other parts of the experiment. Figure 7.8 displays the results for the subjects high in *n* Achievement when they were also either low or high in *n* Affiliation and working under contingent or noncontingent conditions. The motivation to perform in this experiment can be conceptualized as a product of three motivational factors: high *n* Achievement, high *n* Affiliation, and a contingency incentive. For the first point in the curve, only one of the motivational factors (high *n* Achievement) is present. For the second two points in the performance curve, two out of the three motivational factors are present (high *n* Achievement and either high *n* Affiliation or the contingency incentive). For the fourth point in the curve, all three motivational factors are present. Once again, the total strength of motivation shows an inverted U-type relationship to performance. The students solved more arithmetic problems under moderate motivational pressure than under either low or very high motivational pressure.

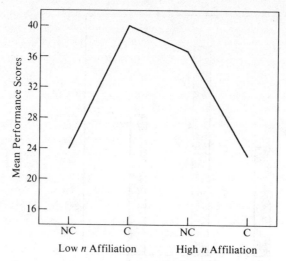

Figure 7.8.

Performance Scores for High *n* Achievement–Low Test Anxiety Subjects in the Noncontingent (NC) and Contingent (C) Conditions Who Are Also Classified as High and Low in *n* Affiliation (after Sorrentino, 1974).

• OTHER CHARACTERISTICS OF PEOPLE WITH A STRONG NEED TO ACHIEVE

Personal Responsibility for Performance

On theoretical grounds, it has always been assumed that subjects high in *n* Achievement would prefer being personally responsible for a performance result, because only under such conditions could they feel satisfaction from doing something better. Horowitz (1961) carried out a simple empirical test of this theoretical expectation. He designed a board game in which the players as salespeople were supposedly crossing the United States and trying to make as much money as possible in encounters they were described as having in various cities. In each encounter the players were asked to choose between two alternatives, each of which gave them a moderate chance ($P_s = .33$) to make a certain amount of money. In one alternative they could do some work—that is, take personal responsibility for the outcome. They could choose to work on an arithmetic problem, the solution to which, they were told, approximately one in three students could reach in the time allotted. If they succeeded in solving the problem in the time allotted, they would be considered to have made the sale and its accompanying financial reward. Or they could choose another option, represented, for example, by the opportunity to invest in digging an oil well, where the chances were also one in three of finding oil. To determine whether or not they won on this alternative, they rolled a die with the understanding that if either of two out of the six numbers came up, they would win. In other words, people who played the game were repeatedly confronted with the opportunity either to take a chance through the roll of a die or to take an equal chance in which they had to work to obtain the result. Under these conditions the subjects high in *n* Achievement chose to take personal responsibility in situations of moderate risk significantly more often than those low in *n* Achievement.

A number of studies have shown that the Atkinson risk-taking model does not apply when the risks involve pure chance rather than personal responsibility. That is, subjects high in *n* Achievement are not more attracted to moderate risks in games of chance such as poker dice (Hancock & Teevan, 1964; Littig, 1963; Raynor & Smith, 1966). However, a study by McClelland and Watson (1973) shows that this is not always the case. They found that in a game of roulette, subjects with high *n* Achievement tended to prefer moderate risks over very short or very long odds, just as if the outcome depended on their performance (see Figure 8.5). Perhaps the tendency to choose moderate risks is so strong in subjects high in *n* Achievement that it generalizes to some situations in which chance only is involved.

The focus on one's own ability to produce a performance result may explain why subjects high in *n* Achievement show less interpersonal sensitivity in the achievement area (Berlew & Williams, 1964). In an experiment, subjects had an opportunity to get to know each other by working on a common problem in five-person groups. At the end of the session the subjects rated themselves on the extent to which they possessed certain characteristics such as being keen, practical, warm, or influential. Each subject was also asked to judge how others in the group would rate themselves. Those high in *n* Achievement, particularly when the experimenters focused their attention on how important the work was for determining leadership ability and intelligence, proved much less able to judge accurately how the others would rate themselves on achievement traits like being keen and practical. In short, they focused so much on doing well themselves that they paid no attention to how achievement oriented the other members of the group were.

Need for Performance Feedback

Theoretically, subjects high in *n* Achievement should prefer working in situations where they get feedback on how well they are doing. Otherwise they have no way of knowing whether they are doing better than others or not. Several different types of studies have confirmed the importance of performance feedback to them. In an early study, French (1958b) introduced two different kinds of feedback to two groups of subjects working on a common task. For one group she drew attention to various things members of the group had been doing that contributed to improving performance on the task. For the other group she drew attention to affiliative behaviors that contributed to the group's working well together. She found that as contrasted with the subjects low in *n* Achievement, those high in *n* Achievement worked subsequently more efficiently after performance feedback than after affiliative feedback. They wanted to know how well they were doing in solving the problems worked on rather than how well they were getting along with other members of the group.

In quite a different confirmation of this point, Kagan and Moss (1962) demonstrated in a longitudinal study that boys with high *n* Achievement were rated more interested in and better at mechanical activities such as carpentry or constructing model vehicles than those low in *n* Achievement. The likely explanation for this finding is that construction activities give very concrete performance feedback. The boys knew how well they had done in terms of whether the model they had constructed worked or whether the pieces of the airplane they were making fitted together evenly. In contrast, social behaviors, or even studying in school, do not give people such immediate direct performance feedback on how well they have done. And children higher in *n* Achievement do not tend to perform better socially or in school than those lower in *n* Achievement.

Another type of very concrete performance feedback is provided by programmed learning, in which a teaching machine gives immediate feedback on the correctness of each step taken to learn something. Bartmann (1965) has shown that subjects high in *n* Achievement profit more under such feedback conditions than subjects low in *n* Achievement.

Money is a common way of giving people feedback on how well they are doing. There is evidence that whereas money is not an incentive for subjects high in *n* Achievement, they do use it as information on how successful their performance has been. For example, in the Atkinson (1958) experiment, some of the results of which are presented in Figure 7.5, the subjects high in *n* Achievement performed better across all levels of expectancy of winning than subjects low in *n* Achievement so long as the money incentive was $1.25. However, if the money incentive was raised to $2.50, the curves for the high and low *n* Achievement subjects across various expectancies of winning were nearly identical, and there was no difference in overall performance. Furthermore, the subjects high in *n* Achievement did not perform significantly better for a $2.50 incentive across all conditions than for a $1.25 incentive. In contrast, the subjects low in *n* Achievement performed significantly better for the larger monetary incentive than the smaller one. This and several other studies (for example, Douvan, 1956) show that offering money rewards to subjects intrinsically high in *n* Achievement does not increase their striving. In fact, as noted earlier, introducing extrinsic incentives to people who are intrinsically motivated for achievement may cause them to work less hard.

In the ringtoss experiment described in Table 7.3, however, the cents to be awarded for a ringer from different distances rises at a more rapid rate for those high in *n* Achievement than for those low in *n* Achievement (see Figure 7.9). This would appear to mean that subjects with a strong achievement motive want a more difficult achievement to be recognized by a larger monetary reward than subjects with a weaker achievement motive. That is, subjects higher in *n* Achievement tend to see money as a measure of success, rather than as an incentive to do better.

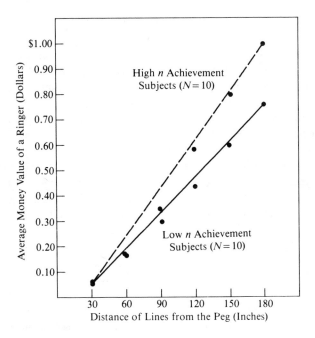

Figure 7.9.

Average Money Reward Assigned for Hits from Different Distances in a Ringtoss Game by Subjects with High and Low *n* Achievement (after Litwin, 1958).

Innovativeness

Doing something better often implies doing it differently from before. It may involve finding a different, shorter, or more efficient path to a goal. It leads to cost-benefit calculations, such as "How can I get the same result with less work?" or "How can the same amount of work produce a bigger result?" In fact, it would be more accurate to call the achievement motive the *efficiency motive,* since the notion of doing things better involves efficiency calculations, whereas *achievement* is a more generic term that can be applied to achieving the goals for any motive.

It follows that individuals high in *n* Achievement should be more restless and avoid routine. They should be more likely to seek out information to find better ways of doing things. They should be more innovative. The very fact that they are always seeking moderately challenging tasks means that they tend always to be moving on from what they had been doing to doing something a little more challenging. Or consider the results shown in Figure 7.6 again. If people high in *n* Achievement find a task unusually difficult, they will not persist in working on it. If they succeed at a moderately difficult task, it will become easier and therefore less attractive to them, so they will move on to doing something else.

A variety of studies support these expectations. When Indian farmers viewed a telecast about a new irrigation technique, those high in n Achievement retained more information from the program than those low in n Achievement (Sinha & Mehta, 1972). In view of this, it is scarcely surprising to learn that farmers in countries as different as India and Colombia adopt more innovative agricultural practices if they are high rather than low in n Achievement (E. M. Rogers & Neill, 1966; E. M. Rogers & Svenning, 1969). In a totally different occupational category, Sheppard and Belitsky (1966) also showed that individuals high in n Achievement were more active in seeking out new information than those low in n Achievement. They found that when blue-collar workers were laid off, those with higher n Achievement started looking for work sooner, and many more of them used at least five of eight different job-seeking techniques, such as checking with a larger number of different companies, going out of town to seek employment, checking newspapers from other towns, and so on. Those with low n Achievement typically sat around waiting for their company to call them back to work.

Using quite a different measure of innovativeness, deCharms and Moeller (1962) showed that the rise and fall of n Achievement scored in popular literature in the United States (see Chapter 11) was closely paralleled by a similar rise and fall in patents issued per million inhabitants (see Figure 11.10 in Chapter 11). If it can be assumed that the amount of achievement imagery in popular literature reflects in a general way the number of persons with high n Achievement in the country, it could be taken as evidence that the larger the number of such people, the more likely they are to come up with innovative ideas for doing something better that get recorded in the patent index.

Seeking short cuts can also lead to cheating, and there is evidence that subjects high in n Achievement are more likely to cheat. Mischel and Gilligan (1964) conducted a study in which children were asked to keep track of their own score in using a ray gun machine while the experimenter was out of the room. Unknown to the children, the machine also kept accurate track of their scores. The children high in n Achievement were more likely than those low in n Achievement to report that they had made more hits than they actually had. McClelland (1961) has argued that this is why entrepreneurial groups high in n Achievement tend to acquire the reputation of being dishonest or tricky; it appears they are so fixated on finding a short cut to the goal that they may not be too particular about the means they use to reach it.

Other studies have shown that individuals high in n Achievement are more restless. They tend to travel more and are more likely to migrate (Kolp, 1965). The tendency toward change shows up even in graphic expression. As noted earlier, Aronson (1958) found that those high in n Achievement produced single, discrete, and different S shapes and diagonals, whereas those low in n Achievement tended to scribble over and over in the same space, producing fuzzy lines and multiple waves. What the graphic designs characteristic of individuals with high *n* Achievement would seem to reflect is the constant search for variety or new ways of doing things.

• SOCIAL CONSEQUENCES OF A STRONG NEED TO ACHIEVE

Occupational Success

Psychologists often seem to expend most of their energy doing research on how college sophomores perform various tasks in the laboratory. The early research on *n* Achievement was no exception to this rule. Out of it came the generalizations that people high in *n* Achievement tend to seek out and do better at moderately challenging tasks, take personal responsibility for their performance, seek performance feedback on how well they are doing, and try new and more efficient ways of doing things. Then it occurred to investigators that these characteristics should have important effects on the way people behave in "real life," in the social world. So a whole line of research was undertaken that led ultimately to the conclusion that the achievement motive is a key factor in economic growth. That story is told in the rest of this chapter and in Chapter 11. For once, psychologists were able to demonstrate that what began as a purely academic or theoretical study of how the achievement motive affects performance had applications in the real world that included an improved understanding of how a basic motive influences the economic well-being of nations.

Very early it was realized that if individuals high in *n* Achievement had the characteristics just reviewed, they ought to behave in ways that, under certain circumstances, would lead to greater success in the real world (McClelland, 1955). For example, Mahone (1960) argued that they should be more realistic in setting occupational aspirations for themselves. That is, they should neither underaspire (prefer low-level occupations relative to their ability) nor overaspire (choose occupations way beyond their ability). Rather, in accordance with Atkinson's risk-taking model, they should aspire to occupations that they stood a moderate chance of succeeding at relative to their ability. Mahone tested this hypothesis by having judges rate the career aspirations of a number of undergraduates at the University of Michigan as to whether they were underaspiring, realistic, or overaspiring relative to the students' intelligence test scores, grade point averages, and major field. The results were striking. Of the vocational choices made by those high in *n* Achievement, 81 percent were confidently agreed to be realistic versus unrealistic, as compared with only 52 percent of the choices of those low in *n* Achievement, a difference that is highly significant statistically. This should give subjects high in *n* Achievement a better start toward occupational success, since they would be more likely to pursue occupations that are realistic in terms of their abilities and performance to date.

Crockett (1962) checked this possibility with a different source of data. Using motive scores obtained from a national sample survey (Veroff, Atkinson,

Feld, & Gurin, 1960), he found that individuals with high *n* Achievement had shown greater upward occupational mobility than those with low *n* Achievement. Figure 7.10 summarizes the results. He determined whether the subjects' occupation had higher, the same, or lower prestige than their father's occupation. Those with high *n* Achievement had more often moved up on the occupational scale, as Figure 7.10 shows. Furthermore, the result cannot be the result of some general "motivational" factor, since no differences in *n* Affiliation or *n* Power scores were obtained for those who were occupationally upwardly mobile. Duncan, Featherman, and Duncan (1972) confirmed Crockett's findings after carefully examining and recoding the occupational classifications.

As would be expected from such findings, another national sample survey conducted in 1976 found that U.S. men high in *n* Achievement are oriented positively toward work (Veroff, 1982). They report more job satisfaction, evaluate their jobs as interesting, do not see work as interfering with family, and prefer work to leisure. Perhaps as a result of their good work adjustment, they report few symptoms of ill health, rate their overall happiness as high, attend church frequently, and do not take drugs to relieve tension. In the same survey, high *n* Achievement was not associated with work satisfaction among women, perhaps because women's jobs are not intrinsically as interesting as men's or because, as Veroff suggested, having been brought up before the women's liberation movement, they were still oriented toward doing well in more traditional

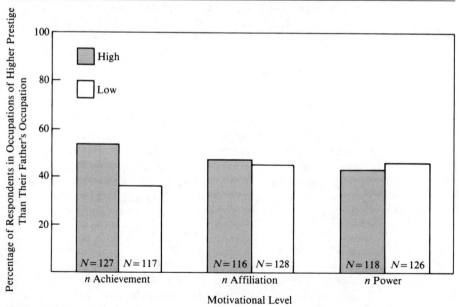

Figure 7.10.

Upward Occupational Mobility of Respondents High and Low in *n* Achievement, *n* Affiliation, and *n* Power (after Crockett, 1962).

women's role activities. For instance, women high in *n* Achievement more often reported participating in challenging leisure activities, perceived their marriages as involving much interaction with their husbands, and worried about whether they were doing well as mothers. Like the men high in *n* Achievement, they also reported a higher sense of well-being, or zest, indicating that they were finding achievement satisfactions in life, if not in work.

Perhaps as a result of the tendency to move upward or to perform better occupationally, men from the middle class generally have higher *n* Achievement scores than those from the lower class (Nuttall, 1964; B. C. Rosen, 1956, 1959; Veroff et al., 1960). At the very highest socioeconomic class levels, *n* Achievement scores tend to drop off somewhat (B. C. Rosen, 1959), perhaps because achievement challenges are less at this high level of prosperity and success. An interesting exception to this trend, which tends to confirm such an interpretation, is provided by U.S. blacks. Their *n* Achievement score is higher the farther they have risen up the socioeconomic class ladder (B. C. Rosen, 1959). There is no dropping off in *n* Achievement among blacks classified as belonging to the two highest classes, as there is among most ethnic groups. But this is quite consistent with the notion that achievement opportunities are still very great even at this socioeconomic class level for an oppressed minority like U.S. blacks. In fact, blacks even at the highest occupational level are not matched in opportunity with others at this level. At the other end of the scale, U.S. blacks of lower socioeconomic status have the lowest average *n* Achievement score, which McClelland (1961) attributes partly to their history of dependency in a slave-holding society and partly to their lack of achievement opportunities.

Several studies have been carried out to investigate the success of individuals high in *n* Achievement in real life. Kaltenbach and McClelland (1958) found that individuals perceived as leaders in small towns had higher *n* Achievement scores than those not so perceived. J. D. W. Andrews (1967) followed the careers of executives in a large company over a three-year period and found that those with high *n* Achievement scores received a significantly larger number of promotions than those with low *n* Achievement scores.

However, this was true only in an achievement-oriented firm in which those who did well were given an opportunity to advance. In another firm ruled in an authoritarian manner by the owner, there was no relationship between *n* Achievement and promotion. Later research demonstrated that *n* Achievement was associated with promotions in a large firm only for managers who did not manage large numbers of other people but who made individual contributions on their own. McClelland and Boyatzis (1982) found that *n* Achievement in managers at the time of entry into the American Telephone and Telegraph (AT&T) Company was associated with promotion up to Level 3 in the company after sixteen years, but not above that point. They reason that at Level 4 and above in the company, the managerial job demands more influencing of other people, and hence a higher *n* Power, rather than doing one's own work particularly well, which is what characterizes individuals high in *n* Achievement. (See Chapter 8.)

Entrepreneurial Success

According to McClelland (1961), high n Achievement should make people particularly likely to be interested in and able to do well at business, for business requires that people take moderate risks, assume personal responsibility for their own performance, pay close attention to feedback in terms of costs and profits, and find new or innovative ways to make a new product or provide a new service. These are precisely the characteristics that laboratory research had shown belong more to the person high than low in n Achievement. McClelland (1961) showed that generally speaking, young men higher in n Achievement are in fact more attracted to business occupations in several countries. Tessler, O'Barr, and Spain (1973) report that this is true even in a non-Western culture, the Kanuri of Nigeria, as it becomes industrialized and its young people learn about business occupations.

Andrews (1966) found that even in college, students with high n Achievement are more entrepreneurial than those low in n Achievement. They do not get higher grades (Entwisle, 1972), but they more often investigate a course's requirements before signing up for it, talk to a teacher about an examination before it is given, contact the teacher about the way an examination was graded, and so forth.

McClelland reported in *The Achieving Society* (1961) that an association between n Achievement and entrepreneurship occurred across cultures. Among preliterate tribes, 75 percent of those with high n Achievement in their folktales were characterized as having at least some full-time entrepreneurs, as contrasted with only 38 percent of the tribes with lesser amounts of achievement imagery in their folktales. He also reported that business executives in three countries (the United States, Italy, and Poland) had higher average n Achievement scores than other professionals of the same educational background.

A further examination of this difference indicated that it was particularly the salespeople from these countries who scored significantly higher in n Achievement than other managers. The explanation for this finding is the same as the one given for the failure of n Achievement scores to predict promotions into jobs where the primary responsibility is managing others rather than one's own performance. Salespeople manage their own performance, whereas general managers manage other people's performance. That is, salespeople must make decisions about what prospects to call on, choose moderate risks, take personal responsibility for making calls, carefully monitor their success and failure in making sales, and find innovative or new ways of persuading people to buy. A strong achievement motive should interest them in doing all of these things and therefore help them to like selling more and to do better at it. General managers, on the other hand, are more likely to spend time trying to influence other people rather than do things themselves (see Chapter 8). As might be expected from these findings, individuals with a strong need to achieve are more interested in investing than in saving money (Regelmann, cited in Heckhausen,

1973) and make better managers of investment portfolios than individuals with low *n* Achievement scores (Wormley, 1976).

Most of these studies are not longitudinal. Therefore, despite the strong theoretical expectation that the achievement motive could be responsible for entrepreneurial success, it is possible that people develop high *n* Achievement because of the entrepreneurial requirements of the jobs in which they find themselves.

However, empirical findings indicate that there may be a causal relationship between *n* Achievement scores and entrepreneurial success. One is the longitudinal study already reported at AT&T in which *n* Achievement at entrance into the company was related to promotion up to Level 3, sixteen years later. Another study involved a fourteen-year follow-up of college students varying in *n* Achievement to see what occupations they entered (McClelland, 1965b). As contrasted with those low in *n* Achievement, those who scored high in college were significantly more often found to be in business—most of them in small business—some fourteen years after they took the test. And Wainer and Rubin (1969) showed that the heads of more successful small research and development companies had higher *n* Achievement than heads of similar, less successful companies.

The most definitive data come from a study by Kock (1965) in which he examined the performance of a number of comparable small knitwear firms in Finland. He found that the *n* Achievement score of the owner-manager (or, in the case of somewhat larger firms, of the three or four top executives) significantly predicted increases in the number of workers for the firm over time, increases in the gross value of output, and increases in the gross amount of investment in expanding the firm (McClelland & Winter, 1969/1971). Furthermore, training in *n* Achievement improves the performance of small business entrepreneurs (Chapter 14).

• RELATIONSHIP OF THE ACHIEVEMENT MOTIVE TO THE PROTESTANT ETHIC AND THE RISE OF CAPITALISM

After studying the entrepreneurial characteristics of individuals high in *n* Achievement, McClelland wondered if the achievement motive might not be the basis for the association between the Protestant Reformation and the rise of capitalism described so eloquently by the German sociologist Max Weber (1904/1930). Weber had argued not that Protestants had invented capitalism, but that Protestant businesspeople and workers were more energetic and entrepreneurial than Roman Catholics. He felt that the Protestants' increased drive was to prove through their own performance that they were not damned, but among the elect. Having broken with papal and church authority, they were more on their own, responsible for their own performance, and less dependent on church authority to grant them indulgences for misbehaviors.

McClelland (1961) observed that the characteristics of Protestant entrepreneurs as described by Weber seemed to be similar to those of individuals high in *n* Achievement, and also that the Protestant reform should have led Protestant parents to stress self-reliance and monitoring one's own behavior more carefully. This, in turn (according to data then available), should have promoted the development of *n* Achievement particularly among Protestant children. Figure 7.11 summarizes these presumed relationships. The connection Weber outlined between Protestant reform and the dynamic spirit of modern capitalism was to be explained, according to McClelland, by greater independence and mastery training by Protestant parents, which promoted the development of the achievement motive, which led to the production of more active entrepreneurs, which should lead to more rapid economic growth. McClelland set about systematically testing the presumed causal links in this chain of events. The relationship between *D* and *E* in Figure 7.11, or between high *n* Achievement and becoming a more active entrepreneur, clearly exists, as has been discussed.

Protestant Reform, Early Independence Training, and the Achievement Motive

What about the connection between *C* and *D* in Figure 7.11—between independence and mastery training by parents and *n* Achievement scores in sons? An early study by Winterbottom (1958) showed that mothers of high *n* Achievement eight- to eleven-year-old boys reported, in response to a questionnaire, having set high performance standards for them at an earlier age than mothers of children with low *n* Achievement scores. The data are summarized in Figure 7.12. Mothers of boys with high *n* Achievement scores say they insisted more often that the boys by the age of five or six be active and energetic, try hard

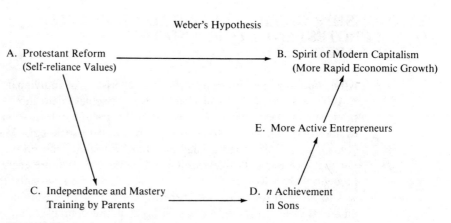

Weber's Hypothesis

A. Protestant Reform
   (Self-reliance Values)

B. Spirit of Modern Capitalism
   (More Rapid Economic Growth)

E. More Active Entrepreneurs

C. Independence and Mastery
   Training by Parents

D. *n* Achievement
   in Sons

Figure 7.11.

Hypothesized Effect of the Protestant Reformation on *n* Achievement and Economic Growth (after McClelland, 1961).

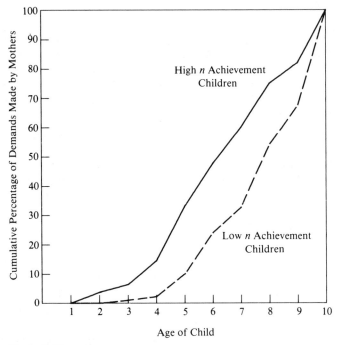

Figure 7.12.

Cumulative Curves Showing the Proportion of Total Demands Made Up to Each Age Level as Reported by Mothers of Children Scoring High and Low on *n* Achievement (McClelland, Atkinson, Clark, & Lowell, 1953, after Winterbottom, 1958).

things for themselves, do well in school, look after their own possessions, and so on.

Later investigations showed that this finding was limited to achievement demands and did not cover caretaking demands, such as being able to undress and go to bed by themselves, and that making achievement demands too early, as well as too late, could be associated with lower *n* Achievement scores (McClelland, 1961). For example, Hayashi and Yamaushi (1964) reported that in Japan among very young children, low achievement motivation is associated with high demands on the mother's part, although this relationship reverses itself among older children. It looks as if the mothers who are promoting the achievement motive tailor their demands to just slightly above what the child can do easily. In other words, they are maximizing the achievement incentives for the children by setting tasks in which the probability of success is neither too low nor too high; the tasks are in the moderate range of difficulty.

McClelland (1961) reports that in Brazil, where on the average mothers make achievement demands on sons early, the *n* Achievement score of sons is positively associated with the age at which their mothers make demands:

the mothers who set later ages for the achievements have sons with higher *n* Achievement scores. The reverse is true in Germany, where the average age set for the same achievements is almost a year later than in Brazil. In Germany, the mothers who expect the achievements at an earlier age have sons with higher *n* Achievement scores. In other words, there is an optimal age for mothers to expect the achievements listed in the questionnaire if they wish to develop the achievement motive. If the mother demands the achievement too early (probability of success too low) or too late (probability of success too high), the child is unlikely to get pleasure out of performing and therefore does not develop high *n* Achievement.

Rosen and D'Andrade (1959) examined the behavior of parents as they observed their sons working on a task. The boys, for example, were asked to stack blocks as high as they could with their left hand when blindfolded while their parents watched. The parents were asked how well they thought their son could do on the task, and then, as the child tried to build the tower, the comments of the parents were recorded and coded. The results are shown in Figure 7.13, with separate curves for the mothers and fathers. Both mothers and fathers of the sons high in *n* Achievement tended to set somewhat higher levels of aspiration for their son's performance than did the parents of sons with low *n* Achievement scores. Furthermore, they expressed more warmth and affection for their sons than the parents of sons low in *n* Achievement. Finally, whereas the mothers of the "highs" were more authoritarian, giving their sons more specific directions than the mothers of the "lows," the reverse was true of the fathers. The fathers of the highs were much less authoritarian than the fathers of

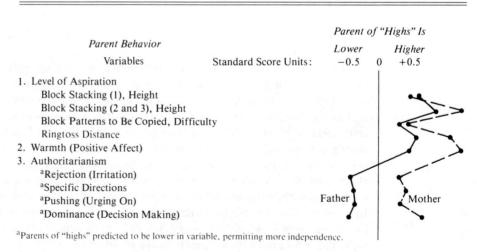

^aParents of "highs" predicted to be lower in variable, permitting more independence.

Figure 7.13.

Mean Differences in the Behavior of Parents of Sons with Low and High *n* Achievement Working in Task Situations (after McClelland, 1961, after B. C. Rosen & D'Andrade, 1959).

the lows. What is important about this finding is that domineering behavior on the part of the mother does not interfere with *n* Achievement, but it does if it comes from the father. In terms of the hypothesis being checked, independence training—that is, allowing the son to proceed on his own—does characterize the fathers of sons with high *n* Achievement scores, but not the mothers.

Other results reported by McClelland (1961) confirm the strong connection between paternal authoritarianism and low *n* Achievement scores. In Turkey, for example, the only businessmen with high *n* Achievement scores were those who had escaped paternal authoritarianism at an early age.

To return to Figure 7.11, what about the connection between *A* and *C*—between Protestantism and independence and mastery training? McClelland, Rindlisbacher, and deCharms (1955) reported significantly later ages at which independence and mastery were expected for Italian and Irish Catholic families as compared with Protestant and Jewish families, and B. C. Rosen (1959) reported similar differences for French Canadian and Italian Catholics versus Protestants and Jews. More careful research demonstrated that these differences tended to disappear in certain groups and may be related to social class differences. McClelland summarizes the research by saying that whereas some traditional Roman Catholic groups have the authoritarian attitudes associated with low *n* Achievement, other Catholic groups have moved toward more general norms for independence and mastery training, so one would not expect an overall Protestant-Catholic difference in *n* Achievement scores at present. In fact, such a difference did not exist in the United States in the 1950s (Veroff et al., 1960) or 1970s (Veroff, Depner, Kulka, & Dowan, 1980).

What seems more crucial is the *spirit of reform* or renewal that originally characterized Protestants in the sixteenth century and that many of the Protestant churches lost as they became more established. For the spirit of reform is likely to translate itself into adherents of the new faith's believing that they are better than adherents of the old way of doing things. This emphasis on being better translates itself into higher standards of performance for themselves and for their children, as well as into higher levels of *n* Achievement. McClelland (1961) found that preliterate cultures tended to have higher levels of *n* Achievement in folktales, which stressed independence training (McClelland & Friedman, 1952), and direct individual contact with the divine rather than contact through established church authority. If people had to set standards for their behavior based on their personal revelations rather than on church authority, they tended to be more achievement oriented and more interested in personally figuring out what was best for them to do.

Furthermore, McClelland (1961) observed what happened in two comparable Mexican villages when one of them had been recently converted to a radical form of Protestant Christianity—a modern replay of the Protestant Reformation. The newly converted Protestants thought of themselves as superior in every way to the "ignorant" traditional folk Catholics in the other village. In order to read the Bible, they had become literate in their own language; they did not worship "idols"; they did not drink and showed more self-control in various ways; and they had become interested in better health and agricultural practices with the help of Protestant missionaries. In other words, they had set for themselves much higher achievement goals than had the people in the traditional nearby village. This achievement orientation had clearly affected the children in the villages, since those from the Protestant village showed evidence of significantly higher *n* Achievement. Thus, Protestant reform from this point of view is simply a special case of any type of ideological movement that helps people set higher achievement goals for themselves. So Weber's hypothesis, or the relation between *A* and *B* in Figure 7.11, translates into a relationship between achievement ideology and more rapid economic growth. Further tests of this hypothesis are discussed in Chapter 11.

However, the findings reported there suggest that reformist ideology is translated so rapidly into the achievement motive, more energetic entrepreneurship, and rapid economic growth that it is highly unlikely the change comes about through the effect of reform on child-rearing attitudes. Thus, in terms of Figure 7.11, *A* (the spirit of reform) must affect *B* (economic growth) directly, as well as *C* (child-rearing) indirectly, which in a generation affects *D* (*n* Achievement), *E* (entrepreneurship), and *B* (economic growth).

The chief value of this investigation lies in the way it was able to translate Weber's argument into measurable variables in terms of which his hypotheses could be scientifically tested. What was concluded in the course of making such tests was that the Protestant Reformation was a special case of an increased social emphasis on excellence or achievement, which, as in other such cases, fostered the achievement motive, entrepreneurship, and economic growth, and may have indirectly influenced child rearing for a time—until the reform became institutionalized. Not all social scientists accept this interpretation of Weber's hypothesis—some because they do not like psychological explanations for complex social phenomena and some because they disapprove of measuring variables and testing their relationships in a scientific way.

• OTHER INFLUENCES AFFECTING THE ACHIEVEMENT MOTIVE EARLY IN LIFE

Several investigators have tried to find the origins of achievement motivation in the earliest years of a child's life. Cortés has suggested that there may be a hereditary factor involved, since he found that mesomorphic boys (with more muscle relative to fat and skin) have significantly higher *n* Achievement scores (and also *n* Power scores) than other boys (Cortés & Gatti, 1972). Their better muscular development should enable them to perform the many motor activities of early childhood with more pleasure and success, building the positive affective associations that make up *n* Achievement through improved performance.

From observing children's success and failure in working at various tasks, Heckhausen (1967) concluded that achievement motivation first appears around the age of three to three and a half, when "the success or failure of one's activity directs the pleasure or disappointment no longer only at the outcome of the activity as such but rather at the self, so that with success the child experiences pleasure about his competence, and with failure experiences shame about his incompetence".

Veroff (1969) agrees that the evaluation of performance is an essential part of achievement motivation and distinguishes it from simple joy in exercising some skill, or what German psychologists had earlier called *function pleasure*. But he sets the time at which this occurs even earlier, somewhere between the age of one and a half to two and a half years, when language develops and children can in effect say to themselves, I did it. He concludes that "autonomous achievement goals generate from repeated experiences of pleasure in the child's new found capacity to do what he was previously unable to do" (Veroff, 1969). He measured the tendency to set such goals by the extent to which children from kindergarten on would choose tasks that were moderately difficult for them, as contrasted with very easy or very difficult tasks. He found that the concept of achievement in comparison to what other children can do develops somewhat later, and that both this concept and feelings of pleasure over performance finally integrate into the *n* Achievement score measured in thought processes, which he found to increase regularly from kindergarten through sixth grade.

There is other evidence that the achievement motive is associated with the development of maturity. Lasker (1978) demonstrated that *n* Achievement scores were strongly associated with stages of ego development, as defined by a measure introduced by Loevinger (1976), in samples from the island of Curaçao and from Chicago. Subjects at Loevinger's earliest, or impulsive and self-protective, stages showed almost no *n* Achievement; those at the middle, or self-protective and conformist, stages had moderate *n* Achievement, whereas those at the highest, or conscientious, level of ego development had high average *n* Achievement scores.

This suggests that only subjects who have matured fully can have really high *n* Achievement scores. Certainly the age trend reported by Veroff supports the notion that *n* Achievement scores increase with maturity. Lasker further demonstrates that this result is partly due to the fact that certain of the scoring characteristics for the *n* Achievement system appear only or primarily in the records of subjects at Loevinger's higher levels of maturity. Lasker divides scoring categories into five sets as follows, beginning with those that appear at the lowest levels of ego development: (*A*) "imagery" and "theme"; (*B*) categories in the form *A* + action and success anticipation; (*C*) categories in the form *B* + need and world block; (*D*) categories in the form *C* + personal block and help; and (*E*) categories in the form *D* + positive and negative feelings and failure anticipation.

Studies by others (for example, Nakamura, 1981) move a few of these categories from one set to the next, but on the whole they confirm Lasker's results. Figure 7.14 shows how scoring categories of the most elementary type begin to appear at the lowest levels of ego development, whereas those of Types B and C appear only at the conformist stages and categories of Types D and E appear only at the highest stages. The explanation for this fact is that thinking about

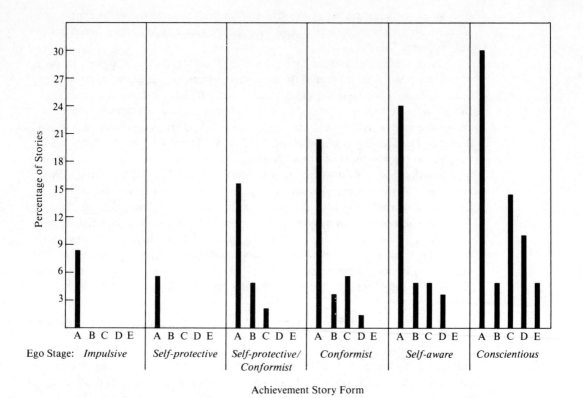

Figure 7.14.

Histogram of Percentage of Achievement Stories of Different Forms by Ego Stage As Defined by Loevinger (1976) (after Lasker, 1978).

possible obstacles in the way of achievement represents a higher level of ego development, and a person's thinking about his or her own characteristics as possible blocks represents an even higher stage of self-awareness. A person's stating how he or she would feel in relation to an achievement event, or even anticipating failure, would represent a still further differentiation of the self from an ongoing story sequence. But whatever the interpretation, the results strongly suggest that the highest levels of *n* Achievement are dependent on overall maturity.

Parental Emphasis on Learning to Control Autonomic Functions

Is there anything that triggers the development of the achievement motive more in some individuals than others? A study by McClelland and Pilon (1983) suggests that parents may have an influence much earlier than was suggested by the studies on achievement goal setting for children by mothers in middle childhood. They administered the standard picture-story test for *n* Achievement to adults at the age of thirty-one whose mothers had been extensively interviewed as to their child-rearing practices twenty-six years earlier by Sears, Maccoby, and Lewin (1957) when their children were five years old. McClelland and Pilon correlated the ratings on some sixty-eight child-rearing practices, as reported by the mothers, with the adult *n* Achievement scores of their children twenty-six years later. Some of the results of this investigation are shown in Table 7.5.

At the top of the table are listed a number of early child-rearing practices that might be supposed to relate to adult *n* Achievement, according to theory or earlier research on middle childhood. None of these practices related consistently to adult *n* Achievement. The only one that fitted with earlier results is that mothers who felt it was very important for their child to do well in school tended to have children—particularly if they were sons and from white-collar families—who had higher *n* Achievement. This is consistent with earlier studies, most of which employed middle-class boys as subjects.

The results for three new child-rearing practices are also shown in Table 7.5, two of which showed significant relationships to adult *n* Achievement across several subsamples of the total population. That is, since these results were not expected and might have been due to chance in the large number of correlations tested, it is necessary to see if they hold up or cross-validate in different samples of subjects. Scheduling of feeding and severity of toilet training are both associated with high *n* Achievement, not only in white-collar and blue-collar families and for males and females, but also for two randomly generated sets of subjects out of the total of seventy-eight. What is curious about this result is that both practices refer to a very early period in the child's life; scheduling feeding normally begins at birth, and toilet training in this sample during the second year of life. This places the origins of the achievement motive earlier than was suggested by Heckhausen or Veroff, although their reasoning that parental emphasis on mastery is important would apply to these areas of behavior as well. Both practices relate to the earliest tasks set for children by the parent—in one case, to regulate their hunger to correspond to the times when they are fed, and in the other, to regulate their sphincters so they are released only in appropriate places.

Two characteristics appear to differentiate what the child learns in these areas as compared with other areas. First, the learning involves control of autonomic functions before the child is capable of much cognitive processing of what is going on, of having much sense of self, or of understanding that "I" did it. These later cognitive additions to affective associations centered around early performance in these areas may have more to do with the value consciously placed on achievement.

Second, the pleasurable experiences in these areas derive from *progressive mastery* of or progressive improvement in timing hunger or eliminating the body's wastes. We hypothesized in Chapter 5 that the need for achievement might derive from the natural variety incentive, from the pleasure people feel in being able to produce a response that confirms a moderate expectation of success. Having many affective experiences of this type based on different expecta-

Table 7.5.

CORRELATIONS OF EARLY CHILD-REARING PRACTICES WITH SOCIAL CLASS AND ADULT *n* ACHIEVEMENT (after McClelland & Pilon, 1983)

Child-rearing practice (Scale: 1–8 or 1–9)	Social Class[a] (N = 78)	Correlations with n Achievement for				
		All Subjects (N = 78)	White-Collar Families[b] (N = 46)	Blue-Collar Families[c] (N = 32)	Males (N = 38)	Females (N = 40)
Early tasks	−.18	−.10	−.05	−.13	−.05	−.15
Mother punishes dependency	.30**	−.12	−.05	−.28	−.01	−.24
Important child do well in school	−.13	.16	.30*	.01	.24	.10
Regular system for earning money	.05	−.12	−.04	−.28	.05	−.37*
Use of reasoning	.24	−.06	−.09	−.07	−.21	.14
Scheduling of feeding	.06	.33**	.25†	.45**	.29†	.38*
Severity of toilet training	−.37***	.41***	.57***	.28†	.43*	.38*
Standards for neatness	−.05	.23*	.39**	.03	.36*	.10

Note: N varies slightly because of missing child-rearing ratings. The *n* Achievement score has been corrected for regression on protocol length. Correlation of *n* Achievement with the social class of the family of origin = .06.

[a]Based on the prestige of the father's occupation and income on a scale of 1 to 9 (Sears, Maccoby, & Lewin, 1957, p. 424; direction here is reversed).

[b]Social class scaled 6 through 9.

[c]Social class scaled 1 through 5.

†$p < .10$ in the predicted direction.

*$p < .05$.

**$p < .01$.

***$p < .001$.

tions should develop a variety motive or a play motive, but not an achievement motive. What characterizes high *n* Achievement is getting pleasure from *progressive improvement* in a particular line of endeavor, not from getting pleasure from several unrelated lines of activity. What parents who stress progressive mastery of autonomic control appear to be doing is placing a constraint on the variety incentive by focusing the pleasure derived from it on increasing probabilities of success in a given area.

We might question whether it is really these early child-rearing practices in themselves that promote the achievement motive. Perhaps they are part of the mother's general attitudes, which continue to shape the child's achievement motivation over the ensuing years. It is true that both of these practices are part of larger strictness-permissiveness syndromes, but neither of these overall syndromes, nor their other components, are related in any way to adult *n* Achievement scores. It is scheduling feeding and toilet training only that appear to be associated with later *n* Achievement (McClelland & Pilon, 1983).

Such a result makes it easier to understand why the presumed early affective learning that shapes the *n* Achievement score is not adequately represented in conscious choices of achievement values, since this learning occurs *before* later cognitive developments represented by achievement values. What seems most likely is that an affective core for *n* Achievement is strongly or weakly established very early from experiences of progressive mastery in learning about feeding and toilet training, and that this affective core gets elaborated—that is, either reinforced or extinguished by later experiences and elaborated by the natural course of cognitive development. Certainly there is no reason not to believe that the achievement goals set by parents in middle childhood cannot also strengthen or diminish the achievement motive core formed earlier in life. Thus, specifically designed educational experiences in adulthood also can strengthen the achievement or any other motive (see Chapter 14). The extent to which a child is taught or learns later to consciously value achievement is seen in this model to be quite independent of the achievement motive based on the pleasure and pain experienced in relation to improving performance in early life.

NOTES AND QUERIES

1. Try scoring the Sermon on the Mount or other sayings of Jesus according to the scoring definition given in Chapter 6 to see if Jesus had high *n* Achievement.

2. Several characteristics of people who have high *n* Achievement are described in the chapter. Try to explain the way they doodle in terms of these characteristics.

3. Would you expect people who work hard and conscientiously to have high *n* Achievement? Why or why not?

4. Generally, students high in *n* Achievement do not get better grades in school. Why do you think this is true? What motives, in your opinion, should lead people to do better in school?

5. Some people just seem to be "born losers"; they keep getting into situations where they have to lose out, or they seem to have a great deal of bad luck. Is there information in this chapter that might suggest why they have so much bad luck and what kind of motivation they might have?

6. Score the imaginative stories you wrote for Chapter 1 for *n* Achievement. Make a checklist of the characteristics a person high in *n* Achievement should show, and decide whether you have shown those characteristic on a number of occasions (recall them specifically). Does the amount of achievement imagery in your stories agree with the number of achievement-related characteristics you have shown? Do you believe you have high or low *n* Achievement? Were there any surprises in the result? Is the value you place on achievement higher or lower than your estimated *n* Achievement score?

7. In Table 7.4 it appears that subjects high in *n* Achievement more often are high in intelligence also, at least in homogeneous classes. Could it be that some students do better in homogeneous classes because they have higher intelligence, and not because they have higher *n* Achievement?

8. Economists often argue that people in general will do what it is in their self-interest to do; that is, they will be guided rationally by the probability of success of various alternatives. For example, if there have been several crop failures in a row, farmers on the whole will give up farming and move to the city, because the probability of success in farming is so low. Explain, in terms of Atkinson's model of the relationship of *n* Achievement and the probability of success, who will be likely to move or not move after crop failures, and under what conditions.

9. Which type of person would be most likely to be happy alone on a desert island—a person high in *n* Achievement, high in *n* Power, or high in *n* Affiliation? Why? What would that person be likely to be found doing?

10. It has been said that whereas money is not everything, it will buy everything in first place. Is this true for a person high in *n* Achievement?

11. Do you think creative writers or inventors would be more likely to be high in *n* Achievement? Why?

12. If any reform movement should promote the achievement motive, should not countries newly converted to Communism be higher in *n* Achievement? (See Chapter 11 for evidence on this point.)

13. In terms of the description of how the achievement motive functions and how it is developed, why do you think U.S. blacks of lower-class background scored low in *n* Achievement in the 1950s?

14. It has been argued that it is absurd to conclude that lower-class blacks have lower *n* Achievement when they obviously want to do many things well, although they may not be the same things middle-class whites want to do well. Comment on this argument. Would the argument have the same force if the achievement motive were called the *efficiency motive*?

15. Why should paternal authoritarianism lower *n* Achievement levels in sons more than maternal authoritarianism?

16. Psychologists have been intrigued by the possibility that cultural "accidents" might have unintended consequences for the development of human motives like the achievement motive. McClelland (1961) speculated that wealthy families in ancient Greece or in the U.S. South might have unwittingly lowered the *n* Achievement levels of their children by acquiring household slaves who spoiled the children, undermining the emphasis on independence and mastery needed to develop high *n* Achievement. Wendt (1961, 1974) has suggested that the tendency for eminence to be associated with birth at certain times of the year might be due to higher levels of *n* Achievement accidentally acquired by eminent people because they learned to walk in the summer months, when there were greater opportunities to get pleasure from independently mastering such an important skill.

Now that it appears that the achievement motive is developed by parental emphasis on strict toilet training, speculate on the possible accidental side effects on n Achievement levels of the introduction of easily disposable diapers. How could your speculation be tested?

17. Under what circumstances could Catholicism be associated with a greater emphasis on performance improvement and higher levels of n Achievement?

8

The Power Motive

• MEASURING THE NEED FOR POWER

Practically every student of personality, from Freud to McDougall to Murray and Cattell, has found that human beings are characterized by a need for power, aggression, or domination. Anthropologists, biologists, and philosophers like Nietzsche have all been impressed by human beings' aggressive urges.

The story of how a measure for the motive involved here was finally derived is considerably more complicated than it was for the achievement motive. An early measure patterned after the scoring system for n Achievement was discovered to have some limitations and was eventually modified, expanded, and refined into the measure generally used today. The account of its development illustrates how science proceeds by trial and correction and, once again, how crucial precise measurement is in science.

The original coding system for n Power was derived by Veroff (1957) from examining the content of stories written by student candidates for office while they were waiting for election returns to be counted. The idea was that students seeking office would be more likely than others to want power and that their power need would be more apt to be aroused while they were waiting to see if they would get power than under more neutral conditions. The stories written when the power motive was aroused contained many more themes about *control of the means of influence* than stories written by comparable subjects under control conditions.

So for scoring purposes, Veroff defined the goal of the power motive as *exerting influence,* and he looked for increases in the subcategories already defined as part of goal-seeking behavior for the achievement motive (see Table 6.4 in Chapter 6). He found such categories as *instrumental activity* aimed at a power goal, or *blocks* interfering with attaining it, to be more frequent in the stories written by those waiting for election returns than by others. However, he did not specifically look for new categories that might be unique to the arousal of power motivation.

The n Power scoring system derived in this way was validated by examining how subjects who scored high in it under nonarousal conditions behaved in a variety of circumstances. For example, Veroff (1957) reported that those who scored high in n Power were rated by their instructors as trying more frequently to convince others than subjects who scored low in n Power. However, as subsequent studies showed, n Power scored in this way sometimes was associated with assertive behavior and sometimes with unassertive behavior. For example, Terhune (1968a, 1968b) found that teams consisting of individuals high in n Power were more assertive, less cooperative, and more deceitful in a multination simulation game than other teams. But Berlew (1959) had previously reported that subjects high in n Power in small discussion groups were *less assertive,* tending to give opinions and suggestions less often than other subjects. Furthermore, sometimes people without social power in society scored high in n Power, and sometimes those with social power scored high.

Does that mean that power motivation measured in this way is aroused by having or not having social status or power? In a national sample, Veroff, Atkinson, Feld, and Gurin (1960) found that men with less education scored higher in *n* Power than those with more education, whereas the reverse was true for women: those with more education scored higher in *n* Power than those with less education. Veroff and Veroff (1972) explained such apparent inconsistencies by reasoning that the *n* Power score was really measuring fear of appearing weak or fear of being deprived of power. Thus, both less educated men and more educated women would be likely to feel somewhat oppressed or relatively weaker in the competition for power in U.S. society. Hence, their high *n* Power scores would represent a kind of defensive reaction to compensate for their relative deprivation or weakness.

The same line of reasoning could explain the inconsistency between behavior in small groups and in the multination simulation game, for in the latter the participants never confronted each other directly. Rather, they wrote notes to each other as diplomats would, and they could appear assertive without the danger of being personally shown up in front of others. In contrast, in Berlew's discussion groups, the individuals were reacting to other people face to face and might have avoided assertive behaviors for fear of being confronted and shown up.

Such an interpretation of the Veroff *n* Power score suggested that it might contain more of an element of anxiety than would be ideally desirable. Certainly the conditions under which power motivation had been aroused included a strong anxiety component: the student politicians wrote the stories while they were waiting for the votes to be counted and were worrying whether or not they were going to win. This suggested that power motivation ought to be aroused in individuals who had more certainty about the outcome of their power impulses. So Uleman (1966) aroused power motivation by appointing students to be "experimenters" in a two-person gambling game for small stakes. The experimenters were told that the purpose of the game was to study the effects of frustration, and they were taught how they could always win the gambling game so that they could frustrate the subjects. As Orne (1962) has pointed out, the role of being an experimenter is an extremely powerful one. Therefore, it was expected that power motivation would be aroused in the students assigned the experimenter role, since they knew how to defeat their subjects. This turned out to be the case. Stories written by the student experimenters were found by Uleman to contain many more themes relating to successful, interpersonal influence than stories written under control conditions. In contrast to Veroff, Uleman looked for new scoring categories not specifically related to the problem-solving sequence involved in the *n* Achievement scoring system and found several new ones, such as more frequent references to the prestige of actors in the experimenters' stories than in those written by others. He developed a coding system called *n* Influence, which has shown some promising correlations with a confident style of interpersonal influence (see Uleman, 1972).

Faced with these somewhat conflicting results, Winter (1967, 1973) undertook a thorough revision of the *n* Power scoring system that includes categories from both the Veroff and Uleman systems and adds some new ones. Winter derived this system by identifying shifts in story content under two new types of power motivation arousal and then checking to see if the same shifts occurred under the Veroff and Uleman conditions for arousing power motivation. In the new arousal experiments, subjects observed a powerful figure in action. In one case, the power figure was a hypnotist behaving in a confident, successful manner and ordering hypnotized subjects to do all sorts of things in front of a class, after which the class members wrote their stories. In the other, the power figure was John F. Kennedy giving his inaugural address as president shown on film to a class of business school students.

In contrast to stories written under control conditions, those written after exposure to the power figures contained more references to a person or persons concerned about having "impact, control, or influence over another person, group, or the world at large" (Winter, 1973). This became the new definition of whether power imagery was present in a story or not. A further explanation of the definition is given in Table 8.1, along with the subcategories Winter found were more frequently present under all or most of the power motivation arousal conditions. Note that he also distinguishes between Hope of Power—an approach component of the motive—and Fear of Power—an avoidance component.

The Winter revised scoring system for *n* Power is the one now in widest use, and it has been employed in most of the studies to be reported in this chapter. It correlates around .44 with the Veroff and Uleman scoring systems (Winter, 1973). Thus, it is not really measuring a different variable, but it represents a refinement and expansion of earlier scoring systems. The kinds of behavior with which it is associated suggest that it is not as related to the fear of weakness as the Veroff *n* Power score is. For example, in national sample surveys conducted in 1957 and 1976, female college graduates scored high in *n* Power less than 50 percent of the time according to the Winter system, in contrast to more than 50 percent of the time according to the Veroff system; this is why Veroff argued that their *n* Power was a reaction to their relative deprivation. Women do score higher in *n* Power, according to the Winter system, in the professions and sales, which are occupations that ought to require more power assertiveness (Veroff, Depner, Kulka, & Douvan, 1980). Furthermore, in the 1976 survey, men high in fear of weakness (the Veroff system) had lower self-esteem (if college educated), drank and took drugs to relieve tension, and attended church less; however, they saw fatherhood as very important and felt good about work competence, which Veroff (1982) interprets as compensation for their underlying sense of weakness. Those high in *n* Power (the Winter system) in the same survey showed none of these characteristics, except the tendency to drink more. (See the discussion of drinking later in the chapter.)

• EVIDENCE THAT THE *n* POWER SCORE MEASURES A MOTIVE

Energizing Function of the Power Motive

According to theory, motives drive, orient, and select behavior. What is the evidence that the power motive as measured this way drives, or energizes, the or-

Table 8.1.

**BRIEF VERSION OF THE *n* POWER SCORING SYSTEM (after
Winter & Stewart, 1978)**

Power Imagery: Scored if some person or group of persons in the story is concerned about establishing, maintaining, or restoring power—that is, impact, control, or influence over another person, group, or the world at large. Examples: (1) Someone shows power concern through actions that in themselves express power. (2) Someone does something that arouses strong positive or negative emotions in others. (3) Someone is described as having a concern for reputation or position.

Subcategories, to Be Scored Only If Power Imagery is Scored:

Prestige: The characters are described in ways that increase or decrease their prestige. Settings, titles, adjectives of status, reputation, and alliance with some prestigeful person or institution are all examples of prestige.

Stated Need for Power: An explicit statement that the character wants to attain a power goal. *Not* inferrable from mere instrumental activity.

Instrumental Act: Overt or mental activity by a character indicating that he or she is doing something about attaining a power goal.

Block in the World: An explicit obstacle or disruption to the attempt to reach a power goal.

Goal Anticipation: Some character is thinking about the power goal, with either positive or negative anticipations.

Goal States: Affective or feeling states associated with attaining or not attaining the power goal.

Effect: A distinct response by someone to the power actions of someone else in the story, or indication of widespread effect on the world at large.

Hope/Fear Distinction:

All stories are scored Hope of Power unless one or more of the following occurs in the story, in which case it is scored Fear of Power: (1) The power goal is for the direct or indirect benefit of someone else. (2) The actor has doubt about his or her ability to influence, control, or impress others. (3) The writer of the story suggests that power is deceptive or has a flaw, as by the use of contrast, irony, or explicit statement. Included are cases in which characters feel happy after power failures and sad after power successes.

Note: This brief version is intended for illustrative purposes only. It is not adequate for actual scoring purposes. A complete version of the *n* Power manual, together with practice stories and procedures for learning the system, is available in Winter (1973, Appendix 1). Scoring system Copyright © David G. Winter, 1973.

ganism? Steele (1973, 1977) conducted an experiment that provides information on this point. He aroused power motivation in student subjects by having them listen to a tape of an actor giving excerpts from famous inspirational speeches, such as Winston Churchill's speech at Dunkirk or Henry V's speeches in Shakespeare's *Life of King Henry* V. In the control condition, subjects listened to some tape-recorded travel descriptions. All students then wrote imaginative stories to pictures. Steele also attempted to arouse achievement motivation before the subjects wrote their stories by having them work on a series of tasks—tasks they were told measured their intelligence and alertness.

He found, as expected, that the stories written after the inspirational speeches contained significantly higher *n* Power scores than those written after the travel tapes. On the other hand, the *n* Achievement scores obtained after the ego-involving instructions were not significantly higher than the *n* Achievement scores obtained after a more relaxed introduction to the tasks, probably because the mean *n* Achievement score under the "relaxed" instructions was not as low as could be expected from comparison with findings in other groups.

Steele measured activation in the subjects either through changes in their moods, as determined from the Thayer Adjective Checklist (1967), or by shifts in the concentrations of epinephrine (adrenaline) in the urine of the subjects from before to after presentation of the speeches. He looked for shifts in epinephrine output because emotional or physiological arousal is regularly associated with activation of the sympathetic nervous system, which increases the output of certain neurohormones—for example, the catecholamines epinephrine and norepinephrine—which are excreted in urine (see Frankenhaeuser, 1978). Table 8.2 presents the results for gains in epinephrine excretion. The biggest average gain occurs from before to after listening to the inspirational speeches. The gains for the other three experimental conditions are lower and about the same. Conspicuously, there is no greater gain in epinephrine excretion for the achievement arousal condition than for its control, which could mean either that the achievement arousal instructions failed or that the arousal of achievement motivation is not associated with catecholamine shifts as closely as power motivation is.

The most striking result in Table 8.2 is that the amount of power imagery present in the stories written after the inspirational speeches correlates highly with gains in epinephrine excretion. In other words, the subjects who showed the greatest signs of physiological arousal were those who injected the highest level of power concern into their stories. Gains in norepinephrine excretion were also highly and significantly correlated with *n* Power scores after the inspirational speeches ($r = .66$; $p < .01$). Note also that shifts in signs of physiological arousal are not significantly correlated with the motivational content of stories under any of the other conditions. It disappointed Steele particularly that gains in epinephrine excretion under conditions of achievement arousal were not significantly associated with *n* Achievement scores after arousal, since he thought that any type of motivational arousal should have the same physiological consequences. The results are not conclusive, because the correlation is in the same direction although insignificant and because Steele may not have succeeded in arousing the achievement motive very strongly. His findings, however, also raise the possibility that catecholamine shifts are more associated with power than with achievement motivation.

An indirect indication that the power motive may be particularly associated with catecholamine function comes from an occasion in which I determined that of those who sat consistently to the right of me in class (from the students'

Table 8.2.

RELATIONSHIP OF EPINEPHRINE INCREASE TO MOTIVATIONAL CONTENT AFTER DIFFERENT TYPES OF EXPERIMENTAL AROUSAL
(after McClelland, 1976, after Steele, 1973)

Condition	N	Mean Gains in Epinephrine Excretion (Nanograms per Minute)	Correlations of Epinephrine Change with Motive Scores	
			n Power	*n* Achievement
Power arousal (stirring tapes)	16	+1.51	.71*	.04
Power control (travel tapes)	14	+0.27	.38	.06
Achievement arousal (ego-involving tasks)	19	+0.35	−.02	.25
Achievement control (relaxing tasks)	14	+0.47	.10	.36

*$p < .05$.

point of view), 66 percent were high in *n* Power as compared with only 25 percent of those who sat to the left of me ($p < .05$). Sitting on the right means students must look more often to the left to observe the instructor. Looking to the left is associated with dominance of the right hemisphere of the brain (see P. Bakan, 1978), and there is evidence that norepinephrine function is concentrated more on the right side of the brain (Oke, Keller, Mefford, & Adams, 1978; Robinson, 1979).

The connection of the power motive and right hemisphere function is further supported by the finding that there is a right hemisphere advantage in recognizing emotional stimuli (Ley & Bryden, 1982) and the finding that *n* Power scores are significantly correlated ($r = .34$; $N = 72$; and $p < .01$) with recognizing better the emotional tone of content-filtered speech in the taped version of Rosenthal's test of nonverbal communication (Rosenthal, 1979). In this test, subjects hear very brief excerpts of a person saying something to someone else that have been electronically filtered so they cannot recognize *what* is being said, although they still can recognize the speaker's emotional tone. They might have to decide, for instance, whether the sounds they hear are of a mother scolding a child or a man making love to a woman. Some people are much better than others at picking the correct response. This should indicate greater right hemisphere dominance, and such people do tend to be higher in *n* Power. So we might infer that those high in *n* Power tend to dominance of the right hemisphere, which is also more associated with norepinephrine output than the left hemisphere.

In a second study, Steele (1977) focused on the adjective checklist measure of activation. In particular, he employed Thayer's measure of General Activation, which covers the extent to which subjects describe themselves as feeling lively, vigorous, energetic, and full of pep. Steele measured the General Activation level and *n* Power before and after some travel tapes and inspirational speeches. As Figure 8.1 demonstrates, the inspirational speeches produced a marked increase both in the *n* Power score and the General Activation level score. Furthermore, he found that for those who heard the inspirational speeches first, the amount of an individual's gain in General Activation level was significantly correlated ($r = .79$; $p < .01$) with his or her *n* Power score in stories written subsequently. This result exactly parallels that shown in Table 8.2 using the epinephrine measure of general activation. Steele also obtained a similar result when he gave the TAT first. That is, those who scored highest in *n* Power on the TAT also showed the largest gain in General Activation when they listened to the inspirational speeches ($r = .65$; $p < .01$). In other words, physiological activation to power stimuli is closely associated with *n* Power in thought content.

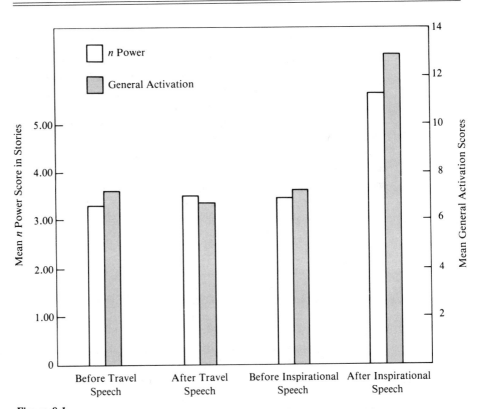

Figure 8.1.

Effects of Inspirational Speeches on *n* Power Scores and General Activation (data from Steele, 1977).

Whereas subjects high in *n* Power are more activated by power-related stimuli, they tend to be sensation avoiders rather than sensation seekers, perhaps for that very reason. In Steele's (1973) study, those whose *n* Power scores tended to be highest in response to the power stimuli of the inspirational speeches described themselves as sensation avoiders. That is, they scored low on Zuckerman's Sensation Seeking Scale (1974; see Figure 5.7 in Chapter 5 of this book). The correlation between *n* Power scores under these arousal conditions and the Sensation Seeking Scale was $-.57$, $p < .05$, whereas there was no correlation under any of the other conditions. A similar result has been reported by Davidson, Saron, and McClelland (1980), who used event-related scalp electrical potentials as a measure of the subject's response to stimulation. In this experiment, as sounds increased in intensity, subjects low in *n* Power reacted with electrical potentials of larger and larger amplitude, as recorded from their scalps. The trend for those high in *n* Power was the reverse. They responded more to a weak sound than those low in *n* Power, but as the sound increased in intensity, their evoked event potentials declined. They were less responsive to stronger stimulation, perhaps because they are already so activated that they react by reducing the response to stimulation from without.

Orienting Function of the Power Motive

Individuals high in *n* Power are more sensitive to power-related stimuli than to neutral stimuli, as demonstrated by findings assessing the electrical responsivity of the brain to various stimuli. In this type of experiment, electrodes are attached to the scalps of human subjects over various areas of the brain to pick up very small changes that occur in electrical potentials due to the response of that portion of the brain to stimulation. In one experiment (McClelland, Davidson, & Saron, 1979) the subjects were shown power-related pictures (for example, a boxer or a car accident) several times interspersed with neutral pictures (for example, an old man standing in a boat or a boy loafing on a bed). The measure of the electrical response to the power and neutral picture exposures was the sum of the amplitude of the first negative deflection (N_1) and the second positive deflection (P_2) in electrical potential. (See Figure 8.2 for an example of how the deflections are identified.)

If there is any difference in the way subjects high and low in *n* Power respond to power or neutral stimuli from electrodes on the scalp, it would be expected to occur first over the occipital area at the back of the head, because that scalp region lies over the portion of the brain where visual sensations are projected. That is exactly what happened. The subjects high in *n* Power, as compared with those low in *n* Power, showed a much larger $N_1 + P_2$ amplitude response (shown by the two dots in Figure 8.2) to power than to neutral pictures over the occipital area, but not over the frontal area. Note that the difference in responsivity to power over neutral stimuli occurs very early—within the first quarter of a second after the stimulus has been exposed. This is presumably before the subjects could have processed the sensations from the pictures very far and reacted more to them perhaps because they evoked power associations.

Rather, those high in *n* Power seem already "preset" to react more sensitively to power cues as soon as they occur.

Figure 8.2 illustrates the difference in electrical scalp potential responsiveness to power stimuli of a subject high in *n* Power and a subject low in *n* Power. For this graph, the $N_1 + P_2$ amplitude of the electrical scalp response to power words (not pictures) is being recorded in the frontal area (Davidson, Saron, & McClelland, 1980). It is greater for the subject high in *n* Power than for the subject low in *n* Power. The difference occurs about 100 to 150 milliseconds after stimulus onset. This response is in the frontal rather than the occipital area, as in the previous study: word meaning is processed more in the frontal area, whereas visual stimuli are processed first in the occipital area. The $N_1 + P_2$ responsiveness was significantly different for subjects high and low in *n* Power in response to power, but not neutral, words when stimulus intensity was low. When the intensity of the spoken words was raised, however, the sensation avoidance characteristic of subjects high in *n* Power appeared.

Selective Function of the Power Motive

McAdams (1982b) has reported that subjects high in *n* Power recall more "peak" experiences that are described in power terms. A peak experience is one a person describes as having had great emotional importance. For instance, a male student, when asked for such experiences, may recall how emotionally

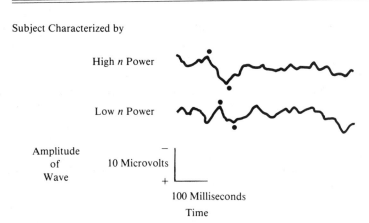

Subject Characterized by

High *n* Power

Low *n* Power

Amplitude of Wave

−
10 Microvolts
+

100 Milliseconds

Time

Figure 8.2.

Event Electrical Response Potentials from Scalp Leads in the Frontal Area in Response to Power-Related Words Spoken at a Moderate Intensity Level for a Subject High and a Subject Low in *n* Power. The electrical response potentials are based on a mean of twenty word stimuli per average. Stimulus onset coincides with the beginning of the wave form. The dots correspond to the first negative (N_1) and second positive (P_2) peaks. This peak-to-peak amplitude was the dependent measure employed (after Davidson, Saron, & McClelland, 1980).

charged he was when he played a part in a play that was loudly applauded by the audience. This would be considered a power peak experience, because he was obviously moved by having impact on others.

Subjects high in *n* Power had more power-related peak experiences to begin with. A more controlled experiment was carried out by McAdams and McClelland (1983) in which the subjects listened to a taped recording of someone telling a story about a picture they were looking at. The story contained thirty facts relating to power, thirty related to intimacy, and fifteen neutral facts. At the conclusion of the story, the subjects filled out a Mood Adjective Checklist and then unexpectedly were asked to recall the story in as much detail as possible. To control for ability in recall, the number of power facts remembered was compared with the number of neutral facts remembered. The subjects high in *n* Power recalled significantly more power facts relative to neutral facts than those low in *n* Power. This difference was shown to persist at least twenty minutes later in another experiment in which recall was delayed and the intervening time filled with other activities.

Selective recall should lead to faster learning of power-related materials by subjects high in *n* Power. An experiment by McClelland, Davidson, Saron, and Floor (1980) reported such a trend. Subjects who participated in the evoked potential experiment previously described were asked to learn to associate either a power or a neutral word to a power or a neutral picture stimulus. That is, when the stimulus appeared, they were given two seconds to say the word before it appeared. After a number of presentations of the twenty picture-word pairs, most of the subjects had learned most of the associations. To test the relative speed with which subjects high and low in *n* Power were learning the different types of associations, the number of correct responses made on Trials 3 and 4 was compared. As compared with the subjects low in *n* Power, those high in *n* Power gave a significantly higher number of correct responses on Trials 3 and 4 to the pairs in which one of the components was power related—that is, either a power-neutral or neutral-power pair. There was not a significant difference in the number of correct responses given by the two motive groups to the power-power pairs—perhaps because these were the easiest pairs for all subjects to learn—or to the neutral-neutral pairs. The faster learning of power words to neutral pictures by subjects high in *n* Power is illustrated in Figure 8.3.

This study also demonstrated a link between *n* Power and catecholamine function, as indexed by the increase in 3-methoxy-4-hydroxyphenylglycol (MHPG) in urine collected before and after the experiment. MHPG is largely a metabolite of brain, rather than peripheral, norepinephrine turnover (Maas, Hattox, Greene, & Landis, 1979). In this experiment there was a significantly greater power pair learning advantage for subjects both high in *n* Power and brain norepinephrine turnover (an increase in MHPG from before to after the experiment) as compared with those low in both measures. Furthermore, the recall of more power than neutral facts from the story in the experiment previously cited is also associated significantly with being high in *n* Power and high in brain norepinephrine turnover during the course of the experiment, as contrasted with being low in both variables (McClelland & Maddocks, 1984). The fact that high brain norepinephrine turnover is not in either experiment connected—in combination with high *n* Affiliation—with better recall of affiliative facts suggests that greater general arousal is not involved, but an arousal specific to power motivational content.

Since the injection of norepinephrine into rat brains increases self-stimulation (see Chapter 4), and since exciting drugs like amphetamines (or "speed") increase norepinephrine at the synapse, it might be inferred that brain norepinephrine represents a physiological reward system—not, as Stein (1975) has argued, for all kinds of drive systems, but specifically for the power motive. To put it in everyday language, suppose brain norepinephrine turnover (as indexed by MHPG in urine) represents the extent to which power stimuli "turn on" subjects, or make them "feel good." Clearly, the pictures used in this experiment would have more turn-on value for some subjects than others. So these results mean that subjects who are high in *n* Power will learn power-related mate-

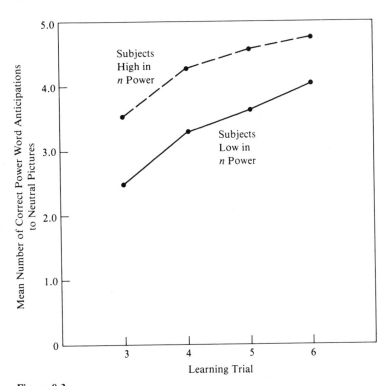

Figure 8.3.

Average Number of Correct Power Word Anticipations to Neutral Pictures on Successive Learning Trials (McClelland, Davidson, Saron, & Floor, 1980).

rials faster if the materials have turn-on value for them than if they do not; in particular, they will learn the power-related materials faster than subjects low in *n* Power, for whom the stimuli have no turn-on value.

The situation is analogous to putting hungry rats in a maze with food at the end that they either like or do not like. The rats who are hungry and like the food will learn fastest, and those who are not hungry and dislike the food will learn slowest. From this point of view, brain norepinephrine turnover can be conceived of as the index of the *reward* or *incentive value* of power-related stimuli. For a related finding at the animal level, see Weiss, Stone, & Harrell (1970). Obviously, such an interpretation is speculative, based as it is at present on two experiments involving relatively few subjects. It is consistent, however, with indirect evidence and theory that link *n* Power to catecholamine function.

• OUTLETS OF THE NEED FOR POWER

Aggressiveness

Just as in the case of the achievement motive, much research has focused on how people with a strong power motive behave under various circumstances. In particular, are they more aggressive? That is a question of special interest to those who tend to define motives in terms of characteristic acts. As it became apparent that high *n* Power did not always lead to aggression, which is tightly controlled and regulated in modern society, the attention of researchers shifted to more subtle ways in which the impulse to assertiveness could express itself.

It might be expected that individuals high in *n* Power would be more competitive and aggressive. Some early results suggested that this was so. Winter (1973) found that college students who had received varsity letters for playing competitive sports scored significantly higher in *n* Power than other men. Competitive sports were defined as those in which there was direct competition between one person and another or one team against another, such as football, tennis, or hockey. McClelland (1975) later confirmed this finding for a sample of older men no longer in school. Those higher in *n* Power voluntarily participated in more competitive sports than those low in *n* Power. Furthermore, in the sample of older men, the *n* Power score was significantly correlated with the frequency with which the men reported they got into arguments.

However, none of these relationships hold for women, which reminds us once again that a motive is only one of the determinants of action. Values and habits or skills also determine whether the power motive will erupt into assertive action. To be openly assertive has been valued for men but not for women, so even if a woman high in *n* Power has the impulse to argue, she might inhibit it because she accepts the sex-role value of being friendly and cooperative.

Nowhere is this clearer than in aggression. Both men and women high in *n* Power confessed to having more impulses to being aggressive that they control at a certain level of maturity than men and women low in *n* Power (see Table 8.6 later in the Chapter). That is, they were first asked whether they had ever felt like carrying out a number of impulsive aggressive acts like yelling at someone in traffic, throwing things around the room, or taking towels from a hotel or motel; then they were asked whether they had ever carried out any of these actions. More men and women high in *n* Power at a certain level of maturity confessed to being angry and to having thought about doing such things, but they did not in fact do them more often than individuals low in *n* Power (McClelland, 1975).

Whether a man actually carries out aggressive actions depends very much on social class values, as Winter (1973) demonstrated. He found that high *n* Power was significantly associated with carrying out more impulsive aggressive acts among working-class men, but not among middle-class men. Thus, there is no simple, one-to-one relationship between *n* Power and aggressive actions. Whether such actions will occur for those high in *n* Power depends on the other determinants of action, namely, the person's skills or habits and values.

Veroff (1982) also pointed out that the power motive is particularly situation dependent, because its goal is to "make a splash" or create excitement, and the way to do this varies markedly with the situation. So what has gradually emerged out of research on the power motive is a picture of a person striving to be assertive in ways that either are appropriate to the situation or that are not and therefore produce feelings of guilt and anxiety over the aggressive impulses. What is not in question is the general conclusion that people high in *n* Power strive to be assertive.

Negative Self-image

The disposition to be aggressive or assertive leads people to view themselves negatively for having what are generally considered to be antisocial tendencies. A sample of adult men and women aged around thirty-one years were asked to fill out the Gough Adjective Checklist (Gough & Heilbrun, 1975). The task is simply to mark any of three hundred adjectives that people think describe themselves. Table 8.3 lists the adjectives checked more often by men and women high in *n* Power as compared with those low in *n* Power. The men with a strong power motive recognized that they felt more assertive—*rebellious, resentful,* and *sulky*—and obviously judged this characteristic rather negatively, as we shall see. The self-picture of women high in *n* Power was similar, although the adjectives used were slightly different. They felt more often *cynical, bitter,* and *resentful.*

What is particularly striking about both sets of the self-descriptive adjectives chosen is that they are so negative. There were many opportunities to pick positive adjectives like *active, adaptable, adventurous, cooperative,* or *courageous,* which could signify an assertive disposition. It is as if the individuals high in *n* Power recognize their aggressive impulses; judge them negatively, just as society would judge them; and have a rather negative self-image in consequence. Aggressive-assertive behavior is punished beginning in early childhood because it is often antisocial, and people learn that it is bad to be aggressive in many—although not all—situations. Hermann (1980) has confirmed these trends in cod-

Table 8.3.

**CORRELATIONS BETWEEN FREQUENCY WITH WHICH SELF-DESCRIPTIVE
ADJECTIVE IS CHOSEN AND *n* POWER SCORE FOR MEN (*N* = 38) AND
WOMEN (*N* = 40)**

	Men		Women	
Adjectives	*Correlations with n Power Score*		*Adjectives*	*Correlations with n Power Score*
Coarse	.47**		Cynical	.35*
Complicated	.42*		Complicated	.35*
Disorderly	.49**		Disorderly	.29†
High strung	.43*		Bitter	.40*
Rebellious	.43*		Self-pitying	.44*
Resentful	.41*		Resentful	.39*
Sulky	.52**		Moody	.35*
Spunky	.39*		Unaffected	.35*
Hurried	.38*			

†$p < .10$.
*$p < .05$.
**$p < .01$.

ing for *n* Power speeches by members of the governing body of the Soviet
Union, the Politburo. She found that those high in *n* Power did not favor
detente with the United States ($r = -.34$; $p < .05$)—that is, they favored
a more assertive foreign policy—and had a more negative self-image ($r = .51$;
$p < .01$).

National sample survey data from the United States also confirm the fact
people high in *n* Power view themselves more negatively (Veroff et al., 1980).
Both men and women with strong power motives report themselves as feeling
more inadequate or dissatisfied with various aspects of their lives and having
problems with drinking or drug taking to relieve tension. (The relation of power
motivation to drinking will be taken up later.) What is clear is that people high
in *n* Power have more emotional problems, a fact confirmed in yet another sample of adults in which high *n* Power among men was correlated with trouble in
sleeping and among women, with more unpleasant dreams (McClelland, 1975).

Entry into Influential Occupations

One of the ways individuals can exercise influence in more socialized ways is
through the occupations they choose to enter. Winter (1973) found that male
students planning to have a career in teaching, psychology, the ministry, business, or journalism had significantly higher *n* Power scores than students plan-

ning to enter other occupations, including law and medicine. These results were for the most part confirmed in longitudinal studies that showed that men who actually entered the first set of occupations had higher *n* Power scores years before as undergraduates than those who did not enter these occupations. The results are summarized in Table 8.4, and they seem to hold up not only in the United States, but also for a small sample of University of Oxford graduates in England.

Winter argues that these results are consistent with theory because the occupations chosen and entered by the men higher in *n* Power all provide more scope for power and influence than the other occupations. More specifically, teachers and the clergy are in a public position trying to influence an audience. Psychologists and journalists have more inside information: they know what other people do not know and are in a better position to influence people through this special knowledge. Sonnenfeld (1975) confirmed the tendency of people high in *n* Power to seek positions of public influence in a study of students who volunteered to work for a college radio station. He found that the correlation between *n* Power scores and the time devoted to the station was .53 ($N = 30; p < .01$). In contrast, *n* Achievement correlated $-.65$ ($p < .01$) with time spent at the radio station, presumably because there was no tangible, lasting product or achievement outcome to display as a result of time spent. In similar fashion, Mueller (1975) discovered that women who perform publicly as musicians score higher in *n* Power than music teachers.

Managers are also in a position to exercise power, although, as we shall see later in this chapter, more is known about the specific kind of power motive syndrome that is related to success in different types of managerial positions. In

Table 8.4.

MEAN *n* POWER SCORES OF COLLEGE MEN ASPIRING TO CERTAIN OCCUPATIONS AND MEN IN THOSE OCCUPATIONS (after Winter, 1973)

	Mean n Power Scores		
Occupation	*Aspirants: Wesleyan T-Scores (N)*	*Occupants: Harvard Raw Scores (N)*	*Alumni: Oxford Raw Scores (N)*
Teaching	53.7[a] (48)	4.85[a] (27)	
Teaching and clergy			10.13[a] (15)
Psychology and clergy	54.1[a] (31)	4.18[a] (17)	
Business and journalism	52.4[a] (34)	6.60[a] (15)	13.86[a] (7)
Law	49.0 (27)	3.59 (29)	
Medicine	46.4 (14)	3.35 (20)	
Other	47.0 (26)	3.06 (65)	5.44 (16)

[a]Significantly higher than all others.

contrast, doctors and lawyers may have influence through their skills rather than their powers of persuasion, although this obviously varies with the type of lawyer. Courtroom lawyers arguing cases should have higher n Power than lawyers involved in settling estates, but Winter's data do not permit such a comparison.

In general, national sample surveys from 1957 and 1976 confirm these results (Veroff et al., 1980). Male professionals (including teachers), as well as laborers and operatives score higher in n Power; farmers and office-secretarial workers score lower in n Power. The results for laborers and operatives suggest that high n Power might lead people to occupations where they have impact on things as well as people, although Winter has argued that the power motive is an *interpersonal* motive. In fact, the scoring definitions include only interpersonal impact. Still, if the power motive develops out of the impact incentive, as suggested in Chapter 4, it might be expected that it would lead to pleasure in having impact over things as well as people. Unfortunately, the results for farmers do not particularly fit in with this line of argument: farmers might also be thought to have wide scope for having power over things, but they score low in n Power. However, they may feel relatively helpless in the face of nature's capricious whims, and they have little scope for interpersonal influence, which could explain why those low in n Power end up in farming. The whole matter deserves more careful study.

Search for Prestige

One way individuals high in n Power can appear powerful in a socially acceptable way is to collect symbols of power, or what Winter (1973) called *prestige possessions.* Both at Harvard and Wesleyan Universities he found that n Power scores were significantly correlated with the number of such prestige possessions owned by undergraduates, such as cars, wine glasses, college banners, a tape recorder, wall hangings, an electric typewriter, and so on. When asked to give their preference in cars, those high in n Power more often chose a foreign car and one that was more maneuverable than did subjects low in n Power. Similar results were obtained for a group of fifty adult males around thirty-three years of age when a different set of prestige items was used that included a color television set, a rifle or pistol, and a convertible car. The n Power score among these men was significantly correlated with the number of such items they owned (McClelland, 1975).

Credit cards are another symbol of prestige. They represent the power to purchase important services, often from prestigious hotels, restaurants, and stores. Winter (1973) reported a significant correlation between the number of credit cards in their wallets and n Power scores among a group of executives in a large manufacturing company. A similar significant correlation was found among men of the lower middle class and working class (McClelland, Davis, Kalin, & Wanner, 1972). McClelland (1975) has reported that the n Power score is significantly correlated with the number of credit cards owned among 115 women, though not among the men in this study. It seems clear that the power motive leads people to collect whatever symbols of prestige are appropriate for the position they occupy in life.

Acting So As to Be Recognized in Small Groups

Grades in school are an important way of gaining recognition for young people, so it is not surprising to discover that a significant correlation has been found (Costa & McClelland, 1971) between n Power scores in eighth grade and twelfth-grade rank in class ($r = -.27$; $N = 64$; $p < .05$). The students with a stronger n Power worked harder to get higher grades and therefore ended up ranking higher when they graduated from high school. The result gains added significance from the fact that n Power is not at all correlated with IQ, the other major predictor of rank in class; from the fact that n Achievement score in this sample, as in many others (see Chapter 6), is not significantly correlated with grades earned in school; and from the fact that the relationship is *predictive*. That is, one might expect people with better grades to be proud of themselves and perhaps develop a higher n Power, but here the higher n Power predicts better grades four years later. The finding is interesting and fits theory, but the same energy should be spent on checking it that has gone into showing there is *not* a relationship between n Achievement level and school success.

Winter (1973) reasoned that in small groups, individuals high in n Power should work to become known and to build alliances. He asked the members of a psychology class to list four friends. He then made up a master list of all these names and submitted it to the members of the class, asking them to check which of the people on the list they knew. A recognition score for each name on the list was obtained by giving it a point for each time the person was recognized by anybody in the class. Winter found that the higher a person's n Power score, the lower the average recognition score of the friends he or she had listed. In other words, people high in n Power (mostly male in this sample) choose as friends individuals who are not particularly well known or in a position to compete with them for prestige. Thus, they seem to surround themselves with lesser known people who can be led.

A more direct confirmation of this characteristic had been obtained by Fodor and Farrow (1979), who arranged a situation in the laboratory in which business school students thought they were supervising three workers in another room. They were told that they could say anything they liked through a two-way communication system to foster the productivity of the workers in making objects out of Tinker Toys. In return, they heard comments from the workers, which in order to standardize the conditions were actually tape-recorded statements. In one condition Worker C made comments aimed at ingratiating the supervisor, such as "You know, I really like your approach. You're going to be a good supervisor." In another condition his comments were neutral. Fodor and Farrow found that subjects high in n Power, as compared with those low in n Power, evaluated more favorably the ingratiating worker in terms of his ability to work, his worth to the company, and their willingness to rehire or promote him. The same difference did not appear for other workers or for Worker C when he made neutral comments. People high in *n* Power like to have people around them who respect them and are loyal supporters.

Furthermore, people high in *n* Power tend to act in a group so as to call attention to themselves. Participants in an achievement motivation training course in India (see Chapter 14) were asked to list the names of those they had known before the course and those they had gotten to know during the course. The gain in the number of times a person was mentioned from before to after the course—the gain in his recognition by others—was significantly correlated with his *n* Power score. Apparently those high in *n* Power behaved in ways that made them more visible to other members of the group (Winter, 1973).

McAdams, Healey, and Krause (1982) have clarified the nature of this behavior further in a study of the nature of friendship episodes engaged in by college students. They found that men high in *n* Power, as compared with men low in *n* Power, reported that they were more often in the company of a group or gang of four or more friends. This would give them more opportunity to stand out in the crowd in some way than if they were in a dyadic relationship. Furthermore, students of both sexes higher in *n* Power more often described their role in the friendship episodes as involving "agentic" striving rather than listening and sharing: "The high-power individual tends to experience friendships in an agentic manner, understanding them in terms of opportunities to take on dominant, controlling, organizational roles. . . . In the agentic mode, relationships are apprehended in power terms. Self and other are understood as separate. . . . The friends take advantage of various opportunities that may arise for self-display and self-expansion within the bounds of the relationship" (McAdams, Healey, & Krause, 1982).

Schnackers and Kleinbeck (1975) demonstrated how exploitations of others occur by having three subjects participate in a con game, one of whom was high in *n* Power. The object of the game was to see which player could get to the goal first by throwing dice and using "power cards" of different values that could be multiplied by the score on the dice. Coalitions could also be formed between two players that, if maintained, would always defeat the third player. But it was also possible to break a coalition at any time after it had been formed. As expected, Schnackers and Kleinbeck found that as compared with the subjects low in *n* Power, those high in *n* Power entered into more coalitions and also broke up more coalitions in order to take advantage of their partners. They also won more points. The results are summarized in Figure 8.4. The correlation between *n* Power scores and points scored in the third round was .45, *p* < .005. Obviously, the subjects high in *n* Power exploited the others in the situation in every possible way in a game that encouraged this type of behavior. Notice that people high in *n* Power, while not more aggressive in all situations, tend to be so when the values governing a social situation favor it.

In a study of small groups of strangers interacting for a while, D. F. Jones (1969) found that those high in *n* Power talked more and were judged to have "most influenced the other participants." However, they were not best liked nor judged as having contributed most "to get the job done and come to a good conclusion" (Jones, 1969). Furthermore, Watson (1974) has reported that men

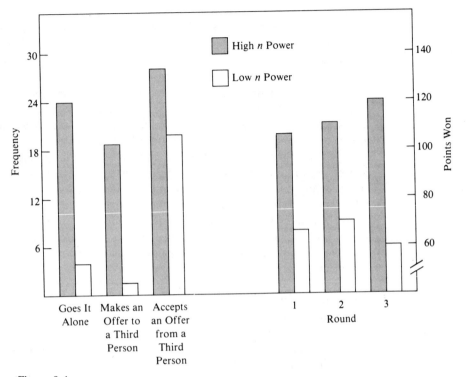

Figure 8.4.

Behavior of Subjects High and Low in *n* Power in a Game. (*Left*) Frequency of three ways of breaking a coalition. (*Right*) Points won in three consecutive rounds (after Heckhausen, 1980, after Schnackers & Kleinbeck, 1975).

high in *n* Power (using its hope of Power aspect, as described in Table 8.1) evaluate other members of the group more often negatively than men low in *n* Power (Winter & Stewart, 1978). Thus, it is not surprising to learn that they are also judged not to be particularly helpful in small group discussions (Kolb & Boyatzis, 1970). In fact, people low in *n* Power have been found to be more helpful in promoting group decision making based on the facts in the case (Fodor & Smith, 1982). Those high in *n* Power are judged to have been more influential by the others in the group, but they are apparently too assertive to be good at bringing other people out.

Other characteristics in combination with high *n* Power are necessary to make a good leader. For example, Constantian (1978) studied one group engaged in studying its own processes in which the behavior of the participants was monitored week by week over a whole semester in terms of the three dimensions Bales has used to classify small group behavior (Bales & Cohen, 1979). Roughly speaking, Bales' upward-downward dimension reflects the amount of dominance behavior a person shows in the group; his forward-backward dimension, the amount of task-related behavior shown; and his positive-negative dimension, the amount of friendly behavior a person displays. At the end of the term, Constantian collected the number of nominations each person in the group received for the position of being "best leader." She then attempted to predict the variance in the best leader nominations from seven determinants: scores on the three dimensions of behavior coded by Bales; the motive scores for *n* Achievement, *n* Affiliation, and *n* Power; plus a measure of inhibition also obtained from the TAT (see the later discussion on the leadership motive syndrome in this chapter). She found that she could predict over 90 percent of the variation of the leadership nomination score from these variables, but that only three variables contributed significantly by themselves to the result. These were the *n* Power score, the positivity of behavior score, and the task orientedness score. In other words, subjects high in *n* Power, in positivity, and in task orientation were most likely to be nominated as best leaders.

What is especially significant about this finding is that the general negativity of subjects high in *n* Power we have mentioned is here canceled out by the requirement that the person behave positively and in a task-oriented manner in the group. In other words, high *n* Power leads to successful leadership if it is combined with the behavior traits of positivity and task orientation. Once again we are reminded that behavior must take into account not only motives, but also values and skills—in this case, two skills (positivity and task orientation) specifically rated by the Bales procedure.

However, when Constantian attempted to cross-validate these findings in another self-analytic group, she obtained quite different results. The same variables no longer predicted the best leader nominations. The explanation lies in the different makeup of the group. Leadership depends not only on personal characteristics, but also on the characteristics of the other members of the group— the environmental determinants in Lewin's well-known equation of behavior as a joint product of the person and the environment. For example, if a group contains a strong abrasive personality, it may not be possible for anyone—no matter how favorable his or her personal characteristics—to assume effective leadership.

Risk Taking

Outward Bound is a training program designed to increase courage and self-reliance by exposing participants to a number of physical dangers they must face and overcome. They have to scale walls, walk narrow planks some distance above the ground, escape from being thrown in the water tied up, and survive for three days alone in the woods with almost no resources. Fersch (1971) found that when adolescents of high-school age, mostly from poverty backgrounds, were sent to this program, a number found the training so rough that they dropped out. But if they were high in *n* Power, they were significantly less likely to drop out. In other words, those with a stronger power motive were more

willing to endure the physical risks and dangers. Furthermore, those whose
n Power score remained high after the program, as reflected in a retest at the
end of the summer, also showed signs of increased social competence in school a
year later.

McClelland and Watson (1973) studied risk taking among seventy-two student volunteers in situations in which the outcome depended either on effort or
on chance. In the first task, the subjects were asked to pick the level of difficulty of a problem they wanted to work on after having had some experience in
trying to solve similar problems. As expected, the subjects high in *n* Achievement, as contrasted with those low in *n* Achievement, preferred to work on
tasks that were moderately difficult for them judged in terms of their prior performance. However, the subjects high in *n* Power were not moved by the
achievement incentive to choose moderately difficult problems, nor were they
more likely to choose extremely difficult problems to solve.

The second task involved deciding what bets to place in roulette, in which
the odds of winning vary all the way from fifty-fifty (placing a chip on red or
black) up to one in thirty-five (betting on a single number out of the thirty-six
available). After the game was fully explained to the subjects, they were told
they would be allowed to place fifteen bets and that they should mark on the
sheet how they wanted to distribute them. These choices were made in private,
without anyone knowing what they were. Then the subjects actually played the
game at the roulette table, choosing any ten of the bets they had previously decided to make. In this condition the bets were made publicly, and wins and
losses could be observed by the others in the group. When the subjects were deciding what bets to make privately, there was a tendency for those high in
n Power to choose more extreme bets, but it was not significant. When they actually played the game publicly, however, the correlation between *n* Power
scores and the riskiness of the bets placed was significant. Furthermore, as contrasted with those low in *n* Power, the individuals high in *n* Power used more
of the extreme bets (seventeen or thirty-five to one) they had chosen in the
private condition. Sixty-one percent of them used all, or all but one, of the
extreme bets, as contrasted with only 34 percent of those low in *n* Power
($p < .05$).

Figure 8.5 shows the distribution of bets according to probability of success
for those high in *n* Power, high in *n* Achievement, or high in *n* Affiliation. The
biggest difference is for the riskiest bet, which only the subjects high in *n* Power
chose most often, in contrast to the other subjects, who tended to choose more
moderately risky bets. The results for the high *n* Achievement subjects are unexpected, since according to theory they should have chosen options with moderate probability of success only when they had a chance of influencing the outcome. However, this tendency may be so engrained in them that they continued
to choose moderate probability of success options even in a chance situation.
The curve for the subjects high in *n* Affiliation only tends to be skewed toward
the safest bets, which suggests that they are not particularly attracted by this
kind of competitive game.

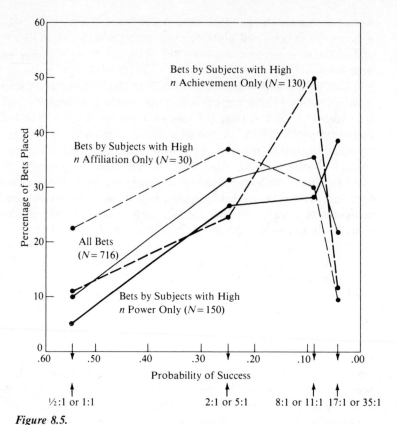

Figure 8.5.

Proportions of Roulette Bets Placed at Various Odds by All Subjects and Subjects High in *n* Power, *n* Achievement, and *n* Affiliation Only (after McClelland & Watson, 1973).

Application of the Atkinson Risk-taking Model to *n* Power

At first, it would appear that subjects high in *n* Power are not behaving as they should according to Atkinson's model (see Table 7.2), which holds that people will be most attracted to options where the probability of success is moderate (P_s = .30 to .50). Whereas Atkinson deals only with the tendency to approach achievement alternatives, the model is stated in terms general enough to raise the question of whether it applies to any kind of motivational choice.

McClelland and Teague (1975) explored the extent to which the model predicted choices of subjects high and low in *n* Power when the alternatives involved exercising power rather than performing better. They asked students to imagine they were a member of a board that had to make a decision on some public issues. Each issue was described in some detail (in one case it had to do with whether to build a coal-fueled electric power plant despite its polluting effect), and four positions the board could take were outlined (for example, build the plant with exacting control specifications, delay its building, build it immediately to promote the economy, or do not ever build it). To provide some control over the probability of success variable, in each case it was indicated roughly how popular each alternative was with the board members. Subjects were then asked to indicate which of the four options they would argue and vote for. They also indicated on a scale of 1 to 10 how likely it was that each position would be adopted by the board (the probability of success variable) and how good they would feel if each of the four positions was adopted (the incentive value of each option for them).

In this instance, the Atkinson model, which states that approach is a function of probability of success times incentive value, did not predict the choice of various alternatives at all well. It failed particularly in predicting the choices of those high in *n* Power, since in their case increased probability of success did not make it more likely that they would choose an alternative. In fact, the reverse was true; the more unlikely they judged an alternative was to be adopted, the more they tended to choose it. They were attracted to extreme risks, just as they were in playing roulette. It is possible that they were choosing unpopular positions in order to stand out more.

This experiment can be criticized, however, on the grounds that the probability of success variable does not represent the probability of *the subjects'* success in a situation in which the outcome depends on a choice they make. So McClelland and Teague (1975) also conducted an arm-wrestling experiment in which all participants were asked whether they preferred to wrestle with someone stronger or weaker than they or about equal in strength. After choosing, the subjects were asked to estimate on a scale of 0 to 10 what their chances of winning were (the probability of success variable), as well as how good they would feel if they won (the incentive value of winning). Unexpectedly, there was no correlation between expectancy of winning (or P_s) and the rated incentive value of winning either among the subjects high or low in *n* Power. This is surprising, because Atkinson assumes in his model that there is a perfect negative correlation between these two variables, that is, that $I_s = 1 - P_s$. It might be expected that the less the probability of winning or the stronger the opponent, the greater the satisfaction would be from beating him or her, but this does not turn out to be the case here.

Furthermore, as might be expected from this result, the probability of beating the opponent seemed to have little effect among those high in *n* Power in determining their choice of how strong an opponent to fight. Their choices were almost perfectly predicted by the incentive value they assigned to winning over the opponent they chose. Including their estimate of their chances of beating the opponent, as in the Atkinson model ($P_s \times I_s$), actually predicted their choices less well.

One possible interpretation of the roulette experiment and these experiments is that the meaning of the probability of success may not be the same for subjects high in *n* Power as it is for subjects high in *n* Achievement: it may not refer to the probability of success or winning through people's own efforts or performance, but to the probability of being considered important in some way.

Thus, it might be possible that Atkinson's model would apply to power choices if it were assumed that in such cases $1 - P_s = P_s$, since the more difficult the task undertaken, the more likely people would be to call attention to themselves for attempting it. Then we might argue that their choices could best be predicted by $1 - (P_s \times I_s)$, although I_s cannot be defined, as it is in the achievement area, by $1 - P_s$. The whole matter needs more careful study, but at the very least we have to be very cautious about applying Atkinson's risk-taking model to choices involving motives other than the need for achievement.

The meaning of the attitude of people high in *n* Power toward risk taking may be made clearer by an example from everyday life. Politicians, if they actively seek office, are generally high in *n* Power (see Winter & Stewart, 1978). They thus are often good at calling attention to themselves, at getting their names in newspapers or on television, and at creating media events that will lead to name recognition. They may identify with a particular issue or take an extreme stand (a low probability of success) in order to get better recognized.

Suppose that a number of them in Congress decide to do something about the problem of alcoholism, which is costing the country billions of dollars annually in terms of highway accidents, treatment facilities, and lost worker productivity. They decide to do something really important and visible—to create a government institute to combat alcoholism in every possible way, for which they succeed in getting $500 million appropriated annually. The probability of success that interests them is whether they can be recognized as doing something big and visible about the alcohol problem. They have a lesser interest in whether the institute so created will actually succeed in decreasing alcoholism. That would be of more interest to individuals high in *n* Achievement. When Congress appropriates the money, those high in *n* Power believe they have done something big about a big problem. Their choice is determined more by the incentive value of having created a big institute than by its probability of success in achieving the goal of decreasing alcoholism. In fact, if later evaluation shows that the institute is not lessening alcoholism, they can only lose prestige, whereas if evaluation shows the institute is being helpful, it only confirms what they said would be true all along. So they tend not to be as interested in performance feedback as individuals high in *n* Achievement are.

• CATHARSIS

It has long been supposed that expressing a motive or an emotion reduces its strength or intensity. The ancient Greeks called this *catharsis* and used the term to refer to the emotional release that occurs from watching terrifying and aggressive scenes in a play. The idea gained further support from the observation that for homeostatic physiological drives like hunger, consummatory behavior like eating reduces the desire to eat. And Freud conceived of instincts or drives as pressures to act in certain ways that could be reduced through achieving their primary aim—or at least they had to be partially satisfied by the achievement of secondary or substitute aims, a process that explains symptom formation or neurosis.

The idea of catharsis has been very appealing to psychologists, but they have had difficulty pinning down exactly in what sense it occurs. At the most general level, it can be taken to mean that any response, once it occurs, is less likely to occur again right away. This built-in refractory phase to repeating a response occurs (see, for example, Telford, 1931) and has adaptive significance, since it prevents the organism from repeatedly making the same wrong response. The principle is considered so basic by Atkinson and Birch (1978) in their model of the dynamics of action that they have stated as a basic assumption that "the consummatory force (C), which reduces the strength of an action tendency (T), comes from expression of that tendency in an activity, from the occurrence of the activity itself."

Most students of catharsis, however, have used the term *catharsis* in the much narrower sense of release or reduction in a motive or emotion, particularly aggression, through some kind of action or action substitute such as fantasy. In particular, people have wanted to know whether watching violence on television increases or decreases aggression. If catharsis occurs from watching people chase and kill each other on television, should not children who watch many such television programs be less aggressive afterward than they were before? Should they not be less aggressive than other children equally aggressive at the outset, who have watched other programs? Or more generally, in terms of the concepts used in this chapter, does finding an outlet for the power motive (a more generalized form of the aggressive motive) decrease power motive arousal at the time or perhaps, if it is continued over time, decrease dispositional *n* Power?

A great deal of research has been carried out in an attempt to answer such questions, but unfortunately, much of it does not bear directly on the question of how expressing a motive affects motive strength in itself. Most studies have found, for example, that children who watch violent television shows often are more aggressive in behavior afterward than other children (Feshbach, 1970; Rubinstein & Sprafkin, 1982). At first this would seem to mean that catharsis does not occur: Experiencing violence through watching a drama does not reduce aggressivity, as the Greeks thought. It increases it. But a closer analysis reveals that such studies do not yield any easily interpretable information about what has happened to the aggressive *motive* as a result of watching violent television shows. This is because motives—as we have repeatedly emphasized—whether dispositional or aroused, are only one of the determinants of the tendency to respond in a certain way (for example, aggressively). Other determinants include knowledge or skills and values.

In a typical study (Feshbach, 1970), one group of children was asked to watch violent television shows for some weeks while another group watched other kinds of shows. When their aggressiveness was measured afterward, it was found that those who had watched the violent shows behaved more often in an aggressive manner. This may have had nothing to do with what happened to their aggressive or power *motives,* since they had obviously learned much more than the other children on *how* to be aggressive: their aggressive knowledge and skill had increased. Furthermore, the fact that some authority figures had told them to watch violent television shows may easily have suggested to the children that such behavior was all right; the value they placed on behaving violently may have been subtly altered. So the increase in aggressiveness may have had nothing to do with changes in the aggressive motive, which could have stayed the same or even decreased while other determinants of the aggressive response increased.

Any number of studies have shown that whether or not aggression occurs and whether one type of aggressive response reduces the likelihood of another type depends on the subjects' cognitive understanding of who is frustrating them and why and whether being aggressive in one way or another helps them to achieve their goals (see, for example, Zumkley, 1978). There are so many non-motivational determinants of whether a person is aggressive or not that in most studies it is impossible to determine how the motive has been affected just from observing changes in aggressive behavior.

A few studies have focused more narrowly on whether catharsis occurs for motives, as they are defined and measured in this book. The classic investigation was carried out by Feshbach (1955). He arranged to insult a number of students, that is, to arouse their power motivation. Some of them then were asked to write imaginative stories to pictures, whereas others performed different tasks supposedly measuring their ability. All students then filled out a sentence completion test and answered questions about their attitude toward the research and the experimenter who had insulted them. As compared with a control group of students who had not been insulted, those who had been insulted included more aggressive themes in the sentence completions and reported themselves to be more angry at the experimenter, so the power motive clearly had been aroused. But the insulted students who had been allowed to fantasize about their anger by writing stories included a significantly lower level of aggressive themes in their sentence completions than the insulted students who had worked at other tasks. This suggested that engaging in aggressive fantasies had had a cathartic effect for subjects whose power motivation had been aroused. However, two criticisms of this interpretation can be made. Perhaps those who wrote aggressive stories felt guilty for doing so, so that they inhibited further thoughts of aggression in their sentence completions. And perhaps writing stories is a more relaxing or interesting thing to do than taking tests, so it subtly improved the subjects' attitude toward the research and made them less angry. That is, the reduction in their aggressiveness might be due not to having expressed it, but to a change in the instigation to aggression.

Feshbach (1961) conducted another experiment in which students who had been insulted either watched a fight film or a neutral film, after which their associations were obtained and scored for aggressiveness. He found that those who had seen the fight film had lower power motivation afterward (gave fewer aggressive associations) than those who had seen the neutral film. It is difficult to see how differences in what the subjects were doing could explain the result, as in the previous experiment, so there was some catharsis for those whose power motivation had been aroused.

Feshbach, however, also found that for subjects who had not been insulted (whose power motivation had not been aroused), the fight film actually increased their power motivation, as reflected in more aggressive associations, as compared with the power motivation aroused after the neutral film. In other words, whereas the fight film reduced power motivation for those in whom it had been aroused, it increased power motivation for those in whom it had not been aroused.

These results have been confirmed for dispositional, as distinguished from aroused, power motivation (McClelland & Maddocks, 1983). Subjects whose *n* Power had been assessed previously in the usual way saw either a power-arousing film about the successes of the Nazis in Germany and their persecution of the Jews, or a neutral film about gardening. Their *n* Power scores then were obtained again from stories written after seeing the films. Just as in Feshbach's power motive arousal study, those who were dispositionally high in *n* Power showed a lower level of *n* Power after seeing the Nazi film than the neutral film, indicating a catharsis effect for them. Those initially low in *n* Power, however, showed a much higher level of *n* Power after the Nazi than the neutral film: their power motive had been aroused. The interaction effect was highly significant. So catharsis does not occur when the motive or emotion is not present or aroused. Quite the opposite occurs. If it is not present, cues that normally arouse it do arouse it. Thus, other things being controlled for, violent television shows for children might arouse power motivation in those who had little to start with, even though it might decrease it for those high in *n* Power.

Attempts have also been made to determine the effects on power motivation of participating in overtly violent activities. Stone (1950, summarized in McClelland, 1951) scored aggression in stories written before and after the football season by football players and other matched male students. He found that whereas both groups had the same average level of concern about aggression before the season, the football players scored significantly lower in thoughts relating to aggression after the season. Apparently, daily participation in sanctioned physical aggression for several months had lowered the level of concern for at least this aspect of power motivation. Unfortunately, other aspects of the power motive system were not scored, so it cannot be determined whether the practice of this type of activity merely shifted power motivation into other channels. As noted earlier, Fersch (1971) also found a decrease in people's overall *n* Power scores after a summer of participating in physically demanding, risk-taking activities in Outward Bound. Unfortunately, however, he did not have a control group, so it cannot be determined whether any group of high-school students would decrease in *n* Power over the summer vacation.

Thus, there is some evidence that outlets for the power motive reduce its strength for those in whom the motive is strong or aroused. The conclusion is not nearly as firm as it should be, however, because most research has focused on testing for cathartic effects on aggressiveness, which has important nonmotivational determinants. Also, very little work has been done on cathartic effects for other motives. For example, does succeeding at a task lower *n* Achievement scores? Atkinson's model in Table 7.2 assumes that to the extent that success changes the probability of success (and, thereby, achievement incentives), it can alter the tendency to perform an act. But what about the effect of success on the motive itself? McClelland, Atkinson, Clark, and Lowell (1953) found that success at tasks was followed by an *n* Achievement level that was somewhat, but not markedly, lower than that obtained after failure at the same tasks. This deserves more careful study to distinguish the effects of catharsis on motives from its effects on behavior.

• ROLE OF THE POWER MOTIVE IN DRINKING

Drinking Conceived as a Means of Reducing Anxiety

From 1940 to 1960, most psychiatrists and psychologists believed that the motive behind drinking alcohol was to reduce tension and anxiety. There were several reasons for this belief. Alcohol is a central nervous system depressant. Therefore, it was reasoned, people would drink it only to depress something that was upsetting them, such as anxiety. Also at this time, the behaviorist model of drive as tension and reward as tension reduction (see Chapter 3) was popular, and alcohol could be conceived as rewarding because it reduced tension. Furthermore, people often say that they drink to "forget their troubles," although this is more common in the United States than in other countries. Finally, a number of clinical studies suggested that alcoholics were anxious because of frustrated dependency needs and drank to feel more comfortable and relaxed (see McClelland, Davis, Kalin, & Wanner, 1972).

Kalin, Kahn, and McClelland (1965) argued that the predominant view of the motive for drinking was biased by the notion prevailing among psychologists at the time that reward was tension reducing, as well as by the view in the general public (which had culminated during Prohibition) that alcohol was bad for people so that the only reason it would be sought was to get rid of something worse. Whereas it is true that excessive consumption of alcohol can lead to deadening thoughts and feelings, most people all over the world drink alcohol in small amounts. Why should most people take only about two drinks at a time? It did not seem reasonable to suppose that such a small amount of alcohol was significantly reducing anxiety.

Furthermore, Kalin et al. (1965) argued that everyone was inferring what was going on in the minds of people drinking alcohol rather than directly studying what was going on in their minds. Finally, they felt that the settings used to study the effects of alcohol were biased against finding any positive effects. Usually the alcohol was consumed in a formal laboratory setting while an experimenter, an authority figure in a white coat, administered alcohol in predetermined doses. To remove the effects of suggestion, the taste of alcohol was often disguised so that subjects would not know what they were drinking. In what was considered an ideally controlled experiment, both the experimenter and the subjects were "blind" as to what the subject was getting, because either alcohol or saline solution was infused intravenously into the subjects. Under these conditions it was scarcely surprising that very few subjects ever reported that they felt good or lively. Such procedures do not "remove suggestion," as was often claimed, but in fact introduce very powerful suggestions derived from the experimenter as authority figure, uncertainty as to what one is drinking, being forced to consume predetermined amounts of alcohol, and the lack of the normal social supports that go with drinking (see McClelland et al., 1972).

Therefore, Kalin et al. (1965) decided that since alcohol has to be consumed in some kind of setting, it would be best to use the settings under which alcohol is normally consumed. Then at least the experimenter would be in a better position to discover the motives for normal social drinking. They ran cocktail parties of the type men usually attended in all-male colleges at which individuals were allowed to drink as they normally would choose to drink rather than as they were told to drink by an experimenter. From time to time during the party the proceedings were interrupted and the participants wrote TAT stories to find out what was on their minds at the time. Other control parties were also run during which stories were collected when good food and nonalcoholic beverages were served. On other occasions alcoholic or nonalcoholic beverages were served as they normally would be during an evening discussion in someone's apartment. To avoid tapping subjects' preconceptions about the effects alcohol is supposed to have, the participants in these experiments were simply told that the researchers were interested in the effects of a party or evening discussion on imaginative thought processes (see McClelland et al., 1972).

Effect of Social Drinking on Thoughts About Power and Inhibition

The early results of these studies showed that as drinking progressed, sexual and aggressive thoughts increased significantly among men over what they were at a comparable time period in the control parties or over what the thoughts had been before the drinking started. Then it was realized that these types of imagery, along with some other types that increased in frequency with drinking, actually represented subtypes of power imagery as it was defined by Winter (1967). A reexamination of the data showed that n Power scores increased as a function of drinking alcohol. It looked as if men were drinking to feel more powerful rather than to reduce their anxiety, at least to judge from their thoughts at the time.

Davis (in McClelland et al., 1972) checked this finding by creating an experience in which men felt they were being required to act more powerfully but were unsure whether they could. He accomplished this by having them lead a blindfolded man through the crowded streets of a city. Davis found that afterward, when the pairs were relaxing in a bar, those who had been under power stress from acting as guides in this somewhat embarrassing way drank more heavily than those who had been blindfolded. In other words, the men who felt somewhat inadequate about the assertiveness and responsibility required of them drank more to feel more powerful.

It was later discovered that women responded differently to alcohol: Their n Power score did not rise while drinking at parties with both sexes present (see Wilsnack, 1974). Instead, drinking made them feel warmer and more feminine. In short, alcohol leads men to feel more powerful (that is, stronger) and women to feel more friendly. At present it is not known whether this difference is due to physiological patterns relating to the interaction of alcohol with different hormonal patterns in men and women, or whether it is due to different social role expectations for the two sexes. There are also ethnic differences in the effects of alcohol (Ewing, Rouse, & Pellizari, 1974).

In the same study, after men had at least four or five drinks, signs of inhibition also decreased significantly, giving some support for the common notion that alcohol releases inhibitions (McClelland et al., 1972). Two such signs were measured. One was called *Time Concern* and was scored whenever a story mentioned time in any way, such as how long it took to do something or when a person did something. There was a significant decrease in the number of individuals mentioning time from the beginning to the middle to the end of a cocktail party. The other measure was called *Activity Inhibition;* it was simply a frequency count of the number of times the word *not* appeared in the protocols. The percentage of protocols showing at least two *nots* declined significantly from the beginning to the end of the party (McClelland et al., 1972).

Thus, drinking had two effects on men: it increased power concerns and decreased inhibitory thoughts. Furthermore, the quality of the power thoughts varied significantly, depending on whether the subjects showed high or low signs of inhibition. On the one hand, if a man was low in Activity Inhibition, his power thoughts much more often focused on personal dominance—on winning at somebody else's expense, as in a zero-sum game ("If I win, you lose"). On the other hand, if a man scored high in Activity Inhibition, power imagery was much more often stated in terms of doing good for others, for humanity, or for some good cause. Furthermore, the power outcome was described in more uncertain terms or with irony.

The contrast is illustrated by the following two plot summaries of stories written to a picture of a boxer:

1. "He is fighting the champ—a chance to win a big purse, retire to a beach in Tahiti."
2. "He is fighting the champ—a chance to win a big purse. His kid is in the hospital and needs an expensive operation."

The first type of power imagery is called *personalized power* (*p* Power), because the goal is exclusively personal. The second type of imagery is called *socialized power* (*s* Power), because the power drive seems to be socialized in the service of others.

Figure 8.6 shows the effects of different amounts of alcohol consumption on the frequency of *p* Power and *s* Power imagery in stories written by participants in the cocktail parties. The curves show the "two-drink effect" the investigators were originally looking for. After about two drinks, the *s* Power curve reaches its highest point and then declines with further drinking. In contrast, the *p* Power curve increases steadily with more drinking. The result is not surprising; it is foreshadowed by the fact that the measures of inhibition decline with heavier drinking, and *p* Power imagery is associated with lower inhibition, just as *s* Power imagery is associated with higher inhibition. Thus, small amounts of drinking in men leads to socialized thoughts of being more powerful—of being big, strong, and important on the job or in the family—but further drinking leads to thoughts of personal dominance—of beating other people in competition or perhaps even beating them up.

Relationship of the Power Motive and Inhibition to Problem Drinking and Other Activities

If it is feelings of power that men get out of drinking, perhaps men who are high in *n* Power to start with drink more. More specifically, those who are high in *p* Power, or high in *n* Power and low in Activity Inhibition, should drink the most. This, in fact, turned out to be the case. In two separate samples of men, a *p* — *s* Power index correlated significantly with a quantity/frequency index of

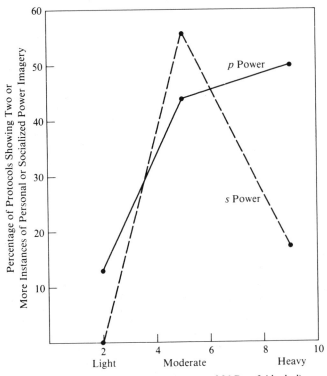

Figure 8.6.

Proportions of Subjects Writing Stories Containing Personal or Socialized Power Imagery with Increasing Alcohol Consumption (after McClelland, Davis, Kalin, & Wanner, 1972).

reported alcohol consumption ($r = .32$; $N = 50$; p $< .05$ and $r = .24$; $N = 108$; $p < .05$).

Figure 8.7 shows the same results in a slightly different format. Subjects in the two samples of men were classified according to whether they were (1) high in n Power and low or high in Activity Inhibition or (2) low in n Power and low or high in Activity Inhibition. Clearly, in both samples the men who were high in n Power and low in Activity Inhibition were much more likely to be classified as heavy drinkers by self-report than subjects in the other three categories. The overall level of drinking reported in the second sample is lower than in the first, but the relative percentages of heavy drinkers in the various categories is similar. It is particularly worth noting that a high n Power results in heavy drinking only if Activity Inhibition is low. If Activity Inhibition is high, the proportion of these individuals reporting heavy drinking is very low.

These studies also demonstrated that a classification by power and inhibition affected activities other than the amount of drinking. Figure 8.8 shows the results of a factor analysis of a number of activities the 108 men in one of these samples said they engaged in. As Chapter 2 explained, factor analysis involves correlating the extent to which people report they engage in pairs of activities (as examples from this study, consuming much wine and also lots of beer, or smoking many cigarettes and spending a great deal of time working). From all

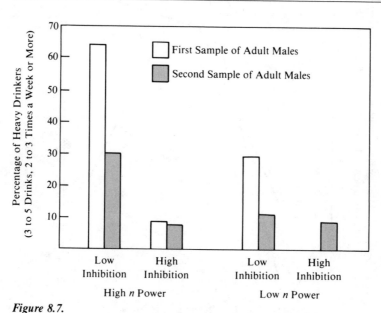

Figure 8.7.

Percentage of Heavy Drinkers Among Men High and Low in n Power and High and Low in Activity Inhibition (after McClelland, Davis, Kalin, & Wanner, 1972).

the intercorrelations of pairs of activities, factors that best account for most of the relationships obtained are extracted by a statistical procedure.

In this case, two independent factors—one characterized by high *n* Power and the other by Activity Inhibition—did a good job of accounting for the intercorrelations of all the variables. For example, beer and wine consumed are not highly related: people who drink a large amount of wine do not necessarily also drink a large amount of beer. Wine-drinking scores load fairly high on the Assertiveness (power) factor and on the Restraint factor, whereas beer drinking scores low on assertiveness and fairly high on lack of Restraint. This way of sorting activities began to make sense of some of the earlier findings on the correlates of *n* Power scores. For example, office holding, as well as wine drinking, loads high on the Assertiveness, or *n* Power, dimension and fairly high on the Restraint, or Activity Inhibition, dimension, whereas the amount of liquor con-

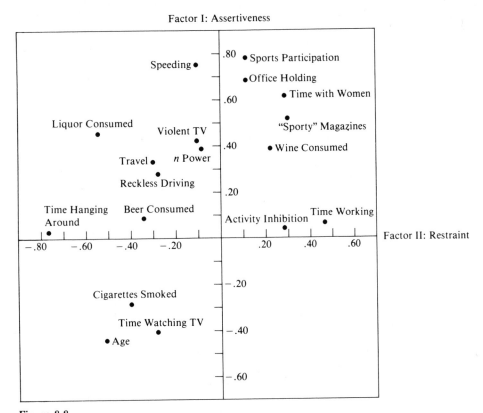

Figure 8.8.

Plot of Drinking and Other Activities Variables on Assertiveness and Restraint Factor Dimensions (after McClelland, Davis, Kalin, & Wanner, 1972).

sumed loads high on the Assertiveness factor and low on the Restraint factor. Similarly, sports participation goes with high *n* Power and somewhat with Restraint but not with lack of Restraint. Driving too fast and getting caught for speeding goes with Assertiveness and lack of Restraint, as would be expected. It became clear from this analysis that inhibition is a very important moderator variable for *n* Power: it determines whether the power motive expresses itself in more socialized, controlled ways or in more reckless attempts to show off as being powerful.

• HOW MATURITY MODULATES THE EXPRESSION OF THE POWER MOTIVE

Deriving a Measure of Social-Emotional Maturity

Even greater clarity in the understanding of the outlets for the power motive was introduced through the discovery that they varied depending on the social-emotional maturity of the person. As Chapter 2 described, Erikson (1963) elaborated Freud's theory of psychosexual stages into a full-blown scheme of stages of psychosocial, or social-emotional, development.

Stewart (1973) decided that if progress were to be made, some method of measuring the strength of various stage orientations had to be developed. She decided to use the approach that had been successful in producing measures of human motives like *n* Achievement and *n* Power. She selected groups of college freshmen, each representing a "pure" stage orientation, in order to compare and contrast the content of the imaginative stories they wrote. That is, she picked out the six freshmen who should be most clearly oriented toward the oral stage, as defined by the criteria of psychoanalysis. These were the students who ate, drank, and smoked much more than other freshmen and who did not score high on any of the behavioral criteria for the other psychosexual stages. She then developed a formal coding system for the content of their stories that differentiated them from stories written by freshmen not clearly in one stage or another. In similar fashion, she picked out the six freshmen most clearly in the anal stage as indicated by the number of self-regulating rituals they performed before going to bed at night, such as taking a shower, emptying their pockets, brushing their teeth, urinating, setting the alarm, opening a window, and so forth. The phallic stage was represented by young men who said they had dated many different girls in high school and who cited "reputation enhancement" and "sex" as the most important motives for dating. Freshmen males were considered to represent the genital stage if they had a steady girlfriend to whom they were faithful and if they reported that on dates they were most likely to study and make love. In this way they satisfied Freud's judgment that "love and work" represent maturity.

Stewart found that the stories of these "pure types" differed from other stories in ways that could readily be predicted by psychoanalytic theory, and this result encouraged her to think that perhaps she had found a way of measuring at least the earliest of Erikson's stages (see Table 2.4). Some of her results are summarized in Table 8.5. The stages are organized in this table according to two dimensions: whether the source of power is outside the self or in the self, and whether the target of power is the self or another.

This classification system generates the four psychosexual stages. In the first, or oral, stage the source of power is another—usually the mother—and the target of power is the self; this defines the dominant modality, which is *intake,* as when a mother nurses a baby. In the second stage the source of power shifts to the self, but the target remains the self, as when children attempt to gain control over themselves in what Erikson calls the stage of *autonomy.* In the third, or phallic, stage the source of power remains the self, but it is now directed toward others, as when a child attempts to influence others. The modality is *assertion.* Finally, in the fourth, or genital, stage the source of power shifts from the self to some higher outside, institutional authority such as the family, the church, or the state, and the individual acts under the influence of higher authority to influence others. As an example of how this highest stage is attained, Erikson (1963) pointed out that after individuals have gone through the "egocentric" Stages II and III of adolescence, they may get married. If they do, they sooner or later discover they are involved in a bond or an "institution" that is bigger than themselves as individuals. The marriage partners do things on behalf of the marriage that perhaps they would not do on their own. The point is even clearer when they become parents and find themselves doing something for the child as parents that perhaps they would not do on their own.

Table 8.5 also briefly lists the themes in stories that uniquely characterized individuals classified as belonging to each of these stages. In the authority area, for example, those in Stage I more often pictured authority as benevolent and providing things for people, whereas those in Stage II saw authority as critical and requiring individuals to control themselves. In Stage III, individuals described rebellion against authority, which should be characteristic of the assertive stage. In Stage IV, authority was described as no longer personal—the direct attempt of one person to influence another—but was characteristically either vague, impersonal, or institutional.

The other thinking characteristics found in the stories of individuals at each stage fitted fairly well with expectations about what people at those stages should be feeling and thinking, according to psychoanalytic theory. Thus, the subjects in the oral stage were pictured as waiting, just as Freud had to wait in his oral dream described in Chapter 2. Those in the anal stage described people clearing disorder, which corresponds to compulsiveness in the Erikson scheme (see Table 2.4 in Chapter 2). Those at the phallic stage described people taking initiative, but also showing guilt from failure and the desire to escape, which can lead to inhibition and hysterical symptoms, according to Table 2.4.

To fill out the picture of each stage, Table 8.5 also lists values that supposedly go with each level of development, as they have been defined by McClelland, Constantian, Pilon, and Stone (1982). Thus, parents would stress the importance of respect for authority in Stage I, the importance of self-reliance in Stage II, the importance of developing skills in Stage III, and the importance of

Table 8.5.
STAGES OF PSYCHOSOCIAL MATURITY (after McClelland, 1975)

Target of Power		Source of Power	
		Other	Self
Self		**I. Psychosexual Stage: Oral**	**II. Psychosexual Stage: Anal**
	Thinking Characteristics[a] — Modality:	Intake	Autonomy
	Formula:	"It strengthens me"	"I control myself"
	Authority:	Benevolent authority	Critical authority
	Relations to things or people:	Gets what he or she wants	Does not get what he or she wants
	Feelings:	Loss, despair	Incompetence
	Actions:	Is passive	Clears disorder
	Values	Respect for authority, decency, obedience To be inspired, healed	Self-reliance, willpower, independence, courage To know
Other		**IV. Psychosexual Stage: Genital**	**III. Psychosexual Stage: Phallic**
	Thinking characteristics[a] — Modality:	Generativity or mutuality	Assertion
	Formula:	"It moves me to serve"	"I have impact"
	Authority:	Impersonal authority	Rebellion against authority
	Relations to things or people:	Differentiates among people	Escapes
	Feelings:	Mixtures of joy and sorrow	Hostility, anger
	Actions:	Schedules work	Action leads to failure
	Values	Understanding of others, tolerance, serving common good To show compassion	Doing well in school and on the job, developing skills, having influence To have power

[a]These characteristics briefly describe the coding system developed by Stewart (1973) to score for various stages of social-emotional maturity. The values are those presumed to be consciously important for people at that stage.

understanding and serving others in Stage IV. From the child's point of view, children would be learning to value inspiration and healing in Stage I, knowledge in Stage II, assertiveness in Stage III, and compassion in Stage IV. McClelland (1975) has attempted to show that powerful figures such as gurus or great spiritual leaders like Jesus have typically been described as having expressed power in all of these valued ways. They healed, showed unusual knowledge, influenced others effectively, and were particularly compassionate.

Alternative Manifestations of the Power Motive as a Function of Maturity

On theoretical grounds, the power motive would be expected to express itself in different ways, depending on a person's level of maturity. If a person is primarily oriented toward Stage I, the power motive should express itself in the intake modality, and if toward Stage III, in an assertive modality.

However, there is no reason to think a person oriented toward Stage III would show behaviors characteristic of other stages. Thus, to sum or average the scores for all possible outlets for the need for power across all stages for a person would be meaningless. If this were done, each person would get a high score for the outlets characteristic of his or her dominant stage and low scores for behaviors characteristic of other stages, and everyone should end up with about the same total or average score. Thus, not much correlation would be expected between *n* Power and the sum total of all possible types of outlets for the power motive characteristic of all stages. Rather, a significant correlation between the *n* Power score and a higher score on any one of the behaviors characteristic of the different stages would be expected.

To test this theoretical expectation, McClelland (1975) chose activities that were theoretically and empirically characteristic of each stage as follows:

1. Stage I (the intake modality): power-oriented reading.
2. Stage II (the autonomy modality): indications of self-control or having many aggressive impulses but not expressing them.
3. Stage III (the assertion modality): frequently expressed anger to people.
4. Stage IV (the mutuality modality): frequent memberships in voluntary organizations.

In a sample of eighty-five adult males, none of these possible outlets for the power motive correlated significantly with the *n* Power score. This is as it should be according to theory, because individuals in Stage I should not join more organizations, and those in Stage IV should not engage in more power-oriented reading. So in a miscellaneous group of men representing all four stages, one would not expect any one of these outlets to be strongly correlated with the *n* Power score. Also, their sum should not correlate highly with *n* Power, because a high score for activities characteristic of the primary-stage orientation would be canceled out by low scores for outlets of other stages. In fact, in this sample of adult males, the correlation of *n* Power with the average expression of these four alternatives was only .19, which is not significant.

However, the correlation of *n* Power with the maximum expression of any of the four alternatives for each man was .32, *p* < .05. That is, scores on each alternative were standardized to make them comparable, and a man was assigned the highest standardized score he got on any of the four activities. Men high in *n* Power generally had a higher standardized score on some one of these outlets than men low in *n* Power. This confirms the fact that high *n* Power leads to greater participation in *some* power-related activity, although which activity a man expresses depends on the presence of a moderator variable, namely, the level of his maturity.

Clinicians have often observed that motives express themselves in alternative ways. Sometimes if a symptom is cured, another one takes its place; this is because the motivational problem remains the same, and if one outlet is blocked it seeks another outlet. In Perry's dream from *In Cold Blood,* discussed in Chapter 2, he first expressed his power motive in terms of the assertive modality—reaching out to grab something valuable. When this outlet was blocked by the snake's swallowing him, he retreated to thoughts characteristic of Stage II, which centered on the problem of self-control. When he was punished for lack of self-control, he retreated to the oral, intake stage and dreamed of an endless supply of delicious food and drink.

The statistical evidence simply confirms what clinicians have long been saying: motives seek alternative outlets depending on the stage of maturity and on whether a particular outlet is blocked or not. In short, motives show *alternative manifestations.* Traits, skills, or habits, however, tend to be quite consistent. A person tends to be consistently shy or late or good at playing the piano. So if someone is cured of shyness, for example, by behavior therapy (see Chapter 12), there is no evidence that he or she will develop other symptoms. Motives, not traits, seek alternative manifestations.

The same results were not obtained for women, perhaps because the outlets most characteristic of each stage were not as appropriate for women as for men (McClelland, 1975). The reason is that values, as well as stages of maturity, affect the way the need for power expresses itself. McClelland found that women's values differed from men's values. Regardless of their *n* Power score, the adult women in his sample were more sociocentric than the men, as other studies have reported. They said they had been taught more sociocentric virtues by their parents than men did. They belonged to a larger number of voluntary organizations. They had loaned material possessions more frequently, and they more often said they would volunteer to look after children because they liked to do it.

As contrasted with women low on *n* Power, those high in *n* Power dieted more often, had a larger number of credit cards, reported a higher average daily fluid intake (of juice, coffee, and other nonalcoholic beverages), and stated they were more willing to donate parts of their body to others after death. This suggests that since the women in this sample valued helping others more than the men did, the power motive in them operates to make them want to have resources to give to others. If their body is disciplined through dieting and kept filled, and they have more credit cards, they should be in a stronger position to help others. They even think of using their body as a resource for others after death. In contrast, because the male role places a value on assertiveness, men high in *n* Power are more assertive or argumentative rather than interested in accumulating more resources to share with others.

Sex Differences in the Outlets for the Power Motive at Different Stages of Maturity

Winter (1982) has made a convincing case for the fact that, in general, the power motive functions in the same way for women as it does for men. It is aroused to the same degree in women and men by observing a hypnosis demonstration or by inspirational speeches. Many of its action correlates are the same for college women and college men. People of both sexes high in *n* Power are more likely to join and hold office in voluntary organizations and to pursue careers like teaching and journalism, where the opportunity for influencing others is great.

The chief difference in male and female behaviors associated with high *n* Power scores lies in the area of what Winter (1982) calls the *profligate expansive impulse.* Men high in *n* Power are more apt to fight, drink, gamble, and try to exploit women sexually. (See the section later in the chapter on the Don Juan syndrome, as well as Table 8.9.) The same is not true for women, because, Winter argues, their power motives are expressed in more socially responsible ways. As evidence, he draws on the cross-cultural studies of Whiting and Whiting (1975), which show that older siblings generally show more responsible behavior because they look after younger siblings and that girls are more often assigned this task, so they grow up to be more socially responsible or sociocentric, as was just noted. Winter has further validated this hypothesis by showing that among members *of either sex* who have had no younger siblings to look after, high *n* Power is associated with the profligate expansive impulse, whereas among those with younger siblings, it expresses itself in more socially responsible ways, such as office holding. Since women in our culture generally, although not always, are taught sociocentric values, their power motive expresses itself less often in profligate, and more often in socially responsible, ways. This line of reasoning illustrates once again the great importance of considering values in trying to predict what activities a motive will be associated with.

Because of differences in sex role values, the outlets for the power motive differ for men and women, as shown in Table 8.6, which has been prepared to summarize how the power motive expresses itself at different stages of psychosocial maturity (McClelland, 1975). The correlations in the table were computed in the following way. Both the *n* Power score and the score for a particular stage obtained from the Stewart coding system were converted to standard scores with a mean of 50 and a standard deviation of 10. Then they were summed, since they then had equal weights, and the sum was correlated with a particular characteristic, such as the number of power-oriented magazines (for example, *Playboy* or *Sports Illustrated*) a person read. Since there were a large number of correlations in this study, and some could have arisen by chance, all the correlations listed in this table were checked in two independent random samples of the total to make sure they were approximately the same. If the *r*'s differed markedly from each other in the two samples, they have been excluded. Thus, the first correlation in the upper left corner of Table 8.6 means that men who scored high in *n* Power and also high in Stage I reported reading more power-oriented magazines than those who scored low on both of these variables.

In another part of the questionnaire, subjects were asked how often they talked to their relatives or friends about matters that are often kept secret, such as health problems, pressures at work, or sexual matters. Men high in *n* Power with a strong Stage I orientation share such information with others. They also tend to be more "intraceptive" in the sense of stating that they feel fantasies are a very important part of their lives, that it is important to understand the underlying motives of other people, and that they sometimes think of natural objects as possessing human qualities. The trend is not significant, but it is theoretically very important, because it fits with the next finding that among the men who can be clearly classified as identifying with their mothers or fathers, those in Stage I more often identify with their mothers. They say they resemble their mothers more than their fathers and prefer metaphors for death like "a compassionate mother," which suggest merging with the divine ground.

This complex is referred to as *pre-oedipal identification* with the mother and fits psychoanalytic theory, since people in the oral intake stage should still be closest to their mothers and should be absorbed in the "omnipotence of thought in which the psychic rather than the material world is the ultimate reality" (McClelland, 1975). It is as if they have not yet quite emerged from the early symbiotic relationship with their mother and are oriented toward maintaining a feeling of unity or oneness with the world, which also expresses itself in terms of sharing more information about themselves.

In Stage II the men with high *n* Power also behave as expected. They report controlling more aggressive impulses, rejecting institutional demands on them, and no longer asking for personal help from their parents. They are expressing their autonomy or independence.

In Stage III they show the typical assertive characteristics Winter (1973) has associated with the legend of Don Juan, the great seducer. They prefer to be free to love several women at once, they lie more, and they drink more and for the wrong reasons (to forget their troubles). They collect valuable objects symbolic of their importance. Not surprisingly, they have little interest in child care.

The picture of how men high in *n* Power behave in Stage IV is not very clear, probably because male values in our culture do not encourage the sharing activities that should characterize people at the Stage IV level of maturity. Nevertheless, they do report sharing more potentially secret information with their wives and list fewer possessions, which should characterize people who have gotten beyond the more egocentric Stages II and III. As for the theoretically most important characteristic, they show only a very weak tendency to join more voluntary organizations, although in other samples this correlation is much stronger.

In view of the sketchiness of the picture of men in Stage IV, it is reassuring

Table 8.6.
OUTLETS FOR *n* POWER AT DIFFERENT STAGES OF PSYCHOSOCIAL MATURITY FOR ADULT MALES (*N* = 85) AND FEMALES (*N* = 115) (after McClelland, 1975)

Correlations with n Power Score Plus Stage Score

	r		*r*
Stage I: Intake		*Stage II: Autonomy*	
Men		**Men**	
Reads power-oriented material	.23*	Controls anger	.22*
Shares more secrets	.31**	Rejects institutional responsibility	.22*
Is more "intraceptive" (psychic minded)	.17	Does not seek personal help from parents	.19*
Has pre-oedipal identification with mother	.35*		
Women		**Women**	
Has stronger male inspiration than female inspiration	.22*	Controls anger	.17*
Would invest a $10,000 gift	.24*	Wants freedom from restrictions on love	.20*
Has more physical symptoms	.19*	Shares less with mother	.16†
Has oedipal identification with father	.29*		
Stage IV: Generativity/Mutuality		*Stage III: Assertion*	
Men		**Men**	
Has many organizational memberships	.12	Wants freedom to love several women	.25*
Has fewer possessions	.19†	Lies more	.22*
Shares more with wife	.20†	Collects valuable objects	.22*
		Reports heavier alcohol consumption	.19
		Drinks for wrong reasons	.27*
		Dislikes child care	.25*
Women		**Women**	
Has many organizational memberships	.30**	Expresses anger to people	.17†
Shares more with husband	.20*	Likes to travel	.19*
		Tries new foods	.25**
		Keeps sex life secret	.20*
		Is more "intraceptive" (psychic minded)	.20*
		Feels "oceanic oneness" with the world	.24*

†$p < .10$.
*$p < .05$.
**$p < .01$.

to know that those who scored higher in Stage IV upon entrance to a large corporation were significantly more likely to be promoted to higher levels of managerial responsibility in the company over the next sixteen years. Among noncollege graduates scoring high in Stage IV, 52 percent had been promoted to Level 3 or above in sixteen years in one company, as contrasted with only 27 percent of those low in Stage IV ($p < .05$; McClelland & Boyatzis, 1982). In other words, their stronger orientation toward serving an institution rather than themselves (as in Stages II and III) had led to more rapid promotion in the company. The difference was not significant for college graduates, because in this company college graduates tended to get promoted automatically because of their background rather than because of their personal characteristics.

The outlets of the power motive for women are quite different. In Stage I, women high in *n* Power are more oriented toward men, just as men in Stage I are more oriented toward women. In McClelland's study (1975), the subjects were asked to list the initials of people who were particularly inspirational to them as they were growing up, to rate the amount of inspiration they received from each one, and then to identify whether the person was male or female. Women high in *n* Power in Stage I report receiving more inspiration (intake) from men and also identified more with their fathers by the same measure used to classify the men as identifying more with their mothers. That is, women high in *n* Power and Stage I say they resented their fathers more and prefer metaphors that describe death in violent terms rather than in terms of union with the divine ground. If given $10,000, these women would prefer to invest it. They list having more physical symptoms. These facts suggest that women high in *n* Power in Stage I are particularly oriented toward thinking of themselves as needing resources to give: they want to have more money to share and are more bothered when their bodies are not functioning perfectly.

In Stage II they also show typical signs of independence. Like the men in this stage, women who score high in Stage II tend to have more aggressive impulses, which they control, than those who score low in Stage II. In love relationships they prefer to go steady with someone but be free to go out with someone else if they desire. They share less with their mothers. In both instances, they seem to be expressing the spirit of independence characteristic of Stage II.

In Stage III, women high in *n* Power express more of their anger openly, travel more, like to try new foods, and keep their sex life a secret. Clearly, they are more assertive, just as the men are in this stage. But what are we to make of the fact that they are also more intraceptive, or psychic minded? If we are right in assuming that psychic mindedness for the men in Stage I reflects a fusion with the maternal source of life, we might infer that women in Stage III are unconsciously beginning to identify with their own sex and to share that feeling of "oceanic oneness" with the world. If Stage III for men high in *n* Power means behaving in an assertive, Don Juan style, the parallel myth for women is surely Diana the Huntress running through the forest with her nymphs and hunting game.

The picture of women high in *n* Power in Stage IV is much clearer than it is for men. They join more voluntary organizations than women who score low in Stage IV, as they should according to theory. They share more secrets with their husbands. Perhaps the expected relationships are stronger for women because values in U.S. culture stress helping others more for women than for men.

It is interesting to note that each sex starts out oriented toward the opposite sex in Stage I, then breaks this dependency tie in Stage II, becomes assertive and identifies with its own sex in Stage III, and then is in a position to return and share with the opposite sex in Stage IV, having firmly established its own identity in Stage III. The picture is very much what one would expect based on psychoanalytic theory. Little boys start out attached to their mothers; they must break this tie (Stage II) and form a firm masculine identity in Stage III, and then they are ready to share, at the most mature stage, on the basis of equality. Women start out dependent on their fathers, break that tie, establish their feminine identity, and return to share on an equal basis with male partners in marriage. Cultural values of the United States tend to emphasize the importance of Stages II and III.

Psychologists, psychiatrists, and school teachers are very concerned about the dependency crisis: they emphasize the crucial importance of people's breaking their ties with their parents and becoming self-reliant and independent. They are also concerned about the crisis involved in going from Stage II to III, because they worry about individuals who stay alone; they insist people must become more extroverted and assertive in the real world. However, there is relatively little emphasis in U.S. culture, except in religious circles, on going from Stage III to Stage IV. In fact, scales developed by other psychologists to measure maturity (Kohlberg, 1969; Loevinger, 1966) tend to stop at Stage III, in which the full actualization of the self is viewed as the highest level of development. Yet in psychoanalytic theory and in all the world's religions, there is a still higher stage in which people sacrifice some of their egotistic concerns for service to others.

How does *n* Power relate to attaining various levels of maturity? It facilitates attaining Stage IV for women and inhibits it for men. The way this was discovered was by correlating either the Stage IV score alone or the Stage IV score plus the *n* Power score with the maximum expression of any one of a cluster of outlets characteristic of that stage. For men, the Stage IV score alone correlated .23 with the outlets characteristic of it, but adding the *n* Power score to the stage score decreased the correlation to an insignificant .14. The reverse was true for women. Adding the *n* Power score to their Stage IV scores increased the correlation with the outlets characteristic of that stage from .24 to a highly significant .39. "If Stage IV represents moving towards mutuality and equality, as the theory maintains, then it is easy to see that a high *n* Power, tending to accentuate the assertive male role, would make it more difficult for men to show behavior characteristic of Stage IV. Just the opposite is true of women: if they are to move towards mutuality, they must behave in a *more assertive* way than is characteristic of traditional women" (McClelland, 1975). Women move out of the stage of being dependent on men and are more able to share with them on an equal basis if they have a high *n* Power.

• CONTROLLED AND IMPULSIVE ASSERTIVENESS IN ORGANIZATIONAL BEHAVIOR

Leadership Motive Syndrome Among Managers

Considerable attention has focused on men whose assertiveness at Stage III is either impulsive (Stage IIIa) or disciplined and controlled (Stage IIIb), for the research on drinking has shown that inhibition is an important moderator of how the power motive expresses itself. Theoretically, men in Stage IIIa should be impulsively assertive and should not make particularly good partners or managers, whereas men in Stage IIIb should be better officers of organizations or managers, since they discipline their power impulses. In a general way, this has turned out to be true. Among service managers in one large organization, 73 percent of those classified as IIIb (high Stage III, high Activity Inhibition) had been promoted to higher levels in the organization, as compared with only 40 percent of those classified as IIIa (high Stage III, low Activity Inhibition). However, the reverse was true of line and sales managers; 88 percent of those classified as IIIa were promoted to higher levels in the organization, as compared with 63 percent of those classified as IIIb. The difference between these differences is significant (McClelland & Boyatzis, 1982). In other words, it depends somewhat on the demands of the managerial job. Service managers need to be more disciplined in managing consumer requests, whereas line managers may need to be more openly assertive.

The more common way of identifying men at the controlled assertive stage is not by using the Stage III score itself, but by using a simpler substitute scoring system that correlates highly with it. Men whose n Power score is high—and higher than their n Affiliation score—and who are high in Activity Inhibition also tend to be high in Stage IIIb, (that is, high in Stage III and high in Activity Inhibition). The correlation between these two sets of scores is .58, $N = 311$, $p < .001$ (McClelland & Boyatzis, 1982). The high n Power, low n Affiliation, and high Activity Inhibition syndrome is called either the *imperial power motive syndrome* or the *leadership motive syndrome*.

The equivalent to the IIIa pattern (high n Power, low n Affiliation, and low Activity Inhibition) is referred to as the *Don Juan* or *conquistador syndrome* (McClelland, 1975). Men characterized by this syndrome tend to make poor husbands, as judged by combined ratings of marital satisfaction and ability of husband and wife to work together (McClelland, Colman, Finn & Winter, 1978). This finding is supported by others showing that high n Power alone in men is associated with poor dating relationships (Stewart & Rubin, 1976) and with being married to wives who are not allowed to compete with them in terms of careers (Winter, Stewart, & McClelland, 1977). On the other hand, husbands who are either at Stage IV or characterized by the leadership motive syndrome (the equivalent of Stage IIIb) tend to have more satisfactory marriages (McClelland et al., 1978).

In a longitudinal study of college students, Winter, McClelland, and Stewart (1982) found that those who showed the leadership motive pattern in school behaved more responsibly in life ten years afterward. They had joined more voluntary organizations, more often held office in them, and participated in more political activities. This was true for both men and women, but only for those *with children*. Thus, it appears that being required to behave more responsibly, as in rearing a child, helps direct the power motive—even in this controlled form—away from a self-expressive mode toward a socially responsible one. This may explain the fact that women high in n Power do not have the same difficulties as men in dealing with interpersonal relationships like dating and marriage, because women tend to be more socialized to be responsible for younger children (Winter, 1982). Thus, they are not as likely as men to use interpersonal relationships to satisfy their power needs.

Several studies (Boyatzis, 1982) have traced the effects of these power motive syndromes on managerial behavior. McClelland and Burnham (1976) showed that male sales managers with the leadership motive syndrome had subordinates who rated the climate of the office higher on such dimensions as the amount of organizational clarity or team spirit. These higher morale scores were significantly associated with more sales, thus indicating that men with the leadership motive profile were more effective sales managers. In contrast, salesmen working for male managers with the Don Juan syndrome gave the office climate lower scores for organizational clarity and felt less sense of personal responsibility, indicating their managers were less effective. The leadership motive syndrome was also found to be associated with greater success as a senior officer in the U.S. Navy. Division and executive officers with the syndrome were rated as performing better than those without it. (See Table 13.2.)

The most definitive study of this sort was carried out on male managers at AT&T whose motive scores were obtained upon entrance to the company (McClelland & Boyatzis, 1982). The careers of the managers were tracked over a sixteen-year period, and the level to which they had been promoted was determined at that time. As the results in Figure 8.9 show, men characterized by the leadership motive syndrome at entrance were more likely to be promoted to higher and higher levels of management in the company over time. Very few of them had remained at Management Level 1, at which they had entered the company, and nearly half of those at Management Level 4 and above were characterized by the leadership motive profile.

By way of contrast, those with high n Achievement peaked in their careers at Management Level 3. The nonlinear trend is significant. The explanation seems to lie in the fact that individuals high in n Achievement are used to doing things by themselves and for themselves, as explained in Chapter 7. They are able to advance in the company so long as their job involves the individual contributions they make. However, at higher levels the focus of the job shifts to influencing others. The greater success of those with the leadership motive syndrome at this level can be explained on the grounds that they are interested in influencing others (the high n Power score), they are not unduly concerned about whether they are liked or not (the low n Affiliation score), and they are self-controlled (the high Activity Inhibition score). If men are high in n Affiliation, they regularly make poorer managers except in very special kinds of posi-

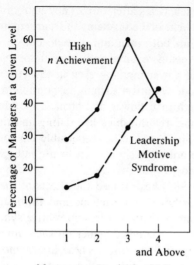

Figure 8.9.

Management Levels Attained After Sixteen Years by Men High in *n* Achievement and with the Leadership Motive Syndrome (after McClelland & Boyatzis, 1982).

tions, such as employee relations managers (McClelland & Burnham, 1976). This is because they are so interested in other people and in maintaining good relationships with them that they find it difficult to make hard decisions that might hurt other people's feelings. Yet success in management depends on applying the same standards of judgment to all people. Managers cannot make too many exceptions in terms of individual needs without making people feel they are unfair, and it is precisely those high in *n* Affiliation who are likely to be most swayed by the needs of particular individuals.

Furthermore, people with the leadership motive syndrome also have other characteristics that should make them good managers. Table 8.7 summarizes these characteristics under four main themes: respect for institutional authority, discipline and self-control, caring for others, and concern for just reward (McClelland, 1975). The correlations were obtained using a slightly different way of identifying which subjects were characterized by the leadership motive or the Don Juan syndromes. The subjects were divided into those that scored either high or low in Activity Inhibition, and then within each group the extent to which a person was higher in *n* Power than *n* Affiliation was correlated with the characteristic in question. Thus, the definitions of the two syndromes are the same. In the first numerical column, those who score higher in *n* Power than in *n* Affiliation and are also high in Activity Inhibition (which defines the leadership motive syndrome) show the characteristics listed. For example, they tend to join more organizations. In contrast, those in the second numerical column who score low in Activity Inhibition and higher in *n* Power than *n* Affiliation (the Don Juan syndrome) join organizations significantly less often, and so on throughout the table. More information on those with the Don Juan syndrome will be provided in Table 8.9 later in the chapter.

In general, individuals with the leadership motive pattern—whether men or women—show more respect for institutional authority, and they favor discipline and self-control. In fact, they like to work. This is particularly interesting, because common sense might suggest that subjects high in *n* Achievement would like to work, which is not really the case. As pointed out in Chapter 7, individuals high in *n* Achievement really like to get out of work by being more efficient. In contrast, those with the leadership motive syndrome, also called the *controlled power motive syndrome,* appear to enjoy work, because it involves being in control of things. They also show more public concern for others. They say they would be more likely to share some of a $10,000 gift with others. And there is some indication that they are more concerned about a just reward in the sense that they tend to feel that the most appropriate metaphors for death signify murder. That is, if they respect institutional authority, discipline themselves, and care for others, they may be led to think that it is quite reasonable that they should get a just reward. In this context, death may seem particularly unjust. As McClelland (1975) points out, institutional religion that strongly favors these themes gets around the problem of "death as injustice" by promising rewards in the afterlife (Christianity) or in terms of being reborn at a higher level (Hinduism or Buddhism). But in the present context it is clear why a belief in centralized authority, hard work, serving others, and justice should make effective managers. In contrast, those with the Don Juan syndrome either do not subscribe to these virtues or behave in ways directly opposed to them, which should mean they would not make very effective managers.

The person high in *n* Power at Stage IIIb is a socially responsible person who manages things well and often assumes a leadership role in organizations or the community. In what sense is such a person not completely mature? The critical difference between Stage IIIb and Stage IV lies in the reasons why such people serve others. Are they doing it on behalf of themselves or truly out of commitment to a higher good? Those in Stage IIIb see the power and authority coming from themselves, and they are serving others to extend their own influence. Thus, they have not achieved the highest level of maturity in which they have become true selfless instruments of higher authority. Jesus characterized such people as praying or performing charitable acts in public so that they could be recognized for what they had done. People truly in Stage IV would not care whether what they had done was recognized or not.

Motive Profiles of U.S. Presidents

As a further check on these findings, Winter (1973) reviewed the managerial effectiveness of U.S. presidents in terms of their motivational profiles. Table 8.8 summarizes the scores for each president since Theodore Roosevelt on *n* Power, *n* Achievement, and *n* Affiliation as obtained by coding the motivational imag-

Table 8.7.

PERSONAL CHARACTERISTICS ASSOCIATED WITH LEADERSHIP MOTIVE PATTERN: HIGH *n* POWER[a] > *n* AFFILIATION, HIGH ACTIVITY INHIBITION[b] (after McClelland, 1975)

Characteristics Among Men	Correlations of High *n* Power[a] – *n* Affiliation When Activity Inhibition Is	
	High[b] (N = 29)	Low (N = 42)
Respect for institutional authority		
Joins more organizations	.25†	−.35*
Prefers psychiatrist for personal help	.29†	−.11
Discipline and self-control		
Feels work is enjoyable	.41*	.03
Keeps feelings to self	.31†	−.12
Caring for others, altruism		
Shares $10,000 gift with charities	.23	−.32*
Taught sociocentric virtues by parents[c]	.30†	−.24
Concern for just reward		
Thinks metaphors for death as murder are more appropriate	.27†	.01

Characteristics Among Women	Correlations of High *n* Power[a] – *n* Affiliation When Activity Inhibition Is	
	High[b] (N = 28)	Low (N = 46)
Respect for institutional authority		
Is elected to more offices	.33*	.05
Accepts institutional responsibility	.37*	−.11
Discipline and self-control		
Feels work is not boring	.40**	.01
Tells no lies	.40**	.04
Caring for others, altruism		
Shares $10,000 gift with friends	.36*	.07
Lists people as among precious possessions	.48**	.02
Concern for just reward		
Thinks metaphors for death as murder are more appropriate	.30†	.20

[a]Score of 3 or more.
[b]Score of 2 or more.
[c]Sociocentric virtues include being kind and friendly to others.
†$p < .10$.
*$p < .05$.
**$p < .01$.

ery in their inaugural addresses (Winter & Stewart, 1978). It might be supposed that the content of these speeches might reflect either the interests of the speech writer or particular issues of importance at the time more than the personal characteristics of the presidents. However, Winter and Stewart's data strongly suggest that this is not so. They found that the general prestige of a president, as well as his strength in action or assertiveness versus passivity as independently rated by Maranell (1970), were strongly positively related to the president's *n* Power score and strongly negatively related to his *n* Affiliation score.

Just by looking at Table 8.8 we can observe that the presidents generally regarded as strong—namely, both Roosevelts, Wilson, Truman, Kennedy, and Johnson—all had *n* Power scores that were relatively high and higher than their *n* Affiliation scores, which is the pattern associated with more effective management if it is also combined with a high Activity Inhibition score (which Winter did not measure). The relatively less effective presidents were either low in

Table 8.8.

MOTIVE SCORES FOR THE TWENTIETH-CENTURY PRESIDENTS USING INAUGURAL ADDRESSES (after Winter & Stewart, 1978)

| President | Standard-scored Motives (Mean = 50; Standard Deviation = 10) | | | |
	n Achievement	n Affiliation	n Power	n Power − n Affiliation
T. Roosevelt	56	45	63	+18
Taft	35	39	33	− 6
Wilson	43	41	49	+ 8
Harding	40	48	41	− 7
Coolidge	38	42	38	− 4
Hoover	47	45	38	− 7
F. D. Roosevelt	52	40	54	+14
Truman	47	41	59	+ 8
Eisenhower	41	55	43	−12
Kennedy	58	58	63	+ 5
Johnson	61	45	56	+11
Nixon	64	58	48	−10
Ford	40	80	46	−34
Carter	63	53	51	− 2
Reagan[a]	62	50	67	+17
Mean score per 1000 words	4.80	3.33	5.53	
Standard deviation	2.53	2.41	2.08	

[a]Scores provided later by David Winter.

n Power, like Coolidge, or higher in *n* Affiliation relative to *n* Power, like Eisenhower, Harding, and Ford.

It is also worth noting that the three presidents who were higher in *n* Achievement than the other two motives and for whom *n* Power was not greater than *n* Affiliation—namely, Hoover, Nixon, and Carter—were all regarded as having difficulty getting things done. They had the characteristics of individuals with high *n* Achievement in that they thought things through on their own and came to good solutions, but they were less effective in managing others and in getting their good ideas implemented than presidents with a higher need for Power. The fact that Nixon was forced to resign for using illegal shortcuts to reach his goals is dramatic confirmation of the tendency of individuals high in *n* Achievement to behave dishonestly if necessary to achieve their goals, as reported in Chapter 7. Winter also showed that the higher a president's *n* Power score (especially relative to his *n* Affiliation score), the more likely it was that the country would go to war during his administration and the less likely that he would favor strategic arms limitation. The same trend is reported for the relation of *n* Power to *n* Affiliation scores in popular literature in Chapter 11.

Finally, a word about Ford is in order, because his *n* Affiliation score is so much higher than that of any other president in the table. Both his *n* Power and *n* Achievement scores are well below average. One might well wonder how he got to be president with this motive profile. The answer, of course, is that he is the only president on the list who did not actively seek the office and who was not directly elected to it. When he pardoned Nixon after succeeding him in office, he made a remark dramatically characteristic of the approach of individuals high in *n* Affiliation. He said, "The man has suffered enough," which was undoubtedly true. From the more universalistic point of view, however, it was also true of many other people who had worked for Nixon and gone to jail for participating in similar activities. This is typical of managers high in *n* Affiliation: they make exceptions to rules in terms of the particular needs of individuals, a style of managing often seen as unjust by others.

Ford became president at a time when the country had suffered a number of setbacks—in the war in Vietnam abroad and the Watergate scandal at home. He responded to the crisis by emphasizing putting the country back together again —stressing the importance of affiliation, as a man high in *n* Affiliation is likely to do. A president with a different motive profile—Franklin Delano Roosevelt, for example—could be expected to respond quite differently to a crisis, just as Roosevelt responded differently to the crisis of the Great Depression in the 1930s with themes of achievement and power, which eventually led the country into World War II.

Motive Profile of Radicals

Rothman and Lichter (1978; Lichter & Rothman, 1982) have carried out extensive studies of the personality characteristics of student and adult New Left radicals as they surfaced in the 1960s. Those who protested against society's oppression of blacks, women, and the poor were generally pictured at the time as being liberated from the power concerns that supposedly activated those who ran the social system. They were described as "flower children" who believed in self-actualization, equality, intimacy, and community; more sympathetically, they were thought to be dedicated to the cause of bringing about a change in the way society was governed so as to provide greater opportunities for oppressed women and minorities. Such concerns would be consistent with having a strong socialized power drive.

However accurate these images may have been in general, they did not characterize radical leaders. Lichter and Rothman (1982) reported that as contrasted with nonradical students, active student radicals scored significantly higher in *n* Power and Stage III assertiveness, as well as significantly lower in *n* Affiliation and the intimacy motive. Non-Jewish radicals scored significantly lower in Activity Inhibition (see also Rothman et al., 1977) than all other student groups. In other words, they showed the Don Juan motive syndrome characterized by impulsive aggressive behavior and a rejection of institutional responsibility. (See the summary of the behavioral correlates of the Don Juan syndrome found in a sample of adult men in Table 8.9.)

Lichter and Rothman also found that adult radicals showed the same pattern, including also a lower Stage IV orientation, indicating an inability to progress beyond Stage III to a more sharing, integrative level of maturity. In other words, if the motive profile of the most successful presidents represents socialized power motivation, which leads to effectiveness in managing the establishment, the motive profile of those most active in opposing the establishment represents the rebellious type of personalized power characteristic of Stage IIIa.

Even here, though, it is important to remember that the action a motive profile leads to depends on other variables in the person-environment interaction. Greene and Winter (1971) found that black student leaders were significantly higher in *n* Power than other blacks, and that among black students reared in the North, a high *n* Power was associated with being directly active in the black community and unwilling to work within the white power system. In other words, high *n* Power in these students led to radical protest. However, among black students reared in the South, a high *n* Power was significantly correlated with being pragmatic or willing to work within the system. Greene and Winter explained the difference as being due to different estimates of the probability of success of alternative strategies depending on past experience with racial discrimination. Northern black students had grown up in a system that was technically integrated and open equally to all, yet they had often felt discriminated against because of their color. So working within the system to them would mean accepting the status quo and little probability of further success in winning their rights. In contrast, black students who grew up in the South would have been exposed to an overtly discriminatory system, so to them a formally integrated, nondiscriminatory system represented a step forward. In both cases high *n* Power led to greater activity, but of different types, depending on their evaluation of how successful one strategy or another would be in advancing their rights.

Table 8.9.

PERSONAL CHARACTERISTICS ASSOCIATED WITH THE DON JUAN MOTIVATIONAL PATTERN IN MEN: HIGH *n* POWER MINUS *n* AFFILIATION, LOW ACTIVITY INHIBITION (after McClelland, 1975)

Characteristics	Correlations of High *n* Power − *n* Affiliation Among Men Low in Activity Inhibition *(N = 42)*
Phallic assertiveness	
Reports more frequent physical fights	.23†
Has higher maximum consumption of any alcoholic drink	.27*
Talks more about sex life	.25†
Does not recall distress for which he was responsible	.28*
Scores higher on Stage III (Phallic) score on Maturity Scale	.33**
Scores higher on any alternative in male Stage III cluster of actions (promiscuity, drinking, lying, collecting valuable objects)	.35**
Rejection of institutional responsibility	
Joins fewer organizations	.35**
Rejects institutional responsibility	.33**
Would not share $10,000 gift with charity	.32*

†$p < .10$ in the predicted direction.
*$p < .05$ in the predicted direction.
**$p < .025$ in the predicted direction.

• INHIBITED POWER MOTIVE SYNDROME AND SUSCEPTIBILITY TO ILLNESS

Cardiovascular Disease

McClelland (1976) observed that individuals high in *n* Power, particularly those with the leadership motive syndrome, behaved in many ways like victims of heart attacks. Friedman and Rosenman (1974) had conducted extensive studies showing that individuals with coronary artery disease were much more likely than normal individuals to be irritable, always in a hurry, hard driving, and tense, often because of repressed anger. They labeled these characteristics *Type A behavior* and contrasted it with *Type B behavior,* which was typical of people who are much more relaxed and easygoing, willing to take things as they come, and unlikely to have heart attacks. They reasoned that the "driven" quality of Type A individuals meant that they had more chronically active sympathetic nervous systems, which in time would put a strain on the cardiovascular system, since chronic sympathetic activation increases heart rate and has other effects, such as releasing epinephrine, that could be damaging to the cardiovascular system. Type A behavior, particularly since it involved suppressed assertiveness, suggested that inhibited power motivation, as represented by the leadership motive syndrome, might lie behind Type A behavior. The implication of the sympathetic nervous system and catecholamine release also suggested that *n* Power might be involved.

The potential importance of the inhibition variable is indicated by the fact that high *n* Power by itself is not related to Type A behavior, nor is high *n* Achievement or *n* Affiliation (Matthews & Saal, 1978). McClelland (1979b) found in three different samples that individuals with the inhibited power or leadership motive syndrome had significantly higher blood pressure, indicating a strain on the cardiovascular system. The most convincing of these studies was longitudinal. Motive scores were coded from TATs provided by adult males some ten years after they had graduated from college. Their blood pressures were checked twenty years after that, when they were in their early fifties. The results are shown in Figure 8.10. Those with the leadership motive syndrome—that is, those with *n* Power higher than *n* Affiliation and those high in Activity Inhibition or self-control—had significantly higher diastolic blood pressure twenty years later than men with other motive combinations. If a diastolic blood pressure of ninety millimeters of mercury is considered indicative of clinically significant hypertension, 61 percent of the men who had the inhibited power motive syndrome in their early thirties showed signs of hypertension twenty years later, as contrasted with only 23 percent of the men in the other three motive classifications ($p < .01$).

Impaired Immune Function and Illness

McClelland, Davidson, Floor, and Saron (1980) reasoned that chronic sympathetic nervous system activation might lead to more susceptibility to infectious disease, because more epinephrine release could damage immune function and thus reduce resistance to infection. In a small sample of male subjects, they found that those with the inhibited power motive syndrome excreted a higher level of epinephrine in urine averaged over two occasions than other subjects, as well as that a higher level of epinephrine excretion was significantly associated with lower concentrations of immunoglobulin A in saliva (S-IgA), a measure of immune function. They further found, as expected, that lower levels of S-IgA were associated with reports of more illness in the past year, particularly from upper respiratory infections or colds. This finding makes good sense, because S-IgA is the body's first line of defense against cold viruses that enter through the mouth and nose.

McClelland and Jemmott (1980) added the important fact that the amount of stress to which the person was exposed combines with the inhibited power motive syndrome to make the person more likely to get sick. Their findings are

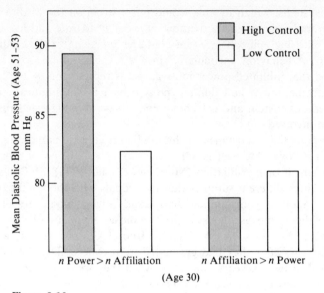

Figure 8.10.

Mean Diastolic Blood Pressure in Men Aged Fifty-one to Fifty-three Classified by their Power Motive Type at Age Thirty (after McClelland, 1979b).

summarized in Table 8.10. Students were asked to list any illnesses they had had in the past year and to rate them for severity on a scale of 1 to 100, "where 100 means you were very very sick with a high fever, nearly died, etc.; 50 corresponds to having a case of the flu that kept you out of circulation for more than three days; and 1 means you hardly noticed the problem" (McClelland & Jemmott, 1980). The illness reports of the subjects were classified according to their motive dispositions (whether n Power was higher or lower than n Affiliation), their Activity Inhibition score (whether high or low), and the amount of power stress they reported in terms of life events in the past year that could be considered power or achievement related, such as failing an examination, involvement in a major sports event, or a major worsening of financial state. As the data in Table 8.10 indicate, all three of these variables contributed to how sick the students reported they had been. The most sick were those who were high in the inhibited power motive syndrome and also high in power stress (mean illness score = 195.5), whereas those subjects who had none of these characteristics had the lowest average illness score (mean = 47.4). The comparisons at the bottom of Table 8.10 show that students with any two of the characteristics reported themselves more sick on the average than the remaining students.

McClelland and Jemmott also found that other motive-stress combinations were not associated with more illness. For example, those high in n Power and

Table 8.10.

MEAN SEVERITY OF REPORTED ILLNESSES AMONG GROUPS DIFFERING IN *n* POWER, POWER STRESS, AND INHIBITION (after McClelland & Jemmott, 1980)

Subject Groups	High Activity Inhibition[a]			Low Activity Inhibition		
	N	Mean	SD	N	Mean	SD
n Power > *n* Affiliation[b]						
High power stress[c]	10	195.5	195.1	8	79.9	56.5
Low power stress	13	103.7	95.9	10	59.3	49.4
n Affiliation > *n* Power[d]						
High power stress	5	66.4	74.8	11	84.5	64.2
Low power stress	10	51.7	40.9	8	47.4	23.8

Sources of variance among versus within groups: $df = 7/67$, $F = 2.32$, $p < .04$.

Planned Comparisons	N	Mean Severity of Illness	F Values
High *n* Power, high power stress, high Activity Inhibition	10	195.5	
Versus low on all three variables	8	47.4	10.1, $p < .01$
Versus all other subjects	65	72.9	13.9, $p < .001$
When Activity Inhibition unknown			
High on *n* Power and power stress	18	144.1	
Versus all other subjects	57	71.9	6.5, $p < .02$
When power stress unknown			
High on *n* Power and Activity Inhibition	23	143.6	11.5, $p < .01$
Versus all other subjects	52	65.2	

[a]Score of 2 or more.

[b]T-score *n* Power $\geq$ 45 and > T-score *n* Affiliation.

[c]Above the median or 4 or more power-achievement life events checked for last year.

[d]T-score *n* Power $\leq$ 50 and < T-score *n* Affiliation.

in affiliative stress (as occurs in falling out of love or the death of a family member) did not report themselves to have been more sick, nor did those high in *n* Affiliation with high affiliative stress. It is the inhibited and stressed power motive that is particularly bad for a person's health.

Some further evidence of this relationship is provided in Figure 8.11, which presents data obtained from male prisoners (McClelland, Alexander, & Marks, 1982). The men higher in *n* Power and reporting an above-median number of power stresses reported more severe illnesses on the average than other subjects (including those low in *n* Power and high in power stress). Furthermore, those higher in *n* Power and in power stress showed signs of impaired immune function, indicated by a lower mean concentration of S-IgA. Thus, the difference could not be due to a tendency of some subjects to complain more about everything, including both illness and stress. Finally, 58 percent of those below the median in S-IgA concentration reported an above-median severity of illness, as contrasted with only 31 percent of those with above-median concentrations of S-IgA ($p < .05$). In other words, the presumption is that stressed high power motivation is damaging immune function, which makes the individuals more susceptible to disease (McClelland, 1982). Another study has shown that the inhibited power motive syndrome is associated not only with lower S-IgA concentrations, but also with another indicator of immune function, natural killer cell activity (McClelland, Locke, Williams, & Hurst, 1982).

One word of caution is in order, however: all the studies involving physiological functions (epinephrine excretion and S-IgA concentrations) have been done on men, and there is at least some preliminary indication that the relationships may not hold in the same way for women. In a further study that showed the usual correlation between high n Power and high power stress and lower

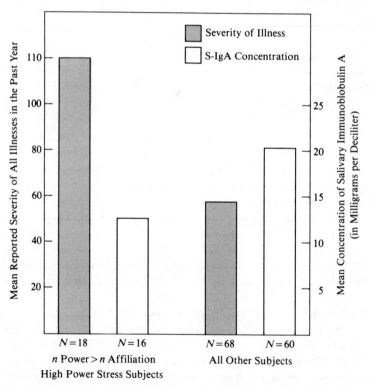

Figure 8.11.

Mean Severity of Illness and Concentrations of Immunoglobulin A in Saliva (S-IgA) Among Male Prisoners High in n Power and Reported Stress Compared with All Other Prisoners (data from McClelland, Alexander, & Marks, 1982).

concentrations of S-IgA in men, no such relationship was found for women (McClelland & Kirshnit, 1982).

• ORIGINS OF THE POWER MOTIVE

Parental Permissiveness About Sex and Aggression

McClelland and Pilon (1983) also examined the child-training antecedents of the adult power motive in the study described in Chapter 7 that investigated the antecedents of the achievement motive. They found that mothers who said when their children were five years old that they were permissive about sex and aggression had children who developed into adults with higher *n* Power scores. The results are summarized in Table 8.11.

The score on permissiveness for sex and aggression is derived from a factor analysis performed years earlier by Sears, Maccoby, and Levin (1957), who conducted the interviews with mothers about child-training practices. Some of the training practices included in the overall factor score are listed in Table 8.11 to better describe what was actually involved. The results for the total factor score are consistent in random subsamples of the total population, as well as for males

Table 8.11.

CORRELATION OF EARLY CHILD-REARING PRACTICES WITH ADULT *n* POWER SCORES (after McClelland & Pilon, 1983)

Child-rearing Practices	All Subjects (N = 78)	Random (N = 38)	Subsamples (N = 40)	Males (N = 38)	Females (N = 40)
Permissiveness for sex and aggression[a]	.31***	.33*	.30†	.28†	.32*
For masturbation	.31**	.39*	.20	.33*	.27†
For sex play	.28*	.22	.35	.37*	.23
For aggression to siblings	.24*	.26	.24	.32*	.17
For inappropriate aggression to children	.12	.04	.18	.06	.14
For aggression to parents	.30**	.39*	.20	.18	.37*
Demands for child to be aggressive	−.05	−.10	.03	−.15	−.01
Encouragement of child to fight back	.16	.08	.25	−.08	.44*
Praise for good behavior at table	−.32**	−.26	−.40*	−.47*	−.23

Note: The *n* Power scores have been corrected for regression in protocol length. Correlation of social class with *n* Power = .30,* and correlation of Social class with Permissiveness for sex and aggression = .59.**

[a]Factor score from Sears, Maccoby, & Levin (1957).

†*p* < .05 in the predicted direction.

**p* < .05.

***p* < .01.

****p* < .001.

and females. They are somewhat less consistent for components of the score, but there is considerable consistency for permissiveness about masturbation and about aggression toward brothers and sisters and parents. Mothers who are relaxed about sexual and aggressive assertiveness are most likely to have children who grow up high in *n* Power.

McClelland and Pilon also found that it is not permissiveness in general that leads to high *n* Power, for Sears et al. also rated permissiveness about feeding, toilet training, bed time, noise around the house, physical mobility, and dependency. Permissiveness in none of these areas was significantly related to adult *n* Power scores.

Why should permissiveness about sex and aggression be especially important? We cannot be certain, but the discussion in Chapter 5 of the natural incentive of "having impact," which presumably underlies the power motive, suggests that the impact incentive may more immediately and regularly be present and result in sympathetic activation in the areas of sex and aggression. If the power motive is served by the catecholamine system involved in sympathetic arousal, as suggested throughout this chapter, then finding that early experiences in the areas of sex and aggression, which also involve sympathetic arousal, lie at the basis of the need for power is entirely consistent with such a viewpoint.

The fact that both sex and aggression are involved is consistent with a great deal of physiological and psychological evidence that these two types of activities are related (Barclay, 1971; Moyer, 1976). The findings suggest that children who are allowed to develop associations around the pleasures from such sexual and aggressive impacts develop a strong *n* Power. If they are punished for these behaviors, they are likely to develop negative associations to having impact in the sex and aggression areas, which would generalize to avoiding impact in all types of situations. The fact that praise for good behavior at the table is negatively associated with adult *n* Power scores suggests that some kinds of inhibition of impulsive-assertive behavior can interfere with the development of the power motive. Furthermore, the use of physical punishment for boys is significantly negatively associated with adult *n* Power scores ($r = -.36$; $p < .05$); this is not true for girls, however, perhaps because physical punishment is less common for girls. It is also noteworthy that positive encouragement for girls to fight back increases their *n* Power scores. In other words, society expects girls to be less assertive and aggressive so that their pleasure from "impact" normally would be more often inhibited, and it takes positive encouragement on the part of the parents for them to develop the associative network that makes up the need for power.

Sources of the Leadership Motive and Don Juan Syndromes

Of particular interest also are the parental training practices associated with the leadership or imperial power motive syndrome and the Don Juan syndrome. As has been noted, the leadership or inhibited power motive syndrome is associated with effective managerial performance, belief in centralized authority, a liking for work, impulse control, and a strong sense of justice. McClelland (1975) has argued that this syndrome in the West is most closely associated with patriarchal authority systems. Boys who grow up to have this syndrome should be reared by strong, self-controlled fathers with whom the boys can eventually identify as adults. In McClelland and Pilon's (1983) sample there is some evidence that this is what happened. In one part of the interview the mothers were asked whether they or the fathers were primarily responsible for the child's upbringing. If the father was reported to have been the most important child-rearing agent, the son was more likely to be characterized by the leadership or imperial power motive syndrome as an adult ($r = .35; p < .05$). The same was not true of daughters, nor was high n Power by itself significantly associated with the father's being more important in child rearing. Father-reared sons are more likely to develop the leadership or socialized power motive syndrome.

There is also evidence that having a younger sibling promotes the kind of socialized power activities characteristic of those with the leadership motive syndrome (Winter, 1982). The reason, as explained earlier, is that having a younger sibling to look after promotes a sense of responsibility for others, which socializes the expression of the power motive. In contrast, those who are only or youngest children are more likely to show the profligate expansive impulse that characterizes the Don Juan syndrome (high n Power and low Activity Inhibition). Unfortunately, no direct test has been made to see whether individuals with the leadership motive syndrome are more likely to have younger siblings.

In discussing the Don Juan legend, which we have associated with high n Power and low Activity Inhibition, Winter (1973) suggests that Don Juan may have been reared particularly by his mother and reports evidence that strong mothers, as indicated by the fact that they were teachers, tended to have sons with higher n Power scores than other mothers. There is also considerable evidence (reviewed in McClelland, 1975) that the absence of the father as a child-rearing agent leads to a son's identifying with his mother and then developing a kind of defensive masculinity in later life to cover up his underlying feminine identification (see Whiting, 1965). The defensive masculinity involves the same kind of impulsiveness-aggressiveness, sexual promiscuity, display, and antiinstitutional activities that characterize the conquistador or Don Juan syndrome (see Table 8.9). This would suggest that mother dominance in child rearing should be associated with a Don Juan syndrome in adulthood. Such is the case in these data. Sons whose mothers said they were the more important child-rearing agent tended more often to grow up with the Don Juan or impulsive power motive syndrome ($r = .46, p < .05$). Again, the same was not true of girls, nor was mother dominance in child rearing associated with higher n Power by itself in their sons.

Some caution is indicated in interpreting these findings, because the numbers of people with the two special power motive syndromes was small in each case, as well as because the results would probably hold only for societies in which families are primarily patriarchal. For example, Ross and Glaser (1970) found the expected relationship between impulsive-aggressive behavior and father absence among Chicano or Spanish American families in the Los Angeles area. They compared the family backgrounds of well-behaved and delinquent boys from the same low-income neighborhoods. Among Chicanos they found that 59 percent of "good" boys had fathers who were the primary decision makers, as contrasted with only 25 percent of the "bad boys," for whom either the mother was the primary decision maker or there was no father present in the home. The same was not true of black families however, where an equal proportion of the good and bad boys came from families with no fathers present. Among blacks, the crucial question seemed to be whether there was a strong mother figure. Seventy-three percent of the good boys had mothers as primary decision makers, as compared with only 39 percent of the bad boys. In other words, impulsive-aggressive behavior of the Don Juan type in boys seems to be associated with the absence of the culturally normal primary authority figure, which is usually, but not always, the father.

Loss of Status and the Development of the Need for Power

To locate child-rearing practices associated with the adult power motive only raises a further question. What would lead parents to behave in those particular ways? In the case of the achievement motive, parents influenced by ideological reform movements seem more likely to emphasize that their children should do things better in contrast to the old ways of doing things (see Chapter 7).

What would lead parents to stress assertiveness or, at least, to not inhibit it? Some indirect scraps of evidence suggest that a loss of or threat to status is associated with a compensatory increase in n Power. Men who have lost a parent through death and black men score higher in n Power than other men (Veroff et al., 1980). In both cases it can be argued that there has been some threat to the men's sense of competency and power. Unemployment should be an even greater threat in the case of men. No direct evidence exists on the n Power scores of unemployed men as compared with others, but McClelland (1976) did find a significant correlation between high levels of unemployment in a given decade in U.S. history and high n Power scores, as coded in popular literature for that decade (see Chapter 11).

More convincing data comes from a study conducted by Heller (1979) on children of the parents involved in the Jewish Holocaust in Europe. He located a sample of Jewish students, all of whose parents had been forced to migrate to the United States from Europe because of oppression by Nazis in Germany and elsewhere. He divided the sample into those whose relatives and immediate family members had died in concentration camps and those whose families had not suffered to nearly the same degree. Many of the parents in what he called the "high-stress" group were themselves concentration camp survivors. He reasoned that those who had personally suffered and whose relatives had died would have been subjected to much greater loss of status than the parents who had not suffered to the same degree. He found that 67 percent of the children of parents who had undergone greater stress scored high in *n* Power, as compared with 44 percent of children of parents who had undergone lesser stress ($p < .05$).

Furthermore, there was other evidence that the higher *n* Power scores were directly related to the highly stressed parents' placing more emphasis on the survival of Jews as a group. The children of the highly stressed parents were not more religious in belief or practice, but they reported that they had been required to learn more about Jewish history and customs, and they had more factual knowledge about such things. Furthermore, many more of them disapproved of intermarriage with non-Jews than did the children whose parents had been forced to emigrate from Europe but had been less threatened. This was particularly true of women. Eighty percent of the daughters of highly stressed parents disapproved of intermarriage, as contrasted with 44 percent of the daughters of less stressed parents ($p < .01$). The finding is especially meaningful because in Jewish culture it is the woman who transmits Jewishness to her children.

In this case we have no direct knowledge of how permissive the parents were in early childhood toward sex and aggression, but there is plenty of evidence that the parents who had felt the most threatened by the possibility of Jews being wiped out were those who insisted that their children be assertive in preserving Jewishness, which led to higher *n* Power. Heller also obtained information directly from the parents and found that those who had been under greater stress also reported that they had placed greater demands on their children to learn about Jewish culture than the parents who had been under less stress.

Incidentally, the children of the more highly stressed parents also had lower *n* Affiliation scores than the children of the less stressed parents: they cared less about liking or being liked by others (see Chapter 9). It is ironic that Germans with the high *n* Power–low *n* Affiliation syndrome (see Table 11.6 in Chapter 11) persecuted Jews in Europe and evoked a similar power motive syndrome in children of those persecuted Jews in the United States. With such a motive pattern, one could certainly expect Jews to fight back, and it is interesting to observe that the leaders in the radical protest movements in the 1960s were overwhelmingly Jewish (see Lichter & Rothman, 1982; Rothman, 1981; Rothman & Lichter, 1978) and were characterized by this particular motive syndrome.

Heller did not measure inhibition directly, but he did employ Winter's hope of Power and fear of Power subscores. Power stories classified as indicating hope of Power center on themes of personal dominance in zero-sum games (see Table 8.1) and are significantly associated more often with high *n* Power and low inhibition (Winter, 1973). Heller found that the children of concentration camp survivors, who had parents under high stress, scored significantly higher in hope of Power than children of Jewish parents under lesser stress. In contrast, there was no significant difference in the scores of the two groups of children on fear of Power, which is associated with themes of expressing power on behalf of others, and with high *n* Power and high inhibition. Thus, oppression may lead to the direct encouragement of a desire to retaliate or strike back in an impulsive-aggressive way rather than to a more socialized type of power motivation. More research is needed on other types of deprivation of status, but preliminary evidence suggests that it leads parents to emphasize or release assertiveness in their children, which allows them to develop strong *n* Power, and perhaps low *n* Affiliation and impulsive or retaliatory assertiveness.

NOTES AND QUERIES

1. Think through the implications of the finding that individuals high in *n* Power seem to be "preset" to register a bigger response to power stimuli. Is this a sign of what Hull meant by the anticipatory goal response? After all, it does not surprise us in terms of learning theory that a hungrier person will salivate more at the sight of a steak than at the sight of a stone. But is an electrical response in a portion of the brain the same as a salivary response? Must greater electrical responsivity be the result of prior learning, or could it reflect some other process?

2. If the power motive is associated with greater right brain dominance, what other behaviors would you expect individuals high in *n* Power to show? Examine the handedness literature, for instance (Gur & Gur, 1974).

3. Why do you think men and women high in *n* Power consider themselves to be *complicated* and *disorderly?*

4. Score the imaginative stories you wrote earlier for *n* Power. Then make a list of each of the common outlets for *n* Power for one of your sex and class background, and check whether or not you generally behave in those ways. Is there agreement between your *n* Power score and the number of behavioral signs of *n* Power you show? Explain any discrepancies, if you can, in terms of other determinants of your behavior, such as values, skills, or opportunities.

5. Design an experiment that would test the hypothesis that the Atkinson risk-taking model applies to people high in *n* Power if *probability of success* means the probability of being noticed rather than the probability of succeeding.

6. Only the men high in *n* Power chose to arm wrestle with opponents who were stronger than they were in the McClelland and Teague (1975) experiment. How would you explain this result either in terms of the Atkinson model of risk taking or any other model?

7. Do you believe men think more about sex, aggression, and power after drinking because they know they are drinking and expect that drinking should affect them that way? In other words, are the effects of social drinking on power thoughts the result of learning, of suggestion, or both? Assemble arguments on both sides of this issue.

8. It is argued in the text that the attempt to conceal from the subjects what they are drinking so distorts the situation that whatever results are obtained

are atypical or meaningless. Is there any other way to distinguish between the effects of alcohol in itself and the effects of the expectations that go with drinking? What about comparing the effects of actually drinking alcohol with the effects when people believe they are drinking alcohol but actually are not? (See, for example, Briddell, Rimm, Caddy, Krawitz, Sholis, & Wunderlin, 1978; Lansky & Wilson, 1981).

9. In Perry's dream described in Chapter 2, when he was frustrated he tended to regress to an earlier stage, whereas in Freud's dream, frustration led to progression to a later stage. Stewart (1978) has confirmed that major life events like marriage or going to a new school tend to lead to regression in stage thinking. Do you think the power motive might modify this tendency in any way?

10. A major unsettled theoretical point is whether the Freud-Erikson stages of maturity refer primarily to stages in development of the power motive or, more generally, to stages in development that could affect how all motives express themselves. Which do you think is more likely to be the case? How could you determine which point of view is correct? (Consult McClelland, 1975.)

11. Have you noticed any evolution in the way your *n* Power has expressed itself over the years that might correspond to changes in your level of maturity?

12. What does it mean that great spiritual leaders, such as Black Elk (see Neihardt, 1932/1972), are described as having powers involving healing, secret knowledge, control over the forces of nature, and bringing people together into an organized nation? How are these characteristics related to expressing the power motive at various stages of maturity? (For a discussion, see McClelland, 1975.)

13. In what type of management positions would you think a higher *n* Affiliation relative to *n* Power might be more important? If you cannot imagine, read Chapter 9.

14. Can you estimate from the figures in Table 8.10 whether stress or inhibition has a greater effect in producing illness for those higher in *n* Power than *n* Affiliation?

15. In view of the various explanations given for the development of either the Don Juan or leadership motive syndromes, what social events would be likely to increase the appearance of each characterological syndrome?

16. Design an experiment that would test whether high *n* Power is associated with the desire to have impact on things as well as on people.

17. Philosophers, psychologists, and sociologists have often assumed that people are inherently selfish—that in the end they are motivated to do whatever is to their advantage. A typical statement of this position is "Man is selfish. Individuals will try to maximize their outcomes" (Walster, Walster, & Berscheid, 1978). Analyze this statement in motivational terms. What could

it mean? In what sense, for example, are individuals high in *n* Power trying to maximize their outcomes by taking extreme risks? Could it be said that individuals high in *n* Achievement are trying to maximize their outcomes more than those high in *n* Power? What outcomes?

18. An advertisement for *Fortune* magazine said: "To make it in business . . . you need all the smarts, guts, and ambition you can muster. Ambition? You bet. It's finally out of the closet. At last you can be frank about your drive for success. That's what the fast track is all about." What motive is being appealed to here?

19. There is some evidence from the study of identical and fraternal twins that assertiveness, aggressiveness, or dominance is determined in part by heredity (see Loehlin & Nichols, 1976). According to the view of the power motive and its biological correlates presented in this chapter, formulate some hypotheses explaining how inherited biological characteristics might make it likely that a stronger *n* Power would develop in some people than others. Review Sheldon's (1942) evidence that mesomorphs with strong muscular development are more assertive, as well as the suggestion in Cortés and Gatti (1972) that mesomorphs may be higher in *n* Power.

9

The Affiliative Motives

• THE MEANING OF LOVE

People appear to have a basic need or desire to be with other people, just as most animals prefer to be with other members of their species. Part of the need is sexual in origin and biologically adaptive, because the two sexes must get together in order to reproduce the species. The need to affiliate with others includes sexual contacts, but it is much broader, including various types of emotional interpersonal attachments that may grow out of natural contact incentives as outlined in Chapter 4. What has always struck observers about this need is how important it is to life and health, how pervasive it is, and how it appears in many different forms. The word *love* is commonly used to describe various types of affiliative ties, and everyone agrees that it is important to satisfy the love need, yet no one is quite sure, in the words of a popular song, "What is this thing called love?" Before we review modern psychology's attempt to answer this question, it will be helpful to turn first to an ancient treatment of the topic in Plato's *Symposium*. The speakers at this banquet, as reported by Plato, managed to mention most of the important themes that have characterized discussions of the psychology of love ever since.

In the *Symposium* some men get together in ancient Athens for an evening of eating, drinking, and entertainment. Socrates joins them, and they look forward to a lively time, for he is known for his ability to challenge their ideas and make them think. The medical man present, Eryximachus, proposes that instead of getting drunk, they spend the evening talking about love, singing its praises, and trying to define and understand it. He contributes to the discussion by arguing that the practice of medicine involves "the knowledge of the principles of love at work in the body," as well as that the good practitioner must be able "to bring elements in the body . . . into mutual affection and love and know how to create love and harmony among the different elements in the body."

He sounds like another doctor, Sigmund Freud, who over two thousand years later also argued persuasively that properly functioning love (or *libido,* in his terminology) was essential to mental and physical health. Both men believed that harmony was an essential aspect of love and health. For Freud, disharmony and disease resulted from the failure of the love instinct to develop normally. For Eryximachus, love was the result of different elements in the mind or body functioning together the way different notes in a chord produce a pleasing sound or different beats on a drum create rhythm. For this reason he thought of music as contributing to creating harmony: "Music, by implanting mutual love and sympathy, causes agreement between these elements, just as medicine does in its different sphere, and music in its turn may be called a knowledge of the principles of love in the realm of harmony and rhythm." We will run into the notion of rhythm and mutual reciprocity again and again in other treatments of love. Remember also that Freud argued that rhythmic repetitive self-stimulation was the cue that naturally elicited the sexual response.

Eryximachus distinguishes between sacred and profane love, or heavenly and vulgar love, for he also realizes that love can cause all kinds of trouble. Love must be disciplined lest it lead to debauchery. Love must be expressed in an orderly manner, for "when inordinate love gets the upper hand . . . it causes widespread destruction and injury." He concludes by arguing that love in general "exercises a multifarious and great, or, to speak more accurately, an omnipotent sway, but it is the love whose object is good and whose fulfillment is attended by sobriety and virtue . . . that possesses the greatest power, and is the author of all our happiness and makes it possible for us to live in harmony and concord with our fellow creatures." Few modern psychologists would disagree with this conclusion, although they have had great difficulty finding ways of measuring love's multifarious influence.

Another participant in the banquet, Agathon, focuses not so much on how love promotes individual well-being, but on how it affects interpersonal relationships: "Love is in the first place supreme in beauty and goodness himself, and in the second the cause of like qualities in others." It promotes "peace among men . . . it is love who empties us of the spirit of estrangement and fills us with the spirit of kinship; who makes possible such mutual intercourse as this." When it is Socrates' turn, he introduces the theme of sublimation, or the changes in the objects to which love is attached. He claims he was taught the mysteries of love by a woman who explained to him that we "first fall in love with one particular beautiful person and beget noble sentiments and partnership with him." Later we "become a lover of all physical beauty" and then discover that beauty of soul is more valuable than beauty of body. Contemplation of examples of moral beauty leads love eventually to attach itself to love of wisdom, or "many beautiful and magnificent sentiments and ideas," until it arrives at its final goal, the "contemplation of absolute beauty," which is unchanging and eternal.

To sum up, the participants in the *Symposium* conclude that love promotes health in body and mind, that it does so by creating harmony among conflicting elements inside the self, that therefore it can be promoted by music and rhythm, that it evokes good qualities in others and promotes peace and happy relationships among people, that in excess or attached to the wrong objects it can cause great distress, and that it starts out in life by being attached to physical objects but then extends its aims to more abstract goal objects. Many of these same themes have been echoed by personality theorists whose contributions were reviewed in Chapter 2. In the rest of this chapter we will review the extent to which these themes have been found to characterize love as modern psychologists have attempted to measure it. Unfortunately, progress in this area has so far been somewhat disappointing. We know much less about the affiliative motives in the scientific sense than we do about the achievement motive, the power motive, or the avoidance motives. The value of reviewing the themes covered in Plato's *Symposium* on love is that it keeps in front of us what psychologists ought to be investigating as we review what they have been investigating.

• THE SEXUAL MOTIVE

The Biological Basis of Sexuality in Males

As both Freud and Socrates suggest, a useful place to start the study of love is with its physical component—with the contact gratifications that make up the sexual response. Sexual arousal or pleasure in this type of contact depends to a considerable extent on the presence of hormones—androgen in the case of men and estrogen and, to a lesser extent, androgen in the case of women. These hormones play an important part in determining sex differences in anatomy and in responsiveness to various stimuli. Embryos containing the Y, or male sex, chromosome in each cell produce a testis that secretes the male sex hormones, or androgens, which promote the development of the male genitalia and secondary sex characteristics. If androgen is not secreted in the prenatal period, the embryonic gonad turns into an ovary, which releases the female estrogen. There have been cases reported of female embryos that have been accidentally exposed to large amounts of androgen (see Money & Ehrhardt, 1972). Whereas children with this prenatal experience grow up as women and are treated as such, they appear more masculinized in several ways. They act like tomboys, prefer traditional male toys, are more aggressive and competitive in sports, and have a lesser interest in children.

The importance of the chief androgen, testosterone, for sexual activity in the male has long been known. Castration in animals, which removes the testis that produces testosterone, greatly diminishes sexual activity in animals, and injecting testosterone subsequently restores it to its former level (see Grunt & Young, 1952). Furthermore, male primates showing more testosterone in blood plasma are more dominant and have more sexual access to females (see Rose, Holaday, & Bernstein, 1971). Yet there is obviously no simple, automatic connection between hormones and sexual behavior, for the brain is also involved in sexual responsivity, and what an animal is experiencing also influences its actions. For example, Rose et al. (1971) reported a case in which a defeat in the struggle for dominance in a primate hierarchy led to lower levels of testosterone excretion. In this instance an experience led to diminished testosterone production, which led to less competitive behavior.

The brain is clearly involved in the complex mechanism by which the body regulates hormone production and sexual responsivity. The hypothalamus, a portion of the midbrain, or limbic system, releases gonadotrophic hormones, which stimulate the gonads to produce testosterone, which feeds back and influences another part of the hypothalamus to increase sexual responsivity. So what the organism experiences influences the hypothalamus at the outset of the cycle, as well as its responsivity at the end of the cycle, when it is affected by the testosterone released (see Klein, 1982).

The influence of higher mental processes is even greater in humans. For example, Bremer (1959) showed that only one half of a sample of males castrated in adulthood lost sexual interest altogether right away. Others remained sexually active for several years. The amount of sexual experience the males had previously had proportionately delayed loss of interest, which suggests that the sexual motive involves learning based on a natural incentive, as we have argued, so that it continues to influence behavior even after the natural incentive is removed. Androgen production increases at puberty in males, as does sexual interest. Because of its association with sexual interest in such biological phenomena as castration and puberty, androgen has been called the "libido hormone"

(Money & Ehrhardt, 1972). But is there any evidence of stable individual differences in sexual drive, as indicated, perhaps, by the fact that some men regularly produce more androgen?

A number of facts raise this possibility, although they do not conclusively establish it. Klaiber, Broverman, and Kobayashi (1967) have reported that the amount of androgen excreted in urine in young males is significantly correlated with various measures of physical size and strength, such as chest, waist, hip, and right biceps circumferences, as well as with body weight. In other words, males who excrete more androgen are bigger and stronger. They are also better at simple perceptual motor tasks, such as naming objects as fast as possible, displaying what Broverman, Klaiber, Kobayashi, and Vogel (1968) call an *automatization cognitive style*. They are less good at tasks that require delay and inhibition, such as finding figures embedded in a complex design. Broverman et al. (1968) do not report on whether the highly androgynized males are more sexually active, but Eysenck (1973), in another connection, has found evidence that suggests they might be. He found that men and women who score high on his measure of extraversion are more sexually active. Table 9.1 summarizes some typical findings showing that among unmarried German students, extraverts are more sexually active than introverts.

Extraverted males appear likely to be more highly androgynized for two reasons: Many of the items on the extraversion scale are similar to the items on Sheldon's Somatatonia Scale (Sheldon & Stevens, 1942), which Sheldon found to be closely associated with the bigger, stronger, mesomorphic body type characteristic of more androgynized males. In other words, both extraverts and somatatonics love physical adventure, need and enjoy exercise, are energetic and assertive, and so on. Furthermore, Eysenck (1973) has shown that extraverts are characterized by adrenergic dominance, as indicated by the "lemon test." He measured the amount of saliva produced by four drops of lemon placed on the tip of the tongue. The glands that produce saliva are innervated both by ad-

Table 9.1.

SEXUAL PRACTICES OF INTROVERTS AND EXTRAVERTS AMONG UNMARRIED GERMAN STUDENTS (after Eysenck, 1971, after Giese & Schmidt, 1968)

Sexual Practice	Males		Females	
	Introverts	*Extraverts*	*Introverts*	*Extraverts*
Masturbation at present	86%	72%	47%	39%
Petting	57%	78%	62%	76%
Coitus	47%	77%	42%	71%
Median frequency of coitus per month (sexually active students only)	3.0	5.5	3.1	7.5

renergic and cholinergic fibers, which act in opposition to each other. Adrenergic stimulation produces "dry mouth" and cholinergic stimulation, a more copious, watery solution. Drops of lemon produce much less saliva from extraverts than from introverts, indicating that in the former the adrenergic control is stronger.

Broverman, Klaiber, Vogel, and Kobayashi (1974) have summarized evidence indicating that adrenergic dominance goes with the automatization style characteristic of highly androgynized males. There is also a strong connection between androgens and adrenergic dominance. For example, injection of testosterone restores adrenergic dominance. Male sex offenders who have been castrated so that their supply of testosterone is shut off show reduced destructiveness and sexual aggressiveness (Hawke, 1950). But injections of testosterone reinstated their destructive aggressive behavior, indicating increased activity of the sympathetic nervous system and adrenergic dominance. So muscular androgynized males seem likely to have stronger sexual motives, because they share temperamental and hormonal characteristics with extraverts, who are more sexually active.

What is not in question here is whether some males are more sexually active than others: Kinsey, Pomeroy, and Martin (1948) demonstrated that long ago. What needs clarification is the role of the androgens in producing these differences in activity, as well as some method of measuring differences in strength of the sexual *motive* that is better than the count of sexual activities. For here, as in every other area of activity we have studied, action is determined not only by motives, but also by habits or skills and expectations or values. Thus, how often a man has sexual intercourse is an imperfect indicator of the strength of his sexual motive. To take an extreme case, it is worthless as an indicator of the strength of sexual drive among monks who have taken a vow of celibacy. All we can conclude so far is that the amount of androgen excreted might be an approximate indicator of the strength of the natural incentive on which the male sexual motive is built.

The Biological Basis of Female Sexuality

Table 9.1 shows that female extraverts, like male extraverts, tend to be more sexually active, yet we argued in the case of males that this might be linked to adrenergic dominance associated with greater production of androgens. Does this imply that androgens might be a factor in the female sexual response? Yes, it does, for there is even better evidence of such a connection in females. After a hysterectomy and removal of the ovaries, or during menopause, women are often given testosterone, which increases their sexual interest (Foss, 1951). The reason seems to be that testosterone is very much like another androgen women secrete naturally—androstenedione—which is produced by the adrenal gland and which is also closely related to women's sexual responsivity (Klein, 1982). It has been speculated that it is the production of this androgen in low levels more or less continuously that makes the human female sexually responsive throughout the menstrual cycle, whereas among lower animals, females are only responsive when estrogen levels are high.

Women's sexual interest and activity are also controlled somewhat by estrogen and progesterone levels. The frequency of sexual intercourse (Udry & Morris, 1968) and of heterosexual dreams (Baron, 1977) is greater during the period when estrogen is building up, reaching a peak approximately fifteen days after the onset of menstruation, at a time when conception is most likely to occur. The levels of both decrease later in the cycle, when progesterone secretion increases. Furthermore, it has been reported that taking a synthetic form of progesterone for birth control decreases sexual desire (Grant & Meyers, 1967).

Is the Sexual Response a Motive?

Not initially. Male infants start having erections the moment they are born, yet it is not appropriate to speak of them as having a sexual *motive* until considerable learning has taken place that ties certain cues to the pleasurable responses evoked by natural incentives. The pleasure, in this case, appears to be mediated by the sex hormones. Initially, rhythmic contact sensations, as from rubbing the genitals or other parts of the body, release the hormones; in time, however, either naturally or through learning, other types of stimulation produce the same effect. Many cues get attached to these sources of positive effect, so among adults it is easy to demonstrate that the sexual response has all the functional characteristics of a motive: that is, it energizes behavior, sensitizes the person to certain stimuli, and causes learning. Many studies have demonstrated that viewing pornographic movies is arousing to most men and women (Mann, Berkowitz, Sidman, Starr, & West, 1974), as indicated by such direct measures as increased size of the penis in males or increased vaginal pulse pressure in females (Wilson & Lawson, 1976b, 1978). Listening to sexually explicit tapes has the same effect (Heiman, 1975). Furthermore, arousal energizes sexual activity when it can occur. Men who were experimentally aroused by erotic stimuli were more likely to engage in sexual intercourse afterward if they were married (Cattell, Kawash, & DeYoung, 1972) or in masturbation if they were not married (Amoroso, Brown, Pruesse, Ware, & Pilkey, 1971).

Increased sensitivity to various tactile and visual stimuli occurs during arousal of the sexual motive. Masters and Johnson (1966), in their detailed study of human sexual behavior, give many illustrations of how this happens through the foreplay leading up to sexual intercourse, but it has obviously been difficult to document with experimental measures just how and to what extent this happens. Other evidence for the sensitizing effect of the sexual motive can be found in the greatly increased interest both boys and girls show in erotic stimuli at puberty.

The sexual motive also selects out appropriate sexual responses, which is what happens when Masters and Johnson (1966) make use of the sexual urge to help partners become sexually more adequate. Furthermore, in adolescence the sexual motive organizes more effective courting behavior and causes married couples to act in ways that are sexually more satisfying. The popularity of books like *The Joy of Sex* (Comfort, 1974) testifies to the fact that the sexual motive stimulates many people to learn better ways of satisfying it.

Homosexuality

Psychologists and other students of human behavior have long wondered why the sexual motive in some people is attached to someone of the same, rather than the opposite, sex. Socrates thought it was perfectly natural and edifying to both parties for men to start out by making love to boys. Freud, the Christian church, and many others thought such attachments were abnormal or a sign of depravity. At the present time no one knows for sure how or why homosexual attachments occur. Biology might play a role. For example, it has sometimes been argued that some kind of hormonal imbalance, particularly at the prenatal level, is responsible for homosexuality (see Bell, Weinburg, & Hammersmith, 1981), and that less androgynized, more feminine males might be less likely to initiate the behaviors that would result in their attracting women. However, at the present time there is no evidence for hormonal differences between adult homosexual and heterosexual males (Meyer-Bahlburg, 1977).

Learning could also play a role. For example, case studies summarized in Bieber et al. (1962) suggest that homosexual males were more likely to have a strong, dominant mother and a cold or absent father. Thus, they grew up fearing women and seeking the love from males that they failed to get from their father. The most obvious flaw in this argument is that cultures in which mothers are dominant and fathers absent—for example, urban black families—do not produce a greater number of male homosexuals.

Learning clearly may play a role, because it occurs quickly in connection with sexual arousal. For example, Rachman (1966) demonstrated that a formerly neutral stimulus could readily acquire sexually arousing properties if it were associated with an erotic stimulus. He had male subjects view pictures of nude females at the same time they were looking at women's shoes. After a few conditioning trials, the shoes acquired the property of producing sexual arousal. Thus, people of the same or opposite sex could become associated in this way with sexual arousal through learning. No one knows whether in fact this leads to homosexual preference, for most boys engage in homosexual activities first, but grow up to be heterosexual.

Storms (1981) has pulled together a number of findings that support the inference that early puberty, with its accompanying changes in sex hormone production, may be responsible for homosexual attachments in males. From the ages of eight to thirteen, boys play predominantly with boys or form homosocial groups. If the sexual drive happens to mature during this period, Storms argues that according to learning theory there would be more opportunities for it to become attached to boys than after age thirteen, when heterosexual groupings are more common. In support of the hypothesis, he notes that 60 to 80 percent of homosexual males report sexual arousal and activity before the age of thirteen, as compared with 20 to 30 percent of heterosexual males. The fact that homosexuality is less common in women (D. H. Rosen, 1974) supports the thesis, since sexual maturity (as represented by orgasm) occurs more often later in women, and at a time when they are no longer playing primarily with girls.

Whatever the explanation for homosexual preference ultimately turns out to be, the learning must be of a very special kind, which is difficult to reverse. Energetic attempts to decondition or decrease the arousal value of homosexual stimuli have, for the most part, been unsuccessful in shifting homosexuals toward heterosexual intercourse (see Birk, Huddleston, Millers, & Cohler, 1971), although pairing homosexual stimuli with shock decreases preference for them.

• MEASURING THE SEXUAL MOTIVE IN FANTASY

Several studies of the effects on fantasy of arousing the sexual motive have been carried out. They show that sexual arousal has an effect on, but does not influence, fantasy in a simple and direct way. Exposing young men to slides of nude females or to an attractive female folk singer *decreased* overt references to sex in imaginative stories they wrote afterward (Clark, 1955; Kalin, 1972). In contrast, when young men were exposed to the same erotic stimulation in a relaxed drinking party, sexual references in fantasy *increased* markedly, suggesting that sexual thoughts had been aroused but inhibited under normal testing conditions.

Mussen and Scodel (1955) demonstrated that exposure to the nude slides evoked more sexual references when the tester was a "young looking, informal, permissive graduate student" rather than a somewhat stern professorial man in his sixties. However, sexual arousal was shown in several studies to increase indirect or symbolic references to sexual activities under less relaxed testing conditions (see Figure 1.4 and Table 5.2). The complexity of these findings has discouraged investigators from developing out of sexual arousal studies a scoring system for the need for Sex (n Sex) that would measure individual differences in the strength of the sexual motive.

May's Scoring System for Sex Differences in Fantasy Patterns

Robert May (1980), however, has developed a scoring system that may fill this need, although he makes no such claim for it. He started with the observation that men and women characteristically tell very different types of stories to a picture of a male and female couple performing as trapeze artists (McClelland, 1963). Here is a typical male story:

> The picture suggests a dynamic, intimate relationship between the man and woman—hence the light is around their bodies and the rest is dark. This picture is a climax to a period in which they have come to understand each other. Both are completely lost in the thought of their union. They are totally occupied. From such heights they can only go down. (McClelland, 1963)

Note that a period of climactic union (which May called *Enhancement*) is followed by "going down" (which May called *Deprivation*). In contrast, in the women's stories the sequence was more often one of Deprivation followed by Enhancement, as this example shows:

> Mary is learning to do a change between trapezes. She is about to swing to the next and her teacher, old Mr. Picken, is going to become instantly ill, and she is going to catch him from falling by a lucky chance. He will then train her to circus stardom. (McClelland, 1963)

The men's stories rise and fall, and the women's stories fall and rise. To establish a scoring system, May first locates in the story the pivotal incident, "the dramatic turning point in the story" (May, 1980). Words or phrases (units) are scored for Deprivation (D) if they refer to physical tension, physical discomfort, harm or injury, exertion or striving, falling, failure, and other unpleasant feelings or outcomes. Units are scored for Enhancement (E) if they refer to physical satisfaction, accomplishment, rising, flying, success, and other positive outcomes. "The numerical scoring of units is done on the basis of their position before and after the pivotal incident, and is arranged such that a story moving from Deprivation to Enhancement receives a positive score ($+1$) and a story moving from Enhancement to Deprivation receives a negative score (-1)" (May, 1980).

Thus, individuals can get very high positive scores, indicating their stories follow the D-E, or female, sequence more often or very high negative scores indicating their stories usually follow the E-D, or male, sequence. Several studies have confirmed the fact that even in very different samples, men's stories yield an average negative score (indicating a predominant E-D sequence) and women's, an average positive score (indicating a predominant D-E sequence), the differences being highly significant (May, 1980).

Furthermore, this thematic difference in sex role style is not limited to our time or our culture, since it occurs in folklore and mythology in other times and places. The E-D sequence has been called the *Icarus complex* by Henry Murray (1955) after the Greek story of the young man who attempted to fly up to the sun on wings made of feathers stuck in wax, only to fall into the sea as the wax melted from the heat of the sun. The D-E sequence has been called the *Persephone complex* by McClelland (1963) after the ancient Greek myth of the young girl who, while playing with her friends, was seized by Hades, the King of the Underworld, who took her down under and kept her there until her mother, Demeter, forced Zeus to have his brother Hades release her. While Persephone was kept a prisoner below, the earth was barren, but after her return there was great rejoicing. It was springtime, and plants and animals began to thrive again—in a particularly dramatic representation of the theme (see McClelland, 1975).

Ogilvie (1967) found that several elements making up the Icarus theme tend to occur together in the myths of preliterate cultures all around the world. Goleman (1976) showed that fiction in the most popular men's and women's magazines in the United States displayed the themes characteristic of each sex. In the stories for men, the hero is an active, adventuring type who is out searching for some treasure like the Golden Fleece, as in the legend of Jason and

Medea. The hero almost succeeds with the help of a woman, but in the end she often betrays him—just as Medea betrayed Jason in the Greek legend—and the hero fails. In the stories for women, a woman finds her hometown and her boyfriend dull and uninteresting. She is attracted to and carried off by a mysterious stranger, who in fact turns out to be a crook and gets her into all kinds of difficulties. In the end she betrays him, returns home, marries her boyfriend, and lives happily ever after. The stories for men follow the E-D sequence, and those for women, the D-E sequence.

But what reason is there to connect these themes with sexuality? In the first place, May points out that they reflect differences between the sexes in their sexual experience. The fact that a man has testicles and a penis

> . . . gives sexual feelings an external and clearly defined locus . . . sensations experienced in the penis, and its tumescence and detumescence, become the barometer of sexual interest. Because it is visible, accessible, and sensitive the penis rapidly becomes the primary bodily focus of attempts to heighten and then resolve tension. . . . Its outward and mobile quality also makes the penis (and testicles) a vehicle for exhibitionistic pride . . . but this same outwardness makes it vulnerable. Concern about the intactness and functioning of the genitals is a convenient metaphor for a variety of fears about physical intactness. Likewise there is a difficult business about will power and control that gets involved. Pride over the activity of the penis is counterbalanced by the eerie recognition that these movements are not under one's conscious control. . . . Put simply, the male genitals function to embody and delineate the themes of external focus, motion, aggressive extension outward, and prideful control versus shameful failure. (May, 1980)

In contrast, May (1980) argues that the female genitals are not so easily known:

> They do not stand out to be seen. They are more likely to be experienced as part of a vital but ambiguous "inside." . . . The difference in sexual anatomy gives the woman more opportunity and incentive to pay attention to and puzzle about what goes on inside her. . . . Possessing a vagina and womb requires imagining, and experiencing, various transactions across that threshold. Menstruation, intercourse, and child birth are all events in which the boundary is crossed—something goes in or comes out.

Often pains or difficulties can lead to pleasure, as in the experience of bearing a child, so "for women the major themes are of internal focus, taking in, and closing and holding, and the need for a faith that things will come out all right" (May, 1980). Thus, the E-D and D-E themes appear to be based on different experiences connected with sex organs. Erikson (1951) had reached a similar conclusion earlier in his study of sex differences in children's play. He found that boys typically built tall towers and worried about their collapse, or made roadways or tunnels along which little cars could move. Girls built more enclosed spaces with typical family scenes that might be threatened by disruption from the outside. He summed up his findings explicitly: "the spatial tendencies governing these constructions closely parallel the morphology of the sex organs: in the male, *external* organs, *erectable* and *intrusive* in character, serving highly *mobile* sperm cells; *internal* organs in the female, with vestibular *access*, leading to *statically expectant* ova" (Erikson, 1951).

Erikson's findings have been criticized, but they have been confirmed recently in a careful replication of the original study by Cramer and Hogan (1975). Some of these differences may be due to social learning. Fathers may encourage their sons to be more interested in cars, and mothers may encourage their daughters to enjoy household activities. Yet it is difficult to attribute all the differences to social role expectations. As May (1980) puts it, "Are girls encouraged to be interested in entrances and boys in towers?" It is even harder to imagine that their parents or others could have socialized them into thinking in E-D or D-E terms.

Evidence That Deprivation-Enhancement Scores Measure the Sexual Motive

Is there any evidence that D-E scores reflect differences in the strength of the sexual motive in men and women? There is some, but it is not conclusive. The sex differences in fantasy patterns become more distinct as children grow older; they approach a peak at puberty, when the output of the sex hormones increases. Cramer and Hogan (1975) tested children a year apart just as they were entering puberty and found that of the twenty-eight whose D-E patterns shifted during the year, twenty of them shifted more in the direction characteristic of their sex. Furthermore, May (1980) reports that homosexual males scored more in the feminine direction than any other group of males tested. However, he did not find that D-E scores varied in women as a function of the sex hormones released during the menstrual cycle. And McClelland and Watt (1968) report that women who work outside the home show less of the D-E pattern than housewives, although it seems unlikely that the former would have a weaker sex drive than the latter.

Probably the most convincing evidence of the link between the D-E pattern and sexuality is provided by a study that demonstrated that the pattern shifted under the influence of a sexually arousing film (Bramante, 1970). As Table 9.2 shows, the film shifted the males toward the male pattern and the females, toward the female pattern. Thus, if we follow the logic employed in other studies of motivational arousal, we might infer that males who think more strongly in E-D terms under normal testing conditions are thinking the way they do when they are sexually aroused, and therefore they have a stronger sexual motive. The same could be said of women who show a stronger D-E pattern. The case is strengthened by findings from two other studies. Kalin (1972) reports that an attractive female folk singer increased sexual and aggressive themes in fantasy for males under disinhibited conditions, and that themes of negative personal aftermath of sex also increased significantly. In other words, sexual arousal in males produced a theme of enhancement followed by deprivation. And Sara Winter (1969) reported that nursing, which produces a form of sexual arousal in women, was associated with an increase in themes of the D-E female type.

Table 9.2.

EFFECTS OF A SEXUALLY AROUSING FILM ON MALE (E-D, −) AND FEMALE (D-E, +) RELATIONSHIP PATTERNS TO TRAPEZE PICTURE (after May, 1980, after Bramante, 1970)

	Mean D-E Score				
	Males		Females		
Kind of Film	N	Mean	N	Mean	*Difference*
Control comedy film (*C;* Laurel and Hardy)	25	−0.59	25	+0.77	1.36
Romantic, sexually arousing film (*A*)	29	−1.89	31	+1.90	3.79
Difference (*A − C*)		−1.30		+1.13	2.43; $p < .05$

If the D-E pattern measures *n* Sex in men and women, it might be expected to relate somehow to sexual activities. Unfortunately, clear evidence for such a connection does not exist, partly because research has not focused on this point and partly because sexual activities are so much determined by nonmotivational factors such as inhibitions and opportunities. May's (1980) case studies of males or females showing scores that are extreme for their sex do fill out the picture of what such people are like. Men who score high in the male direction tend to be more "macho." They value self-conscious toughness and bravado and admire their fathers as tough and competent. However, they are often uneasy about their manliness and worry about whether they can really perform physically and sexually as required: "They envision men as inherently tougher than women and thus properly the leaders and initiators in relations with women" (May, 1980).

Women high in the female pattern, on the one hand, see their mothers as demanding that they be nice and "ladylike," and they resent the passivity that seems to be required of women. On the other hand, they are less concerned about achievement and more with nurturance, succorance, and endurance. In other words, the two extreme scores are associated with extremes in sex role stereotyping—the active, aggressive male and the receptive, nurturing female—together with some doubts and dislike for the pattern they show.

Furthermore, May (1980) reports that "in both sexes the people with the more extreme and traditional fantasy patterns report that they felt isolated, lonely, and cut off from peers in early adolescence." They felt they had failed to establish good affiliative relationships with others. It is not certain just what this means, but one possibility worth exploring is that their stronger sexual drive either caused them to overaspire for satisfactory love relationships or made forming affiliative relationships more difficult for them. May (1980) summarizes Sullivan's view that ideally in prepuberty, children develop a close relationship with a chum or an intimate friend of the same sex with whom they can feel sympathy and uncomplicated love: "The early adolescent transition is difficult. Lust impels one towards someone *different* from oneself. Thus it disrupts the chumship, and also impels one into situations that are intensely anxiety-provoking and fraught with potential humiliation."

If we speculate that extreme E-D or D-E patterns reflect differences in sexual drive, then the alienation and difficulties that men and women with extreme patterns report are understandable in Sullivan's terms. For if, in their case, lust comes too early or in too great strength, it could well cause awkwardness and anxiety in developing normal affiliative relationships. However, such speculation needs to be carefully checked out by further research. Do androgynized males, for example, show the E-D pattern more strongly on May's measure? And are males with a strong E-D pattern more sexually active when opportunities and values permit? May did not regard his score as a measure of sexual drive, but of differences in sex role style, and the suggestion that it might reflect sexual motivation needs much better confirmation than presently exists.

• THE NEED FOR AFFILIATION

People clearly like interacting with other people, and some like it more than others. The conceptual problem is how to get from the physical rhythmic contact sensations characteristic of sexual pleasure to pleasure in more distant, nonphysical types of interactions. A link has been provided by the work of Condon (1979), who has conducted microanalyses of interpersonal interaction in sound motion pictures, frame by frame. He has demonstrated that motion of various body parts is carefully articulated with the speech patterns of the speaker and with the body movements and speech of the listener: "In essence the listener moves in synchrony with the speaker's speech almost as well as the speaker does . . . as rapidly as within fifty milliseconds the whole organization of change of the body motion of the listener reflects the organization of change in the incoming speech" (Condon, 1979).

These interactional patterns have been observed in film sequences from several different cultures and in newborns: "All of the infants exhibited a marked synchronization of body movement with both tape recorded and live human voices. Interactional synchrony thus begins as early as the first day of life" (Condon, 1979). Clearly, rhythm and harmony are involved, just as Plato argued thousands of years earlier. Condon likens interactional synchrony to a kind of dance in which two persons unconsciously engage. If the dance goes well there is pleasure; if interaction goes badly—if the action and reaction are not in synchrony—there is dissatisfaction and, in extreme cases, pathology such as is found in autistic children. Thus, we may conceive of contact gratifications as a specific subtype of a larger set of rhythmic interpersonal interactions that, if they are present and in harmony, produce pleasure, and if they are absent or not in harmony, produce unhappiness or anxiety.

Methods of Measuring the Need for Affiliation

Whether or not it is exactly what people seek in interacting with others, certainly depriving individuals of the opportunity for interaction arouses in them what has been called the *need for affiliation,* or the need to be *with people.* Shipley and Veroff (1952) studied the effects on fantasy of two types of affiliative arousal. In one case students in a fraternity, seated in a group, rated the attractiveness to them of a number of characteristics, such as *argumentative, entertaining, modest,* and *sincere.* Then each member of the group stood up, and the others recorded which two adjectives from the list best described him. This procedure was designed to make more salient for each subject the extent to which he was liked or disliked by other members in the group. In the second instance, thirty-five freshmen were located who had not been chosen for admission to any fraternity in a college in which 95 percent of the freshmen were admitted to fraternities. Thus, these students had been specifically denied the opportunity for interaction of a type that was strongly valued in this particular college. The stories men in these two groups wrote to pictures were contrasted with stories written under control conditions by subjects who had not undergone the sociometric rating procedure just described and who had been accepted by fraternities. The stories written after a concern for affiliation had been aroused contained many more references to rejection, loneliness, separation, seeking forgiveness, or people's changing their ways to preserve an interpersonal relationship.

Similar shifts in story content were found when the concern for affiliation was aroused by the sociometric rating procedure among another group of students at the University of Michigan (Atkinson, Heyns, & Veroff, 1954). These investigators also found shifts in various subcategories related to the problem-solving sequence taken from the scoring system for *n* Achievement (see Figure 6.6). They defined affiliation imagery as the concern over *establishing, maintaining, or restoring a positive, affective relationship with another person or persons.* They also found increases in the aroused over the control group for such subcategories as instrumental activity, anticipatory goal state, and obstacles in the environment to establishing a positive relationship. The frequency with which people include these categories in stories written under neutral conditions constitutes their *n* Affiliation score. Rosenfeld and Franklin (1966) demonstrated that the same type of arousal increases the frequency of the same categories for women. The French Test of Insight described in Chapter 7 also yields an *n* Affiliation score that is very similar in its correlates to the *n* Affiliation score obtained from stories written to pictures (see French & Chadwick, 1956).

Evidence That the Need for Affiliation Score Measures a Motive

Do people who score high in *n* Affiliation behave in the three distinctive ways that indicate they are more motivated for affiliation? While no studies have demonstrated that *n* Affiliation is associated with physiological arousal, those who score high in it are *energized* to act more often in an affiliative way. The best evidence confirming the point is presented in a study by Constantian (1981) and reviewed in Chapter 13. When students were equipped with electronic pagers and were beeped randomly throughout the day for a week, those high in *n* Affiliation, as contrasted with those low in *n* Affiliation, were found to be more often talking with or writing a letter to someone.

The need for Affiliation also *sensitizes* people to affiliative cues. Atkinson and Walker (1956) presented to subjects some slides of objects so blurred that they could not be recognized. Images were projected in each of four quadrants on the slide, and the task was to state in which quadrant the image was clearest. The fuzzy images were either of faces, neutral objects like lamps, or plates about the size of a face. Subjects high in *n* Affiliation saw the quadrant in which the faces appeared as most clear more often, even though they could not recognize the stimuli. This was particularly true if the affiliation motive had also been aroused by the sociometric judging procedure used in previous studies. For subjects high in *n* Affiliation, visual cues related to affiliation or those present in the human face are more salient.

The *n* Affiliation score also passes the third criterion for determining whether it is measuring a motive. As contrasted with individuals low in *n* Affiliation, those who score high tend to *learn affiliative associations faster.* The task that showed this effect involves learning relationships among people. For example, subjects are told that there are four staff members in a library—A, B, C, and D—and they are to learn the relationships among them. After reading about an event involving the staff, they are asked to mark on an answer sheet which of several simple statements such as "A likes B" and "C dislikes B" is correct. If they mark the right answer with a special crayon, a *T* for "true" appears on the sheet telling them that their response is correct. Otherwise, an *F* for "false" appears. They are given opportunities to show their knowledge by repeatedly choosing among such statements about the people involved on successive trials. Subjects high in *n* Affiliation learn the network of social relationships in such tasks faster than subjects low in *n* Affiliation, as Figure 9.1 shows. For a sample of seventy-four adults, the total number of correct responses made in five trials correlated .20, $p < .05$, with *n* Affiliation; $-.08$ with *n* Achievement; and .08 with *n* Power, the latter two being insignificant correlations. The tendency of people high in *n* Affiliation to learn social networks faster is not strong, but it has been confirmed in a second sample of young adults. This is a further example of the fact that a motive facilitates learning only that material specific to achieving its goal. Neither a high *n* Power nor a high *n* Achievement led to subjects' learning social networks faster.

• CHARACTERISTICS OF PEOPLE WITH A STRONG NEED FOR AFFILIATION

Performing Better When Affiliative Incentives Are Present

Individuals with a strong affiliative motive will also perform better on tasks that do not involve affiliative content if the incentive in the situation is shifted from achievement to affiliation. Normally in a laboratory situation, subjects high in *n* Achievement recall more interrupted tasks than subjects low in *n* Achievement (Atkinson, cited in McClelland, Atkinson, Clark, & Lowell, 1953). However, Atkinson and Raphelson (1956) demonstrated that this is true only if the in-

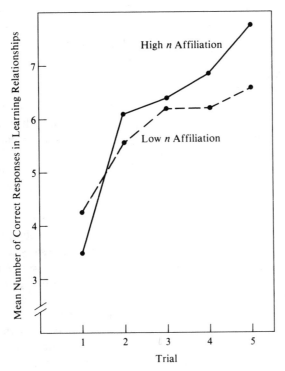

Figure 9.1.

Mean Number of Relationships Correctly Identified on Successive Trials for Subjects High and Low in *n* Affiliation.

structions and approach to the subject suggest the importance of doing well. They deliberately sought to minimize such achievement cues by approaching the subjects in a very relaxed way and simply asking them to help out the experimenters by doing the tasks. In this instance the recall of interrupted tasks was no longer associated with high *n* Achievement, but with high *n* Affiliation. In other words, the subjects for whom the incentive of pleasing the experimenter was more important tended to recall the tasks in which they had failed to please the experimenter by not completing them.

French (1955) reported a very similar result. In presenting a digit-symbol substitution task to a group of officer candidates at a U.S. Air Force base, she varied the incentives for working at the task by giving different instructions to different groups. In general, subjects with high *n* Achievement performed better when the instructions stressed the importance of achievement (see Table 7.1). She also assayed *n* Achievement and *n* Affiliation after the men had finished working on the task and again found that those who scored highest in *n* Achievement had shown the greatest gains in performance previously in two out of the three conditions. However, in the relaxed condition there was no correlation between the postperformance *n* Achievement score and past performance. Instead, there was a strong relationship between the postperformance *n* Affiliation score and having done better at the task previously. She reasoned that this was because, in the relaxed condition, the female experimenter was friendly and asked for cooperation, so those who would have done better in this condition would be those for whom the incentive of cooperating in getting the experimenter's approval would be most likely to be salient. Thus, those in whom affiliation motivation was aroused by the cooperation incentive were the ones who had done better at the task.

The effect on performance of shifting from achievement to affiliation incentives is dramatically shown in Table 9.3. Atkinson and O'Connor (1966) were attempting to confirm once again that subjects high in *n* Achievement and low in Test Anxiety preferred intermediate risks, performed better, and showed less persistence when the odds of success were very small than subjects low in *n* Achievement and high in Test Anxiety. However, the results did not conform to expectations, as Table 9.3 demonstrates. Instead, the subjects high in *n* Affiliation showed the characteristics supposedly associated with high *n* Achievement. They preferred intermediate risks, showed less persistence at a very difficult task, and tended to perform better than subjects low in *n* Affiliation. The researchers reasoned that what had happened was that the way the task to be performed was administered differed from the usual practice. The subjects were all male, and they were tested individually by a female experimenter while she stood by and watched their performance. Thus, an affiliation incentive was introduced in the sense that the subjects would be more likely to want to please her or get her approval than when performing in groups for a male test administrator.

In any case, the results make sense if it is assumed that in this situation, the more difficult the task, the more approval the subjects might expect for performing it. That is, in terms of the Atkinson model presented in Chapter 7, the incentive value of approval equals $1 - P_s$. If this were true for subjects high in *n* Affiliation, multiplying the incentive for approval $(1 - P_s)$ times the probability of success (P_s) would yield the preference for intermediate risk for subjects high in *n* Affiliation—which is exactly what is shown in Table 9.3.

The important theoretical point about such an analysis is that it shows that motives other than the achievement motive not only can lead to faster performance if the incentive is changed, but can also produce other behavioral characteristics like preference for moderate risk, which we have identified as associated with *n* Achievement. We must know not only the motivation of the performers in a situation, but also the incentives for which they are working. Female experimenters seem more likely than male experimenters to introduce affiliation incentives for male subjects. Jopt (cited in Heckhausen, 1980) has also shown that in Germany, a female test administrator produced better performance from male sixteen-year-olds who were high in an aspect of *n* Affiliation than a male test administrator did.

Table 9.3.

RELATIONSHIP OF *n* ACHIEVEMENT AND *n* AFFILIATION TO PERFORMANCE WITH A CLOSELY SUPERVISING FEMALE EXPERIMENTER (after Atkinson & O'Connor, 1966)

Motive	*N*	*Prefer Intermediate Risk*	*Fast Substitution Performance*	*Low Persistence When $P_s = .05$*
n Achievement — Test Anxiety				
High	9	44%	67%	67%
Moderate	19	53%	59%	47%
Low	9	56%	22%	44%
p value		n.s.	n.s.	n.s.
n Affiliation				
High	11	82%	73%	73%
Moderate	12	50%	42%	58%
Low	12	25%	42%	25%
p value		< .05	n.s.	.10 — .05

Gallimore (1981) has reviewed evidence that affiliation incentives are more important to students of Hawaiian ancestry than individualistic achievement incentives are. He has obtained results for this cultural group that are very like those in Table 9.3. Students of Hawaiian ancestry with high *n* Affiliation orient more to teachers, are able to relate to others more effectively, do better at certain types of tasks such as reading achievement, and prefer tasks of intermediate difficulty. In none of these cases is their *n* Achievement score related to these same performance characteristics. All that is needed to explain these results is to assume, as in the case of Table 9.3, that for Hawaiian students the incentive associated with doing more difficult tasks is social approval or affection rather than the achievement incentive.

The way in which affiliation incentives affect the performance of subjects high in *n* Affiliation is dramatically illustrated in Figure 9.2. In this study (McKeachie, 1961), the grades college students received in a course were related to the students' motive scores and characteristics of the teacher's classroom. As the graph shows, students with high *n* Affiliation worked harder and got better grades in a classroom where the instructor was judged to be warm and friendly (taking a personal interest in students, calling them by name, and so forth). Students with high *n* Affiliation, in contrast, did not do as well in classrooms where such affiliation incentives were not present. The fact that students with low *n* Affiliation in less friendly classrooms also did better means only that subjects high in motives other than *n* Affiliation, like *n* Achievement or *n* Power, did better in other types of classroom environments.

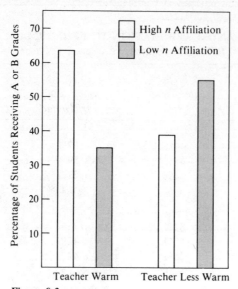

Figure 9.2.

Relationship of Teacher Warmth and *n* Affiliation to Grades in Psychology Class (data from McKeachie, 1961).

Maintaining Interpersonal Networks

Since individuals high in *n* Affiliation learn social relationships more quickly, are more sensitive to faces than to other objects, and engage in more dialogue with others, they might be expected to also show signs of maintaining their connections with other people. This has turned out to be the case. Lansing and Heyns (1959) reported that individuals high in *n* Affiliation make more telephone calls, write more letters, and pay more visits to friends than individuals low in *n* Affiliation. Boyatzis (1972) confirmed, using a slightly different measure of affiliation motivation, that they tend to make more telephone calls. Lundy (1981a) found that high-school students with high *n* Affiliation tended to join more social clubs, although the same relationship does not occur for adults (McClelland, 1975), probably because many voluntary organizations for adults represent special interest groups where the primary incentive is not merely social.

People are very important to individuals high in *n* Affiliation. They prefer friends to experts as working partners (French, 1956), and, when given feedback by the experimenter about how a group is working out, they prefer feedback on how well the group is getting along together rather than on how well they are performing at the task (French, 1958b). In judging welfare clients seen on slides and heard on a tape, they tend to pick more positive adjectives than do subjects low in *n* Affiliation. The correlation between *n* Affiliation and such a positive bias score in adjective descriptions of people in trouble is .22, $N = 134$, $p < .01$ (McClelland & Klemp, 1974).

However, a positive bias toward people is strongly influenced by other factors such as the expectation of success from reaching out to others, as it should be according to the Atkinson model for predicting approach tendencies. Table 9.4 shows the mean percentage of positive acts toward others displayed by women in small groups as a function of their *n* Affiliation score and their expectation that they were in a friendly group (Fishman, 1966). High *n* Affiliation did not lead to more positive acts if a woman thought she was in an unfriendly group that was not likely to reciprocate.

Furthermore, being in a friendly group by itself does not lead to significantly more positive acts, regardless of *n* Affiliation score. If we think of positive sociometric expectancy as equivalent to a high probability of success of an affiliative act, then the Atkinson model applies here, too: the affiliative motive times the probability of success of an affiliative act yields the strongest approach tendency, or the largest proportion of affiliative acts actually emitted.

The importance of other factors can also explain variations in relationships found with the *n* Affiliation score in different samples. For example, Rokeach (1973) reports in a college sample that high *n* Affiliation is associated with a high value placed on *a world at peace* and *true friendship*—both of which suggest the importance to such individuals of positive interpersonal networks. However, in another sample of adults aged thirty-one of a more varied socioeconomic background, these correlations were insignificant (McClelland, Constantian, Pilon, & Stone, 1982). Instead, *n* Affiliation correlated with the value placed on *happiness*. We can only speculate as to the reason for these differences, but it seems possible that the adults, as contrasted to the college students, thought the possibility of *a world at peace* was so low that even those with high *n* Affiliation did not rank it very high in their value scheme. They were reacting

---

Table 9.4.

MEAN PERCENTAGE OF POSITIVE ACTS IN A SMALL GROUP AS A FUNCTION OF *n* AFFILIATION AND POSITIVE SOCIOMETRIC EXPECTANCY, OR PROBABILITY OF AFFILIATION (after Fishman, 1966)

	Female Subjects' n Affiliation		
	Low	*High*	$p_{difference}$
Low positive sociometric expectancy[a]	25.8%	23.4%	
High positive sociometric expectancy	26.1%	36.8%	$< .001$

[a]The extent to which a subject saw others as friendly and thought they liked her; the extent to which they saw her as friendly.

like the subjects in Table 9.4 with high n Affiliation, who did not react positively if they thought they were in an unfriendly environment.

Cooperation, Conformity, and Conflict

Those concerned about other people might be expected to be more cooperative and to conform more to the wishes of others, but the data on this point do not permit clear generalizations. Individuals high in n Affiliation, particularly males, believe that goodwill is more important than reason in solving human problems (McClelland, 1975); women high in n Affiliation responded more to a partner's request to "please slow down" in working on a task together than women low in n Affiliation (Walker & Heyns, 1962), but the same result was not obtained for men.

Attempts to relate n Affiliation to conformity with and without social support or in conflict with the majority have yielded complex results (Hardy, 1957; Samelson, 1958). People high in n Affiliation tend to go along with the opinions of a stranger who disagrees with them so long as the stranger is attractive, but not if the person who disagrees is unattractive (Burdick & Burnes, 1958). Furthermore, both deCharms (1957) and Harris (1969) found that increasing affiliative incentives in the environment increased cooperative performance in a group more for those low in n Affiliation than for those high in n Affiliation. This is reminiscent of Wendt's (1955) finding that pacing work increases performance more for those low in n Achievement than for those high in n Achievement. But what is missing is any clear evidence that individuals high in n Affiliation are generally more cooperative or conforming.

However, many studies demonstrate that they act whenever possible to *avoid conflict.* When subjects were asked to work together to solve a problem, communicating with each other by means of written slips of paper, the participants high in n Affiliation wrote fewer references to potentially disruptive decisions about what the group ought to be doing (Exline, 1962). At a political level, Hermann (1980) found that the n Affiliation score in Russian political leaders' speeches was correlated .47, $p < .05$, with favoring detente with the West: they wanted to avoid confrontation with the West. People high in n Affiliation also want to change people more who disagree with them. Subjects high in n Affiliation made more suggestions for changes to strangers the greater the views of the strangers differed from their own, but the same was not true for those low in n Affiliation (Byrne, 1962).

People high in n Affiliation avoid competitive games such as roulette (see Figure 8.5). When participating in a simulation of international diplomacy, individuals high in n Affiliation tend to be quite passive: they carry out fewer conflicting or cooperative acts, tell fewer lies in newspaper reports, and so on (Terhune, 1968b). The need for Affiliation in males is negatively associated with playing checkers or chess ($r = -.29$; $N = 78$; $p < .05$; McClelland, 1975). Young adults with high n Affiliation avoid joining special interest groups ($r = -.32$; $p < .01$; McClelland, Constantian, Pilon, & Stone, 1982). They also avoid talking about people in negative terms ($r = -.30$; $p < .01$). As would be expected, *n* Affiliation is regularly negatively correlated with *n* Power, which promotes competitiveness. For example, among a sample of 685 mostly older males in business, the correlation is $-.13$, $p < .001$; for a sample of 125 older women, the correlation is $-.32$, $p < .001$.

Managerial Behavior

People who try to avoid conflict and criticism should not make very good managers, and, as findings presented in Chapter 8 have already indicated, men with high *n* Affiliation tend not to succeed in management. They do spend more time with subordinates (Noujaim, 1968), but this may only mean they want to be on good relations with them, which is not always possible for a manager who must make difficult decisions at times. At any rate, young men with high *n* Affiliation tended not to get promoted as often to higher levels of management at AT&T (McClelland & Boyatzis, 1982). Small manufacturing firms or research and development firms headed by men high in *n* Affiliation tended to be less successful (Kock, cited in McClelland & Winter, 1969/1971; Wainer & Rubin, 1969).

The one exception to this general picture is the motivational profile of managerial integrators, among whom Litwin and Siebrecht (1967) found *n* Affiliation scores to be somewhat higher for those judged more rather than less effective. Lawrence and Lorsch (1967) also found that effective integrators had higher *n* Affiliation scores than ineffective integrators. A typical integrative management job is that of the employee relations manager, whose objective is to get management and labor to work together. Obviously, it is functional for a manager in this job to like being with people and to spend time trying to get people to resolve their differences and go along together, both of which are characteristics that would be theoretically expected of a person high in *n* Affiliation. In contrast, more typical management jobs require being competitive, trying to influence others, and making hard decisions that may hurt people's feelings, all of which involve actions difficult for people high in *n* Affiliation to take, since they are primarily interested in avoiding conflict.

In groups that meet to study their own interactions (called *self-analytic groups*), effective helpers had higher *n* Affiliation scores than other participants, which suggests they might make good managers (Kolb & Boyatzis, 1970). *Effective help* was defined as an instance of someone reporting that he or she had tried to help another, who said at the end of the session that the help had been significant. But remember that the goal of such groups is to understand group process, and the behavior of the participants is not aimed at getting work done, as it is in most management jobs. Thus, the skill that those high in *n* Affiliation showed would be more useful in an integrator type of management position. Furthermore, individuals very high in *n* Affiliation were most often classified as nonhelpers—that is, they made no attempt to help other members of the group. It was those with moderate *n* Affiliation who were the most effective helpers.

McClelland (1975) has described the characteristics of a special motivational syndrome in which *n* Affiliation is high but *n* Power is also high and inhibition is low. He calls it the "personal enclave" motivational pattern, because it is characteristic of people in countries like Mexico and Italy, where *n* Power and *n* Affiliation are both high and where paternalistic family firms are also common. Close affiliative ties are maintained within firms, which are often dominated by a single family, and power motivation and competitiveness pit the cohesive unit against outsiders. Men and women with the personal enclave motivational pattern seek strength from inspirational figures, find security in close personal ties, and are unusually aware of threats from the outside. Perhaps managers with this motivational pattern are more successful in countries where high values are placed on affiliation, although no evidence has yet been collected on this point. However, it may be as true in these countries as it is in the United States that high *n* Affiliation leads to making particularistic judgments about people in the firm that are viewed as unfair by others, thus leading to poor morale and less productivity.

Fear of Rejection

Throughout the history of the *n* Affiliation score, investigators have suspected that it represents primarily a fear of rejection (*f* Rejection) for a variety of reasons. As was just noted, individuals high in *n* Affiliation act in various ways to avoid conflict and competition as if they feared negative feedback from others. Furthermore, the methods of arousing the motive in order to develop the scoring system all involved the threat of rejection by peers. The original scoring system focused on rejection and loneliness (Shipley & Veroff, 1952) and was only later expanded to include more positive types of affiliative activities (Atkinson, Heyns, & Veroff, 1954). Subjects who scored high according to the 1954 system were more often judged by their peers to be *approval seeking* and *egotistical,* as well as *self-assertive* and *confident* in contrast to others.

Furthermore, a number of investigators have reported that individuals with high *n* Affiliation are less popular (Atkinson, Heyns, & Veroff, 1954; Crowne & Marlowe, 1964; Shipley & Veroff, 1952). The explanation given for this has been that individuals high in *n* Affiliation are anxious about their relations with others, fear disapproval, and spend time seeking reassurance from others, which makes them unpopular. For example, Mussen and Jones (1957) reported that late-maturing boys, who are anxious about their masculinity, score higher in *n* Affiliation.

Crowne and Marlowe (1964) found that people high in *n* Affiliation tend to score high on a measure of the need for Social Approval, although others have not duplicated this finding (Fishman, 1966; McClelland, Constantian, Pilon, & Stone, 1982). But there is evidence that they are apprehensive about social evaluation. If they are told they are being observed during a performance through a one-way mirror, they are more anxious than individuals with low *n* Affiliation scores (Byrne, 1961a). They also dislike a person more whose views differ from their own (Byrne, 1961b). Presumably they wish to avoid the possibility of coming in contact with someone who disagrees with them. However, if they also have high self-esteem, they are less worried about social contact. Black males high in *n* Affiliation and in self-esteem report less social distance in their relations with whites (Littig & Williams, 1978).

Some theorists, particularly Schachter (1959), have argued that there should be a connection between the motive to affiliate and fear of rejection, because people affiliate in response to threat. He found that threatening female college students with a future shock led them to spend more time with others than alone while they were waiting for the experiment to start. Of course, the tendency to affiliate does not indicate the presence of an affiliative *motive:* spending time talking with others may be simply a means of reducing anxiety. This is discussed further in Chapter 10.

Because of the association of the *n* Affiliation score with fear of rejection, several attempts have been made to get separate scores for approach and avoidance aspects of the affiliative motive (Byrne, McDonald, & Mikawa, 1963; Mehrabian & Ksionzky, 1974). deCharms (1957) simply divided the score into two parts, one of which was the sum of all story categories dealing with positive affiliation themes and the other, the sum of all subcategories for themes dealing with negative, fear-of-rejection themes. The partitioning was logical but not strongly justified by previous research, since arousal studies had shown that both positive and negative themes increased even when the arousal involved primarily fear of rejection (Rosenfeld & Franklin, 1966).

Furthermore, attempts to use these different scores have not produced a particularly meaningful set of findings (Conners, 1961; Fishman, 1966). Laufen (1967) attempted to derive separate scoring systems for the two aspects of the affiliative motive by presenting subjects in advance of the TAT with a questionnaire that focused either on positive or negative affiliative themes (see Heckhausen, 1980). But he found that only the questionnaire dealing with negative affiliative themes (*f* Rejection) succeeded in producing differences that could be scored in the stories written afterward, as compared with what was obtained under control conditions. Boyatzis (1972, 1973) employed a semiprojective technique and an a priori scoring system for distinguishing between *f* Rejection and *n* Affiliation. Subjects were first asked to write a story of the usual type about a person like John mentioned in a brief introductory sentence such as "John has started a new job. He and his family have just moved into a new neighborhood." After writing a story about John, the subjects are presented a number of incidents that might arise in John's life and are asked how they think John would feel about them. For example, "After John received an invitation from Harry and Joanne (some of his new neighbors) for dinner, (a) he was pleased at the opportunity to meet some of his new neighbors (Affiliative Interest), or (b) he wanted his neighbors to like him and hoped that they could become close friends (Rejection Anxiety)."

It was hoped that employing this technique would avoid some of the biases inherent in having the subjects make statements about themselves indicating either affiliative interest or rejection anxiety. Results obtained with this instrument support the notion that these two aspects of affiliation motivation have different correlates. As Table 9.5 shows, in two different studies, those scoring high in Affiliative Interest reported having a larger number of close friends. This was true of both men and women, although in the first study the greater interest in close friends for women was shown only by the measure of the length of time they had spent with their closest friends living away. In contrast, those scoring

Table 9.5.

CORRELATIONS OF AFFILIATIVE INTEREST (AI) AND REJECTION ANXIETY (RA) SCALES WITH REPORTED AFFILIATIVE BEHAVIORS (after Boyatzis, 1972)

Reported Affiliative Behaviors	Males				Females			
	AI		RA		AI		RA	
	Study 1[a] (N = 23)	Study 2 (N = 75)	Study 1 (N = 23)	Study 2 (N = 25)	Study 1 (N = 52)	Study 2 (N = 76)	Study 1 (N = 52)	Study 2 (N = 76)
Number of close friends	.36*	.25**	.17	−.02	.03	.22*	−.05	.01
Length of time seen closest friends living away	.45*	—	.08	—	.37*	—	.13	.17
Attitude similarity to closest friends	−.12	.09	.53***	.25**	−.20	−.03	.25*	.17
Time spent alone	.33*	.13	.08	−.19	.13	−.15	.04	−.21*
Amount enjoy being alone	.16	—	−.04	—	—	.11	—	−.30**

[a]Study 1 included twenty-three males and fifty-two females; Study 2 included seventy-five males and seventy-six females.

*p < .05.

**p < .01.

***p < .001.

high on Rejection Anxiety seemed most concerned about having close friends who had attitudes similar to their own. The inference to be drawn from this fact is that they wanted to be sure their friends agreed with them. Furthermore, they appeared to avoid spending time alone, as if they constantly needed the reassurance of the presence of others. In Constantian's (1981) study discussed in Chapter 13, she found that subjects high in *n* Affiliation, when beeped randomly throughout a week, were significantly less often found to be completely alone.

We will consider further aspects of the fear of rejection in Chapter 10 on the avoidance motives.

• THE INTIMACY MOTIVE

Methods of Measuring the Intimacy Motive

McAdams (1980) decided that a whole new approach was needed to measuring the positive aspects of the affiliative motive, in view of the fact that the *n* Affiliation score seemed to reflect primarily, although not exclusively, the fear of rejection. Returning to the characteristics of love as described by many authors ever since Plato's *Symposium,* he decided that arousal conditions should stress openness, contact, reciprocal dialogue, joy and conviviality, and caring and concern.

He obtained written imaginative stories in four situations that approximated these conditions. In one, new members of a sorority or fraternity in college were being welcomed in a celebration that addressed the goals of togetherness and good feeling for one another. In another, students were obviously having a good time at a dancing party, and those who had not had more than two drinks (to avoid picking up the influence of alcohol) were invited to write stories. In still another condition, undergraduates had just participated in a psychodrama in which they had become acquainted with and interacted with a number of new people under very enjoyable circumstances. Stories written under all these conditions were compared with stories written when the same kinds of individuals were not under the influence of affiliative feelings, as in a classroom setting. Finally, McAdams compared stories written by both members of undergraduate couples who were very much in love (Peplau, Rubin, & Hill, 1976) with stories written by other undergraduates, most of whom were not involved in a relationship.

In searching for scoring categories to characterize the stories written under affiliative arousal, McAdams was much influenced by the writings of Martin Buber (1965, 1970) on the I-Thou relationship, by David Bakan (1966) on the difference between agency and communion, by Maslow (1954) on the distinction between being-love versus deprivation-love, and by Sullivan's (1953) general treatment of interpersonal relationships. McAdams found that the scoring categories listed in Table 9.6 distinguished the stories written under all four arousal conditions from stories written under control conditions. The differences were significant in three out of the four comparisons and in the same direction for the fourth comparison. As can readily be seen, these categories come much closer to the characteristics described by experts in the field from Plato to the present. Note in particular that the categories for scoring for the intimacy motive do not describe aspects of a problem-solving sequence, as did the original *n* Affiliation scoring scheme based on earlier work with *n* Achievement. Instead, the categories reflect more often *states of being,* that is, the *quality* of interactions rather than aspects of getting something done, which is involved in an achievement orientation. This conforms to theoretical expectations, since, as McAdams (1982a)

Table 9.6.

INTIMACY MOTIVATION SCORING CATEGORIES (after McAdams, 1980)

A relationship or *interpersonal encounter produces positive affect* (love, friendship, happiness, peace, or tender behaviors).

Dialogue occurs, as in "swapping stories" or discussing a relationship.

Psychological growth and coping results from an interpersonal encounter.

A character feels a sense of *commitment* and *concern* for another not rooted in guilt or a sense of duty.

Two or more characters are engaged in a *relationship that transcends time and space.*

There is a reference to the *reunion* of people who have been apart.

Characters find they are in *harmony* with each other, "on the same wavelength."

A character *surrenders* to a power beyond the self controlling an interpersonal relationship, as in "they fell helplessly in love."

Characters *escape into intimacy,* to a situation in which they can experience peace, liberation, and so on, together.

There are references to *togetherness with the natural world,* as in "they love the way the air feels against their skins."

---

points out, the active pursuit of intimacy "undermines the striven-for goal state, rendering it less preferable, less intimate. As Buber so eloquently put it, 'The Thou encounters one by grace—it cannot be found by seeking'."

Stories written after intimacy arousal describe people enjoying being together, being committed to each other in a relationship that transcends time and space and in which they show a commitment and concern for each other. Furthermore, they refer to interpersonal harmony just as Eryximachus or Condon (1979) do, as well as to union with each other, with the natural world, or with a power beyond the self. All in all, this scoring system captures the essence of what is meant by love or the positive affiliative motive much better than the *n* Affiliation scoring system does.

Contrast Between the Affiliative and Intimacy Motives

The intimacy motive score obtained by summing the presence of such characteristics in stories written under neutral conditions measures a disposition that differs from *n* Affiliation. The correlation between the *n* Affiliation score and the intimacy motive score is only .32, $p < .05$, as reported in McAdams and Powers (1981).

Table 9.7 compares how people who score high in each motive are rated by their peers (McAdams, 1980). As would be expected, those with a strong intimacy motive are judged to be more *warm, sincere, appreciative,* and *loving* and

Table 9.7.

CORRELATIONS BETWEEN MOTIVE SCORES AND ADJECTIVE RATINGS BY PEERS (after McAdams, 1980)

Adjective	Intimacy Motive	n Affiliation
Natural	.59***	.14
Warm	.54***	.27
Sincere	.50***	.12
Appreciative	.37*	.26
Loving	.34*	.21
Sensitive	.27	.13
Honest	.49***	.21
Calm	.44***	.04
Dominant	−.43**	−.05
Outspoken	−.41**	−.02
Self-centered	−.40**	−.13
Imagination	−.41**	−.25

*$p < .05$.
**$p < .01$.
***$p < .001$.

less *dominant* and *self-centered,* whereas none of these characteristics is as strongly associated with the *n* Affiliation score.

The picture is clarified still further by self-ratings of various characteristics, as shown in Table 9.8. Young adults high both in the intimacy motive and *n* Affiliation regard themselves as more *gentle, natural, loyal, contented,* and *realistic* than subjects low in the motives. In contrast, only subjects high in *n* Affiliation regard themselves more often as *unselfish, cooperative, sociable,* and *thoughtful.* Notice that many of these characteristics involve doing things for others. They imply that such people think they go out of their way to be nice to others. Those who score high in the intimacy motive do not have this opinion of themselves. In fact, as the right section in Table 9.8 shows, they have a rather negative view of themselves as *frivolous, tactless, touchy,* and *cowardly.* The implication is that they have higher standards about their relationships with others and therefore are more likely to regard themselves as having fallen down in their empathy for others' feelings. In contrast, individuals high in *n* Affiliation seem not so sensitive to the feelings of others.

Adjective peer ratings in a later study (McAdams & Powers, 1981) confirm this impression. On the one hand, subjects scoring high in the intimacy motive are considered to be significantly more *nervous,* whereas those high in *n* Affiliation are nearly significantly less nervous. On the other hand, strong intimacy motivation goes with being judged more *sincere, loving,* and *cooperative,* all of

Table 9.8.

CORRELATIONS BETWEEN *n* AFFILIATION AND INTIMACY MOTIVE SCORES AND SELF-DESCRIPTIVE ADJECTIVES CHECKED BY YOUNG ADULTS (*N* = 78)

			Correlations Significant[a] for *n* Affiliation			The Intimacy Motive		
Both Motives								
	r^b	r^c		r^b	r^c		r^b	r^c
Realistic	.39	.40	Unselfish	.31	.05	Self-confident	.11	.27
Contented	.31	.24	Cooperative	.24	.07	Foresighted	.01	.29
Loyal	.30	.22	Patient	.27	.10	Frivolous	−.01	.26
Gentle	.25	.23	Sociable	.37	.12	Tactless	.12	.38
Natural	.23	.27	Stable	.34	.13	Touchy	.11	.28
			Steady	.30	.05	Cowardly	−.03	.27
			Thoughtful	.30	.05			
			Warm	.24	.11			
Positive feelings about self and relationships			Reaching out to others			Sensitive to the feelings of others		

[a]r = .28 at $p < .05$, and $r = .30$ at $p < .01$.

[b]Numbers in this column show correlations with whether adjective is checked and *n* Affiliation score.

[c]Numbers in this column show correlations with whether adjective is checked and intimacy motive score.

which are characteristics less often attributed to those high in *n* Affiliation. In this study the subjects high in *n* Affiliation were considered to be more *enthusiastic* and *expressive* in contrast to those high in the intimacy motive, to whom these characteristics were not attributed. In a study by McAdams and Constantian (1982) it was found that students high in *n* Affiliation who when beeped by a pager were found to be alone more often expressed the wish to be with somebody than subjects low in *n* Affiliation. The same contrast did not appear for those low and high in the intimacy motive. Once again it appears that high *n* Affiliation implies a more active approach to interpersonal relationships, which goes along with the need for contact and reassurance.

Evidence That the Intimacy Score Measures a Motive

Do people who score high in intimacy engage in more energetic intimacy-related actions? Two research assistants observed and coded various behaviors during psychodrama sessions, and most sessions were also videotaped so that other measures could be obtained later from these recordings (McAdams & Powers, 1981). As the findings summarized in Table 9.9 show, students who were higher in either *n* Affiliation or the intimacy motive engaged in more affiliative behaviors. They stood closer to other people, made more "we" references in talking about their scenario, produced more laughter from the group, and issued fewer commands for others to do things. The differences in the effects of the two motives were most apparent in the themes chosen for the scenarios. Participants high as compared with those low in the intimacy motive much more often chose themes of positive interpersonal affect and surrender of control. These and several other indicators in action of the characteristics of the intimacy motive scoring system were summed to get a total intimacy *behavior* index score, which correlated very highly with a person's intimacy score in written stories, but not with the *n* Affiliation score in stories. Perhaps the best indication of the effect of intimacy motivation on behavior involves touching. Even though some of the data were lost due to failure in the videotaping machine, it is apparent that participants with a strong concern for intimacy touched other people more often in an affectionate, nonthreatening way.

To turn to the second type of behavior indicating the presence of a motive, other studies have also confirmed the fact that individuals scoring high in intimacy get involved in deeper relationships with others. Fourth- and sixth-graders with strong friendship motivation (a simplified version of the intimacy motive

Table 9.9.

CORRELATIONS BETWEEN MOTIVE SCORES AND BEHAVIOR IN PSYCHODRAMA SCENARIOS: $N = 43$ (after McAdams & Powers, 1981)

Behavior in Psychodrama Scenarios	Intimacy Motive	n Affiliation
Discrete behaviors		
Physical proximity of protagonist to nearest other	.42**	.35*
Number of "we" references per minute of introductory phase	.39*	.30
Number of outbursts of laughter per minute of scenario	.32*	.31*
Number of commands per minute of introductory phase	−.31*	−.26
Themes of scenarios		
Positive affect	.68***	.33*
Reciprocal dialogue	.55***	.33*
Surrender of control	.45**	.12
Nonthreatening touching[a]	.31†	.08
Total intimacy index	.70***	.27

[a]This theme was judged from videotapes available for only twenty-eight subjects and is not included in the total intimacy index.

†$p < .10$.

*$p < .05$.

**$p < .01$.

***$p < .001$.

score) had more detailed knowledge about their best friend and described the relationship in terms of greater depth than boys and girls low in friendship motivation. Their friendships were also more stable over time (McAdams & Losoff,
1982). When college students were asked to recall in some detail what went on
in a number of friendship episodes, those high in intimacy motivation, as contrasted with those low, more often described a relationship as involving listening
(rather than agentic striving), self-disclosure, and mutual trust (McAdams,
Healey, & Krause, 1982).

McAdams (1979) found that the intimacy motive sensitizes individuals to
people's faces. He exposed subjects to schematic drawings of faces originally employed by Brunswik and Reiter (1938) to show that judgments of personal characteristics changed markedly with variations in the placement of the eyes, nose,
and mouth. McAdams found that subjects high in the intimacy motive showed a
much greater sensitivity to variations in placement of facial features than subjects low in the intimacy motive. Sixty-six percent of the former, as contrasted
with 31 percent of the latter ($p < .01$), varied their adjectival characterizations
of the faces more than the average amount as the configurations changed. This
was true for intimacy-related adjectives like *friendly/hostile* and *sincere/insin-
cere,* but not for adjectives unrelated to intimacy like *intelligent/stupid* or
honest/dishonest.

The result fits well with theories that face-to-face contact is an essential part
of intimate relationships. The quality of face-to-face contact between mothers
and infants is related to the quality of the mother-child attachment a year later
(Blehar, Lieberman, & Ainsworth, 1977). Among adults, the intimacy of a relationship is signaled by face-to-face or eye-to-eye contacts (Argyle & Cook,
1976). Some believe that "eye contact" serves as an innate releasing mechanism
(or natural incentive) for maternal care-giving responses (Brazelton, Koslowski,
& Main, 1974) or for interpersonal intimacy in general (Patterson, 1976). If
this is true, it is not surprising that those high in intimacy motivation are
particularly sensitive to variations in facial cues, even those of schematic
figures.

The intimacy motive also has a *selective effect* on memory. In one study, individuals with a strong intimacy motive recalled more autobiographical incidents
involving intimacy experiences (McAdams, 1982b). In another study, subjects
were asked to listen carefully to stories read to them about each of two pictures,
"because we will return to them later on" (McAdams & McClelland, 1983). The
story to the first picture centered on a group of old college friends enjoying a
twenty-five–year reunion in the woods, and it contained references to friendship,
dialogue, warmth, and interpersonal harmony. The story to the second picture
contained no intimacy themes and dealt with a man who travels from Utah to
Mexico City and eventually comes to own a pizza parlor. The two stories were
approximately equal in length, and each contained thirty-three facts that could
be recalled. After listening to the stories, the subjects engaged in other activities
lasting about one hour and then were asked to recall each of the stories. Intimacy motivation was highly correlated with the number of facts recalled from

the intimacy story ($r = .56$; $p < .001$) but not at all with number of facts recalled from the neutral story ($r = .07$; not significant). The difference between the correlations is highly significant.

In another, similar study, subjects were shown a single picture on a screen and read a lengthy story containing thirty power facts, thirty intimacy facts, and eighteen neutral facts (McAdams & McClelland, 1983). Subjects whose intimacy motive scores were higher than their n Power scores recalled significantly more intimacy facts relative to the power facts they recalled. The reverse was true of subjects higher in n Power. The intimacy motive, like other motives, exerts a selective effect on memory.

Work on the intimacy motive has only recently begun, but two recent studies suggest it may be a very important human characteristic. If the theorizing about love that has been going on for centuries is correct, those who are more capable of love or who love and are loved more should be more mature, healthier, and happier. McAdams (1982a) reports that those scoring higher in intimacy motivation as a measure of the capacity to love and be loved also score as more mature in the Loevinger Sentence Completion Measure of Ego Development (1976) and as having reached a higher stage of commitment in their religious lives.

Furthermore, McAdams and Vaillant (1982) found that the intimacy motive score was significantly related to the lifelong personal adjustment of a group of male college graduates. The psychosocial adjustment of fifty-seven male graduates of a prestigious college was rated when they were about forty-seven years of age. They had originally been tested and interviewed in college, approximately thirty years earlier, and had been recontacted for information every five years since. Thus, it was possible to base the overall rating of adjustment on continuous information over their lifetimes on success in their work (as reflected in income, promotions, and job enjoyment), in nonvocational adjustment (as reflected in regular pastimes and enjoyment of vacations), in marriage (if sustained at least fifteen years with both partners happy), and in avoiding trouble (as reflected in low frequency of psychiatric visits, low number of days of sick leave used, and misuse of alcohol or drugs).

On one of the visits when the men were approximately ten years out of college, they were administered a TAT, which was retrieved and scored for various social motives. Those who scored high on the intimacy motive at age thirty were rated as significantly better adjusted at age forty-seven than those at age forty-seven who had scored low on the motive at age thirty. There was a trend in the same direction for those scoring high versus low on n Achievement at age thirty, but there were no differences approaching significance for those scoring high versus low on n Affiliation or n Power. These findings strongly suggest that the capacity to love, as reflected in the intimacy motive score, enabled these men to live happier, better-adjusted lives in their work, play, and interpersonal relationships. The case for such an inference would have been better if the motive scores had been obtained in college, but as it is they represent a period in the men's lives some seventeen years before the final ratings of adjustment were made, suggesting that the intimacy motive may have helped promote the better adjustment that occurred afterward.

• THE AFFILIATIVE MOTIVES AND HEALTH

Chapter 8 reviewed a number of studies showing that the inhibited power motive syndrome (at least moderate *n* Power that was greater than *n* Affiliation, along with high inhibition) is associated with sympathetic nervous system activation and poor health. For the most part, the opposite result—better health—is associated with the reverse motivational syndrome (*n* Affiliation greater than *n* Power and low inhibition, or the relaxed affiliative syndrome). Some evidence already suggests that the affiliative motives promote better health. In a longitudinal study of blood pressure, the *n* Affiliation score obtained when male college graduates were in their early thirties was significantly *negatively* correlated with diastolic blood pressure twenty years later ($r = -.26$; $p < .05$; McClelland, 1979a). Inspection of Table 8.10 shows that those with the relaxed affiliative syndrome report the lowest average severity of illness score (47.4), which is significantly different from the average severity of illness score for all other subjects (94.2).

Similarly, male prisoners whose *n* Affiliation score was greater than their *n* Power score and who also reported little stress had experienced less severe illnesses than all other subjects (McClelland, Alexander, & Marks, 1982). Figure 8.11 reflects this result in the lower average severity of illness score for all other subjects, for most of whom the *n* Affiliation score was higher than the *n* Power score. Their better health was also reflected in the fact that their immune defense system was in better order: they tended to have higher concentrations of immunoglobulin A in saliva (S-IgA), the body's first line of defense against viral infections, particularly those of the upper respiratory tract.

These same results appeared more clearly in another study (Jemmott, 1982), the results of which are summarized in Figure 9.3. In this case, motive scores were collected from first-year dental students in the summer before they began their academic work. Concentrations of S-IgA and illness reports for the past six weeks were also obtained at different points throughout the year at periods of high and low academic stress. The students were under great pressure in November, April, and June, because they had to pass very exacting examinations in order to continue their work. In general, concentrations of S-IgA declined for all subjects significantly during periods of high academic stress and recovered at the time of a period of low stress in July following the first year. The data for the two most extreme contrasting motivational groups are also included in Figure 9.3. Notice that those with the relaxed affiliative syndrome (higher *n* Affiliation than *n* Power, low inhibition) showed significantly higher concentrations of S-IgA throughout the year, indicating that their immune system was functioning better than those with the inhibited power motive syndrome, who had a lower level of immune defense, which weakened throughout the academic year and failed to recover afterward. As might be expected from this difference, subjects

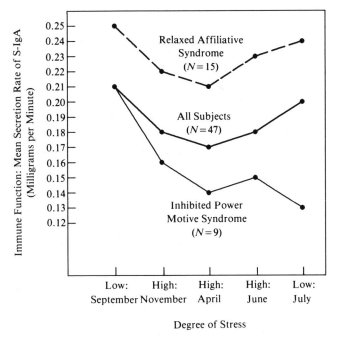

Figure 9.3.

Mean Salivary Immunoglobulin A Secretion Rate During High and Low Stress Periods for All Subjects and for Two Motive Groups (after Jemmott, 1982).

with the relaxed affiliative syndrome reported a lesser increase in the number of colds they experienced in the April-to-June period as compared with those with the inhibited power motive syndrome.

There is other evidence that aroused affiliative states are associated with signs of good health. In a study conducted by McClelland and Kirshnit (1983), subjects' motive scores were obtained on one day (assessment day), along with saliva samples to check on concentrations of S-IgA. A few days later (treatment day), the subjects came to the laboratory in small groups to view films designed to arouse different motivational states. One film, *Triumph of the Axis,* was a documentary showing Hitler's early successes in World War II and his cruel treatment of Jews. It was designed to arouse power motivation and had that effect in imaginative stories written afterward. As Figure 9.4 shows, it did not depress S-IgA concentrations overall. However, it did have that effect for those who were high in the inhibited power motive syndrome to start with.

The other film was a documentary on the life and work of Mother Teresa of Calcutta, a nun who has devoted her life to caring for the poor, the sick, and the dying in the slums of Calcutta. It was designed to arouse the affiliative motives and had that effect in stories written afterward. As Figure 9.4 also shows,

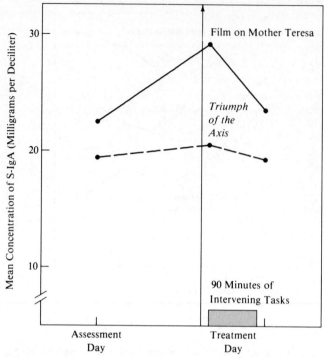

Figure 9.4.

Effects of Two Films on Salivary Immunoglobulin A (after McClelland & Kirshnit, 1982).

it produced a significant increase in S-IgA concentrations immediately, suggesting that Mother Teresa's capacity for loving had evoked a similar response in the viewers, which had a beneficial effect on their body's defense against disease. The finding needs further confirmation and clarification, but it is consistent with the overall picture derived from a number of similar experiments: the affiliative motives, or the capacity to love and be loved, are somehow associated with better health, just as Eryximachus contended over 2000 years ago.

• ORIGINS OF THE AFFILIATIVE MOTIVES

The longitudinal study that discovered child-rearing practices consistently associated with *n* Achievement and *n* Power scores did not succeed in finding any such practices associated with higher adult *n* Affiliation or intimacy motive scores that meet rigorous criteria for cross-validation (McClelland & Pilon, 1983). Only two clues to the origins of these motives turned up. The mother's report when her child was five years old that she used praise more often as a technique of socialization was significantly associated with the adult intimacy motive score. Although the correlation was low ($r = .26$; $p < .05$), it was fairly consistent across subdivisions of the sample (male or female, and middle or lower class), and it is certainly consistent with theoretical expectations that positive encouragement should develop the capacity for loving. In contrast, if the mother reported at the same time that she was unresponsive to a child's crying, this practice was significantly associated with a higher *n* Affiliation score in adulthood ($r = .27$; $p < .05$). This was especially true for individuals from a middle-class background and for girls, although the results were not significant for boys or individuals from a lower-class background. Once again the finding, as far as it goes, is consistent with the belief that high *n* Affiliation is associated with high *f* Rejection, since it might be expected that babies whose mothers refused to go to them when they were suffering would be likely to grow up with a strong unconscious need for reassurance or *f* Rejection. Such an interpretation is also consistent with Youngleson's (1973) report that institutionalized children who receive less mothering than noninstitutionalized children score higher in *n* Affiliation, particularly its negative *f* Rejection aspect.

The fact that findings on the origins of the affiliative motives are so much less definitive than those for *n* Achievement and *n* Power suggests either that later experiences are more important for shaping these motives, or that the Sears' group, which defined the dimensions of child rearing to be investigated, was more "doing" than "being" oriented (Sears, Maccoby, & Levin, 1957). That is, most of the over one hundred dimensions of parent behavior that they rated dealt with something the parent did or failed to do to or for the child. On theoretical grounds we might suppose that it was more the relationship of the parents to the children that would shape the affiliative motives than any particular techniques they employed. Thus, further studies of good parent-child relationships (see Sroufe & Waters, 1977) are needed to get a clearer picture of how the capacity to love develops more in some people than in others.

• RELATIONSHIP OF SEXUALITY TO AFFILIATION AND INTIMACY

There are many reasons for thinking on theoretical grounds that the development of the sexual motive should relate to the development of the affiliative and intimacy motives. The reasons are based on information as diverse as that obtained from case studies of individuals with sexual dysfunctions and those obtained from Harlow's studies of the inabilities to function sexually of monkeys that have been deprived of the early rhythmic, caressing body contact characteristic of normal mother-infant relationships (see Chapter 5). However, empirical studies that confirm these relationships using the methods described in this chapter have not yet been made.

Researchers working with the affiliation and intimacy motive scores have not been interested in examining their relationship to sexual experience or sexual behavior. The closest they have come is the finding in a national sample survey that the reported frequency of a husband's affectionate interaction with his wife (which suggests sexual activity) is not related to his *n* Affiliation score (Veroff, Depner, Kulka, & Douvan, 1980). Nor is a mother's treatment of childhood sexuality related to adult *n* Affiliation or intimacy scores (McClelland & Pilon, 1983), although punishment for masturbation and sex play might be expected to inhibit the development of the intimacy motive. Perhaps the sexual motive is quite independent of the other two despite their supposed theoretical relationship. However, these findings are by no means definitive. They only call attention more sharply to the fact that more work needs to be done on the origins, development, and interrelationship of the sexual and affiliative motives.

NOTES AND QUERIES

1. Freud felt that the libido (or sex drive) underwent various stages in its development, which could be characterized by attachments at the oral, anal, phallic, and genital levels. In Chapter 8 we reviewed the Stewart system for coding the extent to which adults are oriented around one or another of these stages. This chapter suggests that testosterone might indicate the extent of sexual motive arousal in males. Would it be a reasonable test of Freud's theory, then, to examine the amount of testosterone produced in males in response to cues characteristic of the stage toward which they are most strongly oriented, according to the Stewart coding system? For example, would you expect that Stage I–oriented males would be more "turned on," as measured in this way, by power-oriented reading than, say, Stage II males? Or would such a difference appear only for more sexually explicit stimuli, showing, for example, that Stage I males are more turned on by oral sex than Stage II males? What would it mean if there were no differences in testosterone produced by various cues in adults oriented toward one stage or another? Would Freud's theory have been disproved?

2. What does it mean that boys who are late in reaching sexual maturity have a higher *n* Affiliation? Does it establish a connection between sexuality and love, or not? It could mean only that late-maturing boys feel left out and concerned about establishing interpersonal relationships. May also reports that young men with a strong E-D pattern also feel left out. How might these facts be connected?

3. Most people can report when they feel they have gotten along well with somebody. They may say there were "good vibes" in the relationship, meaning much the same as Condon does when he observes harmonious reciprocal voice and movement interactions. Harlow's work with real and substitute mothers discussed in Chapter 5 shows that the ability to establish such harmonious relationships in adulthood depends on good mother-infant interac-

tions. If the affiliative or intimacy motives are built on the pleasure from harmonious interactions, would it not mean that there should be a correlation between good mother-child interaction—as measured by Sroufe and Waters (1977), for example—and adult *n* Affiliation or intimacy motive scores? Speculate on what aspect of the mother-child interaction would be more likely to lead to strengthening the affiliative versus the intimacy motive.

4. Why do you think it has been difficult to get consistent results showing that *n* Affiliation is related to cooperation or conformity behavior? What other factors should influence whether such behavior occurs? Try to design an experiment taking these other factors into account that would show that *n* Affiliation is related to cooperation and conformity.

5. If moderate risk taking characterizes people high in *n* Affiliation under certain conditions, as reported in this chapter, how can it be concluded, as suggested in Chapter 7, that moderate risk taking characterizes people high in *n* Achievement? Does this suggest a reason why types of behavior are seldom good indicators of the motives behind them? Or can you think of behaviors that might pretty uniquely indicate the presence of a motive like the achievement or affiliative motives?

6. If appeal to different types of incentives can produce more approach behavior from people strong in different motives, does it follow that teachers, for instance, can produce better performance from all their students simply by employing a wide variety of incentives? Or does an appeal to one type of incentive facilitate performance for people with one type of motive and inhibit it for others? Review McKeachie's (1961) work mentioned in this and the previous chapter.

7. Chapter 8 stressed the fact that motives show alternative manifestations. Apply this concept to the affiliative motive. For example, a person strong in *n* Affiliation might have many friends, spend a good deal of time with a few friends, or telephone or write letters often. If these were genuine alternative expressions of *n* Affiliation, how would we get a composite measure that would demonstrate this fact?

8. This chapter and the previous one have asserted that managers high in *n* Affiliation would respond more to individual needs and have a harder time sticking to universalistic rules, but this hypothesis has never been empirically tested. Design an experiment that would test it.

9. Explain the fact reported by McAdams and Constantian (1982) that subjects high in *n* Affiliation but not in intimacy motivation more often expressed a wish to be with somebody when they were alone.

10. In examining the reports students gave of what they were thinking and doing when they were paged at random intervals during a week, it was found that women reported having interpersonal thoughts nearly twice as often as men, yet the two sexes did not differ in average levels of intimacy

motivation and *n* Affiliation (McAdams & Constantian, 1982). What could this mean? Which would be the better measure of motive strength—the TAT or the pager reports? What other variables might influence either measure?

11. Meditation has been associated with relaxation (see Benson, 1975) and with an increase in *n* Affiliation (see Alexander, 1982). Would you expect meditation to be connected with an improvement in health? Look for evidence to back up your conclusion.

12. If love and loving are associated with health, would you expect loving couples to be sick less often? How would you test such an hypothesis?

13. An undergraduate once carried out a study in which he found that brown-eyed college males were more sexually aroused (that is, told stories with more sexual content) by a picture of a beautiful blue-eyed woman than by a picture of an equally beautiful brown-eyed woman, and vice versa: blue-eyed males were more aroused by the picture of a brown-eyed woman. If this finding were confirmed, how would you explain it? Does it have any implications for the view that eyes have a special significance in arousing the affiliative motives?

14. Chapters 4 and 5 argued that motives are based on positive and negative emotions of various types. McAdams and Constantian (1982) found that subjects with a strong intimacy motive reported more positive affect when interacting with someone than subjects with a weak intimacy motive. No difference in affect was reported between the two motive groups in noninteracting situations. Does this confirm the hypothesized relationship between motive and affect, or could the relationship found be explained in some other way?

15. In commenting on Wilsnack's study of the effects of drinking on women's thought content, Wilson and Lawson (1976b) state: "However, it is unclear what the sexual content of these dubious projective tests means without validating the tests against appropriate objective measures." In what sense is thought content "dubious"? Their proposed appropriate objective measure of sexual arousal is a vaginal photoplethysmograph, which, when inserted, measures vaginal pulse pressure and blood volume. What if the two measures of sexual arousal do not agree? Can it be assumed that the physiological measure is always a better measure against which the thought measure must be validated? Think of what can happen during rape, for example.

10

The Avoidance Motives

For historical reasons, as explained in Chapter 3, academic psychologists first conceived of motives as efforts to avoid discomfort and to reduce strong stimulation, whether caused by hunger, thirst, pain, electric shock, conflict, or frustration. They found it easy to observe the effects of such strong stimulation on their favorite subjects—namely, animals in the laboratory—and they believed that psychoanalysts working with patients had confirmed their view that anxiety reduction was a kind of master motive. From this point of view it did not make much sense to think in terms of different kinds of avoidance motives: Individuals simply learned different ways of reducing their anxiety, and these might be as varied as the number of people studied. Thus, one person might reduce his or her anxiety by chewing gum, another by jogging, and a third by going to the movies.

It did not make sense to try to define and measure a gum-chewing motive, a jogging motive, or a movie-going motive, so not much attention has been given to sophisticated measurement in this area such as has characterized the work on measuring n Achievement or n Power. In the beginning, scholars were satisfied with simple reports by individuals as to how anxious they felt. Evidence of the existence of other types of more specific avoidance motives began to crop up in the study of approach motives, as noted in the past three chapters. All of this work will be reviewed, but it does not as yet add up to a very clear or coherent picture of what the avoidance motives are and how they should be measured.

• GENERALIZED ANXIETY AS A MOTIVE

Self-report Measures and Their Correlates in Behavior

Many questionnaires have been developed that measure the extent to which people say they feel nervous, anxious, or worried. They include items like "Do you consider yourself rather a nervous person?" or "Do you worry over possible misfortunes?" or "Do you get nervous in places such as lifts, trains, or tunnels?" These items are from Eysenck's Measure of Neuroticism (1957a), an instrument widely used in Great Britain. In the United States the Taylor Scale of Manifest Anxiety (1953) has been the instrument of choice, as noted in Chapter 3. It asks the subject to respond to items like "Every few nights I have anxiety dreams" or "I am easily upset."

Spielberger, Gorsuch, and Lushene (1970) simplified the measure even further by asking subjects to indicate the extent to which they felt nervous, irritable, or anxious versus calm and relaxed. By rating adjective descriptions of such characteristics they indicated how they generally felt—which Spielberger called a measure of *trait anxiety*—or how they felt at the particular moment—which he called a measure of *state anxiety*. He reasons that "anxiety as a personality trait (A-trait) would seem to imply a motive or acquired behavioral disposition that predisposes an individual to perceive a wide range of objectively nondangerous circumstances as threatening, and to respond to these with A-state reactions disproportionate in intensity to the magnitude of the objective danger" (Spielberger, 1966). The distinction is the same as the one made in Chapter 6 between a motive disposition, considered to be a relatively stable aspect of personality, as compared with aroused motivation, a temporary aspect of personality (Zuckerman, 1976). All these instruments, as well as several others, measure the same disposition—the willingness of the person to admit to anxiety in its various forms. They have the same behavioral correlates and correlate highly with each other (see Feij, 1975; Shiomi, 1978). Those who score high on one tend also to score high on the others.

There is also a substantial body of knowledge showing that individuals who score high in Manifest Anxiety display the characteristics that are an essential feature of being more motivated. They are more activated or energized. Particularly when stressed, they show various signs of greater autonomic activity such as pupillary dilation, increased heart rate, increased sweating as picked up in the galvanic skin response, faster breathing, more oxygen uptake, and so on (Eysenck, 1947). However, self-reports of anxiety and physiological signs of anxiety are by no means perfectly correlated. Some people who show all the physiological signs of anxiety do not admit to feeling anxious or nervous (see, for example, Salter, Meunier, & Triplett, 1976). So once again we run into the problem of response bias characteristic of all self-reports of motivation.

More anxious than nonanxious people also show the selective sensitivity characteristic of greater motivation. They report stimulation increasing in intensity to be painful sooner than subjects low in anxiety do (Shiomi, 1978), and they do not see as well in the dark (Eysenck, 1947).

Finally, they display the third essential feature of being more motivated: They learn some types of material faster under certain conditions than people low in anxiety. (See, for example, Figure 3.7.) In general, anxious people are better at learning easy material and poorer at learning more difficult material (see Weitzner, 1965). The explanation of this fact in terms of Hullian theory was that drive (in this case represented by a score on the Manifest Anxiety Scale) was kind of a blind, nondirective force that served to activate whatever responses were already strongest in the situation. If the strongest response happened to favor learning, as in simple tasks, higher drive would facilitate learning, but if the naturally stronger responses were incompatible with doing the task, higher drive would interfere with learning.

However, there were several crucial objections to such an interpretation. To begin with, Eysenck (1957a) reported that increasing another irrelevant drive (namely, hunger) during conditioning did not facilitate acquiring the eyelid response the way higher anxiety did. How could this be true if *any* increase in drive blindly activated the strongest natural response in the situation, which had been demonstrated by the anxiety research to be the eye blink? Also, as Chapter 3 pointed out, Weiner (1966) demonstrated that the reason more anxious subjects did more poorly on difficult tasks was because they failed more often on them.

This led to a new and much simpler interpretation of the learning results. Anxiety is not a blind force, but a directive one. In comparison to nonanxious individuals, more anxious individuals will learn more quickly to do whatever will reduce their anxiety. In the conditioned eye blink experiment, an air puff to

the eyeball is unpleasant, and more anxious subjects learn more quickly to anticipate the puff and to blink their eyes in order to avoid the unpleasantness (Taylor, 1951). In simple learning tasks, more anxious subjects experience much success and continue to learn more quickly in order to reduce the anxiety that
would come from failure. In more difficult tasks, they experience more failure and
respond by trying to avoid doing the task that results in poorer performance.

If the goal of the anxiety motive is some kind of escape, measurement in
this area is deficient, because it concentrates on the anxiety responses rather
than on what relieves them. A motive is better defined in terms of its objective,
or the incentive that it seeks or that would satisfy it. There is some evidence
that what more anxious people seek is some kind of security, or the reassurance
that comes from being told what to do or knowing what to do. For example, if
they are talking to someone who nods or says "Mhm-hm" every time they say a
plural noun, they begin quite unconsciously to say more plural nouns (Doherty
& Walker, 1966). Or if they are standing still with their eyes closed and the experimenter suggests strongly that they are swaying forward, they are more likely
to sway further in response to the suggestion than subjects low in anxiety
(Eysenck, 1947).

The Incentive Value of Being with Others as a Means of Reducing Anxiety

Schachter (1959) carried out a series of experiments that illustrates dramatically
the incentive value of being with others for anxious people. He aroused state
anxiety by having a number of female college students participate in an experiment concerned with the effects of electric shock. In one condition the women
were told by a very formal, authoritative experimenter in a white coat that the
shocks would really hurt but would do no permanent damage. In the other condition the women were told by an informal experimenter that the shocks would
be very mild and would only tickle or tingle. In both conditions the subjects
were then told that they had to wait awhile before the experiment began and
they could either wait in separate rooms alone or with others.

Schachter found that those threatened with severe shock were much more
likely to choose to spend the waiting time with others than those who expected
only a mild shock. In other words, anxiety increased the incentive value of being
with others. He also tried in a variety of ways to find out exactly what was reassuring about being with others and concluded that the subjects wanted to be
with others to talk over the situation and reduce their anxiety and uncertainty
as to how they should react. He did not include a trait measure of anxiety, but
presumably if he had, those higher in trait anxiety would have wanted even
more to be with others. He did, however, locate an indicator of individual differences in anxiety levels. Firstborn or only children chose more often to be
with someone than others did. He reasoned that firstborn or only children are
under more pressure from their parents, tend to be more anxious, and tend to
have been more often and more quickly rewarded by the presence of another
when they cried. For when there are more children in the family, the mother
cannot as readily respond to a child's trouble by going to him or her immediate-

ly. All the evidence points to some kind of need for security, reassurance, or reduction of uncertainty as being characteristic of people with high anxiety levels.

Measuring the Need for Security in Fantasy

Since self-report measures of motives are generally weak, and since the measure of the anxiety motive is particularly weak because it does not mention its incentive, it would seem desirable to develop better measures using the more sophisticated methods of measurement outlined in Chapter 6 and used in other areas. Two such attempts have been made, although neither has been developed very far. As has been described, Walker and Atkinson (1958) had soldiers write stories to pictures under different levels of aroused anxiety created by their nearness to the explosion of an atomic bomb. In the control condition men wrote stories at a remote desert camp before they knew they were to participate in atomic maneuvers. Another group wrote stories at the camp after they had been briefed fully on the fact that an atomic explosion was to take place in ten hours' time. The third group wrote stories just after the bomb had gone off, while the atomic cloud was boiling up directly overhead and while they were in a state of "acute alertness for the wail of a siren" that would announce the declaration of an emergency, meaning that everyone had to leave as soon as possible. Other men wrote stories at times farther removed from the explosion.

A scoring system for the stories was developed based on previous work with the *n* Achievement score. The researchers first identified whether a story was fear or anxiety related in any way, as indicated by the presence of *threat imagery,* which was scored when there was mention of threat of bombing, physical harm, or attack, as well as the emotional response of fear. Table 10.1 illustrates some of the scoring categories they developed to cover various aspects of the anxiety-reduction action sequence. Note that the measure in this case is oriented around relief of fear—wanting to remove threat, doing something to remove it, overcoming obstacles to avoid threat, or experiencing relief from threat. In this sense it is a more adequate measure than the Manifest Anxiety Scale, which focuses exclusively on the threat or anxiety itself.

Furthermore, an overall need for Security (*n* Security) score obtained by summing these characteristics showed validity, as Figure 10.1 illustrates, for it increased in strength as the bomb threat became more salient and decreased as it receded in time.

In addition, this measure should not be subject to the response biases involved in self-reports of anxiety. For example, Epstein (1962) has shown that reports of anxiety vary considerably with the experience of a potentially threatening event like sport parachute jumping. The experienced jumpers report less and less anxiety but do not show a correspondingly regular decrease in physiological signs of anxiety. In other words, their bodies continue to show signs of anxiety, although subjectively they report very little anxiety. Despite the promise of the Walker and Atkinson measure, it has been used only in the one study.

Table 10.1.

SAMPLE SUBCATEGORIES SCORED ONLY IF THE STORY CONTAINS THREAT IMAGERY
(after Walker & Atkinson, 1958)

Category	Brief Definition	Example
Need (N)	Someone wants something that, if attained, would remove the threat of physical harm.	"They want shelter from the bomb."
Instrumental Activity (I)	Someone performs or thinks of performing an act, the function of which is to reduce the threat of physical harm. If the outcome of the act is successful, score I+; if unsuccessful, score I−; and if doubtful, score I?	"They are running away from the fire."
Nurturant Press (NuP)	Forces from the environment provide relief.	"First aid will be given."

The Effect on Behavior of Maslow's Needs for Safety and Self-esteem

A somewhat more widely used measure of *n* Security was developed by Aronoff (1967). He employed a sentence completion test to measure Maslow's hierarchy of needs (see Chapter 2), for he was convinced that two groups of people he was studying on the island of Saint Kitts in the British West Indies differed in the extent to which their basic needs had been satisfied. Maslow's theory argues that basic needs for food, drink, safety, security must be satisfied before higher order needs for love and self-esteem can become salient.

Aronoff observed that most of the men on the island cut sugar cane for a living, and very few become fishermen, despite the fact that there is an excellent market for fish and those who fish make a better living. He thought an explanation for this fact might be that *n* Security on the island was great and was best satisfied by cutting cane rather than by fishing. Certainly working in a cane-cutting gang provides more security than fishing. The men work down the rows in a field like a wedge driven in deeper at one end. They work at a pace set by the head cutter and cannot get ahead or behind the person on either side of them. They need not assume responsibilities for their efforts. They are paid for what the whole group accomplishes, so if they are tired or ill, they will benefit nevertheless from what the other men have cut that day. Furthermore, they get a lot of individual support from each other, as they continually talk and make jokes as they work. There is "little room for individual achievement. It is impossible for a person to decide, by himself, that on a given day or week he will cut more cane, because the pattern of cutting arranges and regulates the speed at which each man works. . . . Even if an individual cutter could cut more on a

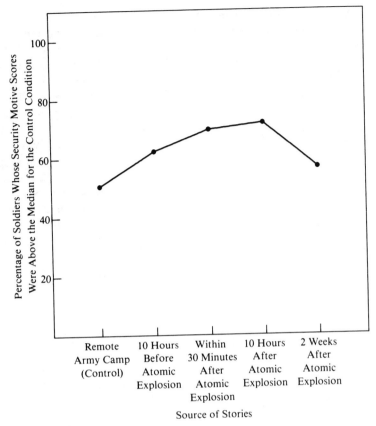

Figure 10.1.

Percentage of Soldiers Scoring High in *n* Security Before, During, and After Exposure to an Atomic Explosion (Form B Results) (after Walker & Atkinson, 1958).

given day, the system of payment is such that he could not benefit exclusively, but would only be augmenting the income of his slower followers" (Aronoff, 1967).

In contrast, the fisherman's income is totally dependent on how much effort he puts out. He must decide how often he goes out, where he fishes, how much he wants to invest in traps, and so on. Aronoff reasoned that men would engage in such activity only if their basic security needs had been met so that, in Maslow's terms, they were now free to pursue needs higher up on the hierarchy, such as the need for greater personal self-esteem. The Sentence Completion Test Aronoff used to examine whether this line of reasoning was correct included cues like "Money is . . ." or "A wife . . ." or "I am sad because I . . ." Safety or security needs were scored whenever the subject mentioned reliance on external authority, the need for care, reciprocity, or safety gratification. Examples of completions in this category are "A wife . . . take care of me" or "A friend . . .

if I need anything he does help me." Completions scored for self-esteem include such statements as the following: "I am good at . . . one and everything" or "I want . . . to live for some purpose before time has expired" or "A wife . . . is the second in the home." Such an interest in who or what is better or worse is very reminiscent of what is scored for *n* Achievement.

Aronoff's results, as summarized in Figure 10.2, confirm his expectations. A much higher proportion of the cane cutters showed a high need for Safety (*n* Safety) or *n* Security than the fishermen, who scored higher in Self-esteem. Furthermore, he found some evidence that might explain why the cane cutters had a greater *n* Security. He recorded the number of men in each occupational group who had experienced the death of a parent by the age of twelve, the death of a large number of siblings in the family while they were young, or both. He reasoned that those who had experienced a higher number of deaths in their family while they were young would be likely to have a stronger *n* Safety. As expected, more cane cutters than fishermen had experienced a severe loss of close family members in childhood.

Aronoff's measure has been used in other studies as well. For example,

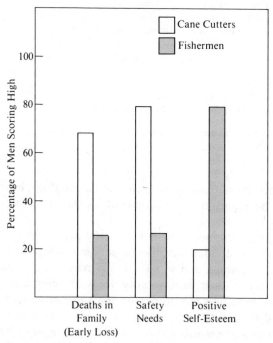

Figure 10.2.

Percentages of Cane Cutters and Fishermen Scoring High in Early Loss, Safety Needs, and Self-esteem (after Aronoff, 1967).

Ward and Wilson (1980) presented to women undergraduates a moral dilemma as if it were a legal case for discussion. The subjects were instructed to read a case and to try to reach a verdict about what to do as if they were members of a jury. They then wrote a two-page essay summarizing the reasons for their particular verdict. Their reasoning could then be coded according to the level of its moral maturity using criteria established by Kohlberg (1969).

Some of the subjects carried through this procedure alone. Others were subjected to group pressure in the following way: After reading the case and stating their opinion, they discussed it with two other women who were confederates of the experimenter and who had been instructed to use the arguments and rationale characteristic of a lower stage of moral reasoning. Thus, each subject was exposed for twenty minutes to strong expressions of opinion and arguments designed to lower the level of their moral reasoning. Then they wrote their final essay giving the reasons for their verdict, just as the subjects did who had gone through the whole process alone.

The subjects had taken the sentence completion test, so their safety and self-esteem needs could be assessed, as in the previous study. As Figure 10.3 makes clear, the women's safety and self-esteem needs interact with group pressure in different ways. Those who score high in *n* Safety lower their level of moral reasoning in response to group pressure, whereas those high in Self-esteem do not. It is clear that those motivated by high *n* Security rely more on others for support and guidance in what they do, just as those who score high on general anxiety scales do.

• FEAR OF FAILURE

Self-report Measures and Their Correlates in Behavior

Much more attention has been given in the motivation literature to a more specific type of anxiety—namely, people's anxiety over whether they are performing well. In his general analysis of motivational determinants of risk taking, Atkinson (1957) conceived of an incentive to avoid failure as the mirror image of the incentive to approach and achieve. So his formula for the motivation to avoid failure paralleled the formula for the motivation to achieve. That is, he conceived of the tendency to avoid failure as a product of the motive to avoid failure times the probability of failure times the negative incentive value of failure, which was conceived to grow larger in direct proportion to how easy the task was at which the person failed. That is, people should be much more unhappy if they failed at easy tasks than at difficult tasks. So the negative incentive value of failing at an easy task should be much greater than for failing at a hard task.

The way the formula works is illustrated in Table 10.2, which is constructed to parallel exactly Table 7.2, which shows how the approach aspect of the achievement motive operates. Notice that for a hard task, where the probability of failure is high, the negative incentive value is relatively slight, so the product

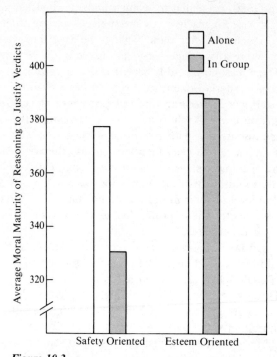

Figure 10.3.

Average Moral Maturity of Reasoning Among Safety- and Esteem-oriented Women When Alone and When Subjected to Group Pressure (data from Ward & Wilson, 1980).

of the variables indicates only a slight avoidance tendency. The two variables have opposite values for an easy task, again yielding a slight avoidance tendency. However, maximum avoidance should occur for tasks of moderate difficulty, just as they should yield the maximum approach tendency for those attracted by the incentive value of success in the parallel case.

To check the applicability of his model, Atkinson needed some way of measuring Fear of Failure (*f* Failure). For this purpose he employed the Test Anxiety Questionnaire developed by Sarason and Mandler (1952). It was made up of forty-two items like the following: "Before taking an individual intelligence test, to what extent are you (or would you be) aware of an 'uneasy feeling'?" or "When you are taking a course examination, to what extent do you feel that your emotional reactions interfere with or lower your performance?" Scores on this test correlate moderately highly with scores on the Taylor Manifest Anxiety Scale ($r = .53$; Raphelson, 1957) and indicate more specifically how fearful the person is about performing in test situations. Atkinson decided that the purest index of *f* Failure would be a high Test Anxiety score and low *n* Achievement, indicating no approach tendencies toward performance. In contrast, the purest

Table 10.2.

AROUSED MOTIVATION TO AVOID FAILURE AS A JOINT FUNCTION OF MOTIVATION (M_{af}), EXPECTANCY (P_f), AND INCENTIVE (I_f OR $-P_s$) (after Atkinson, 1957)

	M_{af}	$\times$	P_f	$\times$	I_f (or $-P_s$)	$=$	*Avoidance*
Task A (hard)	1	$\times$	.90	$\times$	$-.10$	$=$	$-.09$
Task B	1	$\times$	.50	$\times$	$-.50$	$=$	$-.25$
Task C (easy)	1	$\times$	.10	$\times$	$-.90$	$=$	$-.09$

index of an approach- or success-oriented achievement motive would be a high *n* Achievement score and a low Test Anxiety score. So he and many others working in this tradition have regularly classified subjects into four groups, depending on whether they scored high or low on each of these measures.

Our attention in this chapter will be focused primarily on those considered high in *f* Failure because they score high in Test Anxiety and low in *n* Achievement. As one would expect if the measure were adequate, such subjects showed signs of greater physiological arousal when they were performing a difficult eye-hand coordination task than subjects performing the same tasks who were high in *n* Achievement and low in Test Anxiety. That is, the more anxious subjects perspired more during the task, as shown by decreased resistance of the skin to the passage of an electrical current (Raphelson, 1957).

A key question is whether subjects considered high in *f* Failure as measured this way will avoid moderately difficult tasks most, as they ought to according to the Atkinson model. To put it the other way around, would they be most attracted to very easy or very difficult tasks? Obviously, according to Table 10.2, they should avoid all tasks somewhat, but it was further assumed that they would often have to choose among possibilities for extrinsic reasons, and in that case their lesser avoidance of extremes in probability of failure should show up as a positive preference for those extremes.

Several studies supported this expectation. Consider, for example, the evidence summarized in Table 10.3 that subjects high in *f* Failure were much more unrealistic than those low in *f* Failure in choosing the occupations they wished to enter. College students were asked to estimate their own ability, as well as the ability they thought was needed for various occupations (Mahone, 1960). When their own occupational choices were examined, it was discovered that those high in *f* Failure much more often had estimated the ability needed for the occupation to be much higher than their own ability. In terms of the model in Table 10.2, they were expressing a preference for an occupation in which, in their own terms, their probability of failure would be quite high, since they did not have the ability for it. In contrast, as pointed out in Chapter 7, those high in *n* Achievement and low in Test Anxiety more often picked occupations for which there was little discrepancy between the ability they perceived they had and the ability that was required for the occupation. Furthermore, those high in *f* Failure were more often inaccurate in estimating their own ability (as compared with actual academic performance), and they even chose occupations that did not realistically fit in with interests they said they had. All in all, it looked as if they were avoiding realistic choices because they had more negative valence for them, just as the Atkinson model would predict.

Feather (1961) obtained results on persistence after failure that fit the model. The results have been included in Figure 7.6. The subjects classified as low in *n* Achievement in this figure are also high in Test Anxiety, meaning in Atkinson's terms that they are high in *f* Failure. Notice that if the task is considered very difficult and they fail, they are much more likely to persist in working on it than if the task is considered easy and they fail. The reason in terms of the model in Table 10.2 is that if they fail at Task C (an easy task), the probability of failure subjectively increases for them, and it has an avoidance value more like that for Task B, which yields the maximum avoidance. So they would be less likely to keep working at the task. In contrast, if they fail at a very diffi-

Table 10.3.

FEAR OF FAILURE RELATED TO LACK OF REALISM IN VOCATIONAL ASPIRATION
(data from Mahone, 1960)

Occupational Choice Characteristics	Percentage of Subjects in Each Category	
	High f Failure High Test Anxiety, Low n Achievement	*Low f Failure Low Test Anxiety, High n Achievement*
Positive goal discrepancy[a]		
High	61	31
Low	39	69
	$\chi^2 = 5.69; p < .01.$	
Inaccuracy in estimate of own ability		
High	67	44
Low	33	56
	$\chi^2 = 3.52; p < .04.$	
Realism of choice in terms of interest		
Realistic	32	56
Unrealistic	68	44
	$\chi^2 = 3.50; p < .04.$	

[a]The difference between the subject's own estimated ability and perception of the ability needed for the occupation chosen.

cult task like Task A in Table 10.2, it increases the probability of failure but moves the avoidance tendency even farther from Task B, which has the maximum avoidance value for them. So they would be more likely to persist after failure on a difficult than an easy task, according to the model.

However, in the most direct test of the model, subjects high in *f* Failure generally continue to show some preference for moderately difficult tasks, even though considerably less than those high in *n* Achievement and low in Test Anxiety. For example, in the classic study by Atkinson and Litwin (1960) on the distances from the peg at which subjects choose to stand in a ringtoss game (see Table 7.3), about 43 percent of the choices made by those high in *f* Failure (high in Test Anxiety, low in *n* Achievement) are for moderate distances, as contrasted with 21 percent for very close or easy distances and 36 percent for very far or difficult distances. This would seem to be a direct contradiction of the model, which predicts that such people should above all avoid the middle distances. The explanation given for such a discrepancy is either that the subjects were not extreme enough in their *f* Failure, or that extrinsic motivational factors have influenced their choices. Another possibility is that the measure of *f* Failure employed is defective.

So far as actual performance is concerned, subjects high in Test Anxiety act in ways that suggest they are afraid of failure and are seeking to do whatever will reduce the experience of failure. As contrasted with those low in Test Anxiety, they typically do more poorly on laboratory tasks such as digit-symbol substitution (Mandler & Sarason, 1952), but occasionally they perform better if the threat of immediate negative evaluation is remote. Thus, they do less well on aptitude tests but tend to get better grades in college (Mandler & Sarason, 1952). The explanation apparently is that in doing course work they work harder to avoid failure but are not disrupted by the threat of immediate failure, as they are in a timed test situation.

Whether they think they are likely to be negatively judged is very important to subjects high in *f* Failure, as the data summarized in Table 10.4 show. In this experiment the subjects were shown a word every two seconds and were asked to learn to anticipate and say what word was coming up before it showed in the window in front of them. In the control, or neutral, condition, they were simply told how to perform the task. With no particular understanding as to what the task was all about, the subjects high and low in Test Anxiety did not perform differently. However, if the subjects were told that performance on the test would yield a measure of their intelligence, the subjects high in Test Anxiety performed much more poorly than those low in Test Anxiety. In contrast, if they were reassured in advance that "these kinds of lists are hard and so it's no surprise or matter of concern if you progress slowly at first and make mistakes," they performed actually somewhat better than those low in Test Anxiety.

Furthermore, Weiner has shown (as reported in Table 3.2) that subjects high in *f* Failure perform better if they believe they are succeeding. Thus, if they are "ahead of the game" they will perform better, because that is the best way to avoid failure, but if they are behind they do worse, because that seems the best way to get out of the failure situation. The conclusion is similar to the one

Table 10.4.

NUMBER OF CORRECT RESPONSES FOR FINAL TRIAL BLOCK ON SERIAL LEARNING TASK (after Sarason, 1971)

Conditions	High Test Anxiety (H)	Low Test Anxiety (L)	Difference (H − L)
Control (neutral)	47.8	46.7	1.1
Achievement orientation	34.1	65.1	− 31.0**
Reassurance	58.8	42.3	16.5*

*$p < .05$.
**$p < .01$.

reached about the effect on performance of a more generalized type of anxiety, as measured in the Taylor Manifest Anxiety Scale. Individuals will do whatever seems to them to be the best way of avoiding anxiety in a situation.

Critique of the Test Anxiety Measure of Fear of Failure

A number of objections have been raised to using Test Anxiety as a measure of fear of failure. It has the usual weakness of all self-report measures: people who are afraid of failure are not always willing to admit they are. This shows up in the fact that some subjects low in Test Anxiety nevertheless show signs of strong physiological arousal under stress (Salter et al., 1976). Furthermore, as already noted, subjects classified as high in fear of failure by this measure do not actually avoid taking intermediate risks the way they ought to according to theory. Perhaps the most troubling aspect of the way the Atkinson group measures the fear of failure is that it does not allow a person to be high both in *n* Achievement and in fear of failure. By the Atkinson method, in order for people to be very high in fear of failure (H), they must be low in *n* Achievement (L). Such people are classified as LH. To be sure, a person can be classified as high in *n* Achievement (H) and high in Test Anxiety (H), or HH, but, according to the Atkinson scheme, such a person can be neither as high in *n* Achievement as one who is classified as HL or as high in fear of failure as one who is classified as LH.

• MEASURING FEAR OF FAILURE IN FANTASY

The Heckhausen, German Measure

In view of the general superiority of fantasy measures of motive strength, several attempts have been made to break down the scoring categories for *n* Achievement into those that seem more oriented around failure in contrast to those oriented toward success (see deCharms & Davé, 1965; Moulton, 1958). However, none of these scoring schemes seem to work very well.

In Germany, Heckhausen (1963) derived a scoring system based on characteristics of stories told by individuals who either did or did not adopt defensive goal-setting strategies. In the level-of-aspiration experiment, in which subjects set goals for their performance on the next trial after learning their score on the previous one, they are considered to be afraid of failure if they set a goal that is the same as or lower than their present performance. If their goal is somewhat higher than their present performance, they are considered to be activated by a positive hope for success. Heckhausen also included more pictures of authority figures, such as teachers or bosses, who might be considered to be demanding achievement from others.

He found that the stories written by two groups of individuals with contrasting goal-setting strategies differed in characteristic ways. Those who set possible goals for themselves told stories dealing more often with positive urges to achieve, with expectations of success, and with concentrated efforts to achieve success. He summed these categories into what he called a *Hope of Success* (*h* Success) *score,* which for all practical purposes correlates so highly with the *n* Achievement score constructed as explained in Chapter 7 that it can be considered a substitute for it. Subjects who adopted a defensive goal-setting strategy wrote stories that dealt more often with a need to avoid failure, as in the statement "He hopes that the teacher won't notice the mistake." Other scoring categories included instrumental acts designed to avoid failure, negative feelings about work, and criticism or scolding from those in charge of the work. These categories were summed to give an *f* Failure score, which correlated neither with the U.S. *n* Achievement score nor with the German *h* Success score at a very high level.

The German measure of *f* Failure has many advantages over the Atkinson system of measurement through the Test Anxiety Questionnaire. It permits a person to be high both in *h* Success and in *f* Failure. It is not subject to response bias, and, as Figure 10.4 shows, it is associated with marked avoidance of tasks of moderate difficulty, as the Atkinson model predicts. In this experiment, Schneider (1978) took the trouble of varying such extraneous factors as the level of the subject's *n* Affiliation and whether the experimenter was present or absent. Thus, the curve shown is for the pure case in which the person is high in *f* Failure, low in *n* Affiliation, and making his or her choices alone without an experimenter's being present. The result is exactly what the Atkinson model would predict. That is, subjects high in *f* Failure prefer very easy or very difficult tasks and positively avoid choosing tasks of intermediate difficulty.

The behaviors associated with the German *f* Failure measure make a coherent theoretical picture (Heckhausen, 1980). As compared with subjects low in *f* Failure, those who score high in this measure better recall tasks they have completed as compared with those they have failed to complete. They take longer to do their homework, solve fewer problems under time pressure, and have a shorter future time perspective than those high in *h* Success. They also perform better after success feedback, which confirms the expectation developed in the last section that they will work harder whenever that is the most obvious way to

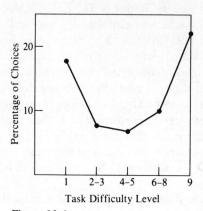

Figure 10.4.

Percentage of Choices of Tasks of Different Difficulty Levels by Subjects Higher in *f* Failure Than *h* Success and Low in *n* Affiliation with Experimenter Absent (data from Schneider, 1978).

avoid the criticism of failure. Furthermore, if they fail at a task they have chosen to do it is less attractive for them, whereas under similar conditions the task is more attractive for those high in *h* Success. Even failure at a task that has been assigned to those high in *f* Failure makes it less attractive for them, although failure at such a task for those high in *h* Success has no significant effect on its attractiveness for them.

The U.S. Measure

The chief drawback of the Heckhausen system for measuring *f* Failure was that it was published in German and therefore was not used by U.S. researchers. Quite independently of Heckhausen, Birney, Burdick, and Teevan (1969) derived a new scoring system for *f* Failure by contrasting stories written when the fear of failure was aroused by performing very difficult tasks. For college students they used a speed-reading machine, in which sentences to be read aloud could be exposed for ever briefer periods of time until the subjects had to fail. For a group of eighth-graders they aroused the fear of failure by giving them a very difficult math test.

Stories written when the fear of failure was aroused in these ways showed a marked increase in what they called *Hostile Press,* defined as reprimands for personal actions; legal or jurisdictional retaliation for actions taken; deprivation of affiliative relationships, "as when a person feels lonely or is afraid of being rejected" (Birney et al., 1969); and hostile environmental forces such as fires or earthquakes. Figure 10.5 shows how the percentage of stories showing Hostile Press increased significantly when the fear of failure was aroused either among eighth-graders or college students. The result is similar to one obtained by the Heckhausen group: When their *f* Failure measure was subjected to a factor anal-

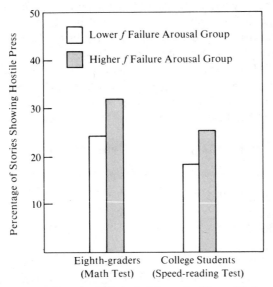

Age Group and Method of Arousal of Fear of Failure

Figure 10.5.

Percentage of Stories Showing Hostile Press Among Groups in Which Fear of Failure Has Been More or Less Aroused (after Birney, Burdick, & Teevan, 1969).

ysis, they discovered two factors, one of which dealt with story content related to avoiding failure, and the other with story characteristics related to criticism for failure. They found that the criticism categories were relatively more frequent among those who scored higher in the overall measure of f Failure (Heckhausen, 1980). Thus, both independent investigations established the fact that high f Failure is strongly associated with being criticized or punished.

The U.S. scoring system also included other categories, such as the desire for relief from Hostile Press, instrumental actions to avoid criticism, and so on. The behaviors associated with the overall Hostile Press score obtained by summing these categories have been examined and found to be very similar to those associated with other measures of f Failure. For example, subjects high in Hostile Press conform more to group pressure, just as subjects high in Manifest Anxiety do. When they were asked to judge which of two lines was longer, after hearing five stooges give the incorrect judgment, they more often also gave the incorrect response, even though it was obviously wrong (Birney et al., 1969).

Characteristics of People with a Strong Fear of Failure

Table 10.5 summarizes some of the relationships found in this study for various types of performance situations. In comparison with those low in Hostile Press, subjects high in Hostile Press took longer to learn to trace mazes correctly when the mazes were presented to them for very short periods. They volunteered less often to play darts "to show how good you are at it." They played an interpersonal game competitively less often than those low in Hostile Press. In this game there are two players, each of whom is trying to collect the maximum number of points. How many points a person can make, however, depends on what the other player does, as well as on what the person's own choices are. The following matrix is typical of the points awarded for different combinations of moves (Birney et al., 1969):

Points Awarded for Player (Player 1, Player 2)

Player 1

		Choice A	Choice B
		Choice A	Choice B
Player 2	Choice A	3, 3	4, 0
	Choice B	0, 4	1, 1

If Player 1 picks Option A, he or she gets either 3 points or 0 points, depending on whether Player 2 picks Option A or B. If Player 1 has picked A, Player 2 gets 3 points for picking A and 4 points for picking B. If Player 1 picks B, he or she gets 4 or 1 points, depending on the option Player 2 picks. Player 2 is faced with a similar set of choices, and neither player knows in advance how the other will choose. The best strategy is for both players to pick the same options, but that means trusting each other, for if one player picks A and the other picks B, one player may lose out altogether. It is possible over a sequence of moves to determine whether a player is primarily defensive—trying to avoid total loss, as when Player 1 picks Option B—or whether the player is actively and competi-

Table 10.5.

PERFORMANCE OF SUBJECTS SCORING HIGH AND LOW IN HOSTILE PRESS IN VARIOUS ACHIEVEMENT-RELATED ACTIVITIES (after Birney, Burdick, & Teevan, 1969)

Activity	Hostile Press Score		p difference
	High	Low	
Average number of trials needed to trace mazes correctly (speeded task)	122.5	102.2	$< .01$
Percentage who volunteer to play darts "to see how good you are"	25%	68%	$< .01$
Percentage who play interpersonal game competitively	21%	43%	$< .05$
Percentage who get above-average grades			
In elementary school	76%	24%	$< .01$
In high school	71%	29%	$< .01$
In college	70%	30%	$< .01$

tively trying to defeat the other person by choosing options that would cause the other player to get 0 points.

Subjects high in the Hostile Press score, indicating a high fear of failure, do not play this game competitively, but more often try to avoid losing. Finally, as Table 10.5 shows, subjects scoring high in Hostile Press more often get better grades at the elementary, high-school, and college levels than those low in Hostile Press. This too is consistent with results obtained with other measures of ƒ Failure.

• COMPARISON OF MEASURES OF FEAR OF FAILURE

Most significantly in terms of Atkinson's theory, individuals who score higher on the U.S. ƒ Failure measure also avoid moderate risks and show preference for extreme probabilities of success. Ceranski, Teevan, and Kalle (1979) reported an experiment in which they used three different measures of fear of failure to see which was most closely associated with this theoretically important prediction. The results are summarized in Table 10.6. The Hostile Press measure of fear of failure is the only measure in these situations that successfully predicts at a significant level which subjects will adopt a defensive goal-setting strategy and show a preference for extreme probabilities of success. A much higher proportion of subjects high in Hostile Press, as compared with those low in Hostile Press, set performance goals that were either the same as, less than, or very much higher than the level they had achieved on a given trial. That is, they set either very easy or very difficult goals for themselves and avoided setting moderately difficult goals. In a different part of the experiment they also showed a distinct preference for working at tasks described either as very easy or very hard. The Test Anxiety measure by itself did not succeed in predicting these preferences, and the Atkinson measure also failed, although the trends were in the expected direction.

The result of all this work is that there are three different measures of fear of failure, all of which show similar relationships to behaviors, such as defensive goal setting, poor performance under some conditions and better under others, avoidance of competition, and susceptibility to positive suggestions from others. The measures also significantly correlate with each other, although at a fairly low level (Birney et al., 1969). Hostile Press scores correlate with the German ƒ Failure measure, as well as with the Atkinson method of determining ƒ Failure scores. The Atkinson method has been used most often because it involves less work, but it is probably the least satisfactory of the three for reasons already given. The German ƒ Failure measure probably is the most carefully worked out and thoroughly tested in terms of its relationships to various behaviors, but it has not been used by U.S. researchers. The U.S. Hostile Press measure has not been used except by those who devised it, and whereas it has clear advantages over the Atkinson measure, it raises some theoretical questions that have never been resolved. One problem is reflected in the fact that one of the scoring categories for Hostile Press involves fear of rejection, or imagery that is also scored

Table 10.6.

RELATIONSHIP OF THREE MEASURES OF *f* FAILURE TO DEFENSIVENESS AND AVOIDING MODERATE RISKS (data from Ceranski, Teevan, & Kalle, 1979)

Measure of f Failure	N	Percentage of Subjects Using a Defensive Goal-setting Strategy in a Scrambled-Words Test[a]	Percentage of Subjects Preferring Extreme Probabilities of Success in Eight Different Tasks[b]
Birney, Burdick, and Teevan measure			
High in Hostile Press	55	62%	53%
Low in Hostile Press	68	21%	9%
P difference		< .001	< .001
Test Anxiety measure			
High in Test Anxiety on Test Anxiety Questionnaire (TAQ)	69	35%	31%
Low in TAQ	63	38%	21%
P difference		n.s.	n.s.
Atkinson measure			
Low in *n* Achievement, high TAQ	33	36%	33%
High in *n* Achievement, low TAQ	37	27%	22%
P difference		n.s.	n.s.

[a]The discrepancy between the goal set for next trial and performance on the previous trial was either negative, 0, or +3.5 or more.
[b]These subjects preferred tasks in which probabilities of success were described as either very easy (.85 to .92) or very difficult (.08 to .15).

for *n* Affiliation. This introduces a significant relationship to the *n* Affiliation score but leaves unanswered the question as to whether this is an artifact of the scoring system or a real relationship between fear of failure and fear of rejection. The German scoring system does not introduce this complication. Another problem lies in the fact that the scoring system for Hostile Press is named for the source of the fear rather than for the incentive that would resolve it. As we have seen, this is a general problem for all anxiety measures. It may simply reflect the fact that we are still unable to specify very precisely what the incentives are for avoidance motives.

• ORIGINS OF THE FEAR OF FAILURE

A question that naturally arises in reviewing the research on *f* Failure measurement is why the self-report approach adopted by the Atkinson group works as well as it does, given the failure of self-reports to measure approach motives adequately (see Chapter 6). The answer may lie in a fundamental difference between approach and avoidance motives. Usually it is some force in the external environment—a parent, a teacher, or a peer—that by punishing a child forms the basis of an avoidance motive. If children do not get food into their mouths properly, their mothers scold. If they do not put their shoes on properly, their nursery-school teachers scold. If they cannot throw a ball, friends may laugh. All of these experiences build up a fear of failure, but they are all based on easily identifiable external events followed by internal responses of feeling upset. So a self-report measure may work better for avoidance than for approach motives because the events underlying the former are more easily identified. The stimulus value of a "moderately difficult task," as well as the satisfactions arising from mastering it that form the basis of the achievement motive, are not so easily identified as a sharp rebuke for performing poorly and the anxiety that immediately accompanies it.

Studies of the origins of the fear of failure support such a hypothesis. Smith (1969) found that mothers of sons who feared failure set higher standards of achievement for their sons and, at the same time, took a less favorable view of their son's ability to achieve those standards than other mothers. They were setting their sons up for criticism and punishment. It is as if they were saying, "You *must* do better, but I know you can't."

Birney et al. (1969) approached the same issue in a different way. They asked both parents and their children how the parents reacted when the children succeeded or failed. They categorized the responses they got into two contrasting patterns. In one the parents reacted neutrally for success but punished the child for failure, and in the other the parents rewarded success and were relatively neutral about failure. Of the students high in Hostile Press or *f* Failure, 83 percent had parents who fell into the first pattern—predominantly punishment for failure—as contrasted with only 54 percent of the students scoring low in Hostile Press, a highly significant difference. Other studies (for example, see Hassan, Enayatullah, & Khalique, 1977) support the general conclusion that parents who are rigid, authoritarian, and punitive tend to produce children with a strong *f* Failure. What such findings also suggest is that the sources of such avoidance motives are external and easily identified by the child, so they can be reported on a Test Anxiety Questionnaire with reasonable accuracy.

• FEAR OF REJECTION

Self-report Measures and Their Correlates in Behavior

Studies of *n* Affiliation reviewed in Chapter 9 strongly suggest that it is primarily a measure of Fear of Rejection (*f* Rejection), whereas the intimacy motive is a better index of positive affiliative tendencies. Nevertheless, some attempts have also been made to get a purer measure of the fear of rejection. Sorrentino and Sheppard (1978) followed the procedure adopted by Atkinson to get a purified measure of *f* Failure. As an equivalent to the Test Anxiety Questionnaire used in that procedure, they turned to a self-report measure of *f* Rejection developed by Mehrabian (1970). It asks subjects to respond to statements like "I prefer not to go to a place if I know that some of the people who will be there don't like me" or "I enjoy discussing controversial topics like politics and religion." A person responding *true* to the first statement and *false* to the second would be scored as high in *f* Rejection. Subjects who score both high in *n* Affiliation and low on this scale were considered by Sorrentino and Sheppard to be low in *f* Rejection (or high in Hope of Affiliation, or *h* Affiliation), whereas those who score low in *n* Affiliation and high on this scale are considered high in *f* Rejection. Subjects with other combinations of scores on these two measures are considered intermediate in *f* Rejection.

Sorrentino and Sheppard were able to carry out a natural experiment that demonstrated that individual differences in *f* Rejection levels made a real difference in the speed with which individuals swam under different competitive conditions. In one instance the swimmers were told to swim as fast as they could, each one having been given a handicap by the coach based on past performance. The goal was to try to beat all other individuals competing. In the other instance the swimmers with the same handicap were told they were part of a team and that the objective was for their team's score to be better than the team scores of other competing groups. As Figure 10.6 makes clear, subjects high in *f* Rejection swam slower when they were working for a team goal than when they were competing as individuals. It is as if their fears that they would be criticized by other members of the group actually interfered with their ability to swim. In contrast, those high in *n* Affiliation (or low in *f* Rejection) swam faster when they were part of a group than when they were competing individually. The differences in swimming times, while small in absolute terms, are highly significant statistically and would have important effects on winning different kinds of races in competitive athletics.

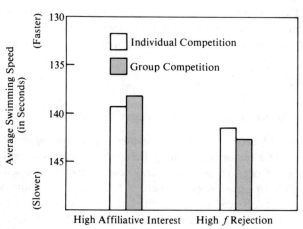

Figure 10.6.

Average Swimming Speeds of Subjects High in Affiliative Interest and in *f* Rejection in Individual and Group Competition (data from Sorrentino & Sheppard, 1978).

A number of other studies have been carried out using a self-report measure of *f* Rejection developed by Mehrabian and Ksionzky (1974), which may be regarded as somewhat valid on the grounds that it reflects an avoidance motive about which individuals may be more aware. Such an assumption seems justified by results obtained with it, such as those illustrated in Figure 10.7. In the experiment shown, student participants were told they were about to take part in a study of how strangers interact with each other. While they were waiting to meet the strangers they filled out a social status survey, which was scored; they were told that in terms primarily of the income level and education of their parents, they were at Positions 2, 5, or 8 on a 10-point scale representing social status. They were all told that the stranger they were about to meet was at Point 5 on the same scale. Thus, they knew whether the stranger was of a higher or a lower status than themselves. Then they chatted for a few minutes with the stranger, who was a confederate of the experimenter instructed to act in certain standard ways. Afterward the subjects reported how much they had liked the stranger on a scale of 1 to 9.

As Figure 10.7 shows, students who were high in *f* Rejection liked the stranger of lower status more than the stranger of higher status. It might be inferred that they were more nervous in the presence of a higher status person because of their fear of being rejected, so they liked the individual less. In contrast, those low in *f* Rejection liked the higher status stranger better. Whereas the Mehrabian and Ksionzky measure of *f* Rejection thus has some promise, its

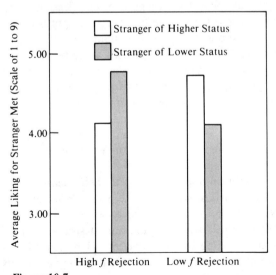

Figure 10.7.

Liking for a Stranger of Higher or Lower Status by Individuals High or Low in *f* Rejection (after Mehrabian, 1971).

exact status is unclear, partly because it is obviously open to response bias and partly because it does not correlate with the *n* Affiliation score (Karabenick, 1977), which has been shown to reflect a fear of rejection.

Relationship Between Fear of Failure, Fear of Rejection, and the Approval Motive

Why should anyone fear failure? If a boy is scolded by his mother for doing poorly in school, why should he care? On theoretical grounds it might be presumed that he is afraid of her disapproval and rejection. In this case, fear of failure simply translates into fear of rejection. There are hints throughout the empirical literature that the two avoidance motives may be connected. Recall the discussion in Chapter 3 of findings that the mere presence of another person can introduce evaluation apprehension that affects performance in ways that look as if the person is simultaneously fearing failure and disapproval or rejection. (See Table 3.3.) Furthermore, the previous sections reviewed several studies showing that reassuring subjects, or even telling subjects what to do, reduced their fear of failure and enabled them to perform better. And Birney et al. (1969) found that arousing the fear of failure experimentally increased thoughts of rejection specifically, so they included these thoughts as a category in their Hostile Press scoring system. Perhaps fear of failure and fear of rejection are closely related, and both derive from a need for social approval.

As Chapter 5 pointed out, Crowne and Marlowe (1964) have developed a measure of the need for Social Approval, so such a hypothesis can be tested. It is conceivable that people who answer items on a questionnaire always in the socially desirable direction may be avoiding making unfavorable comments about themselves because they fear disapproval or rejection. Supportive evidence for such an inference derives from the fact that the approval motive score obtained from such a questionnaire correlates highly significantly with the *n* Affiliation score (Crowne & Marlowe, 1964), which we have determined is primarily a measure of *f* Rejection. Furthermore, the behaviors associated with a high need for Social Approval are very similar to those associated with a strong *f* Failure and a strong *f* Rejection, as measured by the *n* Affiliation score. Subjects who score high on any of these measures tend to engage in defensive goal setting, to yield to group pressure, and to more readily shape what they say in response to the nod and the "Mhm" from the experimenter in verbal conditioning experiments.

But then we run into an apparent snag. If these measures are all tapping the same or similar characteristics, why does the need for Social Approval score correlate *negatively* with the Manifest Anxiety score (Crowne & Marlowe, 1964)? That is, why do those who mention only desirable qualities in themselves score so very low in admitting to any anxieties? They deny they are anxious. That makes sense, but how can we argue then that they are really anxious about being rejected?

At a deeper level the results are not really contradictory. A person who fears rejection may deny being anxious in the search for approval. What is at fault is the self-report measure employed, which reflects more the strategy of dealing with the fear (denial) than a measurement of the extent of the fear itself. So we can only conclude that the fear of failure, the fear of rejection, and the need for approval could probably all be shown to be related to each other, if we only had better measures of each of them that had tested their relationships in a definitive study. One other bit of evidence supports this conclusion. In Germany, Laufen attempted to develop a method of scoring stories for h Affiliation and f Rejection by having subjects first fill out a questionnaire containing statements relating to either n Affiliation or f Rejection. Only the exposure to f Rejection statements produced significant changes in the thought content of stories in the direction of increasing thoughts about rejection (Heckhausen, 1980). The scoring keys for the stories he developed were subsequently used in another study by Jopt (cited in Heckhausen, 1980), who found that f Failure and f Rejection scores summated to produce the best performance from sixteen-year-old male students working for a female teacher. That is, the boys worked harder for such a teacher if they scored high on the Heckhausen f Failure measure and the Laufen f Rejection measure than if they were high on either one of these scales alone. The same result was not obtained when the teacher was male. This suggests that under certain conditions, fear of failure and fear of rejection combine readily to produce an effect, although it does not prove they are aspects of the same characteristic.

• FEAR OF SUCCESS

Measuring Women's Fear of Success in Fantasy

Trained in the Atkinson tradition for studying achievement motivation, Horner (1968) became curious as to why women did not always behave the same way as men in achievement situations and, in particular, why they scored higher in Test Anxiety. She noted that many psychologists believed women had much more anxiety over appearing aggressive and competitive than men did (Horner, 1973). So she designed a test to tap this anxiety by asking subjects to write a story about a verbal lead such as the following: "After first-term finals, Anne finds herself at the top of her medical school class." For men she substituted the name *John* for *Anne* in the verbal lead. She found that women wrote many more negative stories to the *Anne* cue than men did to the *John* cue. The stories written by women dealt with the negative consequences of success or even with denial of the situation described by the cue. Here are some examples:

> Anne is an acne faced bookworm. She runs to the bulletin board and finds she is at the top. As usual "she smarts off." A chorus of groans is the rest of the class's reply.

Well it certainly paid off. All the Friday and Saturday nights with my books, who needs dates, fun—I'll be the best woman doctor alive.

Anne, the girl who swallowed the canary in her younger days, is pretty darned proud of herself. But everyone hates and envies her.

Anne is a code name for a non-existent person created by a group of med students. They take turns taking exams and writing papers for Anne. (Horner, 1973)

In general, these stories indicated that women feared social rejection based on performance success much more than men did. Horner called the score obtained by summing these negative characteristics a measure of *fear of Success* (f Success). She validated the measure by checking whether women who scored high in f Success would in fact avoid winning in direct competition with men. She arranged for a large number of students of both sexes to work at a number of verbal and arithmetic tasks in a group competitive situation to see who could get the best scores. Some of the subjects then worked under noncompetitive conditions. Whereas most of the men did better under competitive than noncompetitive conditions, only 23 percent of the women high in f Success performed better under competitive than noncompetitive conditions, as contrasted with 93 percent of the women low in f Success. Fear of Success did not have the same effect on the performance of men. In other words, the women who had written stories about the negative consequences of success were holding back in competition with men as compared with how they would perform normally when they were not in competition.

Horner's original data showed that 65 percent of the women as compared with only 9 percent of the men, wrote stories that were scored for f Success. However, this sex difference tended to disappear in later replications of her findings (Hoffman, 1974; Zuckerman & Wheeler, 1975). Furthermore, several investigators reported a failure to find the expected relationship between f Success scores and performance of women in a mixed-sex classroom situation (Feather & Simon, 1973). One problem may have been that the original findings on fear of success in women had been widely written up in national magazines, so many college women knew about them. The women's movement was gathering momentum at the same time, and it seemed reasonable to infer that many women were consciously avoiding writing negative stories to the *Anne* cue to prove they were not afraid of getting ahead in the world.

Horner, Tresemer, Berens, and Watson (1973) then developed a new scoring system for f Success based on the stories written after succeeding or not succeeding in competition with a particular male. That is, feedback on performance was manipulated so that each woman in the arousal condition appeared to have beaten her male competitor. In the control condition, similar women wrote stories after working on the same task but not in competition with anyone. The scoring categories that differentiated the stories written under these two conditions had to do with the problematic expression of instrumental performance activity, with problems' being solved without effort (called "relief"), and with approach to other people introduced into the story. These new indicators of *f* Success are less obvious than the old ones and therefore are harder for individuals to change consciously in line with their values. At any rate, perhaps for this reason the results with this measure have been more consistent in picking out those people who will do less well in competition with others.

How Fear of Success Affects Competitive Behavior in Women

Shinn (1973) used the new measure of *f* Success to study the effects of the merger of two formerly single-sex secondary schools. She found that before the merger, when the boys and girls were tested separately in their segregated schools, they did not differ in average levels of *f* Success, nor did the *f* Success score predict who would do poorly in working competitively on a verbal task like anagrams. The girls did do better than the boys on the verbal task on the average, in accordance with a general tendency of women to do better on verbal tasks. However, the results were quite different a year after the merger had taken place, when the boys and girls were in the same classrooms competing with each other. The girls had lost their superiority in performing a similar verbal task—unscrambling words—and their *f* Success score had risen dramatically over what it had been when they were in the single-sex school. The boys had not shown a similar rise in *f* Success scores. Furthermore, after the merger, only 30 percent of the girls high in *f* Success scored above average on the scrambled-words task, as compared with 72 percent of those low in *f* Success, which is a significant difference. In other words, fear of success was inhibiting the performance of the girls now that they were in a situation where they were competing with boys, whereas before, when they were competing with girls, high *f* Success had not inhibited their performance. A similar shift did not occur for the boys. Their *f* Success score was not associated with poor performance. In other words, it looked as if it was specifically the fear of the consequences of competing with boys that inhibited the performance of girls.

Karabenick (1977) showed that high *f* Success diminished performance for women competing with men only when they thought the task was masculine. He described anagrams as related either to masculine or feminine abilities and interest and stated further that either men or women were particularly adept at solving them. Different groups of subjects worked at the task, believing that it was masculine or feminine. They either worked alone or in competition with a member of the same or opposite sex, who was described as performing a little below average on the same task. Thus, the subjects would tend to believe that they had a good chance of beating the other person. The crucial question was whether they performed better under competitive or noncompetitive conditions when they were working against a member of the same or opposite sex on a task they thought was either masculine or feminine. The results showed that the *f* Success score was related to a difference in performance under competitive conditions under only one condition—when women high in *f* Success were competing with men on a masculine task, they tended to perform less well ($r = -.25; p < .01$). If they were working on exactly the same task in competition with men but thought it was a feminine task, their f Success had no affect on their performance. Nor did male f Success scores relate in any way to their performance in competition with women or other men.

The inhibiting effects on performance of fear of success in women shows up not only in laboratory tasks but also in attitudes toward family and career throughout life. Stewart (1975) obtained f Success scores from stories written by women in two different colleges in their freshman year and then observed how these scores related to what the women did over the next fourteen years. Fear of Success scores were significantly higher in College B than in College A, and Stewart found considerable evidence that the women in College B experienced much more conflict about whether pursuing a career would interfere with having a happy marriage and family. In College A the women were much more single-mindedly oriented toward a career, and they were less concerned about marriage. Thus, it was not surprising to discover that f Success scores among College B women were associated significantly with getting married early, with having children soon, with not working, and with "job dabbling," that is, with playing around with working rather than pursuing a consistent career path. Stewart interpreted this as meaning that the women in College B, who were afraid of the consequences of success, were so worried about working and appearing unfeminine that they quickly got married and had children to prove their femininity.

She also found signs that among women who single-mindedly pursued a career without thinking about family, high f Success could be associated with a lack of career persistence. For example, among the substantial number of women from both colleges who had received a Doctor of Philosophy degree, high f Success was associated with *not* working full-time ten years after college, whereas there was no such relationship for women who had attained only a Master's degree. The explanation is that women who are afraid of the negative consequences of success are much more likely to worry about working after having concentrated on a career enough to get a Doctor of Philosophy degree than are women who have not spent so much time in professional development. As another sign of the same trend, Stewart discovered that among women who had never married or not had a child early, high f Success was significantly related to a lack of career persistence; this was not true, however, among women who had married or had a child. She explains the finding as meaning that the women with families had proved their femininity, so their fear of success would no longer hamper them in pursuing a career. On the other hand, single women who feared success would still be worried about whether they were working so much as to exclude the possibility of having a happy married life, so they would keep interrupting their careers in order to give more balance to their lives.

Jackaway and Teevan (1976) reasoned that if fear of success results from a fear of failure in interpersonal relationships, then there should be a positive correlation between the Hostile Press f Failure measure and the f Success measure. They found this to be the case, the correlation being .44 for male and .53 for female high-school students. The relationship was higher for women, as would be expected from the larger number of their stories that mentioned affiliative failure consequent upon success, although the difference between the correlations for men and women did not reach significance. As Jackaway and Teevan (1976) point out, the correlation is due in part to an overlap in the scoring systems, since some of the same events in the stories are scored by the two different systems. In particular, as mentioned earlier, the Hostile Press system scores for affiliative failure, which also is scored in the f Success system. It would be worth checking the correlation with the German fear of failure measure before suggesting, as they do, that "for those people (especially women) whose affiliative and achievement needs are interrelated, fear of failure and fear of success may be nearly equivalent since fear of rejection thus becomes tantamount to fear of failure" (Jackaway & Teevan, 1976).

Fear of Success Among Black Men and Women

Fleming (1974) found that fear of success functions quite differently among black men and women. At the outset, using verbal cues like Horner's, she discovered that only 29 percent of black college women gave f Success story completions, as contrasted with 67 percent of black college males. Thus, the results were the opposite of what Horner had been finding for white college students. The black women were much lower in f Success than white women, and the black men were much higher than white men. She explained this reversal as due to racial discrimination and oppression. Historically black men have been in much greater danger for being assertive and "uppity" than black women. Often, in fact, it was easier for black women to find housework and support the family than it was for black men, who were systematically discriminated against. Thus, black women had no reason to fear the negative consequences of achievement; in fact, they were taught to expect rewards from working hard, whereas among black men, trying to get ahead could often lead to trouble, disappointment, and rage.

However, in later studies using the Horner-type cues, the differences between black men and women tended to disappear, just as the opposite difference had disappeared among whites. Nevertheless, a closer analysis of the stories written by black men and women, as well as application of the new scoring system for f Success, still led Fleming (1975b) to conclude that black men feared success more than black women, although the evidence was not as conclusive as might be wished for. The following are typical stories written by black college men:

> Sam is finding himself. He is out of sight. . . . Sam is thinking that the white boys will obviously without a doubt be uptight.
>
> Sam will be wanted by all of the Wall Street Firms. A lot of white boys will jump out of Holyoke Center. The professors will of course make sure that Sam is not number one the following term. (Fleming, 1975a)

Fleming (1974) found, furthermore, that f Success scores were negatively related to performance when black men were competing directly with white men. First, she obtained f Success scores under neutral conditions and three weeks later had a white male compete directly with a black male on an arithmetic test to see who would do better. She then reported that the black had won, and she administered a second f Success measure followed by further performance alone on the anagrams task. She found that those black men whose f Success scores had increased most after beating a white male opponent did perform significantly less well on the final anagrams test ($r = -.46$; $p < .001$). Their high f Success had interfered with their performance. She also reports that achievement motivation training of the type described in Chapter 14 increased fear of success motivation in black males rather than achievement motivation.

In Fleming's (1974) study the black women competed with black men rather than with white women. She found that high f Success was significantly related to poorer performance in competition with black men only among black women of lower-class background. She felt that this was true because the conflict between career and marriage is more severe among lower-class than among middle-class blacks. For example, among the women of lower-class background, 75 percent of those high in f Success had mothers who were better educated than their fathers, as contrasted with only 38 percent of those low in f Success. This difference suggests that in the families of women with high f Success there was more conflict over what women should be doing—that is, working in line with their better education or taking care of the family. These differences of opinion also showed up in the fact that whereas none of the parents of the women low in f Success were divorced, 38 percent of those high in f Success had divorced parents.

The black students were also asked what values their parents had stressed in bringing them up. Table 10.7 reports the correlations of f Success scores among black men and women with values stressed either by their mothers or fathers. The most striking finding so far as the women are concerned is that those high in f Success had mothers who emphasized one characteristic and fathers who emphasized another. For those of working-class background, the mothers stressed achievement and social assertiveness while the fathers stressed self-reliance. For those of middle-class background, high f Success was associated with mothers who played down self-reliance and whose fathers stressed achievement. In this case it looks as if ambivalence over being assertive (high f Success) derives directly from the fact that they were getting opposite messages about the importance of such behavior from their fathers and mothers.

In the case of black men, the only significant result is that fathers both from the middle class and the working class who insisted on social assertiveness tended to have sons who were *low* in f Success. To put it the other way around, if the fathers cautioned their sons against being assertive or "uppity," the sons tended to grow up with high f Success. This finding supports Fleming's general argument that high f Success in black males is associated with fears of the negative consequences in a white society of being an assertive black man.

What if a black male high in f Success is placed in a competitive white environment? Table 10.8 contrasts how black men high in f Success behave in a predominantly white college as compared with how they behave in a predominantly black college; both of the colleges were located in the deep South (Flem-

Table 10.7.

CORRELATIONS OF *f* SUCCESS SCORES AND SUBJECTIVE REPORTS OF PARENTAL TEACHING EMPHASES AMONG BLACK MEN AND WOMEN IN COLLEGE (after Fleming, 1974)

	Women				*Men*			
	Working-class Background		*Middle-class Background*		*Working-class Background*		*Middle-class Background*	
Parental Teaching Emphases	*Mother*	*Father*	*Mother*	*Father*	*Mother*	*Father*	*Mother*	*Father*
Achievement orientation	.46*	.08	.06	.30**	−.07	.04	−.23	−.14
Self-reliance	−.22	.51**	−.28*	−.04	.22	.16	.04	−.09
Social assertiveness	.36*	—ᵃ	.20	.15		−.38*	—ᵃ	−.43**

ᵃNot enough cases to compute.
*$p < .05$.
**$p < .001$.

ing, 1983). In the white college black men tend to be more successful than usual. They hold more offices in extracurricular activities, they are described as more outspoken, and they think of themselves as more extraverted. In a white environment, their high *f* Success has led to social success. The study suggests that they have been sensitive to the criticism of being too assertive in a white environment and, as a consequence, have been accepted by their white peers. Some blacks more oriented toward the Black Power movement might regard them as "Uncle Toms" who "go along in order to get along." But notice that this behavior also has a cost. The men who are high in *f* Success in a white environment also have needed more medical assistance for psychosomatic disorders. In contrast, black men high in *n* Achievement do not do particularly well in a white college in the South; they find it harder to do well and feel fatigued and disoriented (Fleming, 1983).

Black men who fear success do not behave in markedly different ways in a black college than other men. They are oriented somewhat more toward male domination, perhaps to compensate for the fact that they fear they will be rejected by women if they outperform them. That is, in a black college they are competing with black women—not with whites, as in a white college environment. Thus, their fears over the negative consequences of success have more to do with sex role relationships than with getting along in a white world, where competition among males dominates.

Fleming's studies underline the fact that fear of success has to do with the negative consequences of a person's standing out in some way or being assertive in relation to another group that is perceived as, or that is, more powerful and in a position to reject or punish the person for being assertive. What people are

Table 10.8.

CONTRASTING BEHAVIORS ASSOCIATED WITH HIGH *f* SUCCESS AMONG BLACK MALES IN PREDOMINANTLY WHITE AND BLACK COLLEGES
(after Fleming, 1983)

Behavior	Correlations with *f* Success	
	White College	Black College
Offices held in extracurricular activities	.41**	—
Described as outspoken	.49**	—
Extroverted self-concept	.37**	—
Times medical assistance sought for psychosomatic complaints	.34*	—
Male-dominated career choice	—	.31*
Belief that marriage will help career	—	.31*

*$*p < .05$.
**$**p < .01$.

afraid of and how it will affect their performance depends very much on whether they are male or female and black or white. But in several different types of situations it has been shown that the more recent experimentally derived *f* Success score is significantly related to poor performance in competition with those in a position of greater power.

• FEAR OF POWER

Measuring Fear of Power in Fantasy

For reasons just given, it seems not unreasonable to suppose that fear of success might be related to fear of power of others, another avoidance motive for which a scoring system has been developed by Winter (1973). He was interested in getting separate measures for approach and avoidance aspects of power motivation. He decided to classify any story as representing fear of Power (*f* Power) if it contained any doubts about the direct expression of assertiveness. These doubts could be reflected in any one of three ways: "(1) explicit statement that the power is for the benefit of some other person or cause; (2) guilt, anxiety, self-doubt, or uncertainty on the part of the person concerned with power; or (3) irony and skepticism about power as shown by the story writer's style" (Winter, 1973). The usual scoring system for *n* Power was applied, and if the major theme of any story expressed doubts of this kind, all the categories scored for this story were put in the "Fear of Power" column. If a story did not show any of these doubts, the scoring categories for *n* Power were placed in a "Hope of Power" (*h* Power) column. In general, the *h* Power and *f* Power scores do not correlate significantly with each other, and the *h* Power score correlates so highly with the overall *n* Power score that it might be considered a substitute measure for it. The *f* Power score correlates only moderately (in the range of .30 to .50) with the overall *n* Power score. Thus, it deserves to be studied in its own right. We might wonder also if *f* Power is the same as the socialized power motive (*s* Power) discussed in Chapter 8, since both include power imagery directed at helping others. There is a moderate relationship: the socialized power score and the *f* Power score correlate .49, and the personal power score (*p* Power) and *h* Power score correlate .46 (McClelland & Watson, 1973), but the relationships are low enough to indicate that the measures are not identical and deserve separate treatment.

The Association of Fear of Power with Atypical Role Behavior in Men

Winter (1973) associates high *f* Power with male paranoia. He reviewed clinical evidence that male paranoids feel weak in a conflict with powerful parents and then associate these feelings of weakness and submission with homosexual wishes and fears. Such men want power, which they hope to get from homosexual attachment to a powerful male, but they fear the effects of the desire for power (since it may lead to feared homosexuality) and also fear the power of other people over them. Winter demonstrated that among males, paranoid schizophrenics average much higher on his *f* Power score than nonparanoid schizophrenics or control subjects, whereas there was no difference among these groups in their average *h* Power scores. He further found that high *f* Power was not related to the usual assertive expressions of power motivation, such as having more prestige possessions, holding office more often, or playing with competitive efficiency in a game of cards.

In contrast, high *f* Power did seem to be related to a desire for autonomy as reflected in answers to questions such as how much freedom students should be given in choosing their subjects of study. Also, students who handed their papers in late at the end of a course or requested an incomplete grade scored significantly higher in *f* Power, suggesting to Winter that they resisted being pushed around by course requirements. When he asked students to give the favorite words or phrases they used when swearing, those who used "asshole," some variation thereof, or any homosexual expression scored significantly higher in *f* Power than those who did not use such expressions. Those who used these phrases were if anything, lower in *h* Power. Thus, he concludes that those "high in fear of power have homosexual desires or fears" and that, following Freud, "fear of power seems to result from a reversal in the Oedipal stage. Here the boy identifies with his mother and becomes thereby a sexual object for the father" (Winter, 1973). His conclusions are based on very few subjects and seem rather far-reaching in terms of the data on which they are based, but they are suggestive and deserve to be checked.

Behaviors associated with high *h* Power and *f* Power were examined in a larger sample of adult males of mixed socioeconomic background (McClelland, 1975). The results are summarized in Table 10.9. So far as the supposed lack of competitiveness of men high in *f* Power is concerned, the evidence is mixed. On the one hand, they are not so interested in traveling to new places or playing the field sexually as those high in *h* Power. On the other hand, they do not report playing competitive games like checkers or chess significantly less often and do report getting involved in arguments more frequently, which is not true of those high in *h* Power. Such a correlation does not tell us how effective they are in arguments, so it does not directly disconfirm Winter's finding that they do not play a competitive card game as well.

The evidence for the greater interest in autonomy of those high in *f* Power is somewhat stronger. They report that they have more difficulty getting up in the morning to face the demands of the day, and they also report that they engage in more rituals before going to bed at night. Recall that both Chapter 2

Table 10.9.

CORRELATIONS OF *h* POWER AND *f* POWER SCORES WITH VARIOUS BEHAVIORAL CHARACTERISTICS AMONG ADULT MEN: $N = 85$ (after McClelland, 1975)

Behavioral Characteristics	*h Power*	*f Power*
Assertiveness		
Frequency of arguments	.04	.30**
Frequency of playing competitive games	−.04	−.09
Travel to new places	.20†	.05
Playing the field sexually	.18†	.03
Autonomy		
Frequency of difficulty in getting up in the morning	−.01	.24*
Number of rituals before going to bed	−.09	.19†
n Power score for those predominantly		
At Stage I (intake); $N = 11$	.95***	.78**
At Stage II (autonomy); $N = 12$	.37	.66*
At Stage III (assertion); $N = 13$	.82**	.04
At Stage IV (mutuality); $N = 33$	.80***	.52**
Mystical "at oneness"		
Transpersonal contacts (with God, nature, and so on)	−.04	.32**
Psychological mindedness	−.03	.25*
Preferred metaphor for death as an "infinite ocean"	−.06	.28**
Deviant stature	−.17	.22*

†$p < .10$.
*$p < .05$.
**$p < .01$.
***$p < .001$.

and Chapter 8 pointed out that ritualistic behavior of this type is theoretically associated with the second stage of psychosexual development, which is oriented around breaking away from dependence on the parents and becoming independent or autonomous.

Further confirmation of the orientation toward autonomy is found in the correlations of the total n Power score with the h Power and f Power scores for men oriented predominantly toward each of the four stages of psychosocial maturity. In this analysis, men were assigned to one stage or another, depending on the stage for which they received the highest standard score in Stewart's coding system (see Table 8.5). Thus, twelve men were classified as being oriented primarily toward Stage II (autonomy); the n Power scores of these men were much more likely to be f Power ($r = .66; p < .05$) than h Power ($r = .37$; not significant). The reverse is true for the men at Stage III (assertion). In their case, the n Power scores were nearly all h Power ($r = .82; p < .01$) rather than f Power ($r = .04$; not significant). What this indicates is that f Power is strongly associated with the autonomy stage in psychosocial development and h Power, with the assertive stage in psychosocial development.

What is new in the findings presented in Table 10.9 is the association of f Power scores with various measures of mystical "at oneness." Men high in f Power report having had more transpersonal experiences such as a religious experience of the presence of God; a feeling of being "at one with nature"; or an extrasensory experience, such as communication from someone not present or dead or the feeling of being healed by someone. They also think that one of the better metaphors for death is an "infinite ocean." Finally, men high in f Power score higher on the psychological mindedness scale, which includes such items as "Sometimes I think of natural objects as possessing human qualities" or "The rich internal world of ideals, or sensitive feelings, reverie, of self-knowledge is man's true home." In Chapter 8 the argument was presented that such feelings of mystical union or of psychic reality, being ultimate, are associated with femininity, the mother, or the female life-giving principle. Thus, these results confirm Winter's hypothesis that men high in f Power may have identified more with their mothers. The results also suggest a reason why these men may engage in less agentic striving than is typical of the traditional male role. They may fear that acting assertively in this way would break up their perceived *union* with the environment (nature, the "divine ground," mother).

The final correlation in Table 10.9 suggests that atypical stature in men may have something to do with the development of high f Power. This measure is the absolute deviation of a man's stature from the average stature for men (seventy inches). The correlation means that men who deviated markedly from this average—being either very tall or very short—are more likely to have higher f Power scores. The relationship is not strong, but once again it suggests some kind of inadequacy lying behind the fear of power in men.

Fear of Power Among Women

Among a similar group of adult women of mixed socioeconomic background, f Power scores had no more significant correlates in behavior than would be expected by chance. Fear of Power did correlate significantly with psychological mindedness ($r = .29$; $p < .01$), as it did for the men in the sample, a fact that takes on significance primarily because Stewart (1975) found in a quite independent sample of women that those high in f Power were significantly more likely to mention that problems they had met in life were of a psychological nature. But why should the fear of power turn women inward—or men, for that matter? Perhaps they are afraid of the consequences of assertiveness in the real world, in which it is all too often met with retaliation. So to avoid the push and shove of competitive interaction with people, they retreat to the world of psychic reality, where they have more control over what is happening.

This is reminiscent of the evidence reviewed in the "Fear of Success" section that white women draw back from assertiveness in competing with white men. In one group of subjects, half of whom were men and half of whom were women, there was a significant correlation ($r = .33$; $p < .05$) between the f Power score and the f Success score (McClelland & Watson, 1973). In two samples of adult women college graduates, Stewart (1975) found that f Success was significantly associated with h Power and not f Power. While more evidence is clearly needed to understand the relationship of these two motives, such a result is not inconsistent with the general argument being presented. For it is the women who are most assertive (high in h Power) who might be most likely to fear the consequences of their assertiveness for interpersonal relationships (high in f Success). But the situation is quite different for men, since they have no reason to fear their assertiveness. So among men it may be those who are ambivalent about expressing power (high f Power score)—perhaps for some of the psychodynamic reasons mentioned by Winter—who will also be ambivalent about successful achievement (high f Success score). Both men and women high in f Power and f Success are in conflict over feelings of weakness, compensate for those feelings through assertiveness, and fear the retaliation or rejection that may come from such assertiveness.

• OTHER FEARS

Correlates of Veroff's Need for Power Score as a Measure of Fear of Weakness

As mentioned in Chapter 8, Veroff has interpreted the measure of n Power he developed as indicating anxiety about the ability to exercise power or fear of weakness. His conclusion is justifiable on two grounds. First, to derive his coding system, he obtained stories written while student candidates for office were awaiting election returns, that is, when they were anxious about whether or not they would be able to exercise power. So we might expect his scores to reflect that anxiety. In contrast, the methods of arousing power motivation used by Winter (1973) and Uleman (1972) encouraged subjects to feel confident of their own strength. Second, the characteristics of people scoring high in Veroff n Power suggest they are concerned about being weak.

Table 10.10 summarizes some key results from a national sample survey undertaken in 1976 (Veroff, Depner, Kulka, & Douvan, 1980). So far as the men are concerned, the interpretation seems straightforward. Those scoring high in Veroff *n* Power are more often the sons of blue-collar workers who earn good money themselves, but from a job of low prestige that they do not regard as very interesting. However, they feel good about their competence at work, report that they very often interact affectionately with their wives (which, as Veroff (1982) remarks, "comes close to asking about their sexual activity"), and feel that being a father is very important. In other words, it looks as if they are compensating in the family area for feeling that they lack prestige and importance in the job area. The fact that they stress their competence at work despite its unimportance, as well as in the sexual area, suggests protest masculinity. In effect, they are saying, "Even though my job does not amount to much in my own eyes or the eyes of the world, I am a good worker, make good money, and am a good (sexually competent) husband and father." The fact that they admit to drinking too much and taking drugs also suggests that there is some anxiety about being powerful, since, as we reported in Chapter 8, drinking alcohol is one way men increase feelings of power. None of these behaviors, except drinking, characterizes men who have a score high in Winter *n* Power, who have a more confident approach to exercising power.

The results for women are less clear-cut but can be interpreted in a similar way. Those high in Veroff *n* Power are particularly likely to mention satisfactions obtained from work outside the home (as contrasted with housework), which seems to contribute to their high sense of self-esteem. They do not ex-

Table 10.10.

SELF-REPORTED CHARACTERISTICS OF MEN AND WOMEN WITH A STRONG FEAR OF WEAKNESS: HIGH VEROFF *n* POWER SCORE (after Veroff, 1982)

Area of Assessment	Characteristics of Men (N = 508)	Characteristics of Women (N = 700)
General well-being	—	Rating high in self-esteem
Background	Being a son of a blue-collar worker	
Work	Having a high income Being in an unprestigious occupation Perceiving work as not interesting Feeling good about work competence	Mentioning ego satisfactions from work Preferring work to leisure Feeling high job satisfaction
Family	Having high marital interaction Seeing fatherhood as fulfilling a major value	Feeling low satisfaction with housework
Behavior	Having a drinking problem causing family trouble Taking drugs to relieve tension	Reporting low reliance on informal support in crises

press satisfaction with various aspects of family life the way other women do. And since they do not rely on others for support in crises, they appear more independent than other women, who find more satisfaction in interpersonal relationships. In short, they are strongly work oriented, which could be interpreted as compensation for feelings of weakness or unimportance as a wife and mother or as a worker in comparison with men. That is, since prestige in our society goes with success primarily in a person's occupation, these women may feel inferior in strength in this respect in comparison with men and compensate by concentrating on job success. However, there are no signs of anxiety associated with this focus on the world of work, so the interpretation that it is the result of a fear of weakness is on shakier ground than in the case of men. The most that can be concluded is that the results for women can be interpreted as meaning that high Veroff *n* Power indicates a fear of weakness as a woman, which leads to a compensatory striving for job success, which is not characteristic of women in general.

Fear of Intimacy

Recently Gilligan and Pollak (1982), in a study of themes in fantasy, reported that men's stories more often than women's stories include images of violence in connection with affiliative relationships. They suggest that this may be interpreted to mean that men fear the consequences of intimacy, just as Horner had earlier argued that women feared the consequences of success. The finding deserves further exploration, since it is consistent with the expectation that all social motives have avoidance aspects.

Obviously there are many more specific fears—for example, fear of the dark, fear of high places, fear of being closed in, or fear of school—that have been studied and that might be considered for discussion in a chapter on avoidance motives. They have not been included here on the grounds that the learning associated with them does not qualify as a general motive disposition affecting a variety of behaviors.

• CONCLUSION

The state of knowledge about the avoidance motives is not very satisfactory. Several different avoidance motives have been measured, and individuals who score high in these measures behave in understandably different ways. Yet we do not know which are the most important avoidance motives, how to measure them best, or how they relate to each other. We are not even entirely sure whether avoidance motives differ theoretically in significant ways from approach motives. Much more systematic work needs to be done in this area comparable to the work that has been carried out on approach motives like the need for power and the need for achievement, for which adequate measures have been developed.

NOTES AND QUERIES

1. Make a list of the situations that make you anxious. What do you seek in such situations? Are your goals similar in each situation?

2. According to Aronoff's analysis, what would be likely to happen on the island of Saint Kitts if living and public health conditions improved? After you have made your predictions, consult Aronoff (1971).

3. Construct a model like Atkinson's that accounts more directly for the fact that subjects high in Test Anxiety do better when they think they are doing well and worse when they think they are doing badly.

4. If individuals high in *f* Failure do less well on exams or laboratory tasks, why should they generally get better grades in school?

5. List the grades you want to get for each of the courses you are currently taking. Then list the grades you have received in similar courses in the past, and decide whether your goals for your current courses are defensive, as defined in the chapter, showing a high *f* Failure.

6. Why would subjects high in *f* Failure be more responsive to what others think?

7. If a coach urges a team to do better for "dear old Siwash," what effect is this incentive likely to have on a person high in *n* Achievement, high in *n* Power, high in *n* Affiliation, and high in *f* Rejection?

8. Try to design a study that would show definitively whether or not fear of rejection, fear of failure, and the need for approval are different aspects of the same avoidance motive.

9. Suppose a female executive is asked to play golf with her male boss. Explain some of the motivational factors possibly present in the situation that would affect how well she played.

10. Describe at least two conditions in which a man high in *f* Success could be expected to perform less well.

11. In Chapter 2, homosexuality was associated with oral aggressiveness (late Stage I); in Chapter 9, with early sexual maturity during homosocial groupings; and in this chapter, with Stage II (autonomy strivings). How could all these relationships possibly be true? Is it helpful to think in terms of what might lead to homosexual attachments and what motives might arise after they have been formed?

12. If psychic mindedness in men is associated with identification with the feminine principle and related to high *f* Power, why should psychic mindedness in women also be related to high *f* Power?

13. If high Veroff *n* Power represents a fear of weakness, at least in men, should it not be related to Winter's *f* Power, which also is associated with feelings of inadequacy?

14. Would you expect the Hostile Press score to be more related to the *f* Power score or the *f* Success score?

15. Perhaps all the avoidance motives that have been identified are aspects of the same anxiety, or "tension reduction," motive of such great theoretical importance to the behaviorists (see Chapter 3). One indication that this might be true would be that they all influence behavior in the same way. Review the behavioral correlates of the different avoidance motives to examine the extent to which the behaviors they lead to are the same or different. Is there any single type of behavior characteristic of one avoidance motive that is not characteristic of other avoidance motives, so a case for keeping avoidance motives separate can be made?

Part 4

Contextual Effects on Human Motives

11

Motivational Trends in Society

• ANALYZING THE REASONS FOR THE GROWTH AND DECLINE OF CIVILIZATIONS

Cultures, like individuals, differ greatly not only from each other, but from themselves at different moments in time. Some are peaceful, others aggressive; some rich, some poor; some expansive and mobile, others stay-at-home. Anthropologists, historians, economists, political scientists, and philosophers have often tried to figure out why. Why were the Romans such geniuses at military and civic organization, and the Greeks not? Why were the Greeks so successful economically for some hundreds of years before Christ only to disappear for a time as a nation of importance in world history? Why did the Roman Empire rise and fall? When a second flowering of civilization occurred on the Italian peninsula during the Renaissance, why was it in the arts rather than in military science, as at a much earlier period? What caused the British Empire to expand over the entire face of the globe in the nineteenth century and to decline almost equally rapidly in the twentieth? Why were the British more successful than any other European nation?

Answers by historians to such questions tend to be given in terms of particular events in history, such as a battle that was won or lost, suddenly favorable terms of trade, or the discovery of a new economic resource to exploit. Such events are of great importance, but they appear to become influential because of national aspirations or collective motivations. Yes, the British were favored in the nineteenth century by being relatively free from land invasion, but they were also more enterprising than other peoples. And in the twentieth century they seem to have lost their "drive," although they occupy the same territory and are still free from land invasion. Or consider the ancient Romans. Once they got organized, they operated from a base that had many natural advantages, but first they had to come back from defeat after defeat on land and at sea at the hands of Hannibal and other Carthaginian generals. Why did they bounce back again and again? Scholars inevitably turn to explanations in terms of character or collective motivation. Some nations or cultures appear to be more "motivated"—to be more active in military, economic, or aesthetic spheres—at some times than others. What has psychology had to say about the role of collective motivations in history and society?

Freud on the Motivational Origins of Civilization

The formal discussion was started in a serious way by Sigmund Freud (1930/1958) who asked the most fundamental question of all: Why should people create any kind of civilization? Why should they not live like other animals, in simple social orders in which primitive urges for food, sex, or aggression are directly and immediately gratified? Why do they construct elaborate governmental structures, norms governing interpersonal relations, artistic and intellectual monuments to people's pride?

He found at least part of the answer in a biologically determined sexual urge that a son has to sleep with his mother and to destroy his arch-rival, his father. Freud called this basic motivational conflict the *Oedipus complex* after the Greek mythical hero who did unwittingly kill his father and sleep with his mother. Because he loves his father and for other reasons, every son eventually observes the incest taboo, represses acting out his sexual interest in his mother, and seeks substitute satisfaction for his thwarted sexual drives in work and in creating a social structure through which his urges can be satisfied later and less directly. The son learns that to get what he wants—let us say sex—without destroying himself and the family, he must "grow up," accept the rules on which his parents insist, go to school, learn a trade, and observe the rules of courtship and marriage.

According to Freud, millions of young men acting out this primitive motivational drama succeed in creating the elaborate edifice we call *society.* By this line of reasoning the most complex social institutions are interpreted as the creation of simple motivational urges and the conflicts among them. Capitalism, for instance, which is often seen as the motivational force behind modern economic development, has been interpreted as an acting out of the urge to "accumulate filthy lucre," or more literally, feces (Fromm, 1947). Sexual or libidinal urges in boys get satisfaction first from various parts of the body; then the boys transfer their attachment to the mother (see Chapter 2). Some peoples get fixated at the "holding-on" stage (see Table 2.4), when pleasure is gained especially from accumulating and playing with feces. Such peoples are motivated especially to accumulate and to become capitalists, according to some followers of Freud.

Other theorists have drawn attention to other types of motivations for civilized activities that derive from the unfolding of sexual and aggressive instincts in the nucleus of the family. N. O. Brown (1959), for instance, has argued that the fundamental motive for creating civilization is the fear of death, of one's own mortality. Social institutions become ways of protecting people from thinking about death or guaranteeing immortality. D. Bakan (1966) believes that the fundamental motives for the two sexes differ: Men are agentic, seeking dominion and control. Women, on the other hand, seek communion or the kind of interrelatedness that permits them to rear their children successfully.

Basic Motivational Structure and Culture

But how could such general motivations account for *variations* in culture growth? Ralph Linton (1945), an anthropologist, and Abram Kardiner (1945), a psychoanalyst, reasoned in the 1940s that a certain social or economic condition might favor the development of people of a certain personality type who would in turn create a special type of culture. Child-rearing practices differ greatly from one culture to another and even in the same culture from one period in its history to another. It seemed logical to suppose that some society might stress toilet training, for instance, in a way that would create more people who, when they grew up, would continue to be interested in hoarding and presumably therefore in capitalistic enterprise as a way of satisfying this urge.

Many case studies were written of particular societies (see, for example, Erikson, 1950/1963) that showed that the type of adult motivations that characterized a society did indeed seem to reflect the way children were reared. For instance, Kardiner (1945), in studying the people of Alor, an island in the Portuguese East Indies, found that the adult males seemed to be suspicious and distrustful, primarily because they had been fed irregularly and abandoned by their mothers in their first month of life because the mothers had to go out to work the family garden daily to survive. An economic condition (daily gardening by the mother away from home) created a child-rearing practice (frequent desertion of children) that produced a personality type (suspicious and distrustful) that made it difficult for the Alorese to collaborate and produce a thriving economy.

Wolfenstein and Leites (1950) analyzed family relationships in a number of U.S. films of the 1940s and discovered what appeared to be an unusual variation in the way the classic son-mother-father triangle was pictured. In these films the father figure or older man typically appeared as bumbling and ineffectual, whether as an ineffectual or corrupt sheriff who could not keep order in a Western town or as an ignorant, perhaps immigrant father who did not understand what was going on. The hero or son figure therefore typically had to take over and set things right. The women to whom the hero was attracted often appeared to be "bad women," but on further acquaintance they turned out to be wholesome types who just happened to be substituting for a friend as a nightclub singer for the evening. Thus, the intensity of the oedipal conflict is eased for the U.S. son, because his father is pictured as somebody too ineffectual to be worth hating and because the son is sexually attracted to bad women (not at all like mother), although they really are like mother underneath.

It does not take any great leap of the imagination to explain the participation of male students in the revolts of the 1960s in just these terms. The young men were showing the characteristic U.S. disrespect for authority figures (fathers, policemen, and college administrators), whom they regarded as bumbling and ineffectual and from whom they must take over the reins of power if society were to improve. Similarly, the young men appeared to be consorting with bad women in sex or drug orgies and "be-ins," yet on further examination these bad women turned out to be wholesome types from the next block. Of course, some further explanation would be needed as to why the U.S. version of the oedipal conflict led to student apathy in the 1950s and revolt in the 1960s, but these analysts would argue that to observe that Americans in the family rebel successfully against their fathers is a start at explaining why there is so much distrust of authority in the United States.

A group of scholars used this approach extensively shortly after World War II in an attempt to find the underlying motivation for the rise of Naziism in Germany and particularly the German persecution of the Jews (Adorno, Frenkel-Brunswik, Levinson, & Sanford, 1950). They discovered it in an authoritarian personality syndrome characterized by "dominance-subordination, deference towards superiors; sensitivity to power relationships; need to perceive the world in a highly structured fashion; excessive use of stereotypes; and adherence to whatever values are conventional in one's setting" (Greenstein, 1969). After carefully examining case histories of highly authoritarian and nonauthoritarian people, they stressed the importance of early experiences in the family in developing this particular cluster of traits:

> When we consider the childhood situation . . . we find reports of a tendency toward rigid discipline on the part of the parents with affection which is conditional rather than unconditional, i.e., dependent upon approved behavior on the part of the child. Related to this is the tendency . . . to base [family] interrelationships on rather clearly defined roles of dominance and submission. . . . Forced into a surface submission to parental authority, the child develops hostility and aggression which are purely channelized. The displacement of a repressed antagonism toward authority may be one of the sources and perhaps the principal source, of his antagonism toward out groups. (Adorno et al., 1950)

In other words, children who are reared strictly and rigidly, often in a way that suggests rejection by the parents, turn their hostility away from their respected parents toward outgroups, such as Jews and other minorities. German families were considered to rear their children more often in these ways and therefore to produce the motivational characteristics of the authoritarian personality syndrome, which in turn was responsible for the rise of Naziism in Germany.

Objections to Motivational Analysis of Historical Events

Critics of this type of motivational analysis of collective phenomena have been numerous. They have contended—sometimes quite persuasively—that to attribute psychological motivations to historical or social events is at worst absurd or at best unnecessary and circular. At times motivational analysis of social characteristics does appear circular. The reasoning runs as follows. A society requires a certain personality type for its survival, so parents bring up their children so that they have motives to act in ways required by society. German society required order and discipline; therefore, German parents must have trained children to want order and discipline. In the United States, people are disrespectful of male authority figures. Therefore, the culture must structure the mother-son-father triangle in ways that make sons want to belittle their fathers.

Is anything added to knowledge by such statements? Is not the desire to attribute "motives" to events a primitive, animistic way of thinking, as we pointed out in Chapter 2? In much the same way, a young child might state that an apple fell from a tree because "it wanted to." We might well ask, Why does it "want to" now and not ten minutes ago? Why did the Germans produce Naziism in the 1930s and not before? The trouble with defining motivations as responses to requirements of the social system is that it does not explain change. Motives become "explanations" for whatever happened that cannot be accounted for by other causes.

The only way out of this circularity is to find some independent way of measuring the alleged collective motivation. Then observers can check to see whether the motives in fact existed that they are using to account for social events. They might be able to show, for instance, that some motivational characteristics of the authoritarian syndrome were in fact higher in Germany at the time of Naziism than they had been previously or than they were in other countries, which did not produce Naziism. A study of motives in society avoids the circularity accusation only when motives can be measured and their contribution to what happened in society assessed independently of the events themselves.

Some scholars have argued that independent assessment of motivation is unnecessary even if it can be done. Most economists, political scientists, and historians have managed to discuss quite sensibly what has happened in history without reference to human motivations; at most they make a simple assumption about the desire to pursue rational self-interest, which appears sufficient to account for most of the social events with which they are dealing. For example, Robert Waelder (1960), a psychoanalyst, was once asked by a social scientist studying the rise of Naziism to give his explanation of what motivated this development. He replied that he thought the success of Prussian militarism in bringing about the unification of Germany had much to do with creating faith in strong-arm methods. Furthermore, the Germans had tried the democratic process and found it unable to cope with problems of inflation and disunity in the 1920s. In other words, Waelder was arguing that the immediate past experiences of the German people, combined with a simple motivational theory about people promoting their own self-interest, were sufficient to account for the rise of Naziism. He goes on to say, "I was then interrupted by my host, a noted anthropologist. This was not what I had been expected to contribute. As a psychoanalyst I should point out how Naziism had developed from the German form of child rearing. I replied that I did not think that there was any such relationship; in fact, political opinion did not seem to me to be determined in early childhood at all. This view was not accepted and I was told that the way the German mother holds her baby must be different from that of mothers in democracies" (Waelder, 1960).

Waelder's view that childhood motivations are largely irrelevant for explaining complex political events is widely shared. But they may be irrelevant for several reasons that are worth examining a little further. They may be irrelevant because motives formed in childhood are simply less important in governing adult behavior than motives arising out of the concrete historical situation in which the adults find themselves. Thus, many social scientists who reject childhood analyses of social character are quite willing to accept similar analyses based on contemporary motivational pressures. An economist might argue that certain groups of people were forced to leave the farm and go to the city because of population pressure in the rural areas. They left because there was too little to eat for so many mouths to feed. They did leave. Therefore they must have been forced to want to. Although this form of motivational analysis is much more popular than the childhood form, it is just as circular. It is assumed that population pressure—or scarcity of food—will make people want to migrate. In fact, that is not always the case. Some peoples migrate under such conditions and others do not. What is needed here, as in the study of childhood motives, is some direct measure of what people want. Only then will the observer be able to predict who will migrate and who will not when there is little to eat (see McClelland & Winter, 1971).

Granted that some motivational analysis is ideally desirable and even necessary, is not the easiest way to find out about people's motives simply to ask them what they want? Thus, one implication of Waelder's argument about the German people would appear to be that if a public opinion poll had been conducted in Germany, say in 1930, it would have been quite possible to find out that the German people wanted Naziism in one form or other. Childhood motivations may be considered irrelevant, because just asking people what they want is a better guide to their actions. It is a fact that public opinion surveys have been found useful in identifying wants that have important social effects. For example, such surveys are now routinely used to make economic forecasts, because the number of people who say they want to buy a car will in fact predict how many cars will be bought in the following year—a fact that is of tremendous importance not only to the auto industry, but to economic planners as well. Politicians have also learned to watch attitude surveys to see what their constituents want and to try to shape their campaign promises and public performance in the light of that information.

Here it is useful to distinguish, as explained in Chapter 8, between demands and motive dispositions. A demand is an immediate situational pressure that evokes about the same motivational intent in all people exposed to it. Thus, a hurricane produces a desire to seek safety; an insult, a desire to retaliate; a bank failure, a desire to withdraw one's money; or cutting prices in half, a desire to buy. Such demands create intents that can be accurately reported by people in public opinion polls, and they will predict actions in the short run but not in the long run. So far as individuals are concerned, demands will predict immediate responses, as when an experimenter asks a subject to take off his or her coat, but any given demand will not predict whether a person will usually wear a coat. Measures of motive dispositions are necessary to explain general long-term "drifts" of behavior over varieties of demand situations—who is more likely to wear a coat over the long term or who is more likely to resist a request to take off his or her coat.

Reasoning by analogy, we would expect then that measures of collective motivation would be better at predicting long-term social trends than at predicting what will happen at any particular time and place. Motivational concerns of nations or cultures, like motivational concerns of individuals, should predict aggregates of actions—say, the number of homicides over a five-year period—rather than particular actions, such as a riot in Detroit. To get at the reasons for a riot in Detroit, it might be better to conduct a public opinion poll to find out what people in the area wanted in that particular place at that particular time.

Measuring Collective Motives

As we have seen, individual psychology escaped the charge of circularity in making motivational analyses by not simply inferring motives from actions, but by insisting on checking these inferences independently by studying fantasy or what was going on in a person's mind. Thus, at the individual level, it is not enough to infer that because a person is studying very hard in school, he or she therefore must have a strong need to achieve. Instead, we must observe thoughts or fantasies and see how prominent the theme of achievement is in them. Only then can we state, based on evidence other than the act of studying itself, that a person has a strong need to achieve, for studying hard may be motivated by a variety of motives—the need to achieve; the desire for social approval; or devotion to parents, who are expecting a strong scholastic record. It is impossible to tell from a performance itself what motivated it. And asking people what their motives are may also not always be helpful, because they will often give the answer that appears socially desirable at the moment. Instead, it is necessary to ask individuals to tell a number of stories, which may be coded for a variety of motivational themes, to find out what is generally of concern to them. This was explained in Chapter 6.

The same line of reasoning can be applied to assessing collective motives. It is circular reasoning to assume that because of the Nazi dictatorship, the Germans had a strong need for power. It would have been unsafe and possibly misleading to ask the German leaders or the general public in a public opinion poll what their motives were. Instead, it is necessary to find out what the German people had on their minds by studying their collective fantasies—as they occur in popular plays or novels, stories for children, or often-retold folk tales. Such material has been coded for the three most widely studied individual motives—namely, *n* Achievement, *n* Affiliation, and *n* Power.

The behavior of individuals scoring high in these motives may give some clues as to what nations will be like when their collective fantasies are focused on achievement, affiliation, or power. But we obviously cannot jump from individual to collective psychology in any simple, straightforward way without careful empirical checks. What, in fact, are nations with a high concern for affiliation like? Will they protect civil rights more? Will they be less aggressive toward their neighbors? Will they develop better local transportation systems or faster direct-dialing telephone systems? Will they be more likely to sponsor child-centered forms of education?

A number of empirical studies have begun to provide answers to questions like these. But before we review them, it should be noted that the "need" terminology used to describe motives at the individual level may not be appropriate at the collective level. When a large number of achievement themes are found in children's stories of a given country, it is not altogether clear what the measure reflects in the country. It may mean that because there are a lot of individuals in the culture whose fantasies turn to achievement, some individuals with high *n* Achievement are more likely to be involved in writing children's stories. In this sense, the achievement content of the stories may reflect the mobile or successful personality types in the culture. Or it may be considered not so much a reflection of the motivation of individuals as an index of a prevailing ideology that shapes everybody's thoughts to a greater or lesser degree in that nation. In this sense we might conceive of collective "needs" that bear only an indirect relationship to the distribution of individual needs in the country. Most authors continue to use the "need" terminology to signal the relationship of collective to individual motives, as we shall see, but they do not intend to suggest that the measures have identical meanings or identical effects in action at individual and collective levels.

• THE COLLECTIVE CONCERN FOR ACHIEVEMENT, ENTREPRENEURSHIP, AND ECONOMIC GROWTH

The case best worked out for the influence of motivational levels on society is the one that links the achievement motive to rate of economic growth. It grew out of studies made of the activities of individuals scoring high in *n* Achievement. As noted in Chapter 7, they tend to be attracted to moderately challenging tasks, to do better at such tasks, to take personal responsibility for a job at work, and to seek feedback on the quality of work—all with the goal of constantly trying to do better. It seemed likely that such men would make good business entrepreneurs, because the business role demands taking carefully calculated risks, using feedback to improve the profit picture, innovating to promote efficiency, and so forth. As data summarized in Chapter 7 make clear, individuals high in *n* Achievement in fact are more likely to turn out to be successful entrepreneurs.

It seemed reasonable to infer that if a culture's collective fantasies were oriented around achievement, that culture should contain a larger number of entrepreneurs. The hypothesis was checked by examining the folk tales from thirty-nine preliterate societies (Kulakow, cited in McClelland, 1961). Folk tales in many ways are like the imaginative stories written by individuals and scored for *n* Achievement. They are short, with a beginning, a middle, and an end; they involve fantasy; and they have the added advantage of representing an oral tradition, meaning that they have been told and retold by different individuals from the culture over time. This should mean that if there is a dominant focus on a theme like achievement in the culture, it should get into the stories. The only disadvantage of using folk tales is that they are not as structured as the stories written by individuals, so the subcategories of the scoring system cannot readily be applied. Therefore, only the number of achievement images was counted in the twelve folk tales collected for each culture. Then, from ethnographic records, it was determined whether there were any full-time entrepreneurs in the cultures. Among twenty-two preliterate societies whose folk tales contained an above-median amount of achievement imagery, 74 percent contained at least some full-time entrepreneurs, as contrasted with only 35 percent of the cultures with below-median amounts of achievement imagery, a difference that is highly significant. This was a clear instance of a hypothesis derived at the individual level that was confirmed at the collective level, that is, by comparing a measure of collective motivation with an index of a type of activity in the culture.

A Motivational Explanation for the Growth and Decline of Ancient Civilizations

Another study pushed the reasoning one step further: if collective achievement motivation was associated with the presence of more entrepreneurs, their energetic activity should be associated with signs of greater economic growth. The hypothesis was first tested by examining achievement motive trends and stages of economic development in the history of ancient Greece. Three periods in

Greek history were distinguished—a period of growth, roughly from 900 B.C. to 475 B.C.; a period of climax, roughly from 475 B.C. to 362 B.C.; and a period of decline, from 362 B.C. to 100 B.C. Comparable samples of Greek literature were selected from each of these periods and scored for *n* Achievement. The selections centered around six different themes: the relationship of people to their gods, farm and estate management, public funeral celebrations, poetry, epigrams, and war speeches of encouragement. For example, in connection with the last theme, all instances of a man's encouraging others to fight in Homer's *Iliad* were scored for the early period, a similar speech by Pericles as recorded by Thucydides was scored for the period of climax, and a speech by Demosthenes was scored for the later period. All of these selections, consisting of 8,440 lines or over 80,000 words, were mixed together and scored blindly—in the sense that the scorer did not know from which period the selections came—for *n* Achievement (Berlew, 1956; McClelland, 1958b).

Historians agree that the period from 475 to 362 B.C. represented the peak of Athenian Greek commercial success, leaving out a very brief period of expansion under Alexander later; quantitative support for this consensus was obtained by constructing maps of the area within which Athenian Greece traded in the sixth, fifth, and fourth centuries B.C. (Berlew, 1956). Such maps could be made because Greece traded largely by exporting surplus wine and olive oil in earthenware jars to various places overseas, and these were discarded when empty. Archaeologists have identified places where the remains of such vases have been found and determined which century they represent from markings on them. Locating the distances of these pottery remains from Athens gives a rough index of Athenian trade area, which shows a steep rise in the fifth century B.C. as noted by historians. See Figure 11.1, which plots the average *n* Achievement score per hundred lines of text in the early, middle, and late periods. Note that the *n* Achievement level was highest before the expansion of Athenian commercial civilization and had declined significantly during the period of economic climax, thus foreshadowing the subsequent economic decline in the area. The general hypothesis is confirmed that collective levels of high *n* Achievement precede economic growth, and collective levels of low *n* Achievement precede economic decline.

Independent confirmation of this relationship was obtained in a different way. As noted in Chapter 7, Aronson (1958) discovered that individuals high in *n* Achievement used more S shapes and diagonals and fewer multiple waves in "doodles" or free-line drawings than individuals low in *n* Achievement. Again, by analogy from the individual to the cultural level, it was reasoned that vases in the early period of Greek history should contain more S shapes and diagonals and fewer multiple waves than vases from later periods in Greek history. Examination of 242 vases from the periods of growth, climax, and decline showed the same decline in this index of collective *n* Achievement level as that obtained from scoring literary productions. Approximately 65 percent of the vases from the early period showed an above-median number of diagonals or S shapes, as contrasted with about 45 percent of the vases from the period of climax and 15 percent of the vases from the period of decline (McClelland, 1958b). Figure 11.2

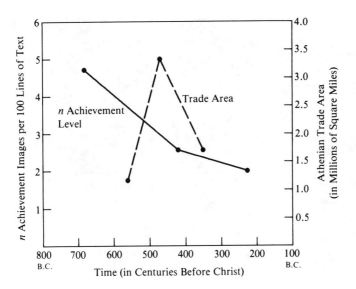

Figure 11.1.

Average *n* Achievement Level Plotted at Midpoints of Periods of Growth, Climax, and Decline of Athenian Commercial Civilization as Reflected in the Extent of Trade Area (after McClelland, 1961).

shows a vase from an earlier period containing many diagonals and S shapes and few multiple waves as contrasted with a vase from a later period showing the reverse pattern.

Davies (1969) subsequently extended this type of analysis to explain the collapse of ancient Minoan civilization on the island of Crete, from which no decipherable written records exist. He obtained an *n* Achievement index score for each pot in three samples of pottery representing three different periods in the history of Minoan civilization. He found once again that by this index, the average level of *n* Achievement was significantly higher in the early period, before the building of great cities and palaces in the middle period (see Table 11.1). There was some rebuilding after great earthquakes in 1640 B.C., but following the eruption of a volcano at Thera in 1450 B.C., which caused tidal waves to flood Minoan seaports, the civilization went into a steady decline. Previous historians have supposed that these external disasters were responsible for the decline of Minoan civilization, but Davies argues that the real cause was loss of the achievement motive, or the psychic energy needed to build and maintain a thriving commercial empire, for the natural disasters such as the tidal waves did not come far enough inland to affect many of the cities directly.

What is especially exciting about such findings is that changes in the collective concern for achievement *preceded* the rise and fall of a civilization. It is common sense to infer that levels of achievement concern were high during the periods of climax of these civilizations, for would that not explain why they

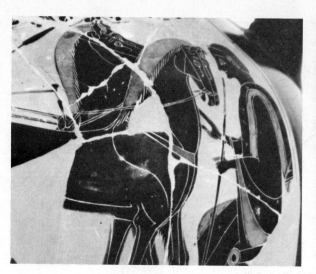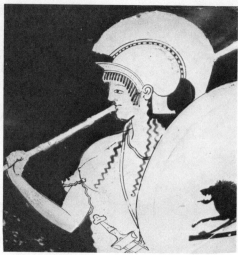

Figure 11.2.

Greek Vases from Earlier and Later Periods Illustrating S Shapes and Diagonals Characteristic of High *n* Achievement (*Left*) and Multiple Waves Characteristic of Low *n* Achievement (*Right*). The left, black-figured Greek vase is from the early fifth century B.C. and the right, red-figured vase, from the late fifth century B.C.

Table 11.1.

MEAN POTTERY INDEX OF *n* ACHIEVEMENT LEVELS FOR THREE PERIODS IN MINOAN CIVILIZATION (after Davies, 1969)

Period	Number of Vases	Mean Pottery Index of n Achievement[a]
Early (2600–1950 B.C.)	37	5.2[b]
Climax (1950–1650 B.C.) Earthquake (1650 B.C.)	67	3.1
Late (1600–1400 B.C.) Eruption of Thera (1450 B.C.) Collapse of Minoan civilization	24	2.7

[a]S shapes plus diagonals minus multiple waves or zigzags.
[b]Significantly higher than for later periods.

were doing so well at that time—expanding trade and building great palaces and cities that could be discovered centuries later by archaeologists? But such reasoning falls into the trap of simply naming a motive to account for a certain type of activity. Actual measurement of achievement motive levels shows that they were higher before the periods of climax and presumably accounted for the increased entrepreneurial activity that accumulated the resources to build the palaces and cities in the period of climax.

Reasons for the Loss of Achievement Motivation and Economic Decline

But why did achievement motive levels decline? Two explanations have been advanced. McClelland (1961) drew on the knowledge gained from studying the behavior of mothers of sons high in *n* Achievement (see Chapter 7) to argue that as Greek merchants accumulated more and more resources as a result of their increased entrepreneurial activity, they used the resources to support household slaves to look after their children. These slaves, particularly the pedagogue who walked the child to school, were so available for child care that it seemed likely they would spoil the children and not make the kind of demands for achievement that mothers make who have sons high in *n* Achievement.

McClelland (1961/1976) advanced a similar argument to explain why the South lost the U.S. Civil War. There too, successful merchants or planters, presumably high in *n* Achievement, acquired household slaves, who might well have spoiled the "young master" to promote their own self-interest, thereby undermining the achievement demands of the parents. This would mean that succeeding generations in the South would have lower *n* Achievement levels than in the North, where there were no household slaves, with the consequence that the South would in time become less developed economically than the North. Most historians agree that this was the case at the time of the Civil War and that one of the main reasons the South lost the war was that it had lesser economic resources to sustain it in the long run.

Unfortunately, such theorizing, while it appears reasonable, has never been directly tested. Another explanation for the decline in *n* Achievement levels following increases in prosperity is simpler and derives directly from Atkinson's model of the aroused tendency to achieve as a function of the probability of success and the incentive value of success (see Table 7.2). According to that model, as the probability of success increases, the incentive value of success decreases, so when tasks are easy or commercial success is assured, the level of aroused achievement interest declines. The model is designed to explain the temporary arousal value of tasks, but it might be supposed that if tasks regularly had little arousal value, the level of dispositional *n* Achievement would also decline. There is some empirical evidence for such a supposition in a study by Andrews (1967) in which he found that levels of *n* Achievement declined over three years for businessmen working in a company that did not present moderate achievement challenges to them. It is difficult to know just how findings at the individual level apply to the collective level, but one simplifying assumption is to suppose that collective concerns also follow the Atkinson model. Then one could argue that the perception of national prosperity from commercial success lowers the collective interest in achievement, just as it does at the individual level.

What is needed to validate such a claim is a systematic study showing that periods of prosperity are followed by a decline in the collective concern for achievement. Several instances of such a relationship are found throughout this chapter, and one careful study has been made of the effect of profitability in a company on lowering subsequent levels of *n* Achievement. (This will be discussed later.) But more attention needs to be given to testing directly the applicability of the Atkinson model at the collective level.

Waves of Achievement Concern and Economic Expansion in the Middle Ages

The explanation for the rise and fall of ancient civilizations was so simple and straightforward, and its empirical confirmation so striking, that other investigators immediately began testing the motivational explanation for economic growth in other times and places. Perhaps the level of achievement concern is important only at very early stages of national development. Could it also account for such complex historical events as the commercial opening up of the New World by the Spanish Conquest in the sixteenth century or the Industrial Revolution in England in the nineteenth century? Did the voyage of Christopher Columbus signify a high level of achievement concern in Spain at the time? Why were voyages not being sponsored by other countries, such as England and France, at the same time? Why did the English voyages come later? Was the English level of achievement concern low earlier, and did it increase? These are the kinds of questions that can be empirically answered using the new methodology of coding popular literature for motivational concerns.

Cortés (1960, in McClelland, 1961) coded popular literature in Spain before, during, and after the period of maximum commercial expansion into the New World. Once again the *n* Achievement levels were estimated by coding a large amount of literary material: about 100,000 words from fifty-six different authors in each of three time periods. As Figure 11.3 illustrates, he found exactly the same relationship as Berlew had obtained earlier for ancient Greece: *n* Achievement levels were high before the period of rapid commercial expansion of Spain into the New World and declined prior to the collapse of Spain's economic empire. The voyages of discovery were sponsored by a country whose *n* Achievement level had been high, giving it the energy and resources to pursue further economic advantage in the New World. And again, prosperity—perhaps particularly the accumulation of gold—lowered subsequent levels of *n* Achievement.

To look for motivational factors underlying waves of economic expansion in England, Bradburn and Berlew (1961) examined a large amount of textual material over a longer period of time, roughly from 1400 to 1830 A.D., representing seven different epochs. They coded 150 pages of comparable text material from forty to fifty authors for each time period, representing usually a half century. Their objective was to select passages from material that had roughly the same form and function throughout the entire historical period studied. So they scored selections from plays (about 2,240 lines per period), accounts of sea voyages (about 2,500 lines per period), and street ballads (about 1,308 lines per period). They chose street ballads to represent the thoughts and feelings of ordinary people who listened to them recited in the streets, and plays and accounts of sea voyages to represent what was on the minds of a better-educated class of people. As in the case of ancient Greece, the amount of achievement imagery

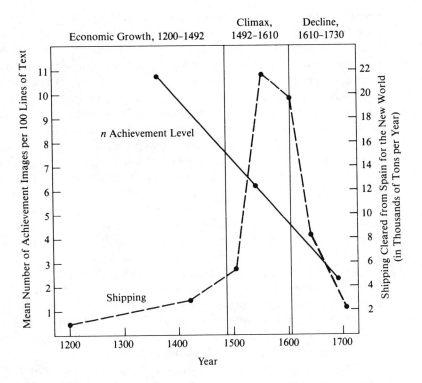

Figure 11.3.

Average *n* Achievement Level in Literature at Midpoints of Periods of Economic Growth, Climax, and Decline in Spain from 1200 to 1700 (after McClelland, 1961).

per one hundred lines for each of these three categories of material was averaged to get an overall index of the *n* Achievement level for that time period.

Then a rough index of economic activity in England was obtained by examining gains in coal imports at London. To get a time series reflecting quantitatively approximate changes in rates of expansion of the English economy was difficult, but Bradburn and Berlew finally found that reports of coal imports at London were the best continuously available figures that would approximately reflect how much fuel the expanding economy was using at different time periods. When the coal figures first become available, coal was important not only for domestic fuel but also for the dressing of meat, washing, brewing, and dyeing—all key activities in the developing English economy. The amount of coal imported increased regularly from the earliest to the latest period considered, and the higher the level of imports, the greater in absolute terms the increase to the next time period.

What the investigators wanted to know was whether the gain was greater or less than could be expected given the level of economic activity in the previous period. To find out, they used a linear regression formula to predict the gain from the previous level and then observed whether the actual gain was more or less than expected in terms of the overall trend. Since this statistical method of estimating *rates* of growth is used throughout this chapter, it is important that it be understood. An analogy may make the point clear. It is common to calculate what a person's expected grade in college should be based on an intelligence or aptitude test score. People with more scholastic aptitude generally get better grades. Given this relationship, it is possible to estimate that a given person, Susan, with her aptitude should be able to get an A. If she gets a B, we say she is an underachiever. She is doing well, but not as well as could be expected given her aptitude. Similarly, Bradburn and Berlew estimated whether the level of economic gain in a given period represented overachievement or underachievement in relation to its starting level, given the general relationship between levels of economic activity at the outset of the periods (analogous to aptitude) and subsequent gains in economic activity (analogous to grades achieved).

As shown in Figure 11.4, according to this measure, gains in coal imports were above expectation in the early period (representing overachievement), then dropped considerably (representing underachievement), and finally rose sharply toward the end of the eighteenth century. The *n* Achievement levels also shown in Figure 11.4 behave as if they are having an influence on subsequent rates of economic growth. They are high in the sixteenth century, preceding the first rapid rate of economic growth; then decline preceding a drop in the rate of economic growth; and finally rise again sharply, predicting the great increase in economic activity in England preceding the Industrial Revolution toward the end of the eighteenth century.

Furthermore, the English *n* Achievement level in the earliest period (1400 to 1550) is lower than later (1550 to 1600), whereas in Spain the *n* Achievement levels dropped sharply over the same time period (Figure 11.3). Thus, a comparison of the *n* Achievement levels in the two countries from 1400 to 1600 predicts that entrepreneurial voyages of exploration should be more frequent in the earlier part of this period for Spain than for England, and more frequent for England than for Spain in the later period. This was actually the case, as shown by the voyages from Spain to South America in the early part of the seventeenth century and the voyages from England to North America in the early part of the sixteenth century.

Findings for England in Figure 11.4 differ from the earlier ones for Greece and Spain in that there are two waves of high *n* Achievement followed by increases and decreases in rates of economic growth. Economic historians have pointed out that the great improvement in the British economy in the early nineteenth century required many concrete changes, such as agricultural improvement through crop rotation; enclosures of land, permitting a marked increase in sheep population; the development of an extensive system of transport through turnpike roads; improved credit; an increase in available capital, and an educational system to turn out the kind of workers needed by industry. Figure 11.4 suggests that a heightened level of achievement motivation in the country as a whole led individuals to make all these changes in various sectors of the so-

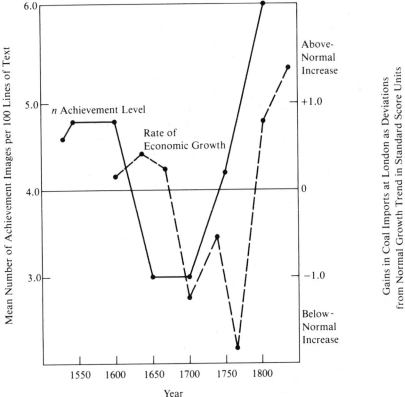

Figure 11.4.

Average *n* Achievement Levels in Samples of English Literature (1500–1800) Compared with Rates of Acceleration and Deceleration in English Economy, Measured by Coal Imports at London (data from Bradburn & Berlew, 1961).

ciety. In other words, the motive measure comes closer to answering the ultimate question as to *why* all these changes were introduced. They were the *means* of improving how the society functioned and were designed to satisfy an increased collective concern for improvement.

How Collective Achievement Concerns Predict Rates of Economic Growth Among Modern Nations

So much for historical changes in rates of economic development. What about modern nations? Can variations in their rates of growth be predicted from levels of collective achievement concern? To test such a possibility, some form of popular literature had to be found that would yield roughly comparable data from countries widely different in level of modernization, industrialization, religious orientation, and so forth. Stories read by children in the public schools were chosen, because they seemed roughly comparable from country to country in purpose, in length, in imaginativeness, and in the extent to which they were relatively uninfluenced by historical events of temporary significance. They seemed comparable to the folk tales used in the study of preliterate cultures in the sense that they often represented an oral tradition in which recurrent cultural themes were shaped by educational authorities to produce stories that everyone would agree should be read by children. Even though the same plot may be present in the textbooks of several countries, such as Aesop's fable of the Fox and the Raven, it is retold in ways that can stress, for example, either achievement or power. Consider, for example, the two versions of the well-known story about the hare and the tortoise in Table 11.2. The plot is the same, but in Portugal the tortoise starts the action by wanting to do better than the hare in a race (*n* Achievement). In England the hare starts the action by boasting of his prowess (*n* Power) and making fun of the tortoise.

In most countries educational authorities take great care to make sure that children read in school what is considered right and proper. What educational authorities think is right for children to read may well represent the motivational ideas uppermost in the minds of people in a country. At least, this was the assumption made in coding children's stories for *n* Achievement, *n* Power, and *n* Affiliation from twenty-three countries in 1925 and thirty-nine countries in 1950 (McClelland, 1961). In each case, twenty-one stories were selected at random from at least three different readers from the second, third, and fourth grades.

As a measure of rate of economic growth, McClelland (1961) employed figures on kilowatt-hours of electricity used, since national income figures were not available in the early period, nor were they comparable from country to country. The advantage of the electricity figures is that they are available in compa-

---

Table 11.2.

ALTERNATIVE VERSIONS OF THE STORY OF THE TORTOISE AND THE HARE

One day the tortoise said to the hare, "Say, Ma'am, *I bet that I can get to that bramble patch first*."[a] The hare replied, "Say, mister, surely you must be off your rocker . . ."

(Portugal)

A hare one day *made fun of a tortoise*[b] because of his slow pace and *boasted of his own great speed*[b] in running. The tortoise only laughed and said, "Let us try a race. I will run with you five miles. The fox will be the judge."

(England)

---

[a]Scored for achievement imagery.
[b]Scored for power imagery.

rable form from country to country, they obviously are a key ingredient in all types of economic activity, and they correlate highly with national income figures where both sets of figures are available. To get an estimate of whether the economy was expanding more rapidly or slowly than expected, the level of electricity consumed at one time period was related to the gain to the next time period across all countries, and the resulting regression equation was used to predict whether a given country was gaining more or less than expected as compared with the average of all countries.

Table 11.3 summarizes the correlations between collective *n* Achievement levels at two different time periods and collective rates of economic growth also at two different time periods. Note first of all that *n* Achievement levels in children's readers around 1925 correlate significantly with the rate of economic growth measured in relative gains in electricity consumed per capita between 1929 and 1950, but not with gains in electricity consumed at a still later time period (1952 to 1958). Furthermore, when stories from a larger sample of countries were coded for *n* Achievement around 1950, the resulting index of collective achievement motive levels predicted gains in electricity consumed between 1952 and 1958 or 1950 and 1967, but not earlier (1929 to 1950). In both cases, high *n* Achievement levels preceded more rapid rates of economic growth. And the *n* Achievement level in 1950 was not the product of more rapid rates of growth earlier (1929 to 1950), meaning that people's *n* Achievement levels did not rise *as a response to* greater economic opportunities, as economists often assume is the case (Papanek, 1962).

A more concrete illustration of just what these correlations represent is given in Table 11.4. Note that many more countries high in *n* Achievement in 1950, like Turkey, Greece, and the Soviet Union, show an above-expected

Table 11.3.

CORRELATIONS OF NATIONAL *n* ACHIEVEMENT LEVELS WITH GAINS IN ELECTRICAL POWER CONSUMPTION IN KILOWATT-HOURS (after McClelland, 1961/1976)

	n Achievement (1925)	*n Achievement (1950)*	*Gain in kwh per Capita (1929–1950)*	*Log gain in kwh (1952–1958)*	*Log gain in kwh (1950–1967)*
n Achievement (1925): $N = 22$	—	.26	.53**	.10	
n Achievement (1950): $N = 39$		—	.03	.43**	.39* ($N = 40$)
Log gain in kwh (1929–1950)			—	.13	
Log gain in kwh (1952–1958)				—	

*$p < .05$.

**$p < .01$.

Table 11.4.

RATE OF GROWTH IN ELECTRICAL OUTPUT (1952–1958) AND NATIONAL n ACHIEVEMENT LEVELS IN 1950 (after McClelland, 1961)

			Deviations from Expected Growth Rate[a] in Standard Score Units		
National n Achievement Levels (1950)[b]		*Country*	*Above Expectation*	*National n Achievement Levels (1950)[b]*	*Country*	*Below Expectation*
High	3.62	Turkey	+1.38			
n Achieve-	2.71	India[c]	+1.12			
ment	2.38	Australia	+0.42			
	2.33	Israel	+1.18			
	2.33	Spain	+0.01			
	2.29	Pakistan[d]	+2.75			
	2.29	Greece	+1.18	3.38	Argentina	−0.56
	2.29	Canada	+0.06	2.71	Lebanon	−0.67
	2.24	Bulgaria	+1.37	2.38	France	−0.24
	2.24	U.S.A.	+0.47	2.33	Union of S. Africa	−0.06
	2.14	W. Germany	+0.53	2.29	Ireland	−0.41
	2.10	U.S.S.R.	+1.62	2.14	Tunisia	−1.87
	2.10	Portugal	+0.76	2.10	Syria	−0.25
Low	1.95	Iraq	+0.29	2.05	New Zealand	−0.29
n Achieve-	1.86	Austria	+0.38	1.86	Uruguay	−0.75
ment	1.67	U.K.	+0.17	1.81	Hungary	−0.62
	1.57	Mexico	+0.12	1.71	Norway	−0.77
	0.86	Poland	+1.26	1.62	Sweden	−0.64
				1.52	Finland	−0.08
				1.48	Netherlands	−0.15
				1.33	Italy	−0.57
				1.29	Japan	−0.04
				1.20	Switzerland[e]	−1.92
				1.19	Chile	−1.81
				1.05	Denmark	−0.89
				0.57	Algeria	−0.83
				0.43	Belgium	−1.65

Correlation of n Achievement level (1950) × Deviations from expected growth rate = .43, $p < .01$.

[a]The estimates are computed from the monthly average electrical production figures, in millions of kilowatt-hours, for 1952 and 1958, from United Nations, *Monthly Bulletin of Statistics,* January 1960, and Statistical Papers, Series J, *World Energy Supplies,* 1951–1954 and 1955–1958.

The correlation between log level 1952 and log gain 1952–1958 is .976.

The regression equation based on these thirty-nine countries plus four others from the same climatic zone on which data are available (China-Taiwan, Czechoslovakia, Romania, and Yugoslavia) is log gain (1952–1958) = .9229 log level (1952) + .0480.

Standard scores are deviations from mean gain predicted by the regression formula ($M = -.01831$) divided by the standard deviation of the deviations from mean predicted gain (SD = .159).

[b]Based on twenty-one children's stories from second-, third-, and fourth-grade readers in each country.

[c]Based on six Hindi, seven Telugu, eight Tamil stories.

[d]Based on twelve Urdu and eleven Bengali stories.

[e]Based on twenty-one German Swiss stories, mean = .91; twenty-one French Swiss stories, mean = 1.71; overall mean obtained by weighting German mean double to give approximately proportionate representation to the two main ethnic population groups.

growth rate in electricity consumed, whereas many more of those low in *n* Achievement, like Uruguay, Belgium, and Switzerland, show a below-expected economic growth rate. The case of Switzerland highlights the fact that we are predicting *rates of gain* in economic activity rather than *levels* of economic activity. Switzerland is a wealthy country with a high level of economic activity, but it shows a slow rate of gain relative to other countries at the same high level, like the United States. The lead time between 1950 achievement motivation levels and subsequent growth is so short—certainly as compared with the lead time in ancient Greece, which was over two hundred years—that we must assume the effect is not taking place through teaching children to be more achievement oriented who later grow up to become active entrepreneurs. (See Chapter 7.)

Other Factors Affecting the Relationship of *n* Achievement Levels to Rates of Economic Growth

Is it not possible that collective *n* Achievement levels merely reflect some other societal characteristic that is really responsible for more rapid economic growth? For example, might they not reflect educational levels of the work force, which in turn produce more rapid economic growth? Perhaps better-educated people understand better the great importance of achievement to improve the standard of living of all the people by economic means. Southwood (1969) has carried out an extensive investigation that checks out such possibilities. He obtained information for each country on such structural variables as occupational stratification, amount of secondary school education, population size, union membership, degree of open political competition allowed among parties, amount of political unrest, and literacy. He correlated each of these variables with *n* Achievement levels, rates of economic growth, and also political unrest, the variable of chief interest to him.

None of the other national characteristics assessed explains away the relationship between collective *n* Achievement levels and rates of economic growth. For example, consider the influence of educational level. The percentage of high-school graduates in a country in 1955 is not related to rate of economic growth from 1952 to 1958 ($r = -.09$) nor to the *n* Achievement level in 1950 ($r = -.22$). If the nations are split in terms of whether they are above or below average in the percentage of high-school graduates, the collective *n* Achievement level relates significantly to economic growth both among better-educated and poorer-educated countries.

However, investment in education does seem to accelerate economic growth if collective *n* Achievement levels are high. McClelland (1966) found that when investment in higher education was high relative to the economic level of a country in 1950, more countries developed rapidly if they were high in *n* Achievement level, but not if they were low in *n* Achievement level. This is important, because policy makers may reason that investment in education is important for promoting economic growth, because more knowledge obviously is required to produce a technologically advanced industrial society. But the data show that simply increasing the knowledge base in a population does not automatically lead to more rapid economic growth: the level of achievement motivation must also be high for people to make more energetic use of such knowledge. Chapter 13 will show how, at the individual level, the contribution of greater skill to performance depends on the level of motivation. Just increasing know-how does not lead to better performance unless motivation for that performance is high. The same principle applies to the economic performance of countries.

Or consider group discrimination. In Southwood's (1969) data, the degree of discrimination against minority groups as of 1965 is significantly correlated with the rate of economic growth between 1952 and 1958 ($r = .38; p < .05$) and with a low level with n Achievement in 1950 ($r = .20$). Could it be that discrimination against minorities forces them into business and increases n Achievement, which increases the rate of economic growth? At first the hypothesis appears reasonable, because many persecuted minorities like the Jews or Quakers in the West, Jains or Marwaris in India, or the Gurage in Ethiopia have been successful in business. Hagen (1962) has argued that it is their loss of status that leads such minorities to try to regain respect through the only channel open to them, namely, increased business activity.

There are two problems with this hypothesis. One is that there is no systematic evidence that discriminated minorities in general counterstrive. As Weber (1904/1930) pointed out, the Catholics in England were a persecuted minority, but they did not become successful in business, and there seem to be as many cases of this type as of the counterstriving variety. Secondly, it is difficult to determine whether the achievement motive is the cause or result of group discrimination. Certainly there is ample evidence that minorities successful in business are persecuted *because* they are perceived as getting rich at the expense of others. McClelland (1961) points out that Hermes, representing the image in myth of the rising Athenian businessman, is pictured as tricky and dishonest, which is exactly the way such businessmen were perceived by the Athenian aristocracy. Such an image has characterized minorities successful in business ever since (see LeVine, 1966), whether they be Jews in the West or the Ibo in Nigeria.

The only systematic way to make sure the n Achievement–economic growth relationship is not the accidental product of its association with other variables is to enter all the variables that predict economic growth into a multiple regression equation and see whether n Achievement contributes to explaining rates of economic growth when the effect of the other variables has been removed. That is, all the factors like group discrimination that are significantly associated with rates of growth are entered into an equation along with collective n Achievement levels to see which factor best predicts rates of growth, as well as whether that factor continues to be significantly associated with rates of growth when the influence of other factors has been partialled out or controlled. When Southwood followed this procedure, he found that the n Achievement variable comes out as being important compared with other factors in predicting rates of economic growth and continues to contribute significantly to the variance in rates of growth after the contribution of other variables has been removed (McClelland, 1961, 1976).

Achievement Motive Levels and Political Protest

High *n* Achievement does not always lead to rapid economic advance smoothly. It can result in violence. Southwood (1969) reasoned that high achievement concerns combined with low opportunities to achieve would produce frustration, anger, and political protest. This, in fact, is what he found, as shown in Figure 11.5, which plots the relationship between collective *n* Achievement levels and a measure of internal war only for countries below average in the proportion of students going to high school. For these countries, the higher the achievement aspiration of the country, the greater the amount of internal violence, presumably because young people with high aspirations do not have the opportunity to advance for lack of education. In contrast, for countries above average in the proportion of students in high school, there is no relationship between the collective *n* Achievement level and domestic violence. In fact, for a somewhat more sensitive index of political disorder—that is, turmoil (the number of strikes, government crises, riots, and demonstrations)—the relationship is even negative with collective *n* Achievement levels. Among the more educated countries, the higher the *n* Achievement level in 1950, the less the turmoil ($r = -.23$).

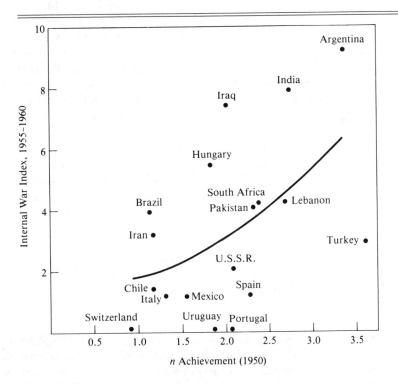

Figure 11.5.

Relationship of Internal War to Collective *n* Achievement Levels (1950) Among Countries Low in High-School Education (data from Southwood, 1969).

Among the poorly educated countries with low educational opportunities, the greater the *n* Achievement level in 1950, the greater the turmoil (*r* = .46; *p* < .05).

McClelland (1975) also found a significant association between *n* Achievement levels and violent protests in the history of the United States. Most of the protest measures involved strikes, riots, or demonstrations over lack of economic opportunity for labor or minority groups being discriminated against. In decades in U.S. history when *n* Achievement levels were high, the index of violent economic protest also was high, and vice versa. A strong urge to get ahead, if it is blocked, tends to lead to violent protest.

The fact that some minority groups with high *n* Achievement levels tend to get ahead faster may lead to discrimination against them, as has been noted. This is vividly illustrated by what happened to the Ibo in Nigeria. LeVine (1966) has shown that Ibo boys report a much higher percentage of achievement dreams than Hausa-Fulani boys, who come from a dominant tribe in northern Nigeria. The Yoruba, another major tribal group in Nigeria, falls in between these two extremes in achievement motivation. The Yoruba were more modernized because of earlier contact with the West. For instance, in the 1920s, of the twelve doctors in the country, eight were Yoruba; four European; and none, Ibo or Hausa-Fulani. By the 1930s forty-nine, or 33 percent, were Ibo; seventy-six, or 48 percent, were Yoruba; and one was Hausa-Fulani. Many have testified to the extraordinary speed with which the Ibo had moved upward in all walks of life in Nigeria, from university professors to poets and novelists. LeVine (1966) comments further: "Apart from this success in becoming a major part of the modernized, professional and governing elite of Nigeria, Ibo entrepreneurs, fanning out all over the country, have also enjoyed a substantial measure of success. The Ibo have a reputation for being willing to take any sort of job, no matter how menial, when they first enter a town and then working their way up, living frugally and accumulating resources until they become wealthy." Ibo people were persecuted and killed, particularly in the Hausa-Fulani part of the country; they protested against the discrimination and ultimately revolted because they felt blocked. They finally seceded from the country, trying to set up the separate state of Biafra. Eventually they were overpowered by the central government of Nigeria. Their history illustrates dramatically the dynamic relationships between *n* Achievement levels, economic advance, discrimination, and violent protest.

• THE COLLECTIVE CONCERN FOR AFFILIATION AND CIVIL RIGHTS

Societal characteristics associated with collective levels of *n* Affiliation have not been extensively studied, but what evidence there is suggests that they are very much what we would expect from knowing how individuals high in *n* Affiliation behave. Table 11.5 lists the main cultural characteristics associated with a high concern for affiliation expressed in folk tales. In such societies, wife beating is uncommon, infanticide is not practiced, daughters tend to live closer to their parents, children are rated to be more often obedient, and adults regularly help each other more. In short, cultures concerned about affiliation show that they care more for people or respect what are generally called *civil rights.*

The analysis of the correlates of national *n* Affiliation levels in children's stories leads to similar conclusions. Countries high in the concern for affiliation tend to have lower psychogenic death rates from homicide, suicide, ulcers, cirrhosis of the liver, and hypertension. Barrett and Franke (1970) correlated children's reader *n* Affiliation scores with national death rates from these causes both in 1925 and in 1950. In nine out of ten time-lagged comparisons (from *n* Affiliation in one period to death rates in the next), the correlations, although small, were negative, suggesting that high *n* Affiliation predicts less violence and the kinds of interpersonal aggravation that accompany heightened psychogenic death rates of this type.

McClelland (1961) also found that national *n* Affiliation levels were associated with a greater interest in having children. As direct evidence for this conclusion he notes that in the countries studied in 1950, collective *n* Affiliation levels were significantly associated with the birth rate ($r = .41; p < .05$). Peoples more concerned about affiliation tended to have more children. However, the relationship was reversed for the 1925 sample of countries: at that time, peoples more concerned about affiliation had fewer children. He explains the shift by demonstrating that infant mortality was a key variable strongly related to the birth rate in 1925 but not in 1950. At the earlier time period, countries with a high birth rate also had a high infant mortality rate, but this was not true by 1950, when public health measures had reduced infant mortality rates everywhere. Countries high in *n* Affiliation in 1925 had a lower infant mortality rate and also a lower birth rate, meaning they had fewer children and took better

Table 11.5.

CROSS-CULTURAL CORRELATES OF *n* AFFILIATION IN FOLK TALES (after data in McClelland, Davis, Kalin, & Wanner, 1972)

Cultural Characteristic	r with Collective n Affiliation	N
Wife beating	$-.50*$	17
Infanticide	$-.50*$	21
Residence distance of daughter	$-.61**$	14
Frequency with which children are obedient	$.33*$	31
Dependency on others for help in adulthood	$.34*$	36

*$p < .05$.
**$p < .01$.

care of them. By 1950, when infant mortality was no longer an issue, peoples concerned with affiliation could express their concern for children more directly by having more of them.

A high collective concern for affiliation appears to have served as a protection of individual rights against violent acts by the government. In *The Achieving Society,* McClelland (1961) observed that ruthlessly totalitarian regimes nearly always have been marked by high collective levels of *n* Power and low collective levels of *n* Affiliation. Children's readers showed this pattern in Germany in 1925, before the rise of Hitler; in Japan before the rise of the military dictatorship in the 1930s; in Russia during the rule of Joseph Stalin; and in Spain both in 1925 and in 1950, when the dictator Francisco Franco was on his way to power or was in power. Of twelve clearly totalitarian regimes, 92 percent showed this motivational pattern, as contrasted with only 18 percent of countries judged not to be controlled by dictators.

Since that time, figures for China have also become available, and they fit the same pattern. In 1925 Chinese children's readers were high in *n* Power (1.50 standard deviations above the mean for all countries) and low in *n* Affiliation (2.01 standard deviations below the mean for all countries), facts that are certainly not at variance with the common judgment that the country was under the control of a military dictatorship at that time. By 1955, after the Communist takeover, China's readers were showing one of the highest *n* Power levels recorded in any country at any time (3.27 standard deviations above the mean), and *n* Affiliation was still below the world average (0.55 standard deviations below the mean). These figures again indicate what most analysts would agree was true—namely, that the Chinese Communist totalitarianism of the 1950s was, if anything, even stronger and more severe than the earlier military dictatorship.

Such findings make good theoretical sense in terms of known correlates of *n* Power and *n* Affiliation at the individual level. As Chapter 8 made clear, individuals with high *n* Power want to be important and to have their way. A strong power motive, however, can be held in check by a high affiliative motive that leads to concern for others' welfare, which might be expected to prevent a government from ruthlessly riding over the rights of individuals. In fact, if high *n* Affiliation is not present, governments can be expected to be violent in trying to get their way. Countries showing a higher *n* Power than *n* Affiliation in their children's readers in the 1950s, such as Iran, are more likely to be politically unstable and have a higher proportion of deaths from domestic violence (Feierabend & Feierabend, 1966). In contrast, countries that have been relatively democratic world powers, such as Great Britain in 1925 or 1950 or the United States in 1950, are characterized by high levels of *n* Power and *n* Affiliation. The desire to impose the national will in these countries is held in check by a concern for the welfare of others. While few social scientists have been willing to place much faith in such indicators of collective motivation levels, high *n* Affiliation in popular literature has considerable utility in predicting that the civil rights of individual citizens of a country will be protected from governmental oppression.

• THE COLLECTIVE CONCERN FOR POWER

The Imperial Power Motive Pattern and Empire Building

Individuals with the imperial power motive profile (high *n* Power greater than *n* Affiliation, and high Activity Inhibition) tend to be more effective managers and empire builders (see Chapter 8). So it seemed reasonable to investigate whether nations characterized by this motive profile are better organized empires or have what political and sociological theorists speak of as greater "system capability." That is, governments vary in the extent to which they extract resources from their members and use them effectively to service individuals or groups in the society or defend it against attack from outside.

McClelland (1975) selected two measures of governmental system capability: the percentage of gross national product (GNP) taken by government away from private expenditure and the percentage of GNP devoted to defense. Table 11.6 shows the proportionate amounts spent in these two ways by various countries, classified according to whether they displayed the imperial power motive syndrome or some other motive combination. Every country with the imperial power motive pattern collected a greater proportion of GNP for government use than the median for all countries in the sample, as contrasted with half of the countries with other motivational patterns, a difference that is statistically significant. Countries with the imperial power motive pattern also spent nearly 5 percent of their GNP on the average for defense, as contrasted with about 3.5 percent spent by other countries. In short, as expected, nations with the imperial power motive pattern showed signs of having developed more system capability than other nations in the sense that they collected more of their GNP in taxes and spent more of it on defense. McClelland (1975) reasons that such countries are typical of expansive, well-organized nations in the past like the great Roman Empire organized in the period after the birth of Christ.

Consequences of the Imperial Power Motive Pattern for Public Health

Since individuals with the imperial power motive pattern also show more susceptibility to cardiovascular disease (Chapter 8), it seemed worth investigating whether nations with such a motive profile showed higher death rates from this cause. The results are summarized in Table 11.7. Once again, a prediction from the individual level is confirmed at the collective level. Countries high in *n* Power and high in inhibition show the highest average death rates from heart disease and hypertension—significantly higher than those low in both factors for hypertension or than those low in *n* Power and high in Activity Inhibition for heart disease. In the latter instance, it appears that higher self-control leads to a more regular life, which protects against heart attacks if *n* Power is also low. The averages for each quadrant should be compared with those for individuals similarly classified in Figure 8.10. There, too, individuals low in *n* Power have lower average diastolic blood pressure, suggesting they should be less susceptible to death due to cardiovascular disease.

Table 11.6.

EXPENDITURES FOR GOVERNMENT (1959–1960) AND FOR DEFENSE (1950s) AMONG COUNTRIES WITH THE IMPERIAL POWER VERSUS OTHER MOTIVE COMBINATIONS (1950) (after McClelland, 1975)

Group	Country	Low Activity Inhibition[a] Percentage of GNP For Government[b]	For Defense[f]	Country (Imperial Syndrome)	High Activity Inhibition[a] Percentage of GNP For Government	For Defense
High *n* Power > *n* Affiliation	Belgium	28.9	3.0	Argentina	31.4	2.6
	Canada	36.5	4.4	China	—	3.6
	Finland	39.5	2.0	Denmark	31.4	2.6
	Iran	—	5.6	W. Germany	41.3	3.8
	Italy	31.8	3.0	India	—	1.9
	Mexico	20.6	0.7	Iraq	38.0	8.2
	New Zealand	34.2	2.2	Pakistan	—	3.9
	Spain	25.9	2.2	Switzerland	36.8	2.9
	Taiwan	29.2	12.3	U.S.S.R.	44.2	10.4
	Union of S. Africa	33.4	0.8	U.S.A.	36.3	9.6
	Mean	31.1	3.62	Mean	37.1	4.95
Low *n* Power or *n* Affiliation > *n* Power	Australia	36.1	2.7	Austria	34.8	1.5
	Chile	17.6	2.8	Bulgaria	30.3	—
	France	33.0	5.9	England	33.3	6.7
	Hungary	27.1	—	Greece	22.2	5.1
	Netherlands	40.0	4.0	Ireland	24.1	1.4
	Norway	40.0	3.5	Israel	28.0	6.3
	Portugal	22.2	3.2	Lebanon	—	2.4
	Sweden	38.1	4.7	Japan	40.5	1.6
	Syria	—	4.9	Poland	30.2	—
	Tunisia	—	1.8	Turkey	23.1	2.4
				Uruguay	—	1.0
	Mean	31.8	3.72	Mean	29.6	3.16

[a]Below or above the median number (46) of the word *not* in twenty-one children's stories.

[b]Reciprocal of the figure for private consumption, after Russett and others (1964), Table 48; median for whole sample = 30.3.

[c]After Russett and others (1964), Table 23; median for whole sample = 2.70.

Table 11.7.

DEATH RATES PER 100,000 INHABITANTS IN VARIOUS COUNTRIES FROM HEART DISEASE (A) AND HYPERTENSION (B) AROUND 1968 AS A FUNCTION OF NEED FOR POWER AND CONTROL (1950) (after McClelland, 1976)

		Activity Inhibition					
		Low				*High*	
Group	*Country*	*A*	*B*			*A*	*B*
	Italy	246.0	33.0	West Germany		252.0	25.9
	Union of	248.0	24.8	Switzerland		247.0	23.6
	South Africa			England		367.0	22.8
	Belgium	320.0	23.9	U.S.A.		339.0	22.8
	Finland	330.0	19.6	Argentina		156.0	22.8
	New Zealand	306.0	13.6	Denmark		363.0	12.5
High	Canada	255.0	13.6				
n Power	Spain	132.0	12.8				
	Taiwan	38.2	8.7				
	Average	*277.4*	*18.8*	Average		*287.3*	*21.7*
	Hungary	302.0	33.0	Austria		326.0	28.4
Low	Sweden	350.0	21.2	Uruguay		189.0	27.2
n Power	Portugal	135.0	18.8	Ireland		374.0	25.2
	Norway	290.0	16.9	Poland		140.0	20.0
	Australia	328.0	15.5	Japan		76.0	18.2
	France	200.0	11.9	Bulgaria		176.0	16.0
	Netherlands	228.0	11.5	Greece		131.0	12.5
	Chile	92.0	8.9	Israel		194.0	11.2
	Average	*240.6*	*17.2*	Average		*200.7*	*19.8*

Note: Mexico is omitted because a very high percentage of deaths was not classified. Mann-Whitney U-tests, heart disease: high high > low high, $p = .07$; hypertension: high high > low low, $p = .04$.

High *n* Power and low inhibition in individuals is associated with heavy drinking (see Figure 8.7). McClelland, Davis, Kalin, and Wanner (1972) also found a similar relationship at the cultural level by examining drinking ratings for cultures classified according to whether they were high or low in *n* Power and Activity Inhibition scores in folk tales. As Figure 11.6 shows, the proportion of heavy-drinking societies is highest in those cultures for which collective power motive scores are high and Activity Inhibition scores are low. Cultures high in *n* Power and high in Activity Inhibition are least often heavy-drinking societies, a result that is also paralleled at the individual level.

In reviewing such studies, we are reminded of early social psychologists who spoke about a "group mind" as if a nation or a group had a mind of its own that led to characteristic group activities. Certainly motive levels as assayed in

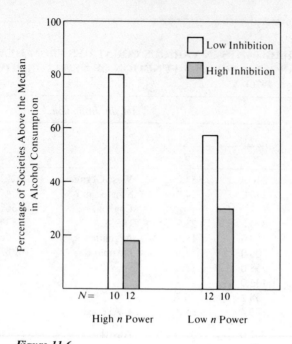

Figure 11.6.

Percentage of Heavy-drinking Societies as a Function of *n* Power and Inhibition Scores in Folk Tales (after McClelland, Davis, Kalin, & Wanner, 1972).

group products—whether of nations or preliterate cultures—are associated with group outcomes very similar to the actions associated with similar motive dispositions assayed at the individual level. The parallels are so close that it seems reasonable to infer that the measures of collective motivation are somehow tapping central motivational or ideological tendencies among individuals in the group.

• HISTORICAL SHIFTS IN COLLECTIVE MOTIVE LEVELS

Motivational Explanations for Events in English History from 1400 to 1830

Several studies have investigated the relationship between historical events and shifts in collective motive levels. The demonstration that high collective *n* Achievement levels preceded periods of economic expansion initiated this mode of analysis. Giliberto (1972, cited in McClelland, 1975) extended it by coding the samples of popular literature collected from various periods in English history for *n* Power (Winter system) and *n* Affiliation.

One of his most striking findings is illustrated in Figure 11.7, which plots average *n* Power scores from 1550 to 1800 obtained from samples of plays and street ballads. Historically this covers a time when there was a power struggle

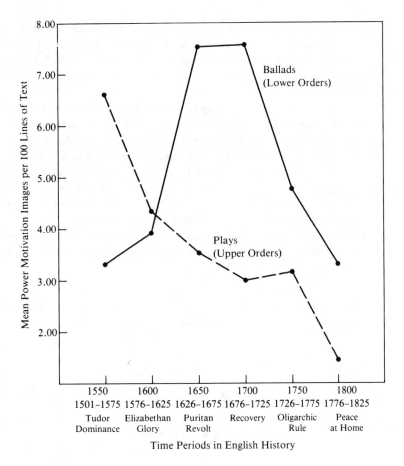

Figure 11.7.

Levels of *n* Power in Lower and Upper Classes: England, 1500 to 1800 (after McClelland, 1975).

going on between the king and his party and Parliament, which was more broadly representative of the people. In the earliest period, the Tudor kings, represented particularly by Henry VIII, had consolidated the power of the aristocracy, which ruled the people in an authoritarian manner. If we assume that the excerpts from plays reflect more the motive levels of the ruling class, labeled the "upper orders" in Figure 11.7, then the power motive level of this class was much higher than that of the "lower orders," as reflected in the street ballads they produced and listened to, during the period of Tudor dominance. Subsequently, the people struggled against the ruling class and succeeded in gaining power during roughly the period of the Puritan revolt (1626 to 1675). The fact that they gained ascendance over the aristocracy is reflected in the much higher level of *n* Power in street ballads around 1650 than in the plays, which presumably reflected the thoughts and feelings of the ruling class. It is not possible to know from these data whether shifts in *n* Power levels led to the successful revolt of the people's party or vice versa, but it is interesting to note that the motivational changes fit well with what was happening in the country, if we assume that the two types of popular literature represent the states of mind of different social classes.

Giliberto pooled the *n* Power scores from all sources and plotted them for various periods in English history along with the *n* Affiliation and *n* Achievement scores, as shown in Figure 11.8. Note first that the collective level of *n* Power is much higher than the level of *n* Affiliation during most of this period, suggesting that there should have been a good deal of internal violence, oppression, and violation of civil rights if cross-national findings are applicable here. This was certainly the case. The famous British historian Trevelyan (1942) describes the period of Tudor dominance in the 1500s as characterized by "senile, ferocious feudalism." Around 1650, during the Civil War and its aftermath, the English were busy killing each other in the name of religion; even as late as

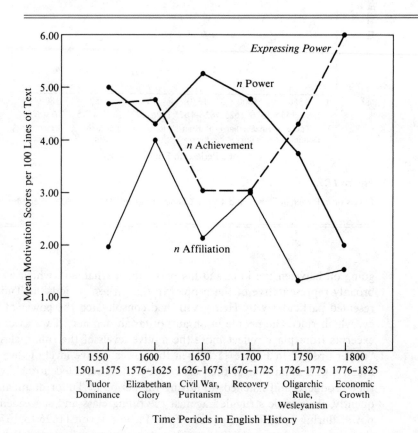

Figure 11.8.

Levels of *n* Power, *n* Affiliation, and *n* Achievement in Popular Literature: England, 1500 to 1800 (after McClelland, 1975).

1750, working-class people were regularly executed for petty crimes such as robbing someone of a shilling or breaking into a house with the intent to steal (McClelland, 1975). According to the motivational data, only the periods around 1600 during the reign of Queen Elizabeth and around 1800 could be described as eras of good feeling in which internal violence should have been less prevalent. In general, historians could argue that these were indeed periods of lesser violence against human life.

The second point Giliberto noted about the curves in Figure 11.8 is that the two sharp rises in *n* Affiliation in 1600 and 1700 were both followed by periods of religious reform on behalf of the oppressed, which were followed by a drop in *n* Affiliation. Such a sequence of events makes sense in motivational terms, because *n* Affiliation at the individual level is strongly associated with a concern for people: if the people were suffering, as they were during the period of Tudor dominance or during the English Civil War, it would seem only natural to those high in *n* Affiliation that steps should be taken to alleviate their condition. In the early period during the Civil War, the steps taken involved putting the champions of the common people in charge in Parliament; at the later period after the Wesleyan Methodist revival, around 1750, the steps involved pushing for laws to protect civil rights and to help the poor.

But notice that while the impulse to help the oppressed may derive from a heightened *n* Affiliation, if it is combined with a high level of *n* Power, the *n* Affiliation level immediately drops. This switch makes sense in terms of the motivational dynamics involved, because acting powerfully on behalf of other people means thinking in terms of what was defined as *socialized power* in Chapter 8, and a high score for socialized power is regularly associated with a low level of *n* Affiliation (McClelland, 1975). In commonsense terms, if there is a powerful concern to help other people, it may become so strong and determined that in the end it overrides sensitivity to whether people are getting hurt. The devotion to a larger good, or social justice, can become so strong that it once again violates individual rights. It was just such a passion for social justice that led the Puritans to kill their English brothers and sisters, or Northerners in the United States to kill their Southern brothers and sisters in the Civil War in the name of protecting the rights of blacks. Such a dynamic sequence is suggested by the English data, although two instances are not enough to demonstrate its generality.

Motivational Factors in the History of the United States from the Founding of the Republic to the Present

McClelland (1975) made a similar analysis of motivational trends in U.S. history on a more fine-grained basis. For every decade from 1780 to 1970, he obtained scores for three social motives from stories in school textbooks, hymns, and popular fiction written during that decade. Since the types of material varied in the frequency with which the motives appeared in them over time—for example, power motive images appeared seven or eight times as often as achievement or affiliation images in fiction—the mean motive scores per decade were converted to standard scores for each type of material (mean standard score = 50;

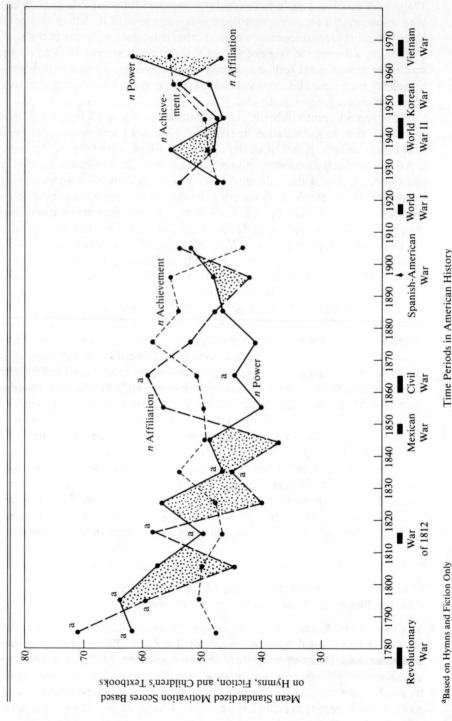

Time Periods in American History

aBased on Hymns and Fiction Only

Figure 11.9.

Levels of *n* Power, *n* Affiliation, and *n* Achievement in Popular Literature: United States, 1780 to 1970 (after McClelland, 1975).

SD = 10), and the three standard scores for a decade were then averaged to give the best estimate of the motive level for that time period.

The results are plotted in Figure 11.9 at the midpoints for each decade. The *n* Achievement curve relates to periods of economic growth, as would be expected. It was consistently high after the Civil War before and during the period of the most rapid economic growth in U.S. history. deCharms and Moeller (1962) had earlier shown that the same rise in *n* Achievement, scored from school textbooks alone, was associated with innovativeness in the general population as measured by the number of patents issued. Figure 11.10 shows how the rise in *n* Achievement in the period from 1870 to 1900 was followed by a sharp rise in the patent index from 1890 to 1930, as well as that the subsequent fall in *n* Achievement from 1900 to 1930 was also followed by a fall in the patent index from 1930 to 1950. The patent index can be considered an index of the entrepreneurial drive to find new and better ways of doing things throughout

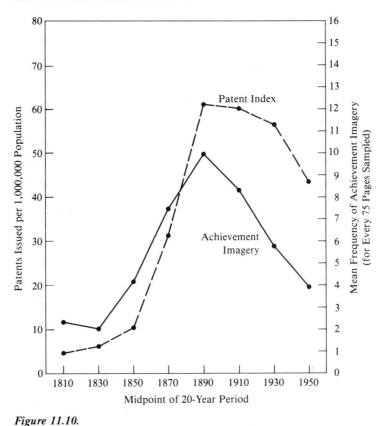

Figure 11.10.

Mean Frequency of Achievement Imagery in Children's Readers and the Patent Index in the United States, 1800 to 1950 (after deCharms and Moeller, 1962).

this time period. The finer-tuned and more comprehensive *n* Achievement levels in Figure 11.9 confirm the deCharms and Moeller findings and also suggest that the low level of *n* Achievement from 1900 to 1930 might have had something to do with the Great Depression in the 1930s. The data also suggest that the recent rise in *n* Achievement may foreshadow a period of relative economic prosperity in the last quarter of the twentieth century.

The shaded portions in Figure 11.9 indicate the periods in which *n* Power was greater than *n* Affiliation. What is notable about them is that they occur regularly before wars in U.S. history. McClelland observed that if one allows a lead time of fifteen years, shaded areas predict war and nonshaded areas, peace, in eleven out of thirteen comparisons before World War I ($p < .05$); one of the "exceptions" was the Spanish-American War, which lasted three months and might not be considered a war at all. After World War II, if the lead time is shortened to around five to ten years, four out of five of the predictions of war and peace are correct. In short, in the history of the United States, there is a statistically significant association between whether or not *n* Power is greater than *n* Affiliation and whether the country subsequently goes to war.

In commonsense terms, this relationship can be interpreted as meaning that when the country is feeling assertive or ruthless (high *n* Power, low *n* Affiliation), it is likely to respond to a challenge or provocation by going to war, whereas the same or a similar challenge when the spirit of the country is more affiliative does not lead to war. Once again, the relationship between the imperial power motive pattern and violence is confirmed at the collective level.

The relationship found in English history between the *n* Power/*n* Affiliation ratio and social reform can also be observed in U.S. history. Table 11.8 lists the decades in U.S. history when *n* Power was at least moderately high (standard score = 46 or more) and *n* Affiliation balanced it (not over ten points higher or two points lower). In the decade following each of these instances, *n* Affiliation dropped markedly, creating the imperial power motive pattern in which *n* Power was greater than *n* Affiliation. This led in the next decade to a wave of social reform, starting with the period of Jeffersonian democracy around 1805 and ending with the crusade for civil rights around 1965.

This is clearer evidence of the dynamics suggested by events in English history. A relatively high *n* Affiliation, if combined with a moderate-to-high *n* Power, leads to a concern for the rights of the oppressed—in the U.S. case including the poor, women, and blacks—which converts into a powerful movement for social reform accompanied by a drop in sensitivity to whether people are getting hurt (lower *n* Affiliation). This then creates the imperial power motive pattern, which has regularly been associated with going to war against an outside enemy. It is suggestive that crusades for social reform have six times followed this motivational dynamic in U.S. history and that crusades for social reform have so often been followed by the country's going to war. McClelland notes that the balanced *n* Power/*n* Affiliation ratio is followed by the imperial power motive syndrome six out of seven times, whereas an imperial power motive pattern develops only once after nine other motive combinations, a difference that would rarely have arisen by chance.

Table 11.8.
MOTIVE PATTERNS, SOCIAL REFORM, AND WAR IN U.S. HISTORY: STANDARDIZED MOTIVE SCORES FROM POPULAR LITERATURE (after McClelland, 1975)

Midpoint of Decade	Balanced		Midpoint of Next Decade	Imperial			Midpoint of Next Decade	Social Reform	Next Time Period of War
	n Power	n Affiliation		n Power	>	n Affiliation			
1785	62	71	1795	64	>	59	1805	Jeffersonian democracy	1812, War of 1812
1815	50	57	1825	57	>	40	1835	Jacksonian populism	1848, Mexican War
1835	46	44	1845	47	>	37	1855	Abolitionism	1860, Civil War
1885	46	49	1895	48	>	43	1905	Muckraking, crusade for social justice	1917, World War I
								Shortened lead time	
1925	47	53	1935	55	>	48	1935	New Deal	1940, World War II
1955	49	53	1965	63	>	47	1965	Crusade for civil rights, War on Poverty	1967, Vietnam War

A final inference to be drawn from Figure 11.9 is that *n* Affiliation appears to rise most often in decades after a war, starting with the Revolutionary War. It makes sense to infer that after people have spent some time killing and getting killed, they should have a heightened concern for the welfare of others. Note in Figure 11.9 that the highest peaks of *n* Affiliation were associated with the Revolutionary War and the Civil War, both of which involved killing brothers, sisters, and friends. In fact, in six out of the eight decades after a war in the history of the United States, *n* Affiliation was high, as contrasted with only two decades out of ten following a period of peace, a difference that is statistically significant. This sets the stage for a new cycle of concern for others, which, if it is accompanied by high *n* Power, will lead in time to the imperial power motive pattern, social reform, and another instance of going to war. While all these relationships need confirmation in the history of other nations, it is noteworthy how much a knowledge of collective motive levels contributes to an understanding of significant events in the history of the United States.

Motive Levels and the Success of Automobile Companies

Nations are not the only kind of collective enterprise. Perhaps indexes of collective motive levels in other types of organizations could predict organizational performance over time. Diaz (1982) reasoned that it might be possible to assess the motivational spirit of a firm by coding the annual letters of the chief executive officer to stockholders in the company. So he coded the annual letters to stockholders for *n* Achievement and *n* Power for two U.S. automobile manufacturers (1952 to 1980) and three Japanese automobile manufacturers (1962 to 1976 and 1980). One of his objectives was to discover whether there was a motivational reason why the Japanese automobile makers seem to be doing so much better than their U.S. counterparts in recent years.

Table 11.9 highlights the differences in efficiency. The Japanese automobile manufacturers come out better in every comparison. Figure 11.11 may explain why. All three Japanese manufacturers (Nissan, Toyota, and Honda) scored higher in collective achievement motive levels at nearly every point in time than their U.S. counterparts, General Motors and Chrysler. All the studies of the *n* Achievement level in individuals and nations suggest that it should translate into greater efficiency and a stronger entrepreneurial spirit, which eventually should lead to a more rapid improvement in company performance. Many explanations have been advanced for why Japanese automobile manufacturers have shown such a large competitive advantage over U.S. firms in recent years, but one of the simplest explanations is that provided in Figure 11.11. The Japanese firms have been activated by a higher level of achievement motivation than their U.S. counterparts.

Diaz (1982) was also interested to see whether *n* Achievement and *n* Power levels within a company could be used to predict rates of growth for the company at different time periods, so he paired Chrysler with General Motors in the United States and Nissan with Toyota in Japan. Since the companies in each pair were directly competing with each other for the same market, he computed for each year the ratio of sales, assets, and return on investment for each pair.

Table 11.9.

COMPARISON OF THE EFFICIENCY OF JAPANESE AND U.S. AUTOMOBILE MANUFACTURERS (after Lohr, 1982, p. 29)

	Japan	*United States*
Manufacturing (machine stamping operations)[a]		
Parts stamped per hour	550	325
Labor power per press line	1	7 to 13
Time needed to change dies	5 minutes	4 to 6 hours
Average production run (days)	2	10
Time needed to build a small car (hours)	30.8	59.9
Personnel (average automobile plant)		
Total work force	2360	4250
Average number absent (vacations, illness, and so on)	185	500
Average absentee rate (percent)	8.3	11.8

[a]Source: Harbour & Associates.

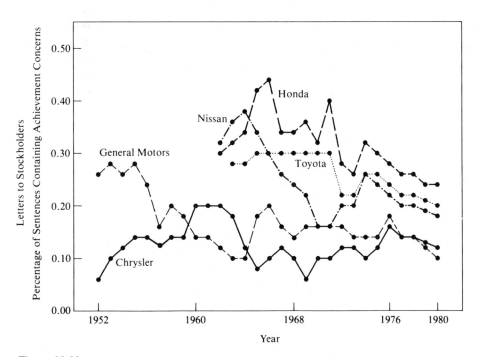

Figure 11.11.

Level of Achievement Concern in Chief Executive Officer's Letters to Stockholders in Japanese and U.S. Automobile Companies over Time (after Diaz, 1982).

Thus, Chrysler's sales fluctuate between 16 and 37 percent of General Motors' sales between 1952 and 1980. What he was estimating was how well Chrysler was doing relative to General Motors. This method of computing comparative performance has the advantage of controlling for changes in demand and market conditions that occur from year to year, since these should affect both companies in the same way. Then he also computed the comparative advantage of Chrysler over General Motors in *n* Achievement and *n* Power levels for each year, smoothed these ratios for adjacent years, and correlated each year's motive ratio score with comparative economic performance scores from all the other years. Thus, for example, comparative *n* Achievement in 1960 would be correlated with the comparative economic performance of the two companies before 1960 and from 1961 to 1980.

The correlations obtained showed a very regular cyclical pattern, as Figure 11.12 shows. If we consider first predicting forward from the motive level in a given year to subsequent performance (here measured in terms of relative assets), it is clear that both comparative *n* Achievement and comparative *n* Power levels predict gains in relative assets maximally about seven years later. The ef-

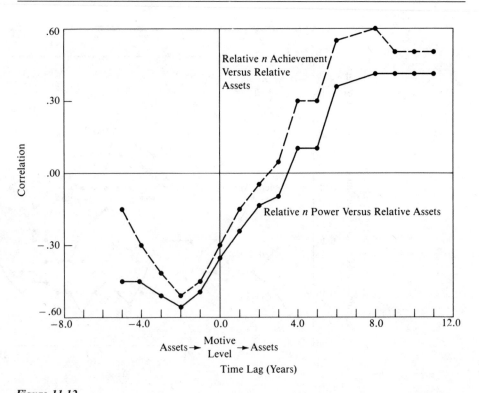

Figure 11.12.

Chrysler and General Motors: Relative *n* Achievement and *n* Power Correlated over Time with Relative Assets (after Diaz, 1982).

fect of comparative motivational advantage is not felt in the near future but has an impact several years later. In fact, the correlation between comparative *n* Achievement levels and relative assets seven years later is .57, $p < .05$. And remember that this correlation is based on every seven-year discrepancy in dates starting with 1952.

Next consider the backward associations: correlations between motive levels and company performance in previous years. It is easier to think of these correlations as the relationship between performance and subsequent motive levels. As Figure 11.12 shows, these relationships are predominantly negative. This means that good performance is associated with low levels of *n* Achievement and *n* Power in subsequent years and vice versa. The maximum negative correlations occur over a two-year period. The immediate effect of comparative advantage in the economic performance of a company is to lower *n* Achievement and *n* Power in the succeeding two years. This fits earlier explanations given for the decline in *n* Achievement. In terms of the Atkinson model (see Chapter 7), as the probability of success increases to a high level, the challenge to achieve decreases.

Figure 11.13 shows a similar curve for Nissan and Toyota, the two Japanese

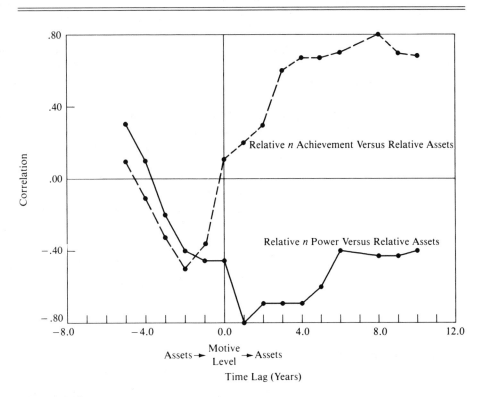

Figure 11.13.

Nissan and Toyota: Relative *n* Achievement and *n* Power Correlated over Time with Relative Assets (after Diaz, 1982).

firms compared. Once again, the relationship of comparative *n* Achievement advantage to comparative economic performance is exactly what we would expect, and it is similar to what was obtained in the United States—with one exception. Comparatively high performance is associated with an immediate drop in *n* Achievement levels over the next two years, and comparatively high *n* Achievement levels are associated with a gain in relative assets in subsequent years, with a peak occurring earlier than for the U.S. companies. Note that the correlation between *n* Achievement levels and relative assets reaches a generally high level after four years in Japan, whereas in the United States at this time lag the relationship is still insignificant. The Japanese high level of *n* Achievement translates maximally into improved company performance after four rather than seven years, as in the United States. Apparently there is less organizational inertia in Japanese companies, so entrepreneurial drive can translate itself into results more quickly.

What are we to make of the fact that comparative *n* Power levels in Japan are *negatively* associated with comparative economic performance in subsequent years rather than positively, as in the United States? Perhaps there is some difference in the way Japanese and U.S. firms are structured or managed such that power motivation promotes organizational performance in the United States and inhibits it in Japan. It is impossible to be certain how this result should be interpreted, but a clue may lie in the difference in the nature of the power motivation expressed in the two countries. As noted in Chapter 8, socialized power motivation (high *n* Power, high inhibition) is associated with management success in the United States. High *n* Power and low inhibition is related to impulsive assertiveness in trying to establish personal control over others and does not go with managerial success.

Diaz also scored the letters to stockholders for inhibition and found that in the Japanese letters to stockholders the word *not* appeared only one half the number of times per hundred sentences as in the U.S. letters. This finding is contrary to the popular belief that the Japanese are a highly controlled people, and it may reflect some translation or linguistic complications; if it is taken at face value, however, it may explain why power motivation has such different effects in the two countries. For if the power motivation in the United States is more socialized, it should lead to better management practices and better performance, whereas if it is less socialized and more personal in orientation in Japan, it should lead to less effective management. And these are the relationships actually found in the two countries. Whatever the meaning of the *n* Power results, those for *n* Achievement are clear and consistent for both countries: high *n* Achievement levels in companies, as in nations and in individuals, lead to more entrepreneurial behavior and better economic performance later.

• ORIGINS OF COLLECTIVE MOTIVATIONS

Ideological Factors Affecting Collective Achievement Concerns

If collective motive levels are important influences on what happens in history, questions naturally arise as to where they come from. Why was Greek literature so much higher in the number of achievement images in early, as contrasted with later, periods? Was it the influence of some person or group of persons in leadership positions who happened to be high in *n* Achievement? It is impossible to know for certain.

Diaz (1982) has shown that motive levels in letters to stockholders of companies shifted markedly depending on who was chief executive officer at the time. So we might infer in this case that it was the achievement or power motivation of individuals that somehow created a climate that changed business performance. If this were generally the case, one might adopt a "great leader" view of history in which happenings in the life of individual leaders would create motive levels that shape the course of history. But unfortunately we do not know the motive levels of the chief executive officers of the automobile companies as tested in the usual way, and it is entirely possible that what they wrote in their letters to stockholders was as much a product of the general climate in the company as it was of their own individual motive levels. Furthermore, the motive levels in letters to stockholders supposedly written by the same man (but perhaps written by an assistant) varied from year to year, which would suggest the chief executive officer was *reflecting* the climate in the company rather than creating it from his own stable motive dispositions. In the case of even larger units such as nation-states, it is even less clear that the motive levels of individual leaders shape the collective motive levels for the society. For example, there is not a close relationship between the motive levels for various decades in recent U.S. history as shown in Figure 11.9 and the motive levels of U.S. presidents during those decades, as summarized in Table 8.8.

If the ideas of an individual leader are not the main determinant of collective motive levels, perhaps major belief systems current in the society have an influence. Attention focused originally on religion as a source of achievement motive levels. The impetus to this idea was provided by Max Weber's (1904/1930) classic analysis of the Protestant origins of the modern capitalistic spirit. He had observed that in countries like England and Germany, Protestant groups seemed to work harder, to save more money, and to enter successfully into business more often than similar Catholic groups. A number of studies have confirmed the fact that in the seventeenth, eighteenth, and even the nineteenth century, business leaders were more often drawn from Protestant than Catholic minorities, particularly from small dissenting groups such as the Quakers or later the Methodists in England (McClelland, 1961). Why should this be so?

Weber found an answer in the doctrines of Protestantism—particularly in its stress on the rationalization of all of life and the devotion to one's calling or vocation. Reformation leaders such as Martin Luther and John Calvin had turned against the authority of the Catholic church in Rome, particularly its authority to guarantee people's salvation by selling them indulgences to make up for past sins by good works. Thus, to a certain extent, Protestant believers were more "on their own" than Catholic believers. They got the impression that "God helps those who help themselves" and that therefore they could in a certain sense, create their own salvation or, more correctly, the conviction that they were saved. They could not gradually accumulate good works to their credit, as in Catholicism, but only by systematic self-control, which at every moment "stands before the inexorable alternative, chosen or damned," could they create the conviction that they were one of the elect of God (Weber, 1904/1930).

Weber argued that such a rigid rationalization of a person's own conduct explains some of the extra determination and vigor with which Protestants pursued capitalistic enterprise. McClelland (1961/1976) observed that the key ideological element may have been the stress on people's continually improving their own conduct, even in small ways, from day to day "till we shall have arrived at a perfection of goodness, which indeed, we seek and pursue as long as we live" (Calvin's *Institutes of the Christian Religion*). Thus, the ideology of the Protestant Reformation may have succeeded in raising achievement motivation among Protestant groups, which in turn led them to develop capitalistic enterprise more successfully than Catholics.

No direct test of this hypothesis has been made by comparing the achievement content of popular literature from Protestant or Catholic sources at critical periods in the sixteenth through the nineteenth centuries. By the twentieth century, however, McClelland (1961) found no consistent differences in n Achievement levels among Protestant and Catholic groups of individuals in the United States and Germany. Nor did children's readers from Protestant and Catholic countries differ in their average n Achievement levels. He concluded, therefore, that the higher n Achievement levels of Protestants could not be attributed so much to the doctrines of the Reformation as to the way in which the Reformation aroused individuals and put them on their toes, so to speak, in their search for salvation in nontraditional ways.

The key element seems to be some kind of an "inner worldly activism," which is supported institutionally by a church that also opposes traditional religious authority. To check this idea, McClelland (1961) studied the religious beliefs and practices of forty-five tribes whose folk tales had already been coded for n Achievement levels. Of the cultures with high n Achievement in their folk tales, 65 percent stressed individual over ritual contact with the divine, as compared with only 23 percent of the cultures low in n Achievement. In other words, in high n Achievement cultures, individuals less often gain favor with the divine by participating in traditional, ritualistically prescribed ceremonies. Instead, they have more direct access to the divine through mystical communion or individualistic interpretations of written traditions. McClelland also found that in high n Achievement cultures, religious experts (priests, shamans, and so on) are much less often *necessary* for the performance of an individual's religious duties. Across cultures, those that stress inner over external religious authority tend to have higher collective levels of n Achievement.

McClelland (1961) also reports an interesting contemporary confirmation of the importance of religious reform in raising n Achievement levels. In the highlands of Mexico in the state of Chiapas, he located a village that had recently been converted to a form of radical Christianity. The new believers acted in many ways like the original Protestants in Europe at the time of the Reformation. They read the Bible in their native language; they burned the Catholic folk images of saints and painted their churches white; they sang hymns; they became more interested in health and schooling; and above all, they felt themselves superior to the traditional folk Catholics in other villages nearby, who had to depend on the priests to make contact with God. Children in this village were tested for n Achievement levels some eight to ten years after most of the adults had been converted. Their scores were contrasted with those of school-children in a nearby village that had remained traditionally Catholic, although it, too, might have received an achievement impetus from the fact that the government had just given the peasants their own land to farm. The children from the village recently converted to Protestantism showed a number of signs of higher n Achievement. At least in this case, religious reform—in its early stages, anyway—apparently had raised n Achievement.

It is not necessary to assume that Protestantism per se is the critical factor. Minority religious groups throughout the world having no connection with Christianity—such as the Jains in India (McClelland & Winter, 1969/1971) or the Gurage in Ethiopia (McClelland, 1977a)—have produced disproportionately large numbers of businessmen and almost certainly have shown higher levels of n Achievement. What seems to be critical is some religious or other reason for believing—perhaps only at the moment of reform—that one's group is superior to more tradition-oriented groups in which authority rests in the institution rather than in the individual, who has become a convert to the new way of life. We can also use such a general interpretation to explain the fact that countries like the Soviet Union and mainland China, which conceive of themselves as originators of the great Communist ideological reform, score significantly higher than the world average in n Achievement levels in school textbooks. On the other hand, Communist countries such as Poland and Bulgaria, which did not originate the reform but accepted it from without, are significantly below average in n Achievement levels. (See Table 11.4.)

Comparable studies have not been made of the possible religious or ideological sources of collective levels of n Affiliation or n Power.

Environmental Factors Influencing n Achievement Levels

In the early twentieth century it was commonly asserted that certain peoples were more energetic or entrepreneurial because of their genetic endowment or because they happened to live in a stimulating climate (McClelland, 1961). Thus, the British, who were very successful economically at the time and who had an empire that stretched around the world, were thought to have the advantage of belonging to the white race and also of living in a temperate climate, which stimulated them to work harder. In contrast, blacks living in Africa were thought to be less successful because they were racially endowed with less energy and because they lived in the enervating tropics. History has already demonstrated the absurdity of such conclusions for the obvious reason that nations of the same racial background and inhabiting the same piece of real estate are much less energetic and successful today than they were two or three generations ago. If we take collective n Achievement levels as indicative of one very important type of psychic energy, it is clear that race and climate can have little to do with national economic success, since *n* Achievement levels have varied widely over time for the same country. For example, collective *n* Achievement in England was well above the world average in 1925, signaling that country's strong economic performance up to World War II, and well below the world average in 1950, foreshadowing its more recent relative economic decline.

A more sophisticated view of the influence of environmental factors on national success has been advanced by Arnold Toynbee (1947), the British historian, after an exhaustive comparative study of the rise and fall of a great many civilizations. He observed that nations tended to rise when the challenge of the physical or social environment was "just right"—neither too great (as in an excessively harsh environment) nor too small (as on the fabled tropical island where everything needed is easy to get). This view comes very close to stating Atkinson's position, as outlined in Chapter 7, that moderately challenging tasks are most likely to arouse achievement motivation (see Table 7.2). Thus, Toynbee's hypothesis seems reasonable on theoretical grounds, and he is able to give many illustrations of how it explains what happened in history. For example, the climatic and social challenge to the Scots in Great Britain was just right, so they did well. But when they migrated to the hills of North Carolina the challenge was too great, and they did less well. The difficulty with the hypothesis is that it is not really testable, because Toynbee proposes no way of measuring the ease or difficulty of the challenge. Sometimes it is social, sometimes economic, sometimes climatic. He had a natural tendency to explain whatever the outcome was in terms of whatever degree of challenge was necessary to explain it.

McClelland (1961) did find some evidence for the hypothesis so far as collective *n* Achievement levels are concerned, if climatic conditions are taken as an index of the degree of challenge. Using data from preliterate tribes, he showed that cultures whose folk tales were high in *n* Achievement were much more likely than those low in folk tale *n* Achievement to live in areas where the mean annual temperature varied between forty and sixty degrees Fahrenheit, where the mean daily or monthly temperature variation was greater than fifteen degrees Fahrenheit, where mean annual rainfall was less than sixty inches, and where the quality of soil was not very good. These findings can be interpreted as meaning that moderate challenge from the physical environment promotes the development of *n* Achievement, but they can also be interpreted to mean that groups high in *n* Achievement tend to seek out such environments.

Several studies point to the importance of challenge in the social structure as a source of achievement motivation, or at least as a necessary complement to it if it is to affect entrepreneurial behavior. Swanson (1967) has demonstrated fairly conclusively that Protestantism won control in the Reformation in those European communities in which the central governing authority was limited or in some way more democratic. Regimes in which power was strongly centralized, sometimes by divine right, tended to remain Catholic. When authority was divided up between representatives of various groups or guilds, the society was more likely to be won over to Protestant reform. If achievement motivation developed in these Protestant centers, as McClelland (1961/1976) has argued, Swanson sees it more as a response to the better economic opportunities provided in a governing system in which more people had a chance to get ahead.

The critical studies have not as yet been made that would show whether changes in *n* Achievement levels occurred before, during, or after the changes in governmental structure.

But certainly an open, competitive structure seems to be regularly associated with higher *n* Achievement levels. For instance, the Ibo of Nigeria, as already noted, have high *n* Achievement. LeVine, who studied them, felt they developed high *n* Achievement because of the most characteristic feature of their status system—the title society: "This consisted in the most developed form of a series of ranked titles, the entry to which was contingent upon acceptance by existing title holders, payment of a set entrance fee and providing a feast for members of the society. Membership was open to anyone of free birth, but the fees and feasts effectively limited title holding to those of some wealth. This was increasingly true as a man progressed to higher titles" (LeVine, 1966). Thus, an Ibo male could attain high status by his own efforts and particularly by accumulating wealth. Parents, knowing this, would be likely to give their sons the kind of achievement and self-reliance training that would develop the high levels of achievement motivation actually found among the Ibo.

In contrast, LeVine noted that the individual Hausa males achieved status primarily by attaching themselves to an important leader who could provide rewards out of the resources he controlled in return for obedience, loyalty, and service. Since Hausa society rewards obedience and loyalty rather than achievement and self-reliance, it is not surprising that the Hausas score low *n* Achievement. Once again, an open, competitive structure in which self-reliance is rewarded, as in the democratically ruled cities at the time of the Reformation, seems to be an important source of encouragement for developing achievement motivation.

One other piece of evidence corroborates this correlation. In preliterate societies, cultures with bilateral kinship systems are more likely than those with other kinship systems to have high *n* Achievement levels in folk tales ($r = .36$; $N = 37$; $p < .05$). The key aspect of a bilateral kinship system from the point of view of the child is that he or she sees both the mother's and father's side of the family as more or less equally important. Thus, children have more options. They are not locked into a patrilineage or matrilineage. They do not have to be what their mother's or father's people expect them to be. At the individual level it is authoritarian upbringing, particularly on the part of the father, that produces low *n* Achievement in sons (Rosen & D'Andrade, 1959). (See Figure 7.13.) For a boy to develop high *n* Achievement, there must be some stress on self-reliance, some opportunity for him to set his own goals. At the societal level the equivalent would appear to be some kind of institutionalization of an open structure that permits people to rise in a variety of ways, balances institutional powers against each other, or at the very least does not restrict the individual to one accepted, traditional way of behaving.

Sources of the Collective Concern for Power

Table 11.10 summarizes what little is known about societal characteristics associated with high *n* Power levels either in the cross-cultural sample employing

Table 11.10.

CORRELATIONS OF SOCIETAL CHARACTERISTICS WITH HIGH *n* POWER
(after McClelland, Davis, Kalin, & Wanner, 1972; Southwood, 1969)

Societal Characteristics	*Correlation with High n Power*
Cross-cultural sample (n Power from folk tales):	
N = 36[a]	
Colder climate	.47***
Percent dependence on hunting	.27*
Percent dependence on agriculture	−.27*
Socioeconomic simplicity scale	.41***
Lineal descent	−.44***
Cross-national sample (n Power from children's textbooks around 1950): N = 38–40[b]	
Gains in electric power use (1937–1954)	.34**
Percent union membership (1966)	−.38**

[a]After McClelland, Davis, Kalin, & Wanner (1972).
[b]After Southwood (1969).
*$p < .10$.
**$p < .05$.
***$p < .01$.

folk tales or in the cross-national sample employing stories in children's text-books. The results make good sense and fit in well with the limited amount known about the origins of the power motive in individuals. What seems to encourage the development of high *n* Power is a demand for individual assertiveness, as in struggling to keep warm or in hunting as contrasted with agriculture, which often relies on collaborative efforts. The socioeconomic simplicity scale in the table is a factor score loading high on such variables as high degree of dependence on hunting, a low degree of jurisdictional hierarchy, impermanence of settlement pattern, and small size of local community. In other words, in such societies, individuals are very much on their own and not part of some large supportive network. A lineal descent pattern is negatively associated with collective *n* Power, presumably because societies oriented around lineal descent are precisely those that maintain a large supportive network dependent on the lineage, so individuals are not expected to be assertive on their own. This pattern of correlations is consistent with the findings reported in Chapter 8 showing that parental permissiveness for assertiveness in the areas of sex and aggression, as well as the lack of tight parental control, are associated with high *n* Power.

The only two societal variables significantly associated with collective *n* Power levels among nations were prior gains in electric power use (positively associated) and the percentage of union membership (negatively associated). Both can be interpreted as consistent with the picture that has emerged so far, for rapid gains in electric power usage means more power is placed in the hands of the individual to make things or to turn on gadgets like radios, light bulbs, irons, or mixers. What technology does is give people more power and encourage their assertiveness in using it, which might promote higher levels of collective *n* Power. On the other hand, union membership provides the kind of solidarity for working people that means they will get support whether they are individually assertive or not. It might be considered the equivalent in the advanced technological world of the lineage system in preliterate society. Both may tend to diminish the need for individual assertiveness and in fact so constrict individuals that they tend toward lower *n* Power. At best, such findings are only suggestive. They need much further investigation.

One other factor associated with high collective levels of *n* Power has been identified (McClelland, 1976). A major challenge to individual assertiveness is unemployment, particularly for men in the period before women entered the labor force in large proportions. In the history of the United States, relatively high levels of unemployment have regularly been followed by higher *n* Power relative to *n* Affiliation scores, as Table 11.11 shows. This table rates employment opportunities from 1820 to 1884 as better or poorer based on whether immigration to the United States was lower or higher than the average for approximately one hundred years. Thereafter the ratings for employment opportunities are based on actual unemployment figures. The *n* Power and *n* Affiliation scores are those shown in Figure 11.9.

In nearly every instance, poorer employment opportunities are associated with a higher *n* Power score in that decade, and better employment opportunities are associated with a lower *n* Power score in that decade. The difference is highly significant. Some figures from national sample surveys of motive levels in the United States confirm and modify this conclusion (Veroff, Atkinson, Feld, & Gurin, 1960; Veroff, Depner, Kulka, & Douvan, 1980). In 1976, 59 percent of black males were high in *n* Power as contrasted with only 48 percent of white males; the difference might be attributed to the fact that there was certainly much more unemployment among black than white males. However, there was not a comparable difference in the 1957 sample. This suggests that an ideological factor combined with a structural one to produce a rise in *n* Power among black males. In 1957, before black consciousness had been raised, unemployment may not have meant the same thing to blacks as it did in 1976, when they felt it to be even more unfair. This serves as an important reminder that environmental factors like unemployment take on meaning in terms of the ideological factors also present at the time.

Sources of the Collective Concern for Affiliation

The only cross-cultural clue to what produces a high collective *n* Affiliation is a positive correlation between signs of male solidarity in a culture and *n* Affiliation levels in folk tales ($r = .36$; $N = 21$; $p < .10$; McClelland et al., 1972). In other words, in societies where men tend to live and work together, affiliative concerns tend to be higher. The only other bit of evidence on this point, as al-

Table 11.11.

**RELATIONSHIP OF EMPLOYMENT OPPORTUNITIES TO RELATIVE STRENGTH OF
n POWER IN U.S. HISTORY (after McClelland, 1976)**

		n Power in That Decade Is	
Epoch	*Employment Opportunities*	*Less Than n Affiliation*	*Greater Than n Affiliation*
1820–1824	Poorer[a]		+
1830–1834	Poorer		+
1840–1844	Poorer		+
1850–1854	Better	+	
1860–1864	Poorer[b]	−	
1870–1874	Better	+	
1880–1884	Better	+	
1890–1894	Poorer[c]		+
1900–1904	Better	+	
1910–1914	?[d]		
1920–1924	Better	+	
1930–1934	Poorer		+
1940–1944	Better	+	
1950–1954	Poorer		+

Note: + = Confirmation of hypothesis; − = Nonconfirmation of hypothesis. The association of competition for jobs with predominance of power motivation is unlikely to be due to chance ($p < .01$).

[a]Estimates are based on whether alien immigration for the five-year period is lower or higher than averages for five-year periods from 1820 to 1913 (Easterlin, 1968).

[b]This estimate may be incorrect, because fewer people migrated to the United States at this time because of the Civil War.

[c]From here on, estimates are based on whether the unemployment rate was 5.5 percent or more in four out of five years, or less. (Easterlin, 1968).

[d]Motivational data are unavailable for this decade.

ready noted, is that killing in organized wars tends to raise collective *n* Affiliation levels, at least in the history of the United States. But overall, the lack of information about sources of the affiliative motive at the collective level is marked and paralleled by a similar lack of information at the individual level.

• DIFFICULTIES IN INTERPRETING MOTIVE TRENDS IN SOCIETY

For ease of exposition, the review of studies of historical trends in collective motive levels has emphasized the findings that can be readily interpreted, but they are only part of the story. In every study, difficulties have arisen that have been resolved in what seems to be a reasonable way that gives meaningful results, but this does not mean the difficulties can be overlooked (McClelland, 1981b). It is worth reviewing some of the problems encountered in this type of research, if only to make it clear that the conclusions reached depend on decisions that are open to dispute.

A major problem arises over the lead times between motivational shifts and subsequent historical events. In the connection between n Achievement levels and subsequent economic growth, the lead time varies from centuries in the study of Ancient Greece to a few years among contemporary nations (Table 11.4). How can the same variable—collective n Achievement level—be supposed to have the same effect after a century as opposed to five years? Part of the difficulty may lie in determining in the studies of remote periods of time just when the n Achievement levels were high. The scores are plotted at midpoints in century-long periods, but that does not really indicate how high the level remained at the end of the period or into the next one. In more recent periods it has been possible to get estimates of motive levels more pinpointed in time; when that is done, the lags to subsequent social changes get shorter, perhaps because the assessment of when the motive level existed is more accurate.

But that explanation does not account for the fact that in U.S. history, the prediction of wars from collective n Power/n Affiliation ratios assumes a lead time of about fifteen years up to World War I and five to ten years thereafter. Is readjusting the lead time just a method of fitting the data to a hypothesis established in relation to an earlier time period? Perhaps, but with increased communication and transportation, motive changes should translate into social changes more rapidly. The comparison of the performance of Japanese and U.S. automobile companies clearly demonstrates that motive levels affect collective performance after different lead times, depending on how well organized a collectivity is. At least whenever adjustments in lead time have been made, they have always been toward shorter lead times in more recent periods.

Another problem arises over how to interpret different estimates of collective motive levels obtained from different sources of popular literature. A major difference in n Power levels obtained from different sources in England between 1600 and 1700 was interpreted in terms of a class difference between the aristocracy and the common people, but no systematic attempt was made to see if differences in other motive levels from these two sources also correlated with differences in other types of behavior between the two classes. We might even question whether it is correct to assume that plays represent the interests of the upper classes more than street ballads.

Furthermore, often differences in motive levels from different sources have not been interpreted. For example, n Achievement level, as estimated from children's textbooks and hymns, appeared to be high in the United States between 1880 and 1900, but according to the fiction sampled it was low (McClelland, 1975). While it may seem reasonable to estimate the level of n Achievement to be high based on all sources, that still leaves the question of interpreting the low level for fiction. Could it be that fiction was read more by women and that their n Achievement level was low? Or that it was read more by the educated classes, who had a lower level of n Achievement than less-educated people, who were participating more in the religious life of the community, showing their higher level of *n* Achievement in the hymns that they wrote and sang and turning more often into successful entrepreneurs? Such questions can only be answered by more extensive research into class and group differences in motive levels reflected in different types of popular literature.

Finally, many questions can be raised about the measures of collective performance that have been used in these studies. Economists interested in measuring the rate of economic growth have never been satisfied with using indexes like coal imports at the port of London or the consumption of electric power. From their point of view, economic growth must be estimated in terms of *all* its constituents, including contributions from agricultural, industrial, and service sectors. When some of these more typical measures of gross national income are used, different results are obtained, and it is not so clear that *n* Achievement levels precede periods of economic growth.

McClelland (1961) argues that aggregate measures of national income levels are not as accurate as index measures, particularly for periods one or two hundred years ago or for underdeveloped countries in the modern period, for which many figures are unavailable. However, there is room for disagreement on this point. Even in the case of the automobile companies, Diaz (1982) employed three different measures of economic performance: sales, assets, and return on investment. The interrelationship between motive levels and assets, as shown in Figures 11.12 and 11.13, was smoothest. The same types of relationship were obtained for sales and return on investment, but more irregularities showed up in year-to-year correlations. It can be argued that assets represent the best overall estimate of the growth of a firm, especially since companies may adjust yearly profits to avoid taxes or to invest more heavily in future products. It can also be argued that sales and return on investment are equally important indicators of a firm's success and that collective motive levels do not associate as closely with such indicators. These matters can only be settled by more studies of this type on other companies and by a closer theoretical analysis of the best way to measure economic success. The studies reported in this chapter have only begun to open a field of investigation that needs further examination to establish more carefully the rules for obtaining data and interpreting them.

The Meaning of Collective Motive Scores

The most important problem in interpreting collective motive scores arises out of trying to understand just what characteristic or characteristics they reflect. The practice of scoring folk tales, speeches, and other types of popular literature for different types of motive imagery grew up as a natural extension of scoring stories produced by individuals. But what do these collective motive scores mean? In what sense can we think in terms of the motive level of a nation or a culture? Do collective and individual motives function in the same way? Do the two types of scores get at the same variable?

Recall that the full motive scoring systems derived for individuals had to be abandoned in scoring speeches or popular literature. Instead, only the number of motive images per standard unit of text are counted. Doesn't that suggest the scores obtained in these two ways are not equivalent? Winter and Healy (1981/1982) refer to imagery scoring as the *running text system* and have systematically examined what kind of results it gives in comparison with more complete scoring systems whenever the two methods have been applied to the same material. They found that the simplified running text system reflects the effects of experimental arousal of motives, although not as well as the full scoring systems. Correlations of the simplified with the full scores for individual protocols run between .40 and .70. Split-half reliabilities for the running text scores vary between .43 and .70 for the various motive systems. Reliability is, if anything, higher for the running text system, probably because such scores are based on larger samples of text than are available in the protocols obtained from individuals. For example, McClelland (1961) found that in the cross-national study of children's textbooks, correlations of *n* Achievement scores in odd and even sets of stories were .67 in 1925 and .59 in 1950. While the odd-even reliability coefficients were considerably lower for *n* Affiliation and *n* Power, these values taken together are higher than those usually obtained for individuals under the set to "be creative." Split-half reliabilities for public speeches and press conferences run in the range of .62 to .77 (Hermann, 1980; Winter & Healy, 1981/1982).

Other methodological issues relate to just how to go about sampling material to get a good estimate of collective motive levels. McClelland (1975) has suggested ten different rules for getting representative and reliable estimates of collective motive levels from popular literature, such as making sure the literature is popular, choosing selections from several different authors and texts, making sure the coding is done blindly so that the coder does not know what time period is represented or what hypotheses are being investigated, and making sure each motive index is based on at least ten sets of one hundred lines or ten thousand words. Figure 11.14 illustrates how two such data sets provide very similar *n* Power data points for different periods in English history. The interpretation of power motive trends would be the same no matter which sample of data had been used.

Winter and Healy (1981/1982) also show that the running text scoring systems predict individual behaviors associated with the motives about as well as the full motive scoring systems do. But they make a further important point: when the running text system is applied to material for which it is designed—in this case, a long intensive interview—the *n* Power score obtained predicts industrial leadership behavior better than the *n* Power score obtained from the standard picture-story exercise. Thus, it is possible that the running text scoring systems may be more reliable and more valid if applied to standardized interviews than the full scoring systems are when applied to protocols obtained under test administration conditions, which are known to influence the results (see Chapter 6).

The main reason for believing that the two types of scores are getting at something similar is that the behaviors associated with collective and individual motive scores are so similar. High *n* Achievement at either level is associated with more entrepreneurial activity and greater economic success; high *n* Power

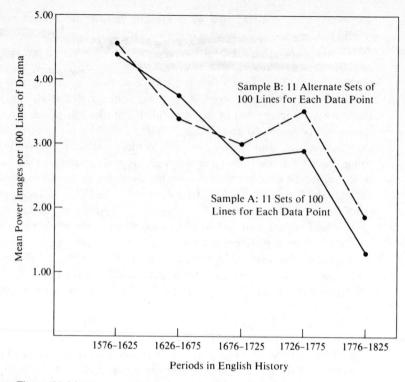

Figure 11.14.

Comparability of *n* Power Scores Obtained from Two Samples of Running Text in Drama at Different Periods in English History (after McClelland, 1975).

plus low Activity Inhibition is associated with heavier consumption of alcohol at either level; high *n* Power plus high Activity Inhibition is associated with empire building at either level; and so on.

What are we to make of such similarities? One possibility is that the collective motive score is an index of the percentage of people in a society or group who are high in the motive in question. An early comparison failed to show a relationship between mean levels of *n* Achievement for groups of individuals in a nation and *n* Achievement levels as coded in children's stories (McClelland, 1961). But the samples of individuals tested were in no way representative.

Veroff et al. (1960) and Veroff et al. (1981) did obtain motive scores from representative samples of U.S. adults in 1957 and again in 1976. The percentage of individuals scoring high in each of the three social motives in 1957 and 1976 can be compared with national motive levels obtained in the 1950s and 1960s from popular literature, as shown in Table 11.12. Only a comparison of shifts in motive levels is meaningful, since the standard scores for popular literature are based on eighteen decades in U.S. history and the samples of individual scores, on only two decades. Both types of measures agree that for both sexes com-

Table 11.12.

COMPARISON OF CHANGES IN MOTIVE LEVELS IN THE UNITED STATES ESTIMATED FROM REPRESENTATIVE SAMPLES OF INDIVIDUALS AND FROM POPULAR LITERATURE (after Veroff, Atkinson, Feld, & Gurin, 1960; Veroff & Veroff, 1981; McClelland, 1975)

Motive Measured	*1957*[a]	*1976*[a]	*Difference*
n Achievement			
Men (percentage high)	47	53	+6
Women (percentage high)	41	60	+19
Popular literature (standard score)	54	55[b]	+1
n Affiliation			
Men (percentage high)	58	39	−19
Women (percentage high)	48	50	+2
Popular literature (standard score)	53	47[b]	−6
n Power[c]			
Men (percentage high)	46	53	+7
Women (percentage high)	48	49	+1
Popular literature (standard score)[c]	49	63[b]	+14

[a]The number of respondents in 1957 was 595 men and 774 women; in 1976 it was 508 men and 700 women.

[b]In 1965, the midpoint of the 1960 to 1970 decade.

[c]Scored according to the Winter (1973) system.

bined, there was a gain after the 1950s in national *n* Achievement levels and in national *n* Power levels and that there was a loss in the national *n* Affiliation level. Furthermore, if the comparison is restricted to the results for men, the two types of measures agree that the gain was largest for *n* Power and next largest for *n* Achievement, and that the loss was very large for *n* Affiliation. However, the popular literature index was poor at picking up a big increase in individual *n* Achievement levels, perhaps because the increase in *n* Achievement for women resulting from the women's movement had not yet affected the popular literature that was being sampled in the 1960s. And the drop in the popular literature *n* Affiliation score did not reflect the fact that women, if anything, increased in *n* Affiliation between 1957 and 1966 (Veroff, Douvan, & Kulka, 1982).

    These findings are based on too few data points to be decisive. Furthermore, there is good reason to believe that the collective motive indexes might not be an index of the percentage of people in the population normally high in the motive at a given time period, for data on individual motive levels summarized in Chapters 7 to 9 suggest that they are reasonably stable over periods as long as fifteen to twenty-five years. Shifts in collective motive indexes are often quite sharp and rapid, so when the standard score for *n* Power in popular literature in the United States goes from 49 in the 1950s to 63 in the 1960s, it seems unlikely that the proportion of individuals stably high in *n* Power had gone up by that much. In fact, the data based on *n* Power scores from representative samples of individuals in Table 11.12 suggest that this was not the case.

However, it is certainly not impossible for the proportions of individuals in a country high in a given motive to change markedly over time, as the data on *n* Achievement for women in Table 11.12 indicate. This is due in part to new cohorts entering the adult population and old ones leaving it through death, and in part to the effect of special forces like the women's movement on special groups within the population. Veroff (1982) reports that the increase in *n* Achievement levels for women from 1957 to 1976 appears to be due to a co-hort effect—to the maintenance of a high level of *n* Achievement among women, as they grow older, who belonged to the generation most affected by the women's movement—and to the dying out of an older generation among whom *n* Achievement had been very low in 1957.

On the whole it seems preferable to think of collective motive scores as more analogous to *aroused motivational states,* which can shift quite rapidly as a result of influences like the women's movement or a period of major unemployment. These aroused motivational states may create effects on group behavior much like the effects produced in individuals by the chronic states of arousal that we have labeled *motive dispositions.* Such states of collective motive arousal may be conceived of as part of the ideology of the collectivity—whether it is a culture, a nation, or a business firm.

Motivational ideology is not explicit in the sense that people can report accurately what it is or answer questions in a public opinion survey that enable investigators to infer what it is. However, it is nevertheless very important in determining actions a group takes, as the evidence reviewed in this chapter indicates.

NOTES AND QUERIES

1. Locate a sample of your doodles and try scoring them for signs of *n* Achievement using Aronson's (1958) coding system. Compare your results with someone else's. Do your results agree with your comparative level of *n* Achievement as determined from coding your imaginative stories?

2. Go to a store, examine carefully a wide variety of vases, decide which ones you like best, and then see if they contain the designs characteristic of high or low *n* Achievement according to the Aronson system. Do the vases you like best contain the same designs you put into your doodles? Explain why the designs you like in a vase might be different from the designs you spontaneously produce.

3. Popular songs can be considered to represent the collective motive concerns of at least those who listen to them. Score for *n* Achievement the lyrics of the ten most popular songs in the United States at two different time peri-

ods, one of which precedes economic growth (say, in the early 1960s) and the other, economic decline (say, in the mid-1970s). Do the expected differences in *n* Achievement levels occur? If not, why not? If the songs reflect the concerns of young people, might the lag in the effect of these concerns be later, after the young people are playing a more central role in society?

4. In the *Communist Manifesto* (1848), Karl Marx and Friedrich Engels state the following:

> The discovery of America, the rounding of the Cape, opened up fresh ground for the rising bourgeoisie. The East-Indian and Chinese markets, the colonization of America, trade with the colonies, the increase in the means of exchange and in commodities generally, gave to commerce, to navigation, to industry, an impulse never before known. . . . Meantime the markets kept ever growing, the demand ever rising. . . . This development has, in its turn, reacted on the extension of industry; and in proportion as industry, commerce, navigation, railways extended, in the same proportion the bourgeoisie developed, increased its capital and pushed into the background every class handed down from the Middle Ages.

Examine critically this motivational analysis in terms of the empirical studies reviewed in this chapter on the motivation behind economic expansion.

5. Make a careful comparison of the motive levels of U.S. presidents in a given decade (see Table 8.8) with the motive levels of that decade as determined from popular literature (Figure 11.9). How much agreement do you find? Try to explain whatever results you obtain. Look also for systematic leads and lags: Do presidents' motive levels regularly precede or follow motive levels in popular literature? You can also make a more detailed analysis by comparing presidential motive levels with motive levels in different *types* of literature (see McClelland, 1975).

6. Try to get figures from Amnesty International for numbers of deaths in a country for political reasons, and correlate these figures (perhaps corrected for population size) with collective *n* Affiliation scores. Is there a relationship? Try to explain any major discrepancies.

7. It is suggested in this chapter that the Roman Empire developed in response to a collective imperial power motive pattern. Design a study that would test this hypothesis. Be specific about what you would do, and construct a table including imaginary numbers that would confirm the hypothesis.

8. Inkeles and Levinson (1954) argue that the term *group mind* should refer to the average or modal psychological characteristics of a representative sample of individuals from the group. Give some alternative explanations of the term, and discuss its possible relationships to characteristics of individuals in the group.

9. Do you think collective motive levels have predictive power for periods of social reform and violence only in democratic countries like the United

States and Great Britain? Why might this be so? Design a study that would test whether similar relationships would hold in another type of country.

10. Compute the relationship between a president's motive levels (see Table 8.8) and the percentage of the national budget he has proposed spending on defense. If there are major discrepancies in what the president asks for and what is voted, can it be explained in terms of discrepancies between presidential motives and collective motives, as determined from popular literature?

11. Design a study that would determine whether changes in *n* Achievement level preceded or followed changes in governmental structure in Swiss cantons, some of which became Protestant and some of which remained Catholic (see Swanson, 1967). How would you interpret the results, however they came out?

12. Collective data suggest that in the United States, major periods of unemployment are followed by a rise in *n* Power in popular literature. Design a study that would test this relationship at the individual level. Be sure to include a way to test for possible sex differences. Would you expect sex differences?

13. In 1982 unemployment levels were higher in the United States than they had been since the 1930s. In terms of findings reported in this chapter on the effects of motive levels in the history of the United States, construct a scenario of how 1982 unemployment might affect motive levels, which in turn might affect collective actions taken in the United States in subsequent years.

14. From a study of country differences (Table 11.6 or McClelland, 1975), from shifts in motive levels in the history of the United States, or from theory, try to construct some hypotheses as to what factors (other than wars) might increase collective concerns for affiliation. Formulating and testing such hypotheses could be very important for the future health and well-being of people. Explain why.

12

Cognitive Effects on Motivation

• COGNITIVE INFLUENCES ON MOTIVE AROUSAL

Several theorists, notably Weiner (1980a) and Heckhausen (1980), have stressed the great importance of cognitive factors in the motivation-action sequence. As Weiner (1979) puts it, "Comprehension stands with hedonism as among the primary sources of motivation." He feels that in motivation theory too much emphasis has been placed on affective arousal and not enough on the understanding the person has of what is happening during a motivation-action sequence, which determines whether affective arousal occurs or not.

A great many empirical studies have been carried out to clarify the relationship between cognition and motivation, but before reviewing them it is worth reexamining Figure 6.1, which identifies the key factors in a motivation-action sequence. Arousal *demands (cues)* typically contact an *incentive,* which, if it relates to an existing *motive disposition,* leads to an *aroused motive* or *motivation* to act. When, how, and whether this motivation gets converted into action is influenced by skills, cognitions (values), and opportunities, which determine whether a particular kind of behavior occurs or not.

As noted previously, Weiner, Atkinson, and others use the term *motivation* to describe the final excitatory potential for an act (the impulse to a given act) *after* it has been influenced by expectations and values, whereas we use the term *motivation* in the more restricted sense to refer to an aroused motive *before* it is influenced by expectations and values that shape preferences for particular acts. In some instances the two uses of the term *motivation* have, for all practical purposes, the same meaning, as when an aroused hunger motive (that is, hunger motivation) is associated with a strong impulse to eat (that is, motivation to eat in the Atkinson sense). But when an aroused motive is not so simply and directly connected with the impulse to act in a particular way, it is important to realize that aroused motivation is different from the impulse to act. For example, power motivation may be aroused by watching a film of John F. Kennedy's inaugural address as president (Winter, 1973), but what kind of impulse to act it is associated with varies from person to person and is shaped in various ways by each person's skills, values, and opportunities.

The distinction is important in trying to understand just how cognition influences motivation, because by definition it influences excitatory potential or the impulse to act, but how it influences or determines the course of motive arousal needs clarification. How experimenters explain a situation to subjects and what the subjects think is going on have important effects on what the subjects want and do, as studies to be reviewed subsequently will show. But to infer that cognition therefore determines motivation is to forget that the experimenter's explanations may have an effect on the subjects' impulses to act in certain ways because most subjects are already motivated to comply in some way with what the experimenter is asking them to do. It is not altogether clear the extent to which explanations or cognitive factors *create* motivation (that is, arouse motives) or merely channel motives that have already been aroused in the situation in the direction of certain acts. So we need to examine how cognitions influence motive arousal as well as later events in the motivation-action sequence.

Cognitive Effects on Incentives

To start with the most obvious effect of cognition, growth in understanding influences what constitutes an incentive (see Chapter 5). At the outset, pleasure is derived from variations around a simple standard to which one is adapted in many sensory or conceptual modalities. As one becomes used to the new variations, more complex variations are needed to give pleasure in music, art, or poetry. Similarly, children get pleasure from simple impacts (for example, from dropping things), but as they grow up the impacts that give pleasure become more and more social and symbolic until some people may get impact pleasure only from influencing the course of national events. Or simple contact gratifications in time become elaborated into the symbolic pleasures of romantic love. The effects of these shifts in what constitutes an incentive or motive arousal are obvious. Giving a child an opportunity to play with a toy car may arouse the achievement motive, but giving the same opportunity to an adult does not. Or watching a film of Kennedy's inauguration arouses the power motive in adults but does not in children, who do not understand what was happening.

Despite such examples, not much empirical work has been done on the capacity of incentives at different levels of cognitive complexity to arouse motives. What has been done has dealt with the effects of performance feedback on the incentive value of tasks for the achievement motive. As noted in Chapter 7, people high in *n* Achievement seek to perform tasks for which there is a moderate probability of success, for only in such tasks do they maximize satisfaction from doing them well. But "moderate probability of success" is a movable standard: it varies as the person gets success or failure feedback in the course of performing a task. How the person evaluates the feedback and consequently adjusts the incentive value of the task should affect the amount of achievement motivation aroused in the situation. That is, if success on a very difficult task that arouses little achievement motivation moves the perceived probability of success at the task into a fifty-fifty chance of success, the task should arouse more achievement motivation to do well on it in the future.

Heckhausen (1975a) carried out an experiment that indirectly suggests that this effect occurs. He arranged for subjects to succeed at a task most of the time. Afterward he asked the subjects to rate the extent to which they thought the outcome was attributable to their own ability on this task, to their ability to perform this task relative to others, or to other factors such as chance or effort. As one would expect, most subjects rated their ability for this task higher after success than they had beforehand. Success changed the incentive value of the task for them, since it altered their perceived probability of success at the task, which in turn should have raised the level of their achievement motivation. This is a direct demonstration of how an understanding of what has happened can modify the incentive value for performing a task, which affects motive arousal.

However, there was one group of subjects for whom this effect did not occur, as Figure 12.1 demonstrates. For subjects low in *n* Achievement (or high

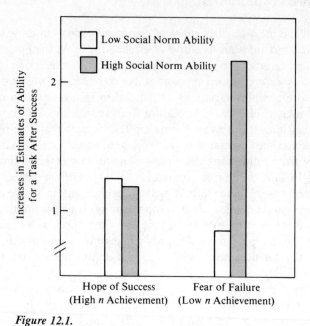

Figure 12.1.

Increase of Ability Estimates (Individual Norm) After Success for Subjects Classified High and Low in *n* Achievement and in Social Norm Ability (after Heckhausen, 1975b).

in *f* Failure) who also regarded themselves as not very good at such tasks relative to others, there was no significant increase in estimated ability for the task after success. We can infer that for them, actual success did not increase their achievement motivation. On the other hand, subjects low in *n* Achievement who felt they were good at the task relative to others were very encouraged by success to believe that they had high ability for the task, which should have raised the level of their *n* Achievement. In other words, both their motive level and their beliefs about their competence relative to others influenced how a successful performance was evaluated, which in turn influenced the incentive value of the task as shown by the judgment of their ability to perform it.

Many studies of this type have been carried out in the achievement area, as we shall see, but most of them have focused on how shifts in perceived probability of success influence the impulse to work hard at a task rather than in how they alter the incentive character of the work situation so as to arouse or diminish achievement motivation. Nevertheless, there is no doubt that alterations in perceived probability of success are affected by the level of *n* Achievement and affect the amount of achievement motivation aroused. (See the discussion later in the chapter in connection with Figure 12.10 of the experiment from which the data in Figure 12.1 were obtained.)

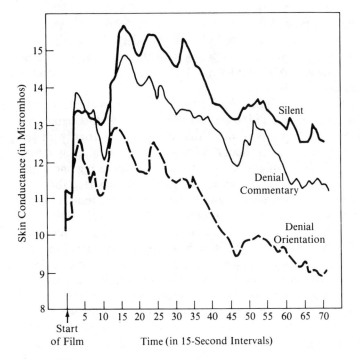

Figure 12.2.

Skin Conductance Curves During Orientation and Film Periods Under Three Experimental Conditions (Weiner, 1980a, after Lazarus & Alfert, 1964).

Cognitive Influences on the Arousal Value of Cues

According to Figure 6.1, the motivational sequence starts when certain stimuli, cues, or demands contact an incentive (or elicit a goal in the mind of the subject), but cognitive factors play an important role in whether or not such contact occurs. Lazarus and Alfert (1964) showed college students a film in which adolescent boys undergo a tribal ritual in which their penises are deeply cut. The students' viewing the film is sufficient to contact the pain incentive, which leads to the arousal of the anxiety motive, as Figure 12.2 shows. In this instance the measure of anxiety is the galvanic skin response, or the increase in electrical conductivity of the skin due to imperceptible sweating from anxiety. The top, "silent" curve shows the great increase in skin conductance reflecting anxiety that accompanies the film when it is presented silently. However, in one ("denial orientation") condition, before viewing the film the subjects received an elaborate explanation on a sound track of the significance of the ritual by an objective anthropologist in which he also stated that the procedure was not harmful. This cognitive orientation significantly reduced the negative incentive value of the film and the accompanying arousal of anxiety. The same denial commentary presented on a sound track along with the film ("denial commentary" condition) also reduced anxiety somewhat, but not as much as reorienting the subjects before they saw the film.

As this experiment demonstrates, a conscious understanding of what is going on can modify the arousal effects of cues. In Chapter 6 a study was reviewed in which it was found that the cues associated with going without food for as long as sixteen hours increased incentive value, as reflected in imaginative stories about getting food rather than actually seeing and eating it (Atkinson & McClelland, 1948). However, Sanford (1937) reported that subjects who consciously fasted for equivalent periods of time did think more about food and eating it as time went along. In other words, knowledge that one was fasting changed the nature of the incentive associated with arousal of the hunger motive. Schachter's (1971b) research on obesity, also reviewed in Chapter 6, demonstrates that other cognitive factors, such as the time of day and the number of external cues available in the environment, significantly affect the degree to which hunger is aroused in overweight people (see Table 6.2). The importance of such contextual understandings for arousal of the sexual drive is illustrated in Table 5.2. In that study the presence of an attractive female folk singer did not increase sexual arousal in young men, even when alcohol was also served, so long as the experiment was conducted in a classroom. However, if the same procedure was followed in an apartment, sexual fantasies were increased. It seems reasonable to infer that the students' understandings of what normally went on in classrooms interfered with the capacity of the sexual cues to contact sexual incentives and motives.

Several studies have demonstrated the way in which cognitive factors can influence the capacity of instructions to arouse the achievement motive. As noted in Chapter 6, when several groups of U.S. women understood that their intelligence and leadership capacities were being tested, their average *n* Achievement score in stories written subsequently did not increase, as it did for U.S. men who had been similarly instructed. Instead, the women's *n* Achievement scores tended to rise when their social competence was being evaluated (see Field, cited in McClelland, Atkinson, Clark, & Lowell, 1953). In other words, for these U.S. women, motivational demands stated in terms of leadership and intelligence did not have the same incentive value as for similar U.S. men. Their cognitive understanding of what was important to them determined whether achievement motivation was aroused or not.

Raynor and Teitelbaum (1982) have shown that even the time orientation in the cues that elicit stories affects the extent of achievement motive arousal. They asked subjects to write stories to sentence leads referring to a person who is thinking about an event that defines "who he or she is becoming," "who he or she is," or "who he or she has been." As Figure 12.3 makes clear, a cognitive orientation toward the future elicits much more achievement motive arousal than an orientation toward the past.

A subject's view of his or her competence for a task displayed in a picture

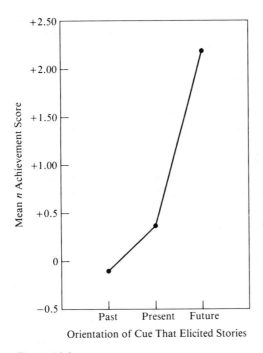

Figure 12.3.

Mean *n* Achievement Score as a Function of Time Orientation of Verbal Cues That Elicited Stories (after Raynor & Teitelbaum, 1982).

cue also affects the amount of achievement imagery in stories written to the picture. Shrable and Moulton (1968) had subjects rate their competence at tasks displayed in various pictures, such as chopping a tree or playing a musical instrument. They found that more intelligent subjects wrote stories with more achievement imagery to pictures displaying a task at which they felt they were competent as contrasted to pictures displaying a task at which they felt less competent. The reverse was true of subjects lower in intelligence. Clearly, people's views of their general competence and their competence at a particular task influence the extent to which particular cues can arouse achievement motivation. What needs to be worked out in this area in more detail is what general cognitive factors have the most influence in modifying the arousal value of demand cues in different motivational areas.

Is Motive Arousal Solely a Function of Cognition?

Several studies have examined the way in which the subject's understanding of a situation influences the degree to which physiological cues are associated with motive arousal. The original impetus for this type of research came as a reaction to the behaviorist tradition, described in Chapter 3, in which drive stimuli were thought to involve physiological sensations that defined the drive. Thus, if an investigator could show that physiological sensations were not automatically associated with drive arousal without a certain type of cognitive appraisal of the situation, the behaviorist position would have been shown to have an important limitation.

Valins (1966) studied the relationship of physiological cues to arousal of the sexual motive. He showed male undergraduates a number of slides of seminude females from *Playboy* along with a tape recording that in one condition purported to be the sound of the subject's heartbeat in response to each picture. The auditory feedback was actually a standard tape recording in which heart rate went significantly up or down to half of the slides and showed no change for the other slides. The slides that supposedly produced a heart rate reaction are referred to as *reinforced,* whereas those that produced no special response are referred to as *not reinforced.* After the experiment was over the college men were asked to rate the attractiveness of all the slides and were allowed to take home the pictures they most preferred.

As Figure 12.4 shows, they rated slides as more attractive that in their own minds they had associated with their heart beat's speeding up or slowing down. They also chose more such slides to take home. In a control condition, subjects observed the same slides and heard the same tape recording, but this time the noises on the tape were explained as being related to something else the subjects were doing. As Figure 12.4 shows, if the subjects did not interpret the increased or decreased noises associated with various slides as their own heart beats, there was no difference in their preference for slides reinforced in this way as compared with those not reinforced. Furthermore, the effect of the sound tape on actual heart rate was the same under both conditions. Thus, physiological cues were not related to sexual arousal unless the subject thought they should be. That is, the subjects reacted to the information that their heart beats were going up or down in response to certain slides by taking it to mean that they were more "turned on" by certain women than others. This cognitive appraisal led to an increase in the desire for these women, as shown by the higher attractiveness ratings the subjects gave them and by their preferences for these pictures to take home. Remember, however, that all the pictures were quite attractive and undoubtedly produced some sexual arousal, so what the cognitive information did was *shift* preferences from one set of pictures to another, not *create* a sexual arousal that did not exist before. It is doubtful if any amount of heart beat information could create a preference for a picture of a witch.

The experiment of this type cited most often by far is one conducted by Schachter and Singer (1962). To produce physiological arousal, they injected subjects with "suproxin," a drug that subjects were told would affect their vision but that was actually either a placebo or a small amount of epinephrine (adrenaline). Then, while the subjects waited for the drug's effects to occur, they were put in a room with another subject who had supposedly received the same drug. Actually, the second subject was a confederate trained to act either in a happy or irritated way. In the "happy" condition the confederate behaved very cheer-

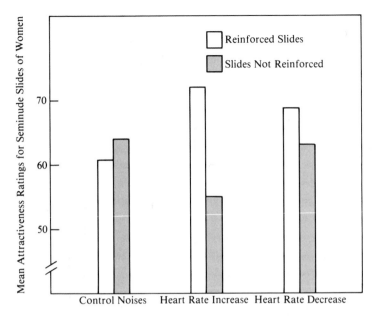

Figure 12.4.

Effects on Attractiveness of Pictures of Women When Changes in Heart Rate Are Associated with Them (after Valins, 1966).

fully, laughing a lot, throwing paper airplanes, playing with a Hula-Hoop, and generally encouraging the real subject to join in the fun. In the "irritated" condition the confederate was filling out a questionnaire for the experimenter that asked a lot of personal questions about sexual or financial matters. The confederate expressed great irritation at having to answer such questions and generally attacked the experiment and the experimenter, again encouraging the real subject to join in expressions of anger.

After this part of the experiment, the subjects filled out rating scales indicating how happy they felt and how irritated they felt. An overall "happiness" score was computed by subtracting the irritation rating from the happiness rating.

As Figure 12.5 shows, the two types of social treatment by the confederate had no differential effect on how subjects felt afterward if they had received a placebo injection. This is a little surprising, since it suggests that the experimenter's attempt to manipulate mood was ineffective. Schachter and Singer explain it on the grounds that perhaps the subjects, after exposure to the angry confederate, did not show an increase in irritation because they were afraid to express their irritation at the experimenter in full.

The effects of treatment on mood were somewhat different if the subjects received an epinephrine injection but were not informed of the physiological ef-

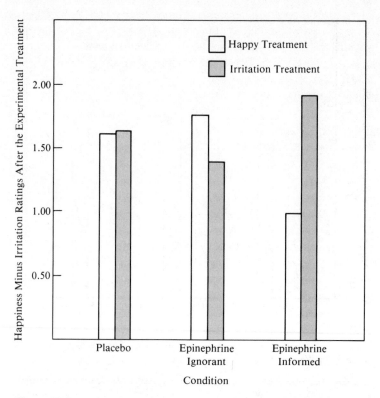

Figure 12.5.

Effects of Social Treatment on Mood of Subjects Receiving Injections Under Different Conditions (after Schachter & Singer, 1962).

fects of the drug. When there is an actual physiological arousal (for example, the increased heart rate from the injection of epinephrine), it looks as if the treatment—representing what the subjects thought the effects should be based on the behavior of another person receiving the drug—had a differential effect on mood. Those exposed to a happy confederate rated themselves as somewhat happier than those who had been exposed to the irritated confederate. The difference shown in Figure 12.5 is not significant, but it was bolstered by coding the behavior shown by the subjects in the waiting room. While being exposed to the angry confederate, they engaged in significantly more acts of irritation than those in the placebo condition, and while being exposed to the happy confederate, they engaged in somewhat more happy acts than those in the placebo condition, although not at a statistically significant level.

Schachter and Singer and others interpreted these results to mean that cognitive appraisal determines entirely the motivational or emotional effects of physiological arousal. A person feels a physiological disturbance, as from an injection of epinephrine, but the emotional label given to the state depends entirely on the subject's understanding of the situation. If people believe the state is associated with happiness, they will feel happy; if they believe it is supposed to be associated with irritation, they will feel irritated. Peoples' observations and inferences about themselves determine their emotions and motivations. As William James put it long ago in describing the James-Lange theory of the emotions, people are afraid because they observe themselves running; they do not run because they are afraid.

The Schachter and Singer experiment has almost universally been cited as support for this inference, although the evidence it provides is by no means conclusive. Marshall and Zimbardo (1979) attempted to replicate the happy treatment effect and found, as had Schachter and Singer, that happiness did not increase significantly after epinephrine injection over what it was after a placebo injection. This raises a real question as to whether the cognition that the drug was supposed to produce happiness in combination with the physiological arousal from epinephrine in fact produced a happier mood than a person would get without the physiological arousal. The subjects, in fact, did not really discover from the euphoric behavior of the confederate the cognition ("I feel happy") to explain their internal arousal.

Furthermore, the biggest change in the effects of social treatment occurred when the subjects were correctly informed of the effects of epinephrine on internal symptoms. At one level this strongly supports the contention that cognitive understandings significantly modify the effects of physiological arousal on emotions, but at another level it raises a major difficulty for the Schachter and Singer point of view. Why should the subjects exposed to the angry confederate feel so much happier after the experiment than those exposed to the happy confederate if they know what the effects of epinephrine are? This is the largest and most significant difference in Figure 12.5, yet Schachter and Singer make little of it, for from their point of view, once the subjects know accurately what the effects of the drug are, the social treatments should have no differential effect or, at any rate, not a *reverse* differential effect, on mood.

What this finding suggests is that there is a bias in a particular direction in the effects of epinephrine on mood. As noted in Chapter 8 on the power motive, there is reason to believe that the catecholamines, of which epinephrine is one, subserve the power motive system. Thus, the stirred-up physiological reactions that go with epinephrine are often associated with anger, aggression, and trying to have impact on others. Once the subjects are allowed to identify correctly these internal reactions—in the informed condition—they can express irritation consistent with those internal cues obtained when they were exposed to the angry confederate. In the ignorant condition they are more confused about the meaning of the physiological signs, and when they act in an irritated way after exposure to the irritated confederate, they are not behaving as consistently with the internal cues as they are in the informed condition. So they feel less satisfied in the ignorant than the informed condition.

We then need only to assume further that expressing anger in a way that is consistent with internal cues has a cathartic effect: the subjects feel better from

having expressed anger that is consistent with their state of physiological arousal, and thus they rate themselves happier afterward. In contrast, exposure to a
happy confederate suggests a reaction that is totally inconsistent with the physiological signs that normally go with anger and irritation, so in the informed
condition subjects remain confused and rate themselves less happy at the end of
the experiment than in the ignorant condition. Admittedly, such an interpretation is speculative and requires further checking, but the results do strongly suggest that the physiological arousal caused by epinephrine—if it is understood—
affects the outcomes of the treatments in a way that suggests that its effects are
biased more in one direction than another. This adds to the skepticism that cognitive appraisal, all by itself, can turn the physiological arousal due to epinephrine into happiness. However, cognition certainly has one important effect:
knowledge of the effects of epinephrine completely reverses the effects on moods
of the two types of treatments in combination with epinephrine arousal.

Alterations in Motive Arousal by Cognitive Dissonance

Later research demonstrated that physiological states were not simply the passive product of cognitive understandings, as suggested by Schachter and Singer,
but could themselves influence cognition. To create cognitive dissonance, Zanna
and Cooper (1974) asked college students to write a brief essay supporting the
view that inflammatory speakers should be banned from the campus. Most students disagreed strongly with this viewpoint, so writing such an essay could
create dissonance because they would find themselves saying things they did not
believe. In one condition the students were told the experimenter realized that
performing the task would involve going against their beliefs, and they were
given a free choice as to whether to do it or not. In the other condition the students were simply asked to perform the task and were not given the choice of
not doing it. At the outset of the experiment they were given a pill, which different groups of subjects were told would either make them more tense, more
relaxed, or have no discernible effects. Ratings of mood states by the subjects
showed that the suggested effects of the pill occurred: those who were told it
would relax them felt more relaxed, and those who were told it would increase
tension felt more tense, even though the pill they received was the same and
should not in reality have had any effects.

Figure 12.6 presents the mean agreement with the view that speakers should
be banned from campus for subjects exposed to various treatments (Zanna &
Cooper, 1974). Consider first the results for subjects on whom the pill had no
effect. Students who freely chose to write a counterattitudinal statement ended
up agreeing more with that viewpoint than subjects who wrote similar statements, but without having freely chosen to do so. Cognitive dissonance can explain the result: Subjects who found themselves *voluntarily* supporting a position
with which they strongly disagreed should be in a state of conflict or confusion.
Why would they do such a thing? To reduce the conflict or dissonance, they
moved toward agreement with the disavowed opinion so that they could feel less
conflict for having endorsed it. Subjects who had not freely chosen to write this

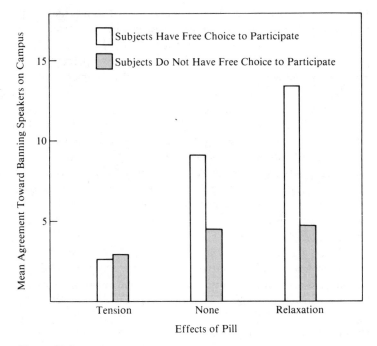

Figure 12.6.

Effects of Meaning of Taking a Pill on Attitudes When Subjects Do or Do Not Have the Free Choice to Participate (after Zanna & Cooper, 1974).

statement felt less dissonance, because they could explain their behavior by saying that they were more or less forced to do it. So they would be under less pressure to change their opinion to explain their strange behavior.

Next, notice what happened when the pill created a state of tension in the subjects: The cognitive dissonance effect disappeared. Now the subjects in the free choice condition had an adequate physiological explanation for their feeling of tension from doing something strange. They no longer needed to modify their attitudes to reduce the feeling of tension, for they perceived that it derived from a physiological source. On the other hand, if the pill produced relaxation, the cognitive dissonance effect was magnified. Now the subjects in the free choice condition had *two* reasons for feeling strange: they were voluntarily doing something inconsistent with their beliefs, and furthermore they were feeling very relaxed about it, which seemed even stranger. So they modified their opinion even more toward a disavowed position because of the much greater feeling of dissonance or inconsistency.

The important inference to be drawn from this experiment is that physiological states, or at least perceived physiological states, modified what the subjects understood was going on. One physiological state (induced tension) destroyed the cognitive dissonance effect obtained when the pill had no psychological effect; another (induced relaxation) enhanced the cognitive dissonance effect. So the conclusion is the same as the one we drew from the Schachter and Singer experiment: physiological cues influence cognitive perceptions, just as cognitive perceptions influence the interpretation of physiological states.

There is no reason to conclude that cognitive factors alone (the knowledge that one is doing something strange voluntarily) create and control the dissonance the subjects are motivated to reduce. Perceived physiological states also contribute to whether the negative incentive of dissonance occurs. Of course, we can argue, as Zanna and Cooper do, that cognitive expectations produced the perceived physiological states so that it looks as if all the effects in the experiment were based on cognitions. However, since the physiological effects were real in the sense that the subjects actually felt relaxed or tense, we can view them as controlling the dissonance effect directly, regardless of how they were produced.

Other cognitive dissonance research has dealt more directly with its effects on the arousal of other motives. In a typical study (Grinker, 1969), subjects participated in an eyelid conditioning experiment in which air puffs are delivered to the eye, causing it to blink. If a tone precedes the air puff slightly, in time the eyelid will blink to the tone before the air puff is delivered. That is, the tone elicits a conditioned avoidance response to the mildly painful air puff. After the subjects were conditioned, they were told that the intensity of the air puff would be increased in the next series of trials. In the control condition this was all the subjects were told, and in the subsequent trials they showed a large gain in the percentage of eye blinks to the tone to avoid the more painful air puffs. In the dissonance condition the subjects were asked whether they wished to continue in this more unpleasant series of trials. All freely chose to do so, but they showed only a very slight increase in the percentage of eye blink avoidance responses to the stronger air puffs. This result indicates that the cognitive dissonance manipulation had directly decreased the pain experienced from the air puffs or decreased the arousal of the fear motive based on the pain. To justify their voluntarily undergoing such an unpleasant experience, the subjects somehow reduced its unpleasantness. A different understanding of what they were doing had decreased the capacity of the cues in the situation to arouse the anxiety motive.

In a more obvious manipulation of drive arousal, Mansson (1969) first created thirst in subjects by having them eat a lot of dry crackers with a hot sauce. After obtaining ratings on how thirsty they felt and other matters, he asked them if they were willing to participate in a further experiment that involved going without water for a period of time. In the low dissonance condition he gave a strong justification for the deprivation procedure, explaining that it was necessary to get good results, and he further noted that the time of deprivation would be short. In the high dissonance condition he gave no justification for the procedure and explained that the time of deprivation would be long. Thus, the subjects in this condition were voluntarily agreeing to remain thirsty for a long period of time for no discernible reason. In the moderate dissonance condition either the justification was strong and the deprivation was long, or the justification was weak and the deprivation was short. Data were also obtained from subjects in a control condition who were not exposed to the dissonance treatment and from subjects who, unknown to the experimenter, had refused to take part in the second experiment.

Mansson then examined many different kinds of responses of the subjects to see whether the cognitive manipulations had affected the thirst drive. He found that subjects in the high dissonance condition, as contrasted with those in the low dissonance condition, gave fewer water-related responses in stories written to pictures, learned thirst-related words more slowly, rated themselves as less thirsty, and actually drank less water when given an opportunity, as shown in Figure 12.7. Note that the thirst manipulation worked: those in the control condition who had eaten salty, highly spiced crackers drank much more than those who had eaten crackers and peanut butter. Yet those in the high dissonance condition drank much less than this, although they too had eaten the highly spiced crackers. Those in the low dissonance condition drank much more than those in the high dissonance condition, as did those who had refused to participate in the experiment. In short, those in the high dissonance condition gave many different signs of being less thirsty than subjects in other conditions. The cognitive pressure to explain their strange, inconsistent voluntary behavior was strong enough to interfere with the capacity of the dry sensations in the mouth (physiological cues, in Figure 6.1) to arouse the thirst motive.

The type of cognitive manipulation involved in dissonance studies is peculiar, but in theoretical terms its effects are no different from examples of similar phenomena described earlier. For instance, in the Lazarus and Alfert genital operation film, the cues arising from viewing what appeared to be a painful operation were blocked or diverted from arousing the fear motive by cognitive explanations that the operation was not so painful and fully justified.

Cognitive dissonance can either increase or decrease motive arousal, depending on other factors. Glass and Wood (1969) had subjects rate another person both before and after they had apparently given the other person a strong electric shock. If they were not given a free choice as to whether they would participate in shocking someone (low dissonance condition), there was no change in their liking for the other person. However, if they voluntarily chose to shock the other person, they disliked the other person more afterward, in order to justify their strange behavior, but only if they were also high in self-esteem. Subjects low in self-esteem in the high dissonance condition actually liked the other people more after shocking them. It is as if they knew they were no good and that shocking another person simply confirmed their negative self-image, so they increased the likability of the other person to justify still further their negative picture of themselves. In contrast, those high in self-esteem found themselves voluntarily doing something very inconsistent with their positive self-image, so they had to increase their dislike for the person to explain to themselves why they were doing it. Here a third variable, self-esteem, interacts with a cognitive dissonance treatment to raise or lower the arousal of the motive to feel aggressive toward another (an aspect of the power motive). Obviously, the effects of cognitive variables on motive arousal are varied and complex.

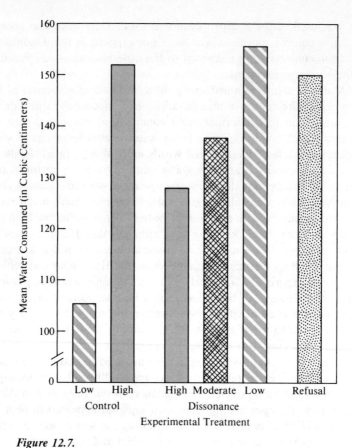

Figure 12.7.

Mean Water Consumption in Cubic Centimeters for the Low and High Control, High Dissonance, Combined Moderate Dissonance, Low Dissonance, and Combined Refusal Groups (after Mansson, 1969).

• MOTIVE-RELATED COGNITIONS

Causal Attributions

Cognitive variables not only influence motive arousal; they also accompany and follow the behavior associated with it. A very extensive research literature has grown up around the explanations people give for what they have done in terms of how such explanations derive from existing motive states or feed back and affect motive states. The interest in this field developed from two sources. One was the research on cognitive dissonance, which showed that if subjects explained or justified their behavior for external reasons, it left their internal motive states relatively unaffected, but if they could not find external justifications, their internal motive states were likely to be altered in significant ways, as in

Mansson's thirst experiment. So explanations for behaviors or causal attributions seem to be important modifiers of motive states. The other source of interest was research on the reasons subjects give for success or failure in an achievement-related context. Taking a clue from an earlier analysis by Heider (1958), Weiner and others (Frieze & Weiner, 1971; J. P. Meyer, 1980; Tasser, 1977; Weiner, 1980a; Weiner & Kukla, 1970) have examined the conditions under which subjects attribute success or failure to ability, effort, task difficulty, or luck.

Table 12.1 lists some of the cues people utilize in making inferences concerning the reasons for success and failure. For example, if people are often successful at a certain type of task, they are likely to attribute the outcome to ability. If performance shows a wide variation, people are likely to attribute it to differences in effort. If they are unexpectedly successful, they are likely to attribute it to luck.

These are not the only reasons given for success and failure, although they are the ones on which the most research effort has focused. Falbo and Beck (1979) suggest that less than half the reasons people give can be classified into these four categories. Subjects typically mention such other factors as calmness, carelessness (which could indicate lack of effort), or personality problems. Factor analyses of all sorts of different reasons people give support the conclusion that there are three general *types* of reasons given for success and failure. One type involves an internal-external dimension. People attribute the outcome either to factors in themselves such as effort or ability, or to external factors such as task difficulty or help from another person. The second type involves a stability dimension. People attribute the outcome either to some stable, relatively unchangeable cause such as ability, or to a variable cause such as effort or luck. The third type involves a controllability dimension. People attribute the outcome to a factor over which they have some control, like effort, or over which they have no control, like luck.

Table 12.1.

SOME CUES UTILIZED FOR INFERENCES CONCERNING THE CAUSES OF SUCCESS AND FAILURE (Weiner, 1980a)

Causes	Cues
Ability	Number of successes, percentage of successes, pattern of success, maximal performance, task difficulty
Effort	Outcome, pattern of performance, perceived muscular tension, sweating, persistence at the task, covariation of performance with incentive value of the goal
Task difficulty	Objective task characteristics, social norms
Luck	Objective task characteristics, independence of outcomes, randomness of outcomes, uniqueness of event

Research on causal attributions linked up with motivation theory when it was discovered that people with a strong or weak achievement motive gave different explanations for success and failure. Weiner (1980a) concluded that those high in *n* Achievement attributed success to ability and effort and failure to bad luck or lack of effort (see also W. U. Meyer, 1973). Those low in *n* Achievement (or high in *f* Failure) perceived success as due to luck and failure as due to lack of ability. Following the lead of others who were defining emotions in cognitive terms, Weiner concluded from these observations that the achievement motive was a cognitive disposition, a pattern of explanations for performance that gives rise to affect. Thus, a woman high in *n* Achievement feels good about performing well, because she attributes her success to high ability, whereas a woman low in *n* Achievement does not feel particularly good after success, because she attributes it to luck. "The achievement motive may be defined as a capacity for perceiving success as caused by internal factors and failure by unstable factors. . . . Thus the achievement motive is a cognitive, rather than affective, disposition. . . . Affect follows cognitive appraisal" (Weiner, 1980a).

The way attributions influence motivation to achieve is described by Weiner (1979) in scenarios like the following. Suppose some students have just received grades on an examination. The first one says to himself, "I just received a D on the exam. That is a very low grade. There really is something lacking in me. What I lack I probably always will lack." As Weiner points out, attributing failure to lack of ability typically leads to hopelessness and a lack of trying to do better, which would seem to characterize people low in *n* Achievement. In contrast, a second student also receiving a D and evaluating it as a poor grade may say to herself, "I didn't really study for the exam. Next time I am going to try harder, and because I know I have the ability, I am sure I will do better." This causal attribution pattern should characterize the person with high *n* Achievement and should also be associated with doing better next time, for Heckhausen (1975a) has shown that effort intended in a subsequent task is correlated .63 with effort actually expended. W. U. Meyer (1973) has demonstrated that subjects who attribute poor performance on the first trial of a task to lack of effort tend to work faster on the second trial (see Figure 12.8). Notice, in contrast, that subjects who attribute failure to the stable factors of low ability or task difficulty do not work harder or do better on the next trial. Weiner reasoned that the differential effect of these causal attributions on performance is similar to the effect expected for individuals high and low in *n* Achievement. Subjects who attribute failure to lack of effort tend to do better, just like subjects high in *n* Achievement; those who attribute failure to lack of ability tend not to do better, just like subjects low in *n* Achievement.

Weiner (1981) has also extended his attributional analysis of motivation beyond the area of achievement. He constructed a number of episodes (Weiner, 1980b) for students to read and react to, such as the following:

At about 1:00 in the afternoon you are riding a subway car. There are a number of other individuals in the car and one person is standing holding on to the center pole. Suddenly this person staggers forward and collapses. The person is carrying a black

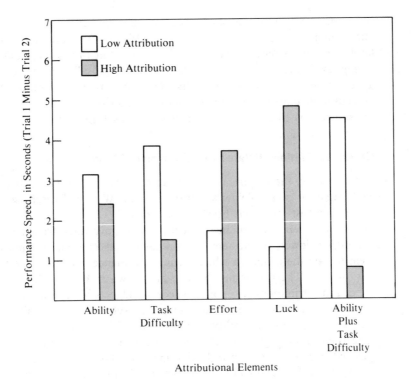

Figure 12.8.

Intensity of Performance, in Seconds (Trial 1 Minus Trial 2) As a Function of Attribution to the Four Causal Elements and to the Combined Stable Factors. High numbers indicate greater improvement in speed (after Weiner, 1980a, after W. U. Meyer, 1973).

cane and apparently is ill. (Alternate form: the person is apparently drunk. He is carrying a liquor bottle wrapped in a brown paper bag and smells of liquor.)

Try to assume that you actually are on the subway and try to imagine this scene. Describe your feelings in this situation.

Then the subjects rated the causes of the person's falling on the dimensions of internal-external, controllability, and stability. In general, it was clear that the students saw the cause of the drunk's falling as internal and controllable, whereas they saw the fall of the ill person as uncontrollable. Furthermore, the ill person elicited emotions of sympathy and desire to help, whereas the drunk elicited disgust and unwillingness to help. In Weiner's view, the subject's cognitive appraisal of the situation (ill or drunk) and the reasons given for it completely determine the emotional response (sympathy or disgust) and the motivation that is subsequently aroused (to help or not help).

In terms of the model of the motivation-action sequence in Figure 6.1, there is no reason to doubt that understanding affects what a person intends to do after a motive is aroused. It may even feed back after an action and affect the level of motive arousal itself, as we have seen. But this is quite different from saying, as Weiner seems to, that the pattern of causal ascriptions *is* the motive. To examine this possibility, it is first necessary to review carefully the evidence on causal attributions of people differing in motive strength and the evidence on the subsequent effects on behavior of such causal attributions.

Causal Attributions Related to Achievement Motive Strength

Unfortunately, the empirical findings in this area are not as clear-cut as one could wish for or as Weiner's theory requires (Weiner, Russell, & Lerman, 1979). The best study has been performed by W. U. Meyer (1973), who asked subjects for their performance goal for a task; gave them feedback of results that was higher, lower, or the same as compared with expectation; and then asked them to rate the extent to which their performance had been due to ability, effort, or luck. The results he obtained are shown in Figure 12.9. Consider first the causal attributions given after success. Subjects high in *n* Achievement (*h* Success), as compared to those low in *n* Achievement (*f* Failure), explained success as more due to ability and effort, and less to luck. So far as failure is concerned, those high in *n* Achievement attributed it more to lack of effort and luck, whereas those low in *n* Achievement attributed it to lack of ability.

Jopt and Ermshaus (1977, 1978) found similar results for intellectual, but not manual, tasks and also reported that subjects high in *f* Failure were more likely than subjects high in *h* Success to attribute failure to task difficulty. Others have found no attributional patterns associated with the achievement motive (Schneider, 1977). Weiner et al. (1971) found a pattern of results that was somewhat different from Meyer's. For instance, they found that subjects high in *n* Achievement attributed *both* success and failure more to ability, and that those high in *n* Achievement attributed failure less, rather than more, to lack of effort, as in Figure 12.9. Some of the findings reported by the Weiner group are complicated by the fact that they regularly use the Mehrabian measure of *v* Achievement as if it were an adequate measure of *n* Achievement, despite the lack of either theoretical or empirical support for such a procedure (see Weiner & Potepan, 1970). Entin and Feather (1982) even found that subjects low in *n* Achievement attributed success to effort and ability in a pattern almost identical to that followed by those high in *n* Achievement. However, the task used involved working only for two minutes on anagrams before performance feedback was given and causal attributions requested. Other studies have typically involved the subjects in much longer, more demanding tasks.

What we must conclude from these results is that a number of variables other than achievement motivation affect causal attributions and that therefore it would be quite unsafe to use the pattern of causal attributions to diagnose *n* Achievement levels, as would seem to be required by a theory that states that the achievement motive is *defined* by the pattern of causal attribution. The most general conclusion that can be drawn is that subjects high in *n* Achievement

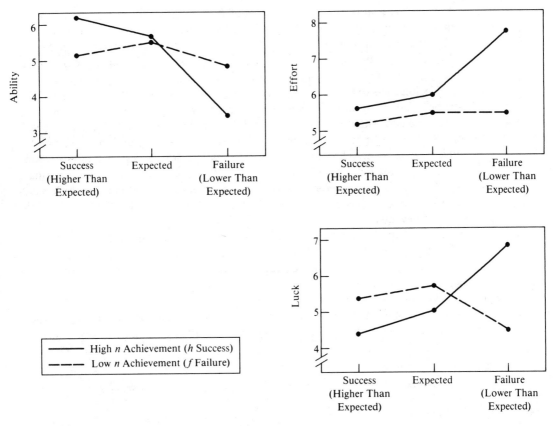

Figure 12.9.

Average Strength of Causal Attributions to Ability, Effort, and Luck for Success- and Failure-motivated Subjects If the Number of Correct Responses Is Higher or Lower Than Expected or as Expected (after Heckhausen, 1980, after W. U. Meyer, 1973).

tend to attribute success to ability and failure to lack of effort, whereas subjects low in *n* Achievement tend to attribute failure to lack of ability (Heckhausen, 1980).

Effects of Causal Attributions on Subsequent Behavior

Most studies of attribution simply ask the subject to think back and try to explain previous performance. Heckhausen (1975a) went a step farther and examined how causal attributions affected what people intended to do next. He first arranged for subjects to be successful on about 50 percent of the trials in performing a task. After a period of rest, subjects were divided into two groups, in one of which success was experienced on about 80 percent of the trials (the success condition) and in the other, on about 20 percent of the trials (the failure condition). They were also led to believe that there would be some further tasks to accomplish. After each phase of the experiment they were asked to give a self-evaluation, their intended level of effort, and their performance goals for the next phase of the experiment.

Heckhausen found that whereas subjects high in *n* Achievement might attribute failure to lack of effort, in this situation neither those high nor low in *n* Achievement showed a gain in intended effort after a period of consistent failure. So there is another weak link in Weiner's presumed causal chain of events: subjects high in *n* Achievement do not necessarily try harder after failure, even though they may attribute their failure to lack of effort. However, their evaluation of themselves depends more on how much effort they think they have made than is true for subjects low in *n* Achievement (see Figure 12.10). If those high in *n* Achievement feel they put out little effort, failing does not lower their self-esteem, but their self-esteem falls if they think they tried hard. In contrast, for the subjects low in *n* Achievement, how much effort they think they put out makes little difference in the general tendency for them to view themselves more negatively after failure.

We could presume that self-evaluation after failure would affect the willingness of the subjects to continue with the task if they had a free choice. On the one hand, subjects high in *n* Achievement who attribute failure to low effort

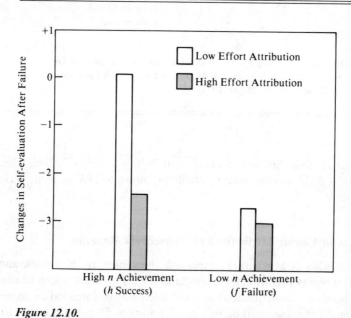

Figure 12.10.

Changes in Self-evaluation of Subjects After Failure as a Function of *n* Achievement Level and Low Versus High Effort Attribution (after Heckhausen, 1975a).

might be more willing to continue working at the task. On the other hand, subjects low in *n* Achievement appear to be just depressed by failure regardless of the reasons they give for it. At times they are even defensively unrealistic. If after failure they say that it means they have *little* ability for the task, they show a significant *gain* in the effort they intend to put out as compared with other subjects low in *n* Achievement who do not attribute the failure to low ability (Heckhausen, 1975a). This is irrational, because if they think they have little ability for a task, they ought to try less hard rather than harder. Apparently, trying hard under such circumstances is reported simply to make them feel better or to make others think better of them for working hard against such enormous odds. Or they are showing the greater attraction to very difficult tasks predicted by Atkinson's model of achieving tendencies (Chapter 7).

In general, causal attributions have more effect on the subsequent behaviors of subjects high in *n* Achievement than on those low in *n* Achievement. Figure 12.11 illustrates the point well (Halisch & Heckhausen, 1977). Six- to eight-year-old children built towers as the experimenter induced different expectations of success. They were scored as high or low in *n* Achievement using Aronson's "doodle" test (see Chapter 7). Toward the end of the experiment, subjects differing in expectations of success were told that they had succeeded or failed. Then the experimenter measured the time between the subjects' picking up a block and putting it on the tower to get an estimate of the enthusiasm with which the child was carrying out the task. Figure 12.11 shows changes in the speed of placing blocks on the tower as a function of the *n* Achievement level, expectation (probability) of success, and success and failure feedback.

The subjects high in *n* Achievement behaved as one would expect: If the probability of success was low, actual success led to greater effort, whereas failure led to less effort. If the probability of success was high, success led to less effort and failure, to more effort. This is exactly what one would expect from Atkinson's expectancy-value model of achievement motivation (see Table 7.2). For subjects high in *n* Achievement, cognitive information on how well they were doing fed back and modified their motive arousal for the next task.

For subjects low in *n* Achievement, however, the situation was quite different. They did not take probability of success into account in relation to success and failure, as those high in *n* Achievement did. Instead, failure simply depressed their performance. So subjects high in *n* Achievement seem more rational: they give explanations for performance that are more realistic, and they adjust their aspirations and efforts according to the feedback they get as to how well they are doing. Subjects low in *n* Achievement take such causal attributions and calculations less into account. When they get failure feedback, they may react quite unrealistically in terms of the amount of effort they put out and the reasons they themselves give for failure.

Evaluation of the Cognitive Theory of Motivation

Cognitive understandings certainly modify behavior and influence motive arousal, but can it be concluded that a causal attribution pattern *defines a motive,* as

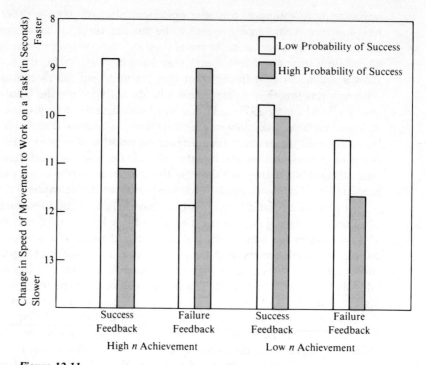

Figure 12.11.

Average Change in Speed of Movement to Work on a Task in Reaction to Success and Failure Feedback as a Function of Low or High Probability of Success and High or Low *n* Achievement (after Halisch & Heckhausen, 1977).

Weiner suggested? Or that the achievement motive is a system for evaluating the self, as suggested by Heckhausen (1980; see also Heckhausen & Krug, 1982)? The redefinition of motives in cognitive terms was part of the general shift in psychology away from emotional variables. At first sight it makes good sense as far as the achievement motive is concerned, because it seems to involve a particular way of people's appraising their own performance. Those with a high *n* Achievement score generally set realistic goals for their performance (with moderate probability of success in terms of their own performance) and tend to attribute success to ability and failure to lack of effort. They therefore maintain a positive attitude toward performance, which facilitates it. Those low in *n* Achievement (high in *f* Failure), in contrast, tend to have a highly negative attitude toward performance; avoid setting performance goals, if possible; set unrealistic, very high or very low goals, if they must set goals; avoid evaluation; and attribute success to luck and failure to lack of ability. Thus, they are caught in a cycle of defensive behavior that prevents them from doing well and feeling good about performance.

So it seems reasonable to conceptualize the achievement motive as a cognitive disposition to judge one's performance in one of these two ways. If this line of reasoning is pushed to its logical conclusion, we might be able to dispense with coding thoughts altogether and measure the strength of the achievement motive from the patterns of goal setting and causal attributions people follow. In fact, Heckhausen (1982) adopts such a viewpoint in discussing the cognitions different students reported while taking a demanding oral examination.

However, the case for the achievement motive's being a cognitive disposition is not persuasive for a variety of reasons. To begin with, the causes people with high and low *n* Achievement assign for success and failure vary considerably, depending on the circumstances. So it would be hazardous to use causal attribution or goal-setting patterns as a way of measuring *n* Achievement strength. For example, as already noted, Entin and Feather (1982) have found that under some circumstances even individuals low in *n* Achievement attribute success and failure to effort and ability. In the second place, while Weiner (1980a) argues that the important effects of achievement motivation on behavior can be explained in attributional terms, this is not always the case. For example, one of the best-supported findings in the attributional literature is that subjects low in *n* Achievement (or high in *f* Failure) attribute failure to lack of ability. So, argues Weiner (1980a), this explains why they "quit in the face of failure" (mediated by the belief that failure is caused by a lack of ability, which presumably is uncontrollable and unchangeable). But subjects low in *n* Achievement do not always quit in the face of failure. If they fail at a task with low probability of success, they are less likely to quit than subjects high in *n* Achievement (see Figure 7.6). Heckhausen (1975a) found in the study just reviewed that subjects high in *f* Failure who attributed their failure to a lack of ability were precisely those who said they intended to try harder next time. Cognitive interpretations of performance vary too much as a function of particular conditions to be considered a reliable index of motive strength.

Figure 12.12 (from Heckhausen, 1975b) provides another illustration of the inability of an attribution pattern to explain the effects of the achievement motive on behavior. As compared with individuals low in *n* Achievement, those high in *n* Achievement prefer working at tasks of moderate probability of success and getting feedback at how well they are doing at such tasks (see Chapter 7). This turns out to be the case for the experimental results reported in Figure 12.12, as shown by the right-hand graph. Subjects high in *n* Achievement prefer to work on tasks of moderate probability of success. Furthermore, one of the best-replicated findings of attribution research is that subjects high in *n* Achievement attribute success to ability. However, as the graph on the left-hand side of Figure 12.12 shows, those who consider themselves to have high ability for a task are *less* likely to prefer feedback on tasks of moderate difficulty than subjects who consider themselves to have low ability. Thus, we cannot predict one of the main behaviors explained by achievement motivation theory if we choose to use people's belief in their own ability as an index of achievement motive strength.

In any case, as pointed out in Chapter 6, if one wants to argue that a particular measure (for example, a goal-setting or causal attributional pattern or a

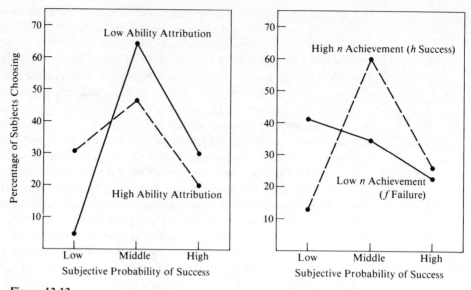

Figure 12.12.

Percentage of Subjects Choosing Performance Feedback on Tasks of Low, Moderate, and High Probability of Success as a Function of Perceived Degree of Ability Possessed for the Task (*Left*) and High and Low *n* Achievement (*Right*) (after Heckhausen, 1980, after Heckhausen, 1975b).

self-evaluative system) is tapping a motive, one must demonstrate that persons high in that measure behave as if they are more motivated—that is, act in a more aroused way, focus more sensitively on some cues than others, and learn relevant responses faster. Thus, for example, it would have to be shown that subjects who generally attribute success to ability or evaluate their performance positively would learn certain types of material more rapidly, just like the subjects high in *n* Achievement do (see Figure 6.13). Such subjects should also be shown to work harder only when an achievement incentive (a moderate probability of success) is present. The fact is that cognitive evaluations of performance have been studied only in the context of an ongoing experiment or episode, so little real attention has been given to whether or not they can be taken as evidence of differences in motive strength. So far, the functional criteria for determining whether a motive disposition is being measured have not been systematically applied to cognitive indexes of motive strength.

Analytically, the difficulty with the attributional model of motivation is that it starts with behavior that is already ongoing and asks the subjects for explanations of it afterward, rather than trying to account for what generated the behavior. A student receives a D on an examination, or a person sees someone fall in the subway. How the person interprets such events has consequences for what the person chooses to do next, but it does not explain why the behavior occurred in the first place. Why did the student take the examination? Why did he or she care about the grade received? What led to the particular causal explanation given? If the student were high in *n* Power, we could readily understand why a D would be upsetting, because it signifies loss of recognition and respect, which are important to the student. Why should a person react with sympathy when observing an ill person fall in the subway? Again, if the observer were high in *n* Affiliation, we would be more likely to expect sympathy than if the person were low in *n* Affiliation and cared not much at all about other people.

Still another difficulty with a wholly cognitive theory of motivation lies in the fact that Nicholls (1978) has demonstrated that causal attributions cannot really be made by children below the age of five. It may seem unreasonable to expect them to verbalize such causal explanations, although they might feel them. In fact, Weiner (1979) attributes causal reasoning to eight-week-old infants, but it seems doubtful that infants, or even young children, have enough sense of self for them even to *feel* attributions like "I should try harder" or "I did well because I am good at this sort of thing." In fact, Heckhausen (1980) assigns the origins of the achievement motive to an age (around two and a half to three and a half years) when a sense of whether one has done well first appears in a child, because he defines the motive as a self-evaluative disposition. But it seems unlikely that the achievement motive depends on a sense of self that develops at this age in view of evidence on the very early origins of the achievement motive as reviewed in Chapter 7.

We must also remember that cognitive understandings do not predict long-term drifts in behavior the way motives do. For example, Chapter 8 reviewed a study by McClelland and Boyatzis (1982) that showed that the imperial power motive pattern predicted the tendency to move upward in the management hierarchy over the long term at AT&T. Yet in the same study, a large number of cognitive variables, obtained from personality inventories, completely failed to predict managerial success over time (Bray, Campbell, & Grant, 1974). For example, *Self-confidence* and *Ascendancy* from the Guilford-Martin Inventory of Factors did not predict managerial success, nor did *v* Achievement, *v* Autonomy, *v* Dominance, *v* Endurance, nor any of the other eleven scales on the Edwards Personal Preference Schedule predict long-term success in management.

It is important to realize that the items that make up these scales refer to just such attributional patterns Wiener claims should motivate behavior. For example, items from the Edwards scale such as "I like to do my best in whatever I undertake" or "I like to work hard at any job I undertake" endorse the importance of effort, and an item such as "I like to supervise and to direct the actions of other people whenever I can" refers to belief in one's ability. Yet beliefs like these, even when aggregated into scales, do not in the long run predict analogous behaviors. They represent factors that can modify or direct power strivings, but they are not the motives themselves. In the short run in experimental situations in the laboratory, the effect of such value statements may be notable, because the experimenter relies on motives that the subject brings to the situation. In life and over the long run, where we cannot assume such motives to generate spontaneous behavior, the cognitive variables have little predictive power. Their chief contribution is in steering behavior once it has been generated by a motive or incentive.

Cognitive understandings, however, play an important role in the motivation-action sequence. Causal attributions, perceived instrumentalities, and self-evaluative systems do generally differ for people high and low in n Achievement, and these cognitive variables explain why they behave differently in various situations—in particular, why people high in f Failure perform in a self-defeating manner. Such cognitive variables modify what a person chooses to do next. They enter in to affect excitatory potential or the final impulse to act in a given situation. They also lead to emotional changes (positive or negative affect over performance), which feed back to alter motive arousal and motive dispositions over time. For example, if people high in n Power get good grades, the fact that they understand they are good grades and are due to their ability and effort leads to the emotion of pride in the recognition that they will receive, which strengthens the incentive character of good grades and perhaps the power motive itself in the long run. Or if a person high in n Affiliation understands that the person who has fallen in the subway is ill, that leads to the emotion of sympathy and the act of helping. The motive comes first, and the cognitive understandings direct or channel it and raise or lower it. It is more correct to say that certain cognitive dispositions characterize a motive than to say they are the motive.

The study of cognitive variables intervening in the motivation-action sequence performed a very important function in clarifying just *how* motives influence performance, as Dweck and Wortman (1982) point out. For example, achievement motivation theory predicts, according to Atkinson's model (Table 7.2), that as people high in n Achievement succeed at a task, it will become less interesting to them (it has a high probability of success), and they will set a higher level of aspiration for that or some other task (with a lower probability of success). But what goes on in their minds as they make this shift? Research on cognitive variables suggests that they view their success as due to ability; this increases their self-confidence, so they choose a more demanding task, perhaps because they want to continue to get information on how capable they are (Trope, 1975). Without information on such cognitive variables, there is a gap in our understanding of how motives get translated into various actions.

Future Orientation and the Achievement Motive

Another cognitive orientation that interacts with the achievement motive has been extensively studied by Raynor and Entin (1982b). They observed that most performances in life are perceived as part of some overall framework and as steps on the way to a goal. This is particularly true for students, for whom writing a successful term paper may be perceived as related to getting a good grade in a course, which is related to graduation, which is related to getting into graduate or professional school and going on to a career as a teacher or a lawyer. Raynor (1968) reasoned that individuals high in n Achievement ought to work harder at a task that they perceived as important for future success than at a task of lesser importance. He asked students to rate the importance/helpfulness of a good grade in an introductory psychology course for future career success (Raynor, 1968). When he sorted out the grades in the course at the end of the semester according to students who were high or low in *n* Achievement and who perceived the course as of low or high importance to them, he obtained the results summarized in Figure 12.13. As expected, the perceived instrumentality of the course made more of a difference to the subjects high in *n Achievement.* They got a considerably higher average grade in the course if they thought it was important than if they thought it was not. The perceived importance of the course made little difference to subjects low in *n* Achievement.

Raynor then moved on to construct a formal extension of the Atkinson achievement motivation model to cover contingent paths in which success in an immediate step is necessary "to earn the opportunity to move on to the next step." As Bandura (1982) summed it up in another connection, "self-motivation is best summoned and sustained by adopting attainable sub-goals that lead to large future ones. Whereas proximal sub-goals provide immediate incentives and

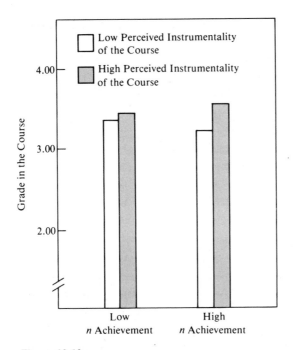

Figure 12.13.

Grades Attained in a Course as a Function of *n* Achievement and Perceived Instrumentality of the Course (after Raynor & Entin, 1982b).

guides for action, distal goals are too far removed in time to effectively mobilize effort or to direct what one does in the here and now." Raynor's model predicted that success in a contingent path should make more of a difference to subjects high than low in *n* Achievement. When subjects were asked to perform three-step arithmetic problems, results were obtained (Entin & Raynor, 1973) that confirmed the prediction, as shown in Figure 12.14. If subjects could not move on to the next step in the task unless they had reached a criterion in performing an earlier step, those high in *n* Achievement performed much better than those low in *n* Achievement. But if the subjects could move on to the next step regardless of how they performed on the first step, there was no difference in the overall performance of subjects high and low in *n* Achievement. The cognitive understanding of what performance means clearly interacts with the motive to determine performance.

The contingent path variable also explains some of the confusion over whether individuals high in *n* Achievement attribute success more to ability than subjects low in *n* Achievement. It turns out that they do, but only in contingent paths (Entin & Feather, 1982). Subjects high in *n* Achievement seem to care less about noncontingent paths, and their ability attribution reflects this fact.

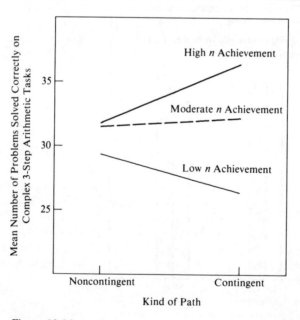

Figure 12.14.

Mean Number of Complex Arithmetic Tasks Solved as a Function of *n* Achievement Level and Whether Moving On Is Contingent on Success at the Previous Step (after Entin & Raynor, 1973).

The greater importance of contingent paths to subjects high in *n* Achievement is also shown by the fact that if on such paths the probability of success declines from step to step, they work much harder than those low in *n* Achievement. The latter tend to slack off as compared with how hard they would work in a contingent path with increasing probability of success (Raynor & Harris, 1982). This result can be explained as being due to the fact that since subjects high in *n* Achievement believe their success is due more to ability, they will continue to work harder even as the task gets more and more difficult; as the task gets more difficult, subjects low in *n* Achievement tend to slacken their efforts, because they believe they have less ability.

To examine how subjects high and low in *n* Achievement engaged in future planning, Pearlson and Raynor (1982) asked students to complete a future plans questionnaire in which the first step was to write in a future goal they sought. Then, on successive pages, they were to write in the steps that would lead to that goal, the activity that constituted each step, the positive and negative outcomes that might result from each activity, the chances of succeeding at each activity, and the importance of the future goal to them. In general, subjects high in *n* Achievement were able to define more steps leading to the future goal. They had a more differentiated cognitive map of how to get from where they were to where they were going, and this was particularly true if the goal was of high importance to them. The importance of the goal, like the contingent path variable, interacts with the achievement motive to influence what the subjects do—in this case, the extent to which they have planned ahead (see also Pearlson, 1982).

Raynor (1982) has extended his analysis to explain the effects of aging viewed as progress toward a closed, contingent path, at least so far as those pursuing careers are concerned. They start out life seeing many steps as leading to a career goal in the anticipated future. Then, as they move through the steps necessary to their achieving their career goal, the probability of success increases—at least to moderate levels—and stimulates achievement motivation. Then, as they approach retirement, they move from "becoming" to "having been": there are no immediate next steps required for attaining a future goal, and their *n* Achievement level declines. There is some support for this model from the two national sample surveys of achievement motivation that were conducted in 1957 and 1976 (Veroff, Atkinson, Feld, & Gurin, 1960; Veroff, Depner, Kulka, & Douvan, 1980), in the sense that *n* Achievement levels are significantly lower for men and women over the age of sixty-five. However, the data do not as clearly support the prediction that *n* Achievement levels should be highest in the middle years. This was not the case for men or women in the 1976 survey.

The virtue of Raynor's analysis is that it calls attention in a variety of ways to the importance of the cognitive context in which the achievement motive interacts with performance. The motive has different effects, depending on what the performance means to the subject, particularly in relation to future goals, as well as what steps, with what success probabilities, are necessary to get to them.

• COGNITIONS AFFECTING THE TRANSLATION OF MOTIVATION INTO THE IMPULSE TO ACT

As pointed out in different sections of this chapter, cognition affects the motivation-action sequence in many different ways. Figure 12.15 attempts to summarize these influences in schematic form. It represents an expanded version of Figure 6.1, and each of the cognitive influences has been given a number to make it easier to identify the relationship to be explained.

1. Cognitions influence the extent to which social or physiological cues contact incentives, which link up with motive dispositions leading to motive arousal. Several empirical demonstrations of this fact were reviewed in the first part of the chapter. A typical example is provided by the finding that references to *leadership* and *ability* do not link up with achievement incentives for certain types of women and thus arouse achievement motivation for them, whereas the same cues do arouse achievement motivation in comparable groups of men. The term *demands* implies a cognitive definition of which actions will obtain the goal implied in the incentive. That is, in mentioning the achievement incentive of doing well in life, the experimenter also states that a person who wants to do well in life should do well on these tasks. Normally, a person accepts this definition of the situation, but it is possible for a person's achievement motivation to be aroused by the incentive of doing well in life and for the person to still not believe that doing well on these tasks is related to that goal. In this case, a cog-

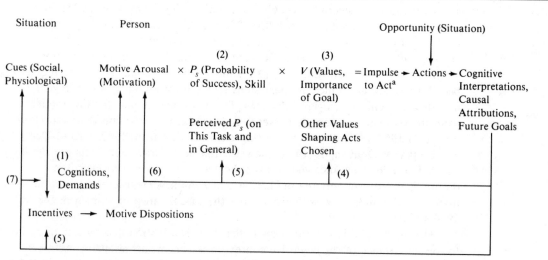

[a]"Motivation," as Atkinson, Weiner, and others use the term.

Figure 12.15.

Role of Cognitive Variables in the Motivation-Action Sequence.

nitive variable does not affect motive arousal (1) but affects instead the relevance of probability of success at this task (2) for the achievement incentive. So the impulse to do well on the task is lowered.

2 and 3. The position taken throughout this book is that an aroused motive combines with two other types of person variables to produce excitatory potential or the impulse to act, labeled *motivation* somewhat confusingly by Atkinson, Weiner, and others. Initially, Variable 2, the probability of success, was defined by the skill a person showed as represented by the number of practice trials in the behaviorist tradition (see Chapter 3). However, in the Atkinson model the variable got redefined in cognitive terms as the *perceived* probability of success. And in its most general form it became self-confidence, social norm ability, or self-efficacy, as we shall see. Variable 3, the value placed on actions related to the motive, is also cognitive. Atkinson's (1957) application of expectancy-value theory to achievement motivation simplified the equation by making the probability of success (P_s) and the value of success (V) completely dependent on each other (that is, $V = 1 - P_s$). This limits the value placed on the activity to difficulty, and whereas there is no question that performing a more difficult task is more valued by most people, many theorists have pointed out that other values also influence the impulse to act. We will consider some of these other values. What it is important to realize here is that both P_s and V are essentially cognitive variables that interact with an aroused motive to produce the impulse to act.

4. In the model, the impulse to act combines with the opportunities to act in the environment to yield a response, which is then interpreted by the person in various ways. These interpretations feed back to influence various aspects of the motivation-action sequence. If a person ascribes failure to lack of effort, it may make the importance of striving harder more salient. Effortful striving is an important value in our culture; according to the model it should therefore influence the impulse to act, but technically it is not part of the motive aspect of the action sequence.

5. If an act is perceived as successful, it feeds back to influence the sequence in two places. At the most direct level it increases the P_s variable, making the act more likely, but it also influences the incentive value of the activity in ways described in Chapter 7. If initial perceived probability of success is low, success increases its incentive value, whereas the reverse is true if perceived probability of success is high.

6. Causal attributions can affect motive arousal directly. Subjects who attributed their enduring thirst to their own voluntary choice showed less thirst than subjects who attributed their situation to external reasons (Mansson, 1969). In a different type of study showing the same relationship, Breit (1969) asked subjects to write essays on how they did (or did not) really control what happens to them. Based on the findings that subjects high in *n* Achievement are more likely to attribute performance to internal factors like ability and effort, he reasoned that subjects who thought about having control over things would have more aroused achievement motivation than those who thought about not having control over things. The results conformed to this hypothesis: the subjects who

had been thinking about having control behaved more like subjects high in *n* Achievement in their liking for occupations of varying difficulty as compared to subjects who had been thinking about not being in control. The findings are not direct confirmation of the relationship, because Breit did not measure aroused *n* Achievement in stories written by the subjects and because the treatment could have affected the P_s or V variables in the equation. However, the findings are consistent with the theoretical expectation that cognitive interpretations can feed back to influence motive arousal directly. Furthermore, Patten and White (1977) have demonstrated that asking a subject to give reasons for failure (a cognitive task) seems to feed back and increase the achievement motivation aroused.

7. The interpretation a person gives an act can also feed back and alter the demands that gave rise to the motivation for performance in the first place. As a simple illustration, consider Raynor's example of a person nearing retirement, which represents the end of a closed, contingent career path. At this point there are no next steps to be taken toward the goal, so the social demand or cue value of the activity giving rise to the achievement incentive declines or disappears.

The research reviewed in this chapter has dealt mostly with cognitive feedback effects on motivation of the type just summarized. Another kind of research deals with how variations in the P_s and V factors interact with motivation to produce different types of performance. Here the findings are not easy to summarize, because they come from a broad field in which studies have not been carried out in a very systematic way. Properly speaking, what is at issue here is the dynamics of action (Atkinson & Birch, 1970), or *the effort to explain action in terms of all its determinants,* only one of which is motivation. The most systematic recent attempt to build a model of how action occurs has been carried out by Atkinson and Birch (1978). To review that enterprise is beyond the scope of this book, but it is worth calling attention to some of the main aspects of the perceived probability of success and value that have been found to interact with motivation to produce behavior.

Self-confidence or Self-efficacy

As the Atkinson model demonstrates, perceived probability of success at a task interacts with aroused motivation to influence what the subject does. The subject's perception of his or her likelihood of success in general in all types of tasks also has an important influence on performance. This important person variable has been called a sense of internal control, feeling like an Origin (deCharms, 1976), mindfulness (Chanowitz & Langer, 1982), self-efficacy (Bandura, 1982), or a sense of personal responsibility. Whatever it is called, it has been shown to facilitate performance under a variety of circumstances.

Some typical findings are presented in Figure 12.16. The research on which the figure is based involves raising the sense of self-efficacy among phobics by enactive mastery of progressively more threatening activities (Bandura, 1982). A typical study involved "severe agoraphobics, whose lives were markedly constricted by profound coping inefficacy that makes common activity seem filled

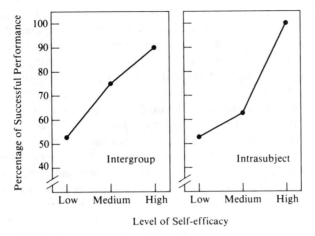

Figure 12.16.

Mean Performance Attainments as a Function of Differential Levels of Perceived Self-efficacy. (The left panel shows the performances of groups of subjects whose self-percepts of efficacy were raised to either low, medium, or high levels; the right panel shows the performances of the same subjects at different levels of self-efficacy (after Bandura, 1982).

with danger. . . . Therapists, who accompanied the agoraphobics into community settings, drew on whatever performance induction aids were required to enable their clients to cope successfully with what they dreaded" (Bandura, 1982). After the treatment, they were able to live successfully through previously dreaded situations such as traveling by automobile, using an elevator, dining in a restaurant, or shopping. At the same time, the perception of self-efficacy increased markedly, and the degree of perceived self-efficacy predicted future successful performance, as Figure 12.16 shows. In fact, the perceived self-efficacy predicted performance better than past performance did, demonstrating that at least under some circumstances the cognitive aspect of the probability of success is more important than its skill aspect.

Heckhausen has increasingly in recent years tended to conceptualize the achievement motive as a self-evaluative system (Heckhausen & Krug, 1982). Those high in *n* Achievement think of themselves as capable (having high self-efficacy or probability of success) and approach tasks with confidence; those low in *n* Achievement (or high in *f* Failure) think of themselves as low in ability or probability of success and act defensively with respect to tasks. This thesis is entirely consistent with the model of the motivation-action sequence in Figure 12.15, in which the perceived probability of success is an important determinant of the impulse to act, but the self-evaluative system is not the motive itself, although it may influence and be influenced by the motive.

Langer and Rodin (1976) have demonstrated the importance of this person variable in another setting. They arranged to have much greater personal responsibility assigned to residents on one floor of a nursing home for elderly people than on another floor where, as is usual in such settings, all decisions were made for the residents by the staff. It was explained to those receiving the special treatment that they really had the responsibility of caring for themselves and of making decisions such as what movie to attend, how they wanted their rooms arranged, how they spent their time, and how the procedures in the home might be changed to suit their needs better. They were also each given a plant to care for. Several measures of attitudes and activities of the residents on both floors were taken one week before the special treatment and three weeks afterward. Those who had been given a greater sense of personal responsibility reported themselves at the later period to be happier and more active than those living in the normal decision-free environment, and they were also rated to be more generally improved and alert by observers. Behavioral measures of time spent visiting with other residents and talking to the staff supported these conclusions. In short, giving these elderly people a sense of personal responsibility or efficacy facilitated actions of all sorts.

What is needed is more investigation of the way in which the sense of self-confidence interacts with motives to produce behavior. One such study is described in the next chapter.

Values

Certain goals are intrinsic to motives. People high in *n* Achievement want to *do better* (which has many cognitive determinants). People high in *n* Power want to *have impact,* which is also defined in increasingly complex ways as people grow older and more sophisticated. People high in *n* Affiliation want to be *with people.* But there are many other factors that combine with these goals to define the *V* variable in the motivation-action sequence. One is simply the importance of any of these goals, as it is consciously defined in the person's world view. Individuals high in *n* Achievement are most "turned on" by tasks with moderate probability of success, because performance in such situations gives them the best feedback on their improvement. However, that does not automatically imply that doing better on such tasks has great importance for them.

As Raynor and Entin (1982b) point out, the *importance* of the goal of a motive has no formal status in the theory of achievement motivation. They had subjects rate the importance of a future goal and also the probability of success of attaining it. They found that more important goals were perceived, on the average, as having $.7\ P_s$, as compared with $.5\ P_s$ for less important goals. This demonstrates the need to distinguish between the goal intrinsic to a motive and the importance of that goal as seen from an extrinsic point of view. A person high in *n* Achievement might conceivably be more attracted to the goal of graduating from law school if the perceived probability of success was moderate ($P_s = .5$) *if no other extrinsic values were involved.* But of course they are involved: graduating from law school may be important for all sorts of other reasons, so the person chooses to go to law school (the action outcome of the motivation-action sequence) only if the perceived probability of success is considerably higher than the .5 P_s theoretically optimal for a person high in *n* Achievement.

It is even possible that the goal state that gives satisfaction to a person's motive is considered completely unimportant by that person. People high in *n* Affiliation are satisfied by being with people, but in the next chapter we will consider the case of individuals high in *n* Affiliation who do not value being with people but prefer solitude. In this case the motive and value conflict and produce an interesting compromise action—namely, writing letters to people.

Most of the research in this area has dealt with extrinsic values, which increase the likelihood that achievement motivation will lead to a particular type of achievement behavior. Heckhausen (1980) has stressed the importance of what might be called the *instrumentality value:* if people see the connection between an outcome or an attribution and an act, they are more likely to perform the act, although this depends also on achievement motive strength and perceived probability of success (Kleinbeck & Schmidt, 1979). Such a result might be explained on the grounds that people have learned that it is valuable to know what leads to what. A feeling of personal control, of being able to do something that leads to a result, is an analogous variable. It is highly valued and facilitates performance, as the nursing home experiment demonstrates. Perlmuter, Scharff, Karsh, and Monty (1980) have even shown that the words people choose to learn are learned faster than words they are simply given to learn.

Value is also placed on effort in our society, so when effort becomes salient, performance improves (see Figure 12.8). In fact, all the causal attribution literature can be reconceptualized in terms of value theory. The dimensions of perceived causation—internal versus external locus of control, controllability, and stability—can be thought of as values (or at least schemata ordering the way things work) that influence performance. In general, the values of internality, controllability, and stability promote successful performance, whereas their opposites diminish it.

Many investigators have been critical of the achieving style, which interpretations of the achievement motive research have suggested is intrinsic to the motive itself. It is sometimes assumed that people high in *n* Achievement energetically pursue their own goals without respect to others, in a kind of caricature of the upward-aspiring, high-achieving Western male. Such an image is incorrect on many counts. At the simplest level it confuses achievement behavior, or the action output variable in Figure 12.15, with a particular motivational input. Obviously, from the model of the motivation-action sequence and from findings reported in earlier chapters, not all achievement behavior (or successful performance) is the result of achievement motivation. As Gallimore (1981) has carefully documented, the *n* Affiliation score among Hawaiians is more closely associated with many types of achievement behavior than the *n* Achievement score is. Hawaiians value interpersonal relations and work hard primarily when they are working together on a project. Thus, obviously a *value* placed on cooperative work in combination with an achievement *motive* ought to lead to different behaviors than if the value were placed on individual accomplishment.

The same point has been made in connection with sex differences by

Lipman-Blumen, Leavitt, Patterson, Bies, and Handley-Isaksen (1980) and Parsons and Goff (1980). Women in our society tend to value relationships more than men do, so for them, achievement motivation tends to be associated with a relational achieving style, whereas for men it is associated more with a direct achieving style. Thus, women are more likely to achieve in a vicarious way or in a contributory or collaborative relationship than men are (Lipman-Blumen et al., 1980). Parsons and Goff (1980) describe much the same difference in terms of Bakan's model of agency (which characterizes the direct achieving style of men) and communion (which characterizes the collaborative style of women). Both groups of researchers have developed value questionnaires to determine the extent to which individuals subscribe to direct or collaborative orientations in the achievement area. This is obviously a step in the right direction in accordance with the motivation-action sequence as outlined in Figure 12.15, for it is only as motives are studied in combination with other determinants of action like self-confidence and values that psychologists will begin to account for the various ways in which people behave.

Research in this area has not advanced very far, because people have confused motives and values and not treated them as separate determinants of action. Many more studies are needed that examine how important values interact with motives to produce action—in particular, studies of how they interact with the affiliative and power motives, which have tended to be neglected in favor of an almost exclusive concern with achievement behavior. What is also needed is a paradigmatic study of just how the three major determinants of action (motives, probability of success, and values) interact to produce performance. That is the topic of the next chapter.

NOTES AND QUERIES

1. Different incentives arouse achievement motivation in different groups of people: References to money rewards arouse more *n* Achievement in working-class than middle-class people (Douvan, 1956); references to social acceptability arouse more *n* Achievement in some groups of women than men. Does this mean that achievement motivation is solely determined by people's understanding of a situation? For example, it has been argued that it is wrong to conclude that lower-class blacks have lower average *n* Achievement than middle-class blacks or whites (B. C. Rosen, 1956), because lower-class blacks are just as achievement oriented, but their achievement motivation is aroused by different incentives. Evaluate this argument. Be sure to distinguish between motive arousal and dispositional level of *n* Achievement. Think about a person whose achievement motivation could be aroused only by one peculiar situation. Would you expect this person's dispositional level of *n* Achievement to be high or low?

2. An extreme version of the Schachter and Singer or James-Lange theory would seem to argue that moods associated with physiological arousal are

solely determined by the meaning people attribute to the arousal. Suppose you had a headache. Can you imagine an understanding of the situation that would lead you to feel really happy about the headache? What limits do you think may exist in our ability to feel what our understanding tells us we should feel?

3. Design a cognitive dissonance experiment that would lower the level of aroused achievement or power motivation the way Mansson's experiment lowered the level of thirst.

4. What kind of cognitive dissonance, if continued over time, might lower *dispositional n* Achievement? (If necessary, consult Andrews, 1967).

5. Try explaining Shrable and Moulton's (1968) finding that picture cues relating to an individual's competencies have differential effects for arousing achievement motivation for individuals of higher and lower intelligence. In other words, could the results have anything to do with perceived probability of success?

6. So far no one has studied the causal attributions of individuals high and low in *n* Power or *n* Affiliation. Make some predictions as to how motive strength in these areas might affect causal explanations for success or failure in gaining power or being loved. Would different types of causes be involved than those important in the achievement area?

7. Think of a successful experience you have had recently. Write out the reasons why you think you were successful. Try classifying these reasons according to the three dimensions discovered in previous research. Do the same for a recent failure experience. Are the reasons you gave related to your motive profile in ways that would be expected from previous research?

8. One can easily imagine how people high in *n* Achievement would develop a positive proactive image of themselves with respect to performance from observing how they behave over time. Similarly, people low in *n* Achievement develop a defensive self-image and style where performance is concerned from observing how they behave. In these instances the self-picture and motive syndromes are consistent and logically related, so it may look as if one is equivalent to the other. But sometimes motive systems and self-images are quite inconsistent with each other. Under what circumstances is such a state of affairs likely to occur? How would you know it existed, and what conclusions would you draw about the person?

9. Do you believe the contingent path model would apply to individuals varying in the strength of motives like *n* Power? Why or why not? Design an experiment to test the hypothesis that subjects high in *n* Power work harder to attain a goal when attaining it opens up the opportunity to attain a more important goal.

10. Construct a theoretical explanation for why contingent paths might not affect the behavior of individuals high in intimacy motivation.

11. If *n* Achievement is more related to time cognitions—that is, the interrelatedness of acts over time—can you think of reasons why *n* Power might

be related to space cognitions (to how they and others are placed in space)? Design an experiment to test this hypothesis.

12. Figure 12.15 has been constructed in a way that shows that relatively stable motive dispositions in a person are an important determinant of the motivation-action sequence. But it is possible to argue that such motive dispositions either do not exist or can be ignored. Such an approach would explain individual differences in aroused motivation solely in terms of cognitive variables like probability of success, values, understandings of what leads to what, and incentives. Try leaving motive dispositions out of the model. Do you run into any difficulties in explaining certain types of behavior when you do so?

13. Take each of the relationships labeled 1 through 7 in Figure 12.15 and try to find an experimental result showing the existence of such a relationship for the power motive or the affiliative motives. Do you run into any particular difficulties?

14. Heckhausen's value of *instrumentality* appears to be related to Raynor's conception of contingent paths. Both suggest that perceived means-end relationships are an important determinant of action. Yet when people are asked why they succeeded or failed, they seldom reply that it was because doing well on the task was (or was not) important for something else they wanted. Why not? Does this throw doubt on the causal attribution method of arriving at values (what is important to people) or on the importance of the value of instrumentality?

15. Heider argued strongly for the importance of cognition in determining motivation. Consider, for example, the following statements:

> If you want to persuade an individual *(p)* he should attack *o* (an "other" person), try to convince him that *o* harmed him, that *o* is much better off, etc. *O* must be portrayed as the unjustified aggressor, the frustrator, etc., and that he is determined to harm *p*. It is a matter of beliefs; if you control beliefs, then you control emotions.
>
> One information, one change in belief, affects motivation, affect, etc., and these direct effects have further effects on action. (Heider, cited in Benesh & Weiner, 1982)

In terms of the schema presented in this chapter for the determination of action, in what sense can it be said that beliefs control emotion or determine motivation? Are beliefs the only determinants of the impulse to attack? If so, how could one explain the greater tendency of the United States to attack at some times in its history than at other times (see Chapter 11)? If it is a question of the extent to which one nation believes another nation *deserves* to be attacked, for the reasons Heider gives, why is a nation more likely to believe such cognitive information at one point in its history than another?

16. Heider is also critical of the way in which psychologists like Murray think in terms of aggressive or power motives, because they leave out the cogni-

tive elements involved in choosing a target or goal for the motive: "Othello does not want just to kill anybody; he does not have a general need to kill, only the need to kill Desdemona" (Heider, cited in Benesh & Weiner, 1982) because of a lot of beliefs he holds about her. How is Heider's legitimate concern for what determines the specific goals of a motive in a given situation handled by the schema for the multiple determination of action presented in this chapter? Make a model based on Figure 12.15 that shows some of the key determinants in Othello's impulse to kill Desdemona.

13

How Motives Interact with Values and Skills to Determine What People Do

Ever since psychologists observed that motivated people or animals learn faster, they have been interested in how motives combine with other variables to increase the probability that a response will occur. In more general terms the question is, What factors in what combinations will best predict what response will be made, or if made, how often and how strongly it will be made?

All psychologists except a few association theorists like Guthrie (1935) assume that motives, rewards, or reinforcers are one of the determinants of response strength, and that there are also several other determinants that need to be taken into account. To begin with, the environmental situation is obviously important. A hungry rat will run faster through a maze or learn the correct turns more quickly than a satiated rat, but only if there is food in the goal box, and only if the rat can get into the maze. In other words, if one is interested in predicting the strength of the maze-running response, it is helpful not only to know how hungry the rat is, but also that the rat has access to the maze and that there is food available at the end of it. Response strength is jointly determined by a motivational variable in the organism and certain environmental variables.

In similar fashion it has been shown that individuals high in n Achievement will perform better than those low in n Achievement, but only if the environment provides them with a moderately difficult task incentive (see Clark & McClelland, 1956; French, 1955). If the task is too easy or too difficult, they do not work harder than those with low n Achievement. The environment has to provide them with an opportunity to do better in order for the motive to increase response strength. As noted in Chapter 8, McKeachie (1961) reported that men high in n Power will work harder (get better grades) than men low in n Power in classes in which there are many opportunities to speak, as contrasted with classes in which there is little opportunity to speak. An environmental variable—the opportunity the instructor provides for speaking in class—combines with a motive disposition to predict performance. Several personality theorists, notably Endler (1981) and Magnusson (1976), have stressed the importance of taking into account interactions between the person and the environment in explaining behavior.

• DRIVES, HABIT STRENGTH, AND INCENTIVES AS DETERMINANTS OF RESPONSE STRENGTH

Chapter 3 summarized the attempt made by Clark Hull (1943) and others (for example, Spence, 1956) to predict response strength or performance from two variables in the organism, ignoring the environmental contribution for the moment. One determinant was motivation or drive. The other was habit strength. Hull's formula was $_sE_R = D \times {_sH_R}$. In other words, excitatory potential, or the tendency to make a response ($_sE_R$), is a function of drive strength (D) multiplied by habit strength ($_sH_R$). What Hull meant by habit strength was the amount of reinforced practice the animal had had in making the response previously, or in more general terms, the skill the animal had acquired in making the response.

Obviously, both determinants of the tendency to make a response are important, and Hull argued—partly for empirical and partly for theoretical reasons—that multiplying the two determinants gave the best prediction of response strength. Empirically the two curves draw apart as practice or habit strength increases, indicating a multiplicative relationship. Theoretically it seemed reasonable to assume that if either drive or habit were reduced to zero, there would be no response, which is the prediction the equation yields if the two variables are multiplied by each other. In commonsense terms, people might be quite skilled at playing the piano, but if they do not want to, they will not play. And no matter how much they want to play, if they do not have the skill to play, they also will not play.

As noted in Chapter 3, later Hull (1952) added a third variable to his equation to take into account the effects of incentive value on performance. Rats run a maze faster for food that they like (for example, bran mash) than for other foods, like sunflower seeds, that they do not particularly like. Or they run faster for sixteen pellets of food in the goal box than for one pellet. So the formula was expanded, again multiplicatively, to read as follows: $_sE_R = D \times {_sH_R} \times K$.

Spence (1956) agreed that incentive value (K) was important, but he felt it should not be combined multiplicatively with the other determinants but instead should be added to drive strength and the sum of these two multiplied by habit strength. In his formulation, the presence of either drive or incentive would lead to some behavior if habit strength existed, whereas in Hull's formulation, if either incentive or drive were zero, there would be no tendency to act.

The intricacies of just what was meant by these terms and how various empirical studies can be interpreted using the alternative formulas need not concern us here. What is important is the identification of the types of variables that need to be taken into account to explain response strength and their application to human performance. McClelland (1951), for example, applied the same set of three variables to explain complex human behavior by arguing at the level of personality structure that motive strength is equivalent to drive strength; traits or skills, to habits; and schemata or values, to incentives. This general model has been used throughout this book in trying to explain how motives combine with other variables to produce the impulse to act. (See Figure 6.1 and Figure 12.15.)

• MOTIVES, EXPECTANCIES OF SUCCESS, AND VALUES AS DETERMINANTS OF PERFORMANCE

As Atkinson (1964) and Weiner (1980a) pointed out, and as we noted in Chapter 1, Lewin's model of motivated behavior identified three variables very similar to those used by behaviorists like Hull and Spence, although Lewin defined them in phenomenological or cognitive terms. Thus, he spoke of need or tension, which is equivalent to drive strength; properties of the goal object, which is equivalent to incentive value; and psychological distance, which is a kind of phenomenological equivalent of the skill or habit variable in terms of how easy or how hard it is to get from the need to the goal.

These ideas were formalized first by Atkinson (1957) and later by Atkinson and Birch (1978) into the best-known contemporary theory of the determinants of action. The formula arrived at was very similar to Hull's except that the variables in it were defined in cognitive terms and operationalized in measures obtained from human subjects rather than animals. As reviewed in Chapter 7, the initial formula read as follows: $T_s = M_s \times P_s \times I_s$. That is, the tendency to achieve success (T_s) is a multiplicative function of the motive to achieve success (M_s), expectancy or probability of success (P_s), and the incentive value of success (I_s). It was further assumed that the incentive value of success could be defined as $1 - P_s$, meaning that the more difficult the task (the less the probability of succeeding at it), the greater the reward value would be of succeeding at it. As we noted in Chapter 7, the multiplicative model worked fairly well in accounting for the general tendency of subjects to choose to work at tasks of moderate difficulty, since $P_s \times (1 - P_s)$ is greatest when $P_s = .50$.

Later, Atkinson and Birch (1978) shifted from what they called the *traditional episodic view of behavior* to a stream of behavior paradigm in which the central problem became not how an act is initiated, but how one act replaces another. That is, they argued that the organism is always doing something, and the problem is to explain how it happens to shift from doing one thing to doing another thing. They identify a number of factors that are responsible for changes in activity, such as instigating force (F), which is very like the old concept of drive; consummatory force (the weakening of a tendency by expressing it); and inhibitory force. Without going into the details of how the variables in their new model are defined and relate to each other in determining action, it is clear that they emphasize at least one variable that had not previously been part of models of the determinants of action. For reconceptualizing the motivational problem in terms of shifts in the stream of behavior calls attention to the great importance of other instigating forces in the situation. Thus, Atkinson (1980) argues that it is important not only to know the strength of *n* Achievement in a situation, but the strength of other motives as well. In its simplest form, this equation can be stated as follows:

$$\text{Percentage of time spent in Activity A} = \frac{M_a}{M_a + M_b + \ldots + M_n}$$

That is, the tendency to spend time thinking about achieving is a function of the ratio of the motive to achieve (M_a) to all motives ($M_a + M_b + \ldots + M_n$) present in the situation. Thus, Atkinson (1979) points out the following:

> . . . [T]wo individuals who differ greatly in absolute strength of achievement motive (the numerator) might, nevertheless, obtain the same thematic apperceptive *n* Achievement score *if they also differ in a certain way in number and/or strength of competing motives (the denominator).* For example, the ratio of
>
> $\dfrac{1}{1 + 1 + 1}$ is equivalent to $\dfrac{3}{3 + 3 + 3}$. Both equal 1/3 and imply the same percentage time thinking about achievement, yet the strengths of the achievement motive are 1 and 3.

Since Atkinson and Birch's new model of the dynamics of action emphasizes shifts in the stream of behavior, it also focuses attention more on the percentage of time spent on various activities, as in these equations, rather than on
the initiation and acquisition of responses, choice, latency, resistance to extinction, or persistence, which are the more traditional indicators of response
strength. In this respect they follow Skinner (1966), who maintains that the
probability of an operant response's occurring represents what is commonly
called *purpose*. That is, the frequency with which a rat presses a bar to get food
when no stimulus that elicits the response is easily identifiable could be seen as
representing the strength of the rat's purpose in seeking food as opposed to
doing other things (scratching itself, sniffing, and so on).

The Atkinson-Birch model developed as a highly formalized attempt to express the ideas in what has come to be called loosely *expectancy-value theory*,
defined as follows:

> A general class of theories that relate tendencies either to perform particular actions
> or not to perform them to the strength of *expectancies* that these actions will lead to
> specific outcomes and the *valences* or subjectively perceived values of those outcomes
> for the person. . . . The expectancies and valences are usually assumed to combine
> multiplicatively to determine the strength of tendencies. (Feather, 1975)

Habit Strength as Expectancy of Success

Atkinson translated the expectancy term in the equation to predict response
strength into probability of success, but probability of success has come to have
two somewhat different meanings. On the one hand, it is a function of the availability of the response: the probability of success is lower if a person cannot
make a response very well. In this sense it has the same meaning as the habit
strength or skill variable in Hull's (1943) or McClelland's (1951) equations. The
importance of the skill variable in predicting response strength subsequently has
tended to be ignored in much motivational research either by using very over-
learned responses, such as canceling *e*'s and *o*'s in a series of letters, or by subtracting across successive trials to "correct" for individual differences in skill.
Thus, in a study that will be discussed at length later in the chapter, Patten and
White (1977) deal entirely with improvements in performance from one trial to
the next. However, improvements get greater and greater the more practice the
subject has with a task, indicating that the subject is getting more skillful, as
well as that the better the performance on one trial, the better it is likely to be
on the next. Skill itself—even in routine tasks—tends to be a product of motives
and expectancies plus practice, but no one doubts that skill is a major determinant of the probability of success and hence contributes in a major way to predicting response strength.

On the other hand, perceived probability of success as a cognitive variable is
different. It is determined in a major way by *beliefs* about the efficacy of making
a response, which may be somewhat independent of a person's skill in making

it. As pointed out in Chapter 12, two types of such beliefs have been studied extensively. One type has to do with the efficacy of effort in bringing about a consequence through a particular response in a given situation. The other type has to do with the generalized confidence people have that they can bring about outcomes through activities of any kind. We have reviewed elsewhere (see Chapter 12) the evidence that a belief in the importance of effort facilitates performance. For example, W. U. Meyer (1973; see also Weiner, 1980a) found that those who attributed their failure to lack of effort tended to show more improvement on the next trial. And Dweck (1975) and Chapin and Dyck (1976) reported that children with learning difficulties who were trained to believe that their failures were due to lack of effort tended to do better subsequently. We can conceptualize these studies as meaning that subjective probability of success was increased through the expectation that greater effort would be more likely to produce a desired outcome.

As also reviewed in Chapter 12, the importance for predicting response strength of generalized beliefs about personal efficacy has been demonstrated in a variety of studies. Perlmuter, Scharff, Karsh, and Monty (1980) have summarized evidence showing that giving subjects a choice of what to do improves their performance over what it would be if they were made to do it. They argue that giving subjects a choice gives them a perception of control over the situation, which enhances performance. Seligman (1975) has summarized a number of studies showing that animals and human beings can "learn helplessness." If they are put in a situation where they are repeatedly exposed to inescapable shock, they will learn to give up trying to do anything about it and will fail to try to escape in a new situation in which they actually could avoid the shock. In other words, their expectancy of the probability of success from taking action has been lowered in general, and a measure of their sense of helplessness should predict performance in a variety of situations.

In contrast, deCharms (1976) demonstrated that teaching junior high school students to act like Origins—to believe that they could personally cause things to happen—significantly improved their grade placement, test scores, and the proportion of boys receiving such training who graduated from high school (see Chapter 14). And Bandura's (1982) self-efficacy training, reviewed in Chapter 12, is similarly effective in helping people get over phobias. Just as Seligman's subjects learned that there was little or no relationship between doing something and success, deCharms's and Bandura's subjects learned that there was a connection between the two. In all these instances, perceived probability of success—whether high or low—is strongly related to subsequent response strength or performance.

The Achievement Incentive and Other Incentives Affecting Achievement

A major misunderstanding has occurred in the discussions of achievement motivation theory because of the failure to distinguish between the incentives specific to the motive and allied incentives or other values affecting the valence of success. The misunderstanding has arisen in part because of Atkinson's terminology. He defines the incentive value of *success* (I_s) as $1 - P_s$. But there are obviously many factors other than task difficulty that determine the incentive value of *success* broadly conceived. He was writing within the context of achievement motivation studies and was trying to explain the preference of subjects high in *n* Achievement for tasks of moderate difficulty, but he used terminology that has been taken to have a more general significance.

Maehr (1974) has been particularly vigorous in criticizing achievement motivation theory for not taking into account cultural variations in the meaning of achievement and success. He and his colleagues believe they have shown that "the traditional conception of achievement motivation results in an ethnocentric bias" (Maehr & Kleiber, 1981), because it has become associated with individualistic, rather than cooperative, achievement; with the Protestant work ethic; and generally with upward occupational striving (see also Duda, 1980).

But strictly speaking, the incentive for the achievement motive relates to such outcomes—if at all—only indirectly and in combination with other values. It is quite specific and limited and can be defined in general terms as the pleasure derived from doing something better. Many studies have demonstrated that if a task is too easy or too difficult, the incentive is not present and subjects with high *n* Achievement do not perform better (see Chapter 7). If something like getting time off from work is the incentive for successful performance, they also do not do better than subjects low in *n* Achievement (French, 1955). Obviously, whether the pleasure derived from performing better gets connected with upward occupational striving or individualistic versus collaborative achievement depends on other values to which the person is exposed. As noted in Chapter 12, it is quite proper to ask what kinds of achievement are valued by older people, by people from other cultures (Gallimore, Boggs, & Jordan, 1974), or by women so long as it is not assumed that these values directly alter the incentive for the achievement motive, which remains doing something better. *What* a person decides to do better will obviously vary, depending on other values. In motivational expectancy-value theory, values are *independent* determinants of response strength or the tendency to act.

Weiner (1980a) and others have created further terminological confusion by referring to measures of achievement values as if they were measures of achievement motives. A generation ago deCharms, Morrison, Reitman, and McClelland (1955) established that valuing achievement (*v* Achievement) as measured in an attitude questionnaire not only does not relate to the *n* Achievement score as obtained from coding thought samples, but also has quite different behavioral correlates. Nevertheless, as noted in Chapter 6, ever since that time, a number of investigators have tried to develop "objective" measures of *n* Achievement through attitude questionnaires, although none of them has correlated consistently with the *n* Achievement measure or predicts better performance in a moderate risk situation when the achievement incentive is present.

The most popular and best validated of these *v* Achievement measures is one developed by Mehrabian (1969). Unfortunately, Weiner (1980a) and others refer to scores obtained from this instrument as measures of *n* Achievement, with the result that the interpretation of much empirical research in this area in recent years is confused and misleading. The disagreement here is not simply a matter of arguing over which measuring instrument is better. Rather, using the Mehrabian instrument as a measure of motives blurs the distinction between motives and values, which leads to just the kind of objections Maehr and others have made to achievement motive theory as it has been developed by some people. Motives appear to be present and function in much the same way in men and women (Stewart & Chester, 1982) and in various ethnic groups, but since the extent to which these groups subscribe to achievement values differs, it may well appear that only the groups that subscribe to achievement values have any achievement motivation—which is patently untrue. For example, certain groups of women do not value strongly the typical achievement values of agentic striving, but there is no evidence they are lower in *n* Achievement.

The Distinction Between Motives and Values

At several points throughout the book we have pointed to differences between motives and values. Values are normally measured by asking people to indicate what is important to them. In the measure of values developed by Rokeach (1973), subjects are simply asked to rank order the importance to them of terminal values represented by words like *freedom, equality,* and *true friendship* or instrumental values like *independent, intellectual,* or *ambitious* (see Chapter 5). There is a strong cognitive, self-conscious component in these judgments. Subjects know what they are doing. They are reporting what is important to them. In contrast, motives are measured from coding operant thought content; subjects do not know what aspect of their thinking is of interest, so they normally cannot consciously shape their thoughts to score high on various motives.

The correlation between these two types of measures is quite low. Beyond this, Rokeach (1973) has reported that while some of his value rankings correlate with motive scores in a meaningful way, others do not. For example, *n* Achievement scores correlated significantly with the value ranking for *independent* and *intellectual* but not with *sense of accomplishment, ambitious,* or *capable.* This is typical of results from a number of studies showing that value attitudes do not correlate with motive scores obtained from coding spontaneous thought (see Child, Frank, & Storm, 1956). The most reasonable interpretation of such findings is that these two types of measures are essentially independent, as they ought to be on theoretical grounds, and that when occasional correlations appear between them, they are the product of a peculiar set of circumstances related to the particular group being tested.

In contrast, both motives and values can influence choices or the valence of one outcome over another, as Feather (1975) has pointed out: "Like motives, values can influence valences. Money, for example, may be a potent incentive for people who assign a very high priority to *a comfortable life* in their value systems" (p. 302). And under certain circumstances, money can also have high valence for those high in *n* Achievement—when it can be used as a measure of how well the person is doing (see Chapter 7).

Motives and values are also both associated with affect. A person who values *freedom* is happy when given freedom and unhappy when it is taken away. Similarly, subjects with high *n* Achievement feel good when thinking about achievement goals and feel bad when thinking about failure (McClelland, Atkinson, Clark, & Lowell, 1953).

There appears to be a difference about when the affect occurs. Zajonc (1980) has summarized evidence indicating that the affective response to a stimulus often occurs before the stimulus is recognized. Before subjects understand consciously what stimulus is being presented, they react to it with positive or negative affect (see Chapter 2). The affect associated with motives appears to be of this kind, since motives operate often without clear cognitive understanding of what is going on. For example, as noted in Chapter 8, subjects high in *n* Power react more sensitively to power cues—when sensitivity is measured in terms of electrical responsivity of the brain—within a quarter of a second after presentation of the cue and before one might presume that the person had recognized or understood the meaning of the stimulus (Davidson, Saron, & McClelland, 1980). In other words, subjects high in *n* Power are reacting very quickly, automatically, and strongly to power cues as contrasted with other cues, and as contrasted with subjects low in *n* Power. In contrast, affect associated with values comes *after* understanding of the situation, since values are made up of such understandings. A man is angry after he understands his freedom has been taken away.

Values are much more affected than motives by social norms and by societal and institutional demands (Feather, 1975; Rokeach, 1973). Thus, values clearly affect choices, serving to direct the energies of a motive into one channel or another. It is at this point that the complaints of Maehr (1974) and others about the limitations of traditional achievement motivation theory make sense. The point can be made very simply from a study carried out by French and Lesser (1964) in which they discovered that the energies of women high in *n* Achievement went into different activities, depending on their values. The data are summarized in Table 13.1.

If the women were intellectually oriented, those high in *n* Achievement did better at an intellectual task, but not at a task involving social skills. In contrast, among women who valued the traditional female role, those high in *n* Achievement tended to perform better at a social skill than those low in *n* Achievement. Both groups of women high in *n* Achievement did better at something, but what they did better at depended on their values. Note also that what is involved in this experiment is not *v* Achievement—that is, the extent to which the women valued achievement consciously—but quite a different set of values related to what women should be doing. Thus, values quite outside the achievement complex can influence the valence of various activities, shunting motivational energies in one direction or another.

• HOW THE ACHIEVEMENT MOTIVE, SKILL, AND ACHIEVEMENT VALUES AFFECT PERFORMANCE

While it is clear that values affect choices and shunt motivational energies in one direction or another, it is not yet clear that they energize behavior and lead

Table 13.1.

RELATIONSHIP OF *n* ACHIEVEMENT SCORES TO TWO TYPES OF PERFORMANCE DEPENDING ON WOMEN'S VALUES (after French & Lesser, 1964)

	Correlations of *n* Achievement with	
Value Orientation of Women	*Intellectual Skill*[a]	*Social Skill*[b]
Traditional	.04	.59*
Career oriented	.55*	.32

[a]Performance on an anagrams test.

[b]Performance on a number of questions such as, If you were a stranger in town, how would you make friends?

p < .05.

to faster learning of related activities the way motives do. The best evidence on this point comes from a number of studies that have shown that subjects high in *v* Achievement measured in various ways do not ordinarily perform better than subjects low in *v* Achievement. Since the point is an important one, it is worth examining in some detail through a recent study. Patten and White (1977) designed an experiment patterned after an earlier one conducted in Germany by W. U. Meyer (1973). Subjects were asked to complete four rows of digit-symbol substitution in one minute. On the second trial, the subjects in the failure condition were interrupted on the fourth row because time was up so that they failed to complete the task in the time allotted. Then they were asked whether they had failed because of lack of effort, lack of ability, luck, or task difficulty. The measure of response strength was the improvement in time taken to complete the first three rows of digit-symbol substitution on the next trial. As a control, some subjects were run through the experiment without experiencing failure. Although Meyer had originally used a measure of *n* Achievement obtained in the usual way, Patten and White (1977) switched to a measure of *v* Achievement obtained from the Mehrabian questionnaire, although they refer to it as a measure of achievement motivation. They also ran some subjects under ego-involved conditions (without failure) when the achievement motive has been shown to be aroused (McClelland et al., 1953).

Some of the main results of this carefully designed experiment are shown in Figure 13.1. The improvement score represents a decrease in the number of seconds from the first trial to later trials. Note first that when the achievement motive had been aroused experimentally by failure, subjects gained significantly more in the second block of trials than they did in the first block of trials. No such improvement occurred for subjects in the neutral, no-failure condition. Furthermore, W. U. Meyer (1973) had shown that for the same task, subjects who

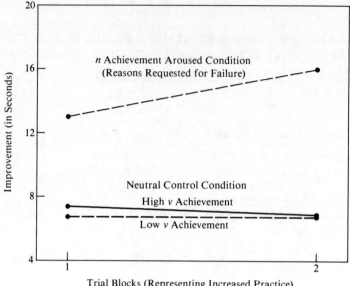

Figure 13.1.

Effect of Aroused *n* Achievement and Differences in *v* Achievement on Group Mean Block Improvement Scores (after Patten & White, 1977).

scored higher in *n* Achievement, if success oriented, behaved like those in whom the achievement motive had been experimentally aroused: they gained more from the first to the second block of trials than those low in *n* Achievement (Heckhausen, 1980). This is a crucial point, because it shows that the effect of increased motive strength is the same whether it is the result of individual differences or situational manipulations. To put it a different way, those who score high in *n* Achievement behave chronically like those whose achievement motive has been situationally aroused.

Technically, this confirms the following relationship in terms of Hull's equation or Atkinson's reformulation of it:

Hull: $_sE_R = D \times {_sH_R}$.
Atkinson: $T_s = M_s \times P_s$.

Freely translated, the tendency to work hard on the task (or performance) is a function of motive strength (represented by the *n* Achievement score) times skill (represented by the number of practice trials).

Note that a similar relationship does *not* hold if the *v* Achievement measure obtained from the Mehrabian questionnaire is used to estimate differences in *n* Achievement levels. This is one more confirmation of many similar results showing that the Mehrabian measure cannot be considered a measure of the achievement *motive*.

Let us assume instead that it is a measure of the incentive value of success (or I_s, in Atkinson's terms). Then we can write the following: T_s (or $_sE_R$) $\neq I_s$ (or K) $\times P_s$ (or $_sH_R$). Freely translated, the tendency to work hard on the task is not a function of the incentive value of success (represented by the v Achievement measure) times skill (represented by the number of practice trials). There is no greater improvement with practice for those high in v Achievement than for those low in v Achievement.

The failure of value attitude measures to predict performance the way motives do exists not only for laboratory tasks like this one, but for outcomes in real life. For example, McClelland and Boyatzis (1982) have reported that the leadership motive syndrome (high n Power higher than n Affiliation, and high Activity Inhibition) is associated with people's greater effort and managerial success in a large company after sixteen years, whereas no value measures obtained from questionnaires like the Edwards Personal Preference Schedule significantly predict managerial success over the same period of time (see Bray, Campbell, & Grant, 1974, as well as Chapters 8 and 12 of this book).

However, it makes good sense to regard v Achievement as a measure of incentive strength, for Hull would also argue that if drive strength were zero, the product of incentive and habit would not increase the tendency to make a response. That is, no matter how much practice a rat has had in pressing a bar to get food, nor how large the incentive, the rat will not press the bar if it is not hungry. This corresponds in the Patten and White experiment to the neutral, no-failure condition in which no achievement motive is aroused, although there are variations in the extent to which people in that condition *value* achievement.

In contrast, as the Hull formula would predict, if the achievement motive is aroused, then incentive value does make a difference. As Figure 13.2 shows (Patten & White, 1977), when the achievement motive was aroused through ego-involving instructions, subjects for whom the incentive value of achievement was high (high v Achievement) performed much better than those for whom the incentive value of achievement was low (low v Achievement). This is analogous to a *hungry* rat's responding more when the reward is large than when it is small. It is as if valuing achievement increases the push to do better in this situation, once the subject's achievement motivation has been aroused. Figure 13.2 also confirms the fact that the difference in v Achievement has no effect on performance in the neutral condition, when the achievement motive has not been aroused.

Furthermore, there is evidence in the Patten and White experiment for the joint effect of all three variables on response strength or the impulse to work hard at the task. If the top curve in Figure 13.1 is broken down and plotted separately for those high and low in v Achievement, it appears that those high in v Achievement gain significantly more with practice when the achievement motive is aroused through failure than those low in v Achievement under similar conditions. In other words, $T_s = M_s \times P_s \times I_s$, or the tendency to work hard equals n Achievement times practice times v Achievement. Patten and White (1977) were not interested in making such a multivariate prediction of performance, but their results support the inference that all of these variables should contribute to predicting response strength in some combination or another.

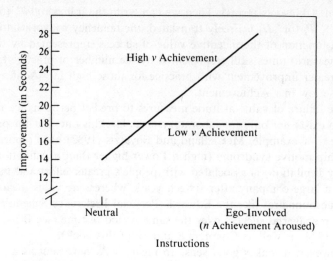

Figure 13.2.

Total Group Mean Improvement Scores, as a Function of Achievement Classification and Instructional Conditions (after Patten & White, 1977).

Patten and White (1977) were also able to show that subjects who attributed their failures more to lack of effort showed a greater improvement in performance by the fifth trial, even when the effects of skill on previous trials and *v* Achievement scores were controlled. In contrast, those who attributed their failures to a lack of ability or task difficulty did not show a greater improvement on any of the trials after failure. In other words, the belief or expectancy that effort would make a difference led to a greater improvement in performance.

In terms of the model, this belief contributes to perceived probability of success in the same way prior practice does. However, this contribution may occur only under conditions of achievement motive arousal, because Patten and White also found that simply asking people for reasons why they failed increased their performance, as contrasted to not asking subjects to give reasons for failure. They argue that asking for causal attributions may simply be another way of arousing achievement motivation. Thus, when they report a significant correlation between *v* Achievement levels and improvement scores in an experiment in which causal attributions were asked for, the result is essentially the same as that shown on the right-hand side of Figure 13.2: when achievement motivation is aroused, high *v* Achievement leads to better performance.

Patten and White also argue that Weiner's theory cannot be correct that *v* Achievement leads to people's attributing failure to lack of effort, which leads to better performance. For under conditions of achievement motive arousal, high *v* Achievement is significantly associated with better performance no matter what causes people assign for failure. There is no indication that the effect of high *v* Achievement is mediated by attributing failure to lack of effort. Once again, the data support the model which states that the incentive value of success, here represented by *v* Achievement, contributes to response strength independently of the perceived probability of success (here represented by the belief that effort will make a difference in the outcome).

HOW MOTIVES, SKILLS, AND VALUES JOINTLY DETERMINE SUCCESS AS A NAVAL OFFICER

What is needed is more research demonstrating how all these variables combine to predict response strength. McClelland (1981a) reported one investigation in which he was able to show that motive, schema or value, and trait or skill variables all contributed independently in a multiple regression to predicting superior performance among commanding or executive officers in the U.S. Navy (see Table 13.2).

The variables tested were not chosen to check on the model being discussed here, but it was possible to show that motive variables, schema or value variables, and skill or trait variables each contributed to predicting officer success. For example, the leadership *motive* pattern (see Chapter 8), the belief that power must be used in the officer's job (a belief or *value*), and scheduling *skill* all contributed significantly to the multiple correlation predicting a person's success as a commanding or executive officer in the Navy. Furthermore, combinations of any two of these types of predictors improved the multiple correlation coefficient *(R)* still further, whereas using all three types of determinants produced the rather substantial multiple *R* of .68, which is considerably higher than is usually found in studies of this type.

McClelland uses this argument to answer Mischel's (1968) complaint that relationships found in personality study are generally low, hovering around correlations of .30. This is true, McClelland argues, primarily because researchers typically focus on single variables rather than on the multivariate determination of response strength. While Table 13.2 makes the point about the importance of multiple determinants of an outcome in a general way, a much more carefully designed investigation is needed to discover what variables in what combinations best predict response strength or performance.

FACTORS INFLUENCING AFFILIATIVE ACTS AND CHOICES

Constantian (1981) has carried out an experiment that has several advantages for testing various ideas that have been put forward about the way motives, values, and skills determine response strength. First, she worked in the area of affiliation rather than achievement. This is an advantage, because previous models proposed are supposed to be general, although they have all been derived from achievement situations. Second, she obtained a measure of the frequency of operant or spontaneous affiliative acts over time, thus adopting a procedure that is a crucial part of the Atkinson and Birch model, although they have never em-

Table 13.2.

CHARACTERISTICS RELATED TO SUPERIOR PERFORMANCE AMONG COMMANDING OR EXECUTIVE U.S. NAVY OFFICERS: $N = 72$ (after McClelland, 1981a)

Tested Variable	Unique Variance Contributed (Percent)	p
Motives:		
1. Leadership motive pattern (n Power $> n$ Affiliation, high Activity inhibition)	6	.01
2. Low entrepreneurial interest[a]	10	$< .01$
Schemata or values:		
3. Ideal climate: responsibility organizational, not personal	5	.02
4. Ideal climate: reacting against bureaucratic inertia	9	$< .01$
5. Use of power required in job	10	$< .01$
6. Use of affiliation not required in job	2	.11
Traits:		
7. Manages by optimizing	12	$< .01$
8. Low on manages by helping	5	.02
9. Has scheduling skill	7	$< .01$

Multiple $R = .68$, $p < .001$, for all nine variables. Regression stopped when additional variables added less than .01 to R.

	Motives Alone	Schemata Alone	Traits Alone	Motives Plus Schemata	Motives Plus Traits	Schemata Plus Traits
Multiple R	.24	.40	.30	.47	.39	.52
p	.12	.02	.095	.01	.05	.001

[a]From Strong-Campbell Vocational Interest Blank.

ployed it in their empirical work. To obtain this measure, Constantian adopted a method reported earlier by Larson and Csikszentmihalyi (1978). Subjects who were summer-school students were asked to wear electronic pagers, or beepers (of the type doctors use), for a week. They were beeped randomly seven times a day between the hours of 9:00 A.M. and 11:00 P.M., in sets of two-hour periods (9:00 to 11:00 A.M., 11:00 A.M. to 1:00 P.M., and so forth). When they were beeped, they were to fill out a brief checklist explaining what they were thinking and doing at the time. The measure of operant affiliative activity was the proportion of times beeped when the person reported he or she was conversing with someone or writing a letter to someone.

Constantian (1981) also obtained a more conventional measure of peoples' preferences for doing things with people, which we will call the Affiliative Choice Measure. Subjects were asked to indicate on a scale of 1 to 7 how much they would like doing fifteen different types of things with friends, such as working at a job, doing errands, visiting a museum, living in an apartment, and so on.

The key question is how the affiliative motive combines with other factors to determine the strength of either operant affiliative acts or affiliative choices. Constantian obtained a measure of *n* Affiliation coded in the usual way (see Heyns, Veroff, & Atkinson, 1958) from stories written to six pictures. To obtain a measure of the value subjects placed on affiliation, she added up the number of positive reactions and subtracted the number of negative reactions to being with people. This will be referred to as the *v Affiliation measure.* Finally, a measure of the perceived probability of success in social situations was obtained in the following way. Subjects rated themselves on a scale of 1 to 7 on a number of items such as "How often do you feel that you have handled yourself well at a social gathering?" (on a scale of *almost never* to *almost always*) and "How sure of yourself do you feel among strangers?" (on a scale of *not at all sure* to *extremely sure*). The mean rating on these items represents subjects' estimates of their degree of *social skill,* or their perceived probability of success in social situations.

How the Situation Combines with the Affiliative Motive and Affiliative Values to Predict Affiliative Choices

The subjects were also asked to rate how much they liked doing various activities alone and with friends (Constantian, 1981). Indirectly this gives an indication of how often activities are in fact carried out alone or with others, as Table 13.3 demonstrates. People report that they like reading for pleasure much more by themselves than with others and that they like dining out with others rather than by themselves. This simply confirms what all theorists have argued— namely, that the environmental situation is a very important determinant of behavior. Whatever peoples' motives, values, and social skills in the affiliative area are, some activities like shopping and dining out provide more opportunities for affiliative behaviors than other activities like reading for pleasure or working on a hobby. Any observer wanting to predict whether a person will be with a friend should first take into account the situation in which the behavior is supposed to occur. People in restaurants are much more likely to be with others than people reading a book.

Person variables also interact with situations differently, as Table 13.3 also shows. Note that people high in *n* Affiliation are significantly more likely to like doing errands, exploring a new city, or shopping with friends, but they are not more likely to like to read, do a hobby, or cook with friends. Those who *value* affiliation strongly like doing almost any activity more with friends except running errands or cooking. The contrast in the results for participating in a hobby or doing errands with friends is particularly interesting. For *n* Affiliation is positively associated with doing errands with friends and *v* Affiliation is not, whereas the reverse is true for participating in a hobby with friends.

The difference between the two activities is that doing errands is compulso-

Table 13.3.

MEAN LIKING FOR DOING VARIOUS ACTIVITIES ALONE OR WITH FRIENDS: $N = 111$ **(after Constantian, 1981)**

Activity	Mean Liking (Scale of 1 to 7)		Correlations with	
	Alone	With Friends	n Affiliation	v Affiliation
Reading for pleasure	5.77	3.43	.07	.19*
Doing art or hobby you enjoy	5.17	4.79	.08	.29**
Doing errands	4.19	4.56	.24*	.09
Cooking	4.07	4.77	.06	.10
Dining out in a restaurant	2.02	6.41	.14	.21*
Exploring a new city	3.47	6.10	.21*	.20*
Shopping	3.96	5.02	.20*	.37***

*$p < .05$.
**$p < .01$.
***$p < .001$.

ry, whereas participating in a hobby is completely voluntary. Thus, the results suggest that high *v* Affiliation, but not high *n* Affiliation, leads to liking to do things with people that are normally done alone, such as reading for pleasure or participating in a hobby. One may doubt that in fact they will read more often with friends and suspect they are just responding in a stereotyped way to the *idea* of doing things with friends. In contrast, subjects high in *n* Affiliation appear to like to do things with friends that they have to do anyway, such as running errands. Of course, some activities are liked more by those both high in *n* Affiliation and *v* Affiliation, like shopping or exploring a new city. The point of this analysis is that personal characteristics interact with different situations in different ways. Thus, it is not enough to know whether a situation calls for more or less affiliative activity. We must also know whether it is a required or completely voluntary activity. If it is the former, people with high *n* Affiliation are more likely to do it with friends, whereas if it is the latter, people high in *v* Affiliation are more likely to do it with people.

The relationship of situation and person variables to behavior in combination is illustrated by Table 13.4. In this analysis, the situation is represented symbolically when subjects are asked how much they would like doing something either alone or with friends. Note that in Section A of the table, the *situation* is very important in predicting how much the students will like working. If they are with friends, they will like working much more than if they are alone. The person variable is also important: those with high *n* Affiliation like work

Table 13.4.

RELATIONSHIP OF A PERSON AND A SITUATION VARIABLE ON LIKING (SCALE OF 1 TO 7) VARIOUS ACTIVITIES: $N = 111$ (after Constantian, 1981)

A. Mean Liking for Working at a Job

	Person Variable		
Situation Variable	Low n Affiliation (N = 54)	High n Affiliation (N = 57)	Combined
Alone	3.7	2.8	3.2 (Difference = 2.3; $p < .001$)
With friends	<u>5.4</u>	<u>5.6</u>	5.5
Combined	4.5	4.2	

Difference = 0.3; $p = .02$

Interaction of motive and situation variables: $p = .03$.

B. Mean Liking for Doing Errands

	Person Variable		
Situation Variable	Low n Affiliation (N = 54)	High n Affiliation (N = 57)	Combined
Alone	4.7	3.7	4.2 (Difference = 0.3; n.s.)
With friends	<u>4.1</u>	<u>4.9</u>	4.5
Combined	4.4	4.4	

Difference = 0; n.s.

Interaction of motive and situation variables: $p = .001$.

less than those with low n Affiliation, presumably because the "highs" would prefer socializing with people to working. The person and situation variables also interact: High n Affiliation has opposite effects on liking for work, depending on the situation. If they are working alone, those high in n Affiliation like work less than those low in n Affiliation; if they are with friends, they like work more than those with low n Affiliation.

In Section B of Table 13.4, neither the person variable nor the situation variable by itself is associated with liking to do errands more or less. But the interaction is very significant: those high in n Affiliation like errands less if they are alone and more if they are with friends, in contrast to those with low n Affiliation. To predict successfully how much a person will like running errands, it is necessary to know the situation variable (whether he or she runs them alone or with friends) and the person variable (n Affiliation score), as well as how they interact. Those who are high in n Affiliation and doing errands with friends will like doing errands most (mean = 4.9), whereas those who will like running errands least are those high in *n* Affiliation and doing them alone (mean = 3.7).

How Values Affect the Way the Affiliative Motive Expresses Itself

Constantian's study was designed to get at the interactive affects of the affiliative motive and affiliative values. According to theory, the affiliative motives involve affectively toned associative networks built on natural incentives connected with early contact gratifications. In contrast, as people grow up, they form concepts relating to their experiences with people, which become conscious values (see Chapters 5 and 9). These values are much influenced by parental and societal inputs as to the importance of affiliative activities; therefore, people's affiliative values need bear no necessary relationship to their affiliative motive dispositions, that is, to the affective experiences they have actually had with people, especially early in life. In Constantian's (1981) study, for example, the correlation between the *n* Affiliation score, which is not under conscious control, and the *v* Affiliation score, which is, is .21, $N = 111$, $p < .05$. In other words, there are almost as many people high in *n* Affiliation and low in *v* Affiliation as there are those who are high in both measures. This means that motives and incentives could turn out to be relatively independent determinants of response strength, as expected according to theory.

How do motives and values interact? Constantian (1981) also obtained a measure of the extent to which people valued solitude using an exactly parallel method except that she substituted the phrase *being alone* for *being with people.* Liking for solitude and liking for being with people were not highly correlated ($r = .14$; not significant). So there are about as many people who feel positive both about being alone and being with people as who prefer one state to the other. However, it proved possible to get two groups of people nearly equal in size who either valued solitude more than affiliation or vice versa. Table 13.5 shows that liking to do things with friends (that is, the summary score for all activities) is jointly increased by the affiliative motive and affiliative values acting in concert. Those who are high in both characteristics have the highest average score (mean = 52.0), much higher than those who are low in both characteristics (mean = 47.0). Both independent variables contribute significantly to liking for doing things with friends, but there is no interaction between them showing that they combine additively.

In contrast, when Constantian (1981) asked the subjects in another part of the questionnaire to indicate what they thought the good effects of a prolonged period of being alone would be, the results were quite different. Those high in *n* Affiliation mentioned increased peace and self-awareness significantly more often than those low in *n* Affiliation, and so did those *valuing solitude* more than affiliation. The result here is that high *n* Affiliation combines with the value for *solitude* (not for affiliation) to produce a stronger response of this type.

Table 13.5.

**DIFFERENT EFFECTS OF VALUING AFFILIATION AND SOLITUDE ON CORRELATES OF
n AFFILIATION SCORES (after Constantian, 1981)**

A. Mean Liking for Doing Things with Friends:[a]

	Values		
		Affiliation Less, Solitude	
	Affiliation	More	
Motive Classification	More		Mean
High *n* Affiliation	52.0	50.2	51.0
Low *n* Affiliation	50.9	47.0	48.9
Mean	51.4	48.6	
Analysis of variance			
Motive source	$p = .05$		
Value source	$p = .01$	Interaction insignificant	

B. Mean Frequency of Mentioning Peace and Self-awareness as Values of Prolonged Solitude:[a]

	Values		
	Affiliation	Solitude	
Motive Classification	More	More	Mean
High *n* Affiliation	49.6	53.2	51.4
Low *n* Affiliation	47.0	50.2	48.6
Mean	48.3	51.7	
Analysis of variance			
Motive source	$p = .03$		
Value source	$p = .01$	Interaction insignificant	

[a]T-scores (mean = 50; SD = 10).

What this finding illustrates is how values can shift the way a motive expresses itself. That is, if people high in *n* Affiliation value affiliation, they seek being with people more; if they value solitude, they may seek the peace and self-awareness that comes from being alone more.

The point is made even more dramatically in Figure 13.3. Note first that valuing affiliation more than solitude had little affect on liking for taking a country walk with friends for those low in *n* Affiliation (left side of the figure). However, for subjects high in *n* Affiliation, if they also valued affiliation, they reported that they liked much more taking a country walk with friends. This is the same result as is shown in Section A of Table 13.5 for doing all types of activities with friends.

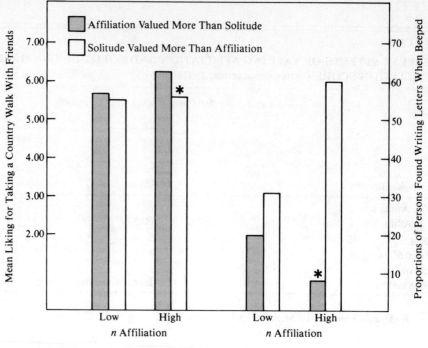

*Difference significant at $p < .05$.

Figure 13.3.

Effects of Differing Values on the Outlets of High *n* Affiliation (data from Constantian, 1981).

The right side of Figure 13.3, however, shows quite a different result, this time for the proportions of persons found to be writing letters when they were paged. In general, those who valued solitude were more likely to be found writing letters, but the difference did not even approach significance for those low in *n* Affiliation. For those high in *n* Affiliation, however, a significantly higher proportion of those valuing solitude more than affiliation were found to be writing letters than those valuing affiliation more than solitude. To put the question in a somewhat different perspective, we might ask what it is that a person high in *n* Affiliation might do to establish contact with others if he or she valued solitude more than being with people. One answer clearly is writing letters, because it is an activity that involves contact with people but that a person can do alone.

In short, values can readily shift the way the affiliative motive expresses itself in various activities. It is precisely this point that the critics of the *n* Achievement literature have failed to recognize in arguing that *n* Achievement is too individualistically defined. It may be defined that way in some cultures but not in others, just as for some people, valuing being with people is more important than valuing solitude. Such people, if they have high *n* Affiliation, will be more likely to do things with friends. But there are other people (just as there are other cultures) who value solitude more, and in those instances the outlet for relating to people, if people have high *n* Affiliation, will be by contacting them in some way like writing letters that does not involve joining with them in activities.

The Joint Effect of the Affiliative Motive, Social Skill, and Affiliative Values on Affiliative Acts and Choices

As theory would predict, the presumed personality determinants of affiliative behaviors do not correlate very highly with each other. As Table 13.6 shows, the *n* Affiliation score is correlated with the *v* Affiliation score only at a barely significant level, and not at all with people's estimates of their social skill. The *v* Affiliation and social skill scores are much more highly correlated, because both are influenced by the subject's self-concept. In the one case, people are asked how much they like being with people, and in the other, how successful they are when interacting with people. It seems reasonable to assume that judg-

Table 13.6.

CORRELATIONS OF PERSONALITY DETERMINANTS WITH EACH OTHER AND WITH AFFILIATIVE ACTS AND CHOICES: $N = 111$, EXCEPT FOR AFFILIATIVE ACTS COLUMN (data from Constantian, 1981)

Personality Determinant	*Motive*	*Value*	*Skill*	*Operant Affiliative Acts (N = 48)[a]*	*Respondent Affiliative Choices[b]*
Motive:					
n Affiliation	—	.21*	.05	.42**	.21*
n Affiliation ratio[c]		.17	−.04	.45***	.19*
Value:					
v Affiliation		—	.45***	.17	.41***
Skill:					
Social skill			—	−.14	.06
Operant affiliative acts (*N* = 48)					.33*

[a]Percentage of times found conversing with others or writing letters when beeped.

[b]Mean liking for carrying out fifteen activities with friends.

[c]T-score *n* Affiliation/T-score *n* Affiliation + T-score *n* Power + T-score *n* Achievement + T-score Activity Inhibition.

*$p < .05$.

**$p < .01$.

***$p < .001$.

ments about social skill would be related to liking for being with people. Individuals who feel they are shy and awkward are unlikely to respond by saying that they like being with people. Ideas about skill and liking are part of people's general understanding of their relations to people.

In this light, it seems surprising that liking to do things with friends (affiliative choices) is not related to perceived social skill ($r = .06$). The reason may be that the social skill items have more to do with dealing with strangers or unfamiliar situations, as well as that some people who think they have poor social skill prefer doing things with friends precisely for that reason. This would reduce the expected positive association between the two variables.

The strength of the affiliative motive, as Table 13.6 shows, is strongly related to the frequency of operant affiliative acts reported by the person beeped. Neither the value placed on affiliation nor the estimate of one's social skill is related significantly to the operant affiliative act measure. In contrast, the v Affiliation measure is much more strongly related to the affiliative choices score than the n Affiliation score is. The social skill measure does not seem to be a determinant of affiliative choices, either.

Why should the n Affiliation score be more related to the operant affiliative acts score and the v Affiliation measure be more related to the affiliative choices score? The key to understanding the difference lies in the realization that the acts score does not involve the subjects' conscious perception or judgment. That is, it is not based on the subjects' report of what they did, which is influenced by all sorts of cognitive factors such as memory distortions, beliefs about the self, or ideas as to what they should be doing. The affiliative choices score does reflect just such cognitive variables. Motives affect the frequency with which people do things that are not passed through conscious cognitive filters. Values, on the other hand, represent the usually conscious conceptions in terms of which people organize their experience and preferences. If people answer in one part of the questionnaire that they like being with others, they should be more likely to answer in another part of the questionnaire that they would prefer doing things with people. Both answers are determined by the value the person places on affiliation.

In contrast, the affiliative motive score is not conscious and therefore does not automatically elicit the value people consciously place on affiliation. It leads instead to more operant interactions with people, because pleasure has been obtained from that type of interaction in the past. Many of the relationships of motive dispositions to operant activities have been missed by psychologists, because they typically use self-report measures in which there is a large cognitive element, which is not part of the motive disposition. As Table 13.6 makes clear, motives are more important for predicting what people *will spontaneously do,* whereas values are more important for determining what they will cognitively decide should be done.

Having emphasized the main result, we may still wonder whether the determinants of operant action do not influence each other. Does it not seem likely that consciously valuing affiliation might strengthen the motive to affiliate (or vice versa) and increase the tendency to interact with others? The data do not permit an unequivocal answer to the question, for there is a slight but significant positive correlation between *n* Affiliation and *v* Affiliation scores, which could mean either that the value promotes the motive or the motive promotes the value. Only longitudinal studies or attempts to change values or motives through education could answer definitely what influences what. And, whereas valuing affiliation is not associated with more operant affiliative acts, we might argue that the affiliative choices measure is an alternative way to get at the value people place on being with people—at least on being with friends. This value indicator does correlate significantly with the affiliative acts score ($r =$ .33), perhaps because in college students can often chat with roommate friends. Thus, it is not surprising to find that there is some relationship between subjects' saying they like to do things with friends and finding that they are more often conversing with people (often roommate friends).

Even this relationship between a cognitive judgment of one's interests and actual act frequency is thrown into doubt by the fact that the choices measure is related to the *n* Affiliation measure, which is in turn related to the affiliative acts frequency. If a partial correlation is calculated to remove the influence of the joint relationship to *n* Affiliation, the correlation of the choice indicator of affiliative values with affiliative acts frequency is reduced to insignificance. The overall conclusion remains the same: estimates of the cognitive value students place on affiliation do not relate to operant affiliative acts as well as operant motive thoughts do. This may be because neither operant thoughts nor acts are directly influenced by the kind of cognitive factors that determine choices.

Table 13.6 also presents the results for the *n* Affiliation ratio to check the prediction from the Atkinson-Birch model that it is not so much the absolute strength of the motive as its strength relative to other motives in the situation that will predict the frequency of acts related to it. Constantian (1981) also scored the TAT stories for *n* Power; *n* Achievement; and Activity Inhibition, a measure reflecting a concern for controlling one's behavior (see McClelland, 1975). The motive ratio is the strength of *n* Affiliation relative to all motivational tendencies present in the person. Its correlation with the affiliative acts score is slightly higher in line with prediction, although not significantly so.

How the Determinants of Affiliative Acts and Choices Interact with Each Other to Produce Their Effects on Behavior

By using the technique of multiple correlation, we can determine the combined effects of motives, values, and perceived skill on predicting affiliative acts or choices. In other words, how much of the variation in frequency of affiliative acts can be predicted by taking all three of its possible determinants and their combinations into account? Table 13.7 gives the relevant results. The affiliative acts measure was available on only forty-eight subjects, but the correlations based on the total number of subjects were used in the analysis wherever possible. This procedure seemed better than limiting the sample just to the forty-eight subjects for each correlation, because the beeper sample was chosen by Constantian (1981) to represent extremes in attitudes toward being alone or with others. This exaggerated correlations between variables in some cases. The partial correlations represent the "pure" contribution of a given determinant to affiliative behavior, with the influence of other variables removed.

The results shown at the top of Table 13.7 simply confirm in a purer form what was previously shown in Table 13.6—namely, that the *n* Affiliation score is the sole significant contributor to predicting the affiliative acts score, and the *v* Affiliation score is the sole significant predictor of the affiliative choices score, once the effect of other variables has been removed. The effect of all three variables taken together is to increase slightly the ability to predict affiliative behavior over and above a prediction obtained from any one of the personality determinants. The multiple *R*'s in Table 13.7 are slightly higher than the single-variable *r*'s in Table 13.6.

Atkinson (1957), Hull (1943), and Spence (1956), have made specific predictions as to how these determinants will interact in affecting behavior, so the interaction terms in Table 13.7 are of particular interest. They show that only the motive times the perceived skill interaction contributes significantly to predicting the affiliative acts score, as the theoretical models would predict. In fact, the ad-

Table 13.7.

PREDICTING FREQUENCY OF AFFILIATIVE ACTS AND CHOICES FROM PERSONALITY DETERMINANTS

Personality Determinant	Affiliative Acts (N = 48)[a]			Affiliative Choice (N = 111)[b]	
	Partial r	p		Partial r	p
Motive *(M)*:					
n Affiliation	.39	<.001		.14	n.s.
Value *(V)*:					
v Affiliation	.19	n.s.		.40	<.001
Skill *(S)*:					
Social skill	−.24	n.s.		−.14	n.s.
Multiple *R* = .48		<.01	.45		
Interactions:					
M × *V*	−.19	n.s.		−.07	n.s.
M × *S*	.41	<.01		.09	n.s.
V × *S*	−.12	n.s.		.10	n.s.
Multiple *R* = .60		<.01	.46		<.01
Gain in *R* by adding in interactions		<.05			n.s.

[a]Percentage of times found conversing with others or writing letters when beeped.
[b]Mean liking for carrying out fifteen activities with friends.

dition of this interaction raises the multiple correlation from .48 to .60, a significant increase.

Its meaning is more clearly illustrated by Figure 13.4, which shows that perceived social skill contributes to predicting affiliative acts frequency only if *n* Affiliation is high. The subjects with low *n* Affiliation showed no increase in the frequency with which they were found conversing with another person the greater they perceived their success to be in social situations. Figure 13.4 plots the relationship between perceived social skill and affiliative acts when *n* Affiliation is assumed to be high (half a standard deviation above the mean) or low (half a standard deviation below the mean). To put it a different way, people's believing that they are likely to be successful in social interaction does not lead to more interaction unless they are motivated to use the skill. This is the same type of conclusion Hull came to in observing rats in mazes. Even though the rats knew how to run in the maze from previous practice, they would not do so unless motivated by hunger. But if the rats were motivated, their previous experience in running the maze (conceptualized as probability of success) would greatly increase the speed and success with which they could now traverse the maze. Likewise, if people *want* to affiliate, perceived skill in affiliating will greatly increase the likelihood that they will be found conversing with others.

This result is the same as that obtained in the achievement area in the Pat-

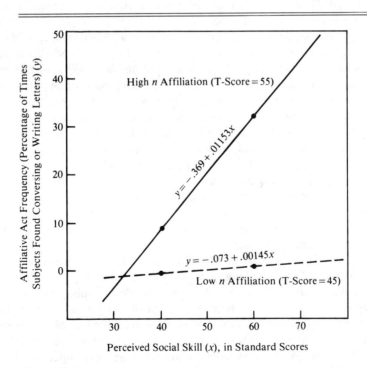

Figure 13.4.

Interaction of Affiliative Motive Strength and Social Skill in Predicting Affiliative Act Frequency.

ten and White (1977) experiment, where a different motive (*n* Achievement) and measure of skill (number of practice trials) were employed. That is, the top line in Figure 13.1 shows that people in whom *n* Achievement is higher gain more from practice. In that instance and in the Constantian experiment, motive and skill combine to increase response strength, defined in the affiliation experiment as response probability.

In the Constantian study, too, there is no significant interaction of the value and skill measures. Subjects high in *v* Affiliation do not engage in more affiliative acts the greater their perceived social skill. This is analogous to the finding in the Patten and White (1977) experiment that subjects high in *v* Achievement with increased practice (or probability of success) do not perform better. (See the bottom two lines in Figure 13.1.) This finding may seem contrary to common sense, because we often assume that if we think something is important— like getting enough exercise—we would be more likely to do it if we were more skillful at doing it, that is, at getting exercise by jogging, playing tennis, and so on. But the findings in these two experiments suggest this is not the case. Exercise would have to satisfy some motive for us to do it more often, and then greater skill would lead us to exercise more often.

The results for the third interaction—between motive (*n* Affiliation) and value (*v* Affiliation)—are not the same as in the Patten and White experiment, in which high *v* Achievement improved performance if the motive was aroused or high. Here the trend is in the opposite direction, although it is not significant: it takes less *v* Affiliation to lead to an affiliative act if *n* Affiliation is high. So we cannot draw a firm conclusion as to whether valuing something and also being motivated for it combine to increase the likelihood that a person will be found doing it. Perhaps it makes a difference *how well* someone can do something, as in the Patten and White experiment, versus how often he or she will do it, as in the study of affiliation acts frequency (Constantian, 1981). Perhaps values combine with motives to improve performance but not to increase the frequency with which the performance is undertaken—which is largely a function of motive level and the combination of motive and skill level.

Where M = motives, S = perceived social skill, and V = incentive value, the $M \times S$ combination does not contribute to predicting the affiliative choice measure, nor do the two other interactions ($M \times V$ or $V \times S$) contribute significantly to predicting that measure. In other words, values do not combine with perceived social skills the way motives do, nor is the effect of multiplying motives times values significant.

If Atkinson's (1980) motive ratio variable is substituted for the *n* Affiliation score, the effect is striking. The multiple correlation goes from .49 for the affiliative acts score without the interactions to .76 including the interactions, a highly significant gain. Again, there is no effect of using a motive ratio for predicting the affiliative choices score. And once more, the effect of the motive times skill interaction makes a highly significant contribution to the multiple R for the affiliative acts measure, as does the motive times value interaction. That is, valuing affiliation has less effect in increasing affiliative acts for those with high *n* Affiliation relative to other motives than for those with low *n* Affiliation relative to other motives. Since such an interaction is the opposite of what would be theoretically predicted and is not significant when the *n* Affiliation ratio is not used, it needs further confirmation.

Next, we should examine the third-order interactions directly, since both Hull's and Atkinson's models assume that the three determinants of response strength multiply with each other. Thus, we would like to see the effect for predicting affiliative behavior of multiplying $M \times S \times V$, but it is not possible to do so meaningfully with these data because of what statisticians call *multicolinearity*. Roughly speaking, this means that multiplying the variables two at a time has taken up so much of the explanatory power of the determinants that there is none left over to be accounted for by multiplying all three together.

There is an approximate way to test the applicability of the Hull and Spence models. It will be recalled that Spence argued that if either incentive (here called *value*) or drive (here called *motive*) were present, some behavior would result, whereas in the Hull model, if either of these variables were reduced to zero, the equation would predict no response. Thus, Spence suggested that M and V should be added rather than multiplied, as in the Hull model. Table 13.8 shows the effects of adding or multiplying the M and V variables. That is, we can treat either the sum or the product of these two determinants as independent variables in a multivariate prediction of affiliative behavior. Then we can see whether either the product $(M \times V)$ or the sum $(M + V)$ times perceived social skill (S) contributes significantly to predicting affiliative behavior.

As Table 13.8 shows, in this instance the Hull formula works and the Spence formula does not. That is, both the sum and the product of M and V contribute significantly to predicting affiliative acts or affiliative choices, but only the $(M \times V) \times S$ interaction adds nearly significantly to the multiple R, and contributes significantly to predicting the affiliative acts score. The $(M + V) \times S$ interaction does not contribute significantly to predicting the affiliative acts score or to increasing the multiple R.

At first glance the results for the $M \times V$ interaction term in Tables 13.7 and 13.8 may seem contradictory, for it contributes negatively to predicting affiliative acts in Table 13.7 and positively in Table 13.8. However, the difference lies in the fact that the contribution of $M \times V$ in Table 13.7 is assessed *after* the contribution of M to the multiple correlation has been taken into account, whereas in Table 13.8 the contribution of M is *included* in the $M \times V$ term. This means that once the effect of M by itself has been removed, the remaining interaction of $M \times V$ may contribute negatively to the multiple correlation.

The Hull-Atkinson formula, however, is not stated this way: it is more nearly represented by the formula $(M \times V) \times S$, which predicts fairly well the affiliative acts score ($R = .57$). To this extent, the results may be taken as confirmation that a multiplicative relationship among these three determinants represents a reasonable way of combining them to predict response strength. However, as good a prediction of affiliative acts can be obtained from the determinants listed in Table 13.7, consisting largely of M and $M \times S$ ($R = .60$). So multiplying all three determinants is not the only, or even the best, way of predicting response strength in this situation.

Table 13.8.

COMPARISON OF HULL AND SPENCE FORMULAS FOR PREDICTING AFFILIATIVE ACTS AND CHOICES; MOTIVE = n AFFILIATION, VALUE = v AFFILIATION

Alternative Formulas for Predicting Behavior		Affiliative Acts[a]		Affiliative Choices[b]	
		Partial r	p	Partial r	p
Hull formula ($M \times V \times S$):					
Social skill		−.29	n.s.	−.06	n.s.
Motive × value (affiliation)		.46	<.01	.39	<.01
	$R = .47$			.39	
($M \times V$) × S		.37	<.01	.12	n.s.
	$R = .57$		<.01	.41	<.01
Gain in R			<.10		n.s.
Spence formula ($M + V$) × S:					
Social skill		−.30	.05	−.06	n.s.
Motive + value (affiliation)		.48	<.01	.39	<.01
	$R = .49$		<.01	.39	<.01
($M + V$) × S		.13	n.s.	.11	n.s.
	$R = .50$		<.01	.40	<.01
Gain in R			n.s.		n.s,

[a]Percentage of times found conversing with others or writing letters when beeped.
[b]Mean liking for carrying out fifteen activities with friends.

Neither Hull's nor Spence's model for interactions of the variables improves the multiple R for the affiliative choices measure of response strength (see Table 13.8). What this analysis shows above all is that it is vitally important to distinguish between operant and respondent indicators of response strength and, in trying to predict these indicators, to include measures of motives, skill, and values as independent determinants of action tendencies. Personality theorists have repeatedly confused these variables and talked about them as if they were interchangeable, just as Weiner (1980a) refers to v Achievement as if it were a measure of the achievement motive. Or what is worse, they have argued that personality is inconsistent because the measures do not correlate highly with each other (Mischel, 1968), when, according to the theory outlined here, they should be independent and *therefore* uncorrelated with each other. If we accept the fact that motives, skill, and values are three nearly independent personal determinants of response strength, they can, taken together, account for a surprising amount of the variation in spontaneous or operant behavior.

In the Constantian study, if the n Affiliation ratio is used as a determinant, it together with affiliative values and skill and their interactions accounts for over 75 percent of the variation with which people engage in affiliative acts over time (see D'Andrade & Dart, 1982, for a discussion of the importance of accounting for variation rather than variance in behavior). This is quite impressive in view of the error undoubtedly involved in sampling people's behavior at different times during a week. The remaining 25 percent of the variation could easily be accounted for by situational factors controlling the *opportunity* for interaction. For example, it is practically impossible for a person to be conversing with someone if he or she is sleeping, in class, or riding the subway when beeped.

In contrast, the determinants do not combine as expected to increase the predictability of affiliative choices. This confirms the importance of the distinction Skinner (1966) made between operants (strength measured by response probability) and respondents (strength measured by amplitude, latency, persistence, and so on), as well as his inference that operants more readily show the influence of "purpose," or motivational factors. Affiliative choices as responses to contrived stimulus situations represented by questionnaire items are determined almost entirely by values deriving from the same cognitive source as the choices. People carry around with them cognitive schemata that organize their feelings, attitudes, and choices in a particular area such as affiliation or achievement. These schemata are often part of their self-image, although they are not coextensive with self-relevant values. They influence behavior, particularly when the nature of the situation in which the behavior occurs is clearly defined in cognitive terms—that is, when a situation is seen to be affiliation or achievement related.

When people are asked whether they would like doing something "with friends," the question taps a value associated with liking for people, which determines how they answer the question. In contrast, the frequency with which people converse with someone else is not determined by the value placed on affiliative activity, but on the pleasure they unconsciously get from such interactions, as reflected in the strength of the affiliative motive.

The distinction between conscious cognitive values and relatively unconscious affectively toned associative networks or motives can also be invoked to explain the differences Silverman (1976) has found in the reactions of people with various personality disorders to emotionally toned phrases or pictures relevant to their pathology when the stimuli could or could not be consciously recognized and processed (see Chapter 2). That is, if a phrase like *go shit* was presented to stutterers too fast to recognize, it touched off affective associations that produced more stuttering. But if the same phrase was presented slowly enough to be recognized, it was processed in terms of cognitive schemata (here called *values*) that filtered out its effect on stuttering.

Just as Hull's and Atkinson's theoretical models have stated, social skill, or a person's perceived probability of success in an interaction, will contribute to the frequency of the interactive behavior *only* if the person is motivated to affiliate. People's being good at doing something does not lead to their doing it more often unless they are really interested in the activity—an obvious point perhaps, but one that has often been overlooked. Even people's valuing a type of activity or its end result does not lead to their doing it more often unless they are motivated to do it. What is needed are more studies of this type that show the joint effects of several determinants on what people do and that also make the distinction between predicting operant acts and cognitively based choices.

• THE DISTINCTION BETWEEN MOTIVES AND INTENTS

At the very beginning of our consideration of what the term *motivation* means in Chapter 1, we distinguished between conscious intents, such as are contained in statements like "I want to go talk to my friend," and unconscious intents, deduced from the fact that I am often found talking to my friend or from a behavioral fact such as a person seeks out a friend in a crowd of people even though the person reports having had no conscious experience of wanting to talk to a friend. Freud deduced unconscious intents from unusual or symptomatic acts; we have just deduced an unconscious intent to affiliate with people from the operant frequency with which people are found talking with others when beeped at random times throughout a week. In other words, a motive behaves like a dispositional unconscious intent, since it is unlikely that the students beeped had made a lot of conscious choices to talk to people when they were found to be doing so. deCharms (1982) is so impressed by the difference between thinking of people as being moved by motivational forces and as intending to do things that he believes the two ways of looking at people involve wholly different perspectives: "Objects are moved by causes, organisms behave from motives, and persons act with intention." He argues that talking about motives as if they were biological forces moving behavior neglects the all-important experience of choice and intention.

From the perspective of this and other chapters, the distinction between a motive and an intent is clear and obvious, and it does not require a major shift in perspective. A motive is a largely unconscious determinant of spontaneously generated behavior, and an intent is a largely conscious preference for doing something that should be determined jointly by motive strength, probability of success, and values associated with doing it. The conscious-unconscious aspect of this distinction is not essential to it: what is essential is the difference between choice of what to do—what Atkinson calls *motivation,* or the tendency to approach or avoid alternatives when they confront people in a respondent situation—and the operant frequency with which people act in certain ways. For people may be conscious of their need for affiliation or may choose an alternative without the choice's being conscious. Nevertheless, the conscious-unconscious distinction catches what characterizes the two types of behavior most often and helps explain why deCharms feels "organisms behave from motives"—for example, are moved unconsciously to do something without consciously intending to do it.

In the Constantian study, conscious affiliative choices or intents turned out to be determined largely by affiliative values, a little by the affiliative motive, and not at all by perceived affiliative skill. However, the choices involved, like going to a movie with a friend, did not require much affiliative skill. One can safely assume that if the choices had required much skill—that is, if they had dealt with *making friends,* for example—the subjects' perceived affiliative skill would have played more of a role in affecting their intent to make friends.

It cannot be emphasized too often that a motivational intent or choice—whether conscious or not—is a product of several determinants, including at least two nonmotivational ones: probability of success and values. Operant trends in behaviors, in contrast, appear to be the product of largely unconscious motives and skill, or probability of success if it is combined with a strong motive. Conscious values play less of a role in determining operant behaviors.

NOTES AND QUERIES

1. In this chapter the similarity is noted between skill and perceived probability of success. Normally we would expect these variables to be closely related: if people know they can do something well, they are more likely to estimate they can do well at it. But think of a situation where this would not be true. Which of the two variables would be a better predictor of behavior? Would it depend on the kind of behavior—whether it was respondent (as in solving a problem) or operant (as in the frequency with which a person turned to solving problems)?

2. The French and Lesser experiment (Table 13.1) shows the joint effect on behavior of motives and values. Redesign the experiment in a way that would also show the effect of skill or the probability of success on behavior.

3. Think through the implications of Patten and White's (1977) conclusion that asking people the reasons for their failure arouses achievement motivation. Does this mean that attributing failure to lack of effort improves performance only when achievement motivation is aroused? Is there any way to examine this question by getting causal attributions without arousing achievement motivation? Individuals high in *n* Achievement might believe that in general effort is important, but would you expect that belief to improve performance in a particular situation if their motivation to achieve was not aroused? Is this analogous to asking if probability of success or self-confidence will improve performance if there is no motivation to perform?

4. Weiner (1980a) would appear to argue at times that a motive has its effect on performance only through causal ascriptions and at other times that the pattern of causal ascriptions is the motive. Evaluate each of these hypotheses in terms of existing findings and design research that would shed further light on the issues involved.

5. One problem with the approach examined in this chapter is that so many different aspects of people's understanding of a situation or the values they bring to it have been identified that it seems impossible to reduce them to a manageable number in trying to predict different kinds of behavior. Cognitive consistency is important, but so is a sense of control, internality, instrumentality, and a flock of other values like cooperativeness, autonomy, and social approval. Rokeach (1973) has listed eighteen instrumental and eighteen goal-state values that might influence behavior. In the study of Navy officers summarized in Table 13.2, four values were measured that do not relate particularly well to any of these values. Do you see any way to determine what the most important values are that must be taken into account, or will the relevant ones be specific to each situation?

6. In Constantian's beeper study, what do you think people high in *n* Achievement and *n* Power would be most likely to be thinking and doing when paged at random intervals throughout a week? Would you expect sex differences? If so, why?

7. Design a treatment study that would determine whether increasing the value placed on being friendly would increase the affiliative *motive*.

8. Our culture values people's being friendly to others, so there is congruence between *n* Affiliation and *v* Affiliation scores. This is less true in the power area, since our culture is ambivalent about people's consciously wanting to be dominant or powerful. So there should be many people high in *n* Power who are low in *v* Power. How do you think their power motive would be most likely to express itself? The analogy is with people discussed in the chapter who are high in *n* Affiliation and low in *v* Affiliation.

9. It is suggested in the text that the reason the $M \times V$ interaction has different effects in the achievement and affiliation studies may be because in the former, improvements in performance are being predicted and in the latter, increased frequencies of an act. Can you think of other possible explanations? Do you think the findings in the affiliation area would be the same as in the achievement area if the behavior to be predicted were shifted to performance on a task of learning relationships among people (as in Figure 9.1)? That is, in that situation, would increases in *v* Affiliation in combination with high *n* Affiliation lead to better performance, as opposed to the result shown in Table 13.7, where the reverse result was obtained? That is, in Table 13.7, the higher the *n* Affiliation, the less *v* Affiliation is needed to get an increase in the frequency of affiliative acts.

10. In the end, the frequency over time of affiliative acts turns out to be much more predictable (multiple *R* as high as .76) than the average liking for fifteen types of affiliative activity (multiple $R = .46$). Why do you think this turned out to be the case? Might it be due to the fact that a larger number of responses was being recorded in the first than the second instance (fifty versus fifteen), to the fact that some appropriate determinants were left out in the second instance, or to the fact that operants are easier to predict than respondents? Design experiments that would answer such questions.

11. Apply the model for predicting behavior explained in the chapter to national behavior. Under what circumstances would a country be most likely to go to war or commit frequent aggressive acts? Chapter 11 summarizes some of the evidence on motivational determinants of such behavior. What other key determinant of this behavior is suggested by the equations tested in this chapter, and how would you measure it?

14

Motivation Training

As it became evident in the 1960s that human motives were related to important human endeavors like entrepreneurship and management, investigators turned their attention to methods of changing motives to improve performance. Since the emphasis was on performance output rather than on motive change in itself, these efforts to produce change can best be understood in terms of the formula for predicting response output presented in previous chapters. According to that formula, response output, given environmental opportunity, is a function of motive strength (M) times probability of success (P_s) times incentive value (V). Technically, response probability can be increased by changing environmental opportunity or any one of the three person variables in the equation. Early efforts to introduce change focused on affecting the probability of success variable. School learning or skill acquisition affects this variable. If people learn how to do something better, it by definition increases the probability of their succeeding at that activity and makes it more likely that they will carry out the activity if they are also motivated to do it and they value it. But motive development courses approached probability of success in a different way. They manipulated the *perceived* probability of success without teaching skills directly.

The Pygmalion Effect

Impetus was given to this approach by Rosenthal's (1966) demonstration that an experimenter's expectation or bias strongly influenced the way subjects behaved in a variety of different types of situations. Of particular importance was the evidence summarized in Rosenthal and Jacobson's book *Pygmalion in the Classroom* (1968) leading to the conclusion that simply giving a teacher the expectation that certain randomly picked pupils in their classes were of high ability was sufficient to improve greatly the academic performance of those pupils. A large number of studies on this Pygmalion effect were carried out, and while some of them were open to criticism (see Elashoff & Snow, 1970), there seems little doubt that the phenomenon exists (Rosenthal & Rubin, 1978).

A typical result is illustrated in Figure 14.1. This study was carried out on inner city black boys aged seven to eleven in second to fifth grade, most of whom were not doing very well in school. The teacher for each grade was given the real ability test scores for a random half of the class and ability test scores that were one standard deviation higher than their actual scores for the other half. In other words, the teachers were led to believe that half of their pupils were much brighter than their test scores showed they actually were. At the end of the school year these students showed a much larger gain in reading and arithmetic achievement test scores than the pupils whose true ability scores had been given the teachers. The difference in score gain for the two types of pupils occurred for each grade, but obviously there were also differences from grade to grade. Thus, in third grade the pupils in the control group also gained greatly in test scores, although those the teachers thought were particularly bright gained

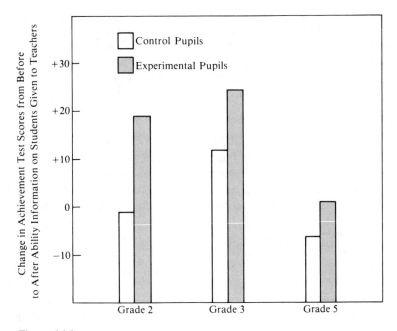

Figure 14.1.

Effects on Pupil Achievement Test Scores of Telling Teachers Their Actual Ability Scores (Control Pupils) or Scores Considerably Higher Than Actually Attained (Experimental Pupils) (after Keshock, 1970).

even more. The pupils in the control group in fifth grade, in contrast, actually lost ground, whereas those from whom the teachers expected better work only managed to hold their own. So it looks as if there are important teacher effects over and beyond what they expect from their students, but however good the teachers are, if they think certain pupils are smarter, those pupils tend to perform better.

Increasing Perceived Probability of Success

What is the mechanism by which teacher expectations affect pupil performance? Heckhausen (1974, 1980) reasoned that the mechanism involves the pupils' perceived probability of success as it is influenced by the reasons assigned by teachers and pupils for success and failure. Teachers who know their pupils lack ability will attribute failure to lack of ability rather than to other causal factors such as lack of effort, luck, or task difficulty (see Chapter 12). This leads the teachers to act very differently toward the pupils than they would if they thought they were of high ability, as Brophy and Good (1970) have demonstrated. For example, they found that if a child gives a wrong answer, the teacher is much more likely to rephrase the question or give the child a clue to the right answer if the teacher regards the child as having high ability rather than low ability. Children of low ability much more often get no feedback from the teacher—whatever they do or say—as contrasted with those of high ability, to whom the teacher nearly always responds somehow. In time, certain children begin to respond in ways that confirm the teacher's expectation that they will perform poorly. For instance, they are much less likely to raise their hands in class than those considered to be of high ability. In short, the teacher conveys to the child that he or she is of low ability and is not expected to perform well; this, in time, creates exactly the same impression in the child's mind, which lowers the child's perceived probability of success and, according to the general formula for predicting response output, decreases the likelihood of successful performance. Raising teachers' expectations about children's ability reverses this trend.

Heckhausen (1974) checked this possibility directly by instructing teachers of underachieving students to attribute failure to lack of effort rather than lack of ability. There were three to eight underachieving target students in each of several classes of fourth-graders, and their teachers were simply told that they should say to these students when they did not do very well, "You could do better if you try harder." There were also other underachieving pupils in each classroom who served as controls. The pupils were given several tests before the experiment started, as well as four and a half months later. All the students in the classes improved on a number of these measures, perhaps because the teachers did not limit their comments about effort only to the target pupils.

However, it was possible to get another control group from the classrooms of two teachers who had not attended the session in which they were instructed to attribute failure to lack of effort. In comparison with the pupils from these classes, the targeted pupils from the experimentally treated classes were significantly more likely to attribute failure to lack of effort rather than to lack of ability; their Test Anxiety scores decreased significantly; and they scored higher on primary mental ability tests involving speed of performance. However, they did not show significant gains in arithmetic performance or the expected gain in the h Success aspect of n Achievement.

These results are consistent with those obtained by other investigators. For example, Dweck (1975) had children perform a number of tasks during training, on most of which they succeeded but on some of which they failed. Whenever they failed they were told, "You got only ——— right. That means you should have tried harder." Other children were given only success feedback. Those who had received training in attributing failure to lack of effort performed better after training and were less disrupted by a failure experience than those who failed and had not had the training.

It took Dweck twenty-five training sessions to produce this effect, but Andrews and Debus (1978) found they could produce a similar change after only one hour of training. As subjects performed a task, they were asked after each trial to give causal attributions for the outcome. Whenever they gave an effort attribution—that is, attributing success to extra effort or failure to lack of effort—they were strongly reinforced by the experimenter by statements like

"OK!" or "Good!" The investigators found that this type of training increased persistence in the face of failure afterward and also increased the likelihood that the subjects would make effort attributions. However, when the subjects were retested sixteen to seventeen weeks later, while those who had been trained continued to make more effort attributions, the effect on persistence had disappeared. In terms of the formula for predicting response strength, what these experiments are doing is increasing the subjects' perceived probability of success by training them to believe that more effort leads to greater success. To put it the other way around, attributing success to greater effort decreases the expectation of failure that comes from attributing it to stable factors like lack of ability or task difficulty. (See Chapter 12.)

Stamps (1973) tested the direct effect on fear of failure of increasing the perceived probability of success. There were three groups of subjects, two of which received treatment of different types and one of which served as a no-treatment control group. In one treatment group, the subjects worked on various arithmetic problems for two weeks, rewarding themselves with tokens exchangeable at the end for prizes, in accordance with how well they were doing. This was called the *Self-Reinforcement Group.* It was designed to increase self-confidence in doing work of this type or, in terms of the formula, to increase perceived probability of success. The other treatment group received a kind of group therapy in which the subjects played various games as the experimenter commented on their performance. The goal of these training sessions was to make the subjects feel positive about their performance, so they were greatly encouraged for effort, and whenever they failed the experimenter either gave a neutral response or encouraged them to do something else.

Both types of treatment significantly lowered fear of failure as measured by the Hostile Press score discussed in Chapter 10. One might suppose that lowering f Failure would have some long-term effects on performance of a similar type, although this was not tested in this experiment. In fact, all any of these experiments show is that it is relatively easy to change perceived probability of success in an experimental situation so far as that particular situation is concerned. This change may have effects that are long-term and generalize to other situations (see the Bandura research on self-efficacy mentioned in Chapter 12), but it is not yet known exactly under what conditions such major effects occur.

Increasing Understanding of and Control over One's Own Performance

Heckhausen (1974, 1980; Heckhausen & Krug, 1982) reports a number of more ambitious attempts to change academic performance through exercises derived from achievement motivation theory. By and large, they focus on the cognitive aspects of performing better, because Heckhausen was thinking largely in terms of how people high and low in *n* Achievement evaluate themselves differently. So he designed the training to help those low in *n* Achievement to think, plan, and evaluate the self like a person high in *n* Achievement, that is, to set moderate rather than unrealistic goals for performance and to attribute success to ability and failure to lack of effort rather than low ability.

Typically, the approach involved teaching students to set moderate goals in tasks varying from ringtoss to school subjects, giving students feedback on the extent to which they had achieved their goals, teaching them to monitor their own performance and reward themselves for doing well, training them in causal attribution so that the importance of effort could be clearly seen, and trying to generalize what they had learned in the training sessions to everyday life. Furthermore, the pupils observed the experimenter as he displayed the characteristics of a person high in *n* Achievement: "He spoke out loud what went through his mind while setting a standard, planning his actions, calculating effort expenditure, monitoring performance, evaluating performance outcome, weighing causal attributions and administering self-reward" (Heckhausen, 1974). Then the students took turns doing the same thing, first speaking aloud and then silently to themselves as they went through the achievement motive thought sequence. There were two control groups of students, one of which received no training and one, another kind of training that was announced as a "program for improving motivation to learn," although the games and activities in it were irrelevant to motive change. This group was included to see whether any effects obtained were due purely to suggestion or expectation that something was being done to improve the students' performance.

After fourteen weeks, those trained in achievement motive practices had gained in a number of ways over those in the other two groups. They showed a larger gain in their *h* Success score as contrasted with their *f* Failure score, as measured by a semiprojective test (Schmalt, 1976) in which a person picks out of several alternatives the one most likely to describe what is going on in a picture. Their goal setting had become more realistic, and their level of aspiration tended realistically to go up after success and down after failure. Also, "self-reward after success had gone up whereas there was no difference in self-punishment after failure . . . last but not least, the gain on the scholastic achievement test exceeded the other two groups." (Heckhausen, 1974). The only area in which an expected shift did not occur involved causal attributions after success and after failure, for which there were no differences among the groups or from before to after the training.

Improvements in goal setting, causal attributions, and *h* Success were found after such training in several studies, although none of these changes had any long-term effects on school grades (Heckhausen & Krug, 1982). Heckhausen (1980) interprets the results in terms of the cognitive characteristics of the achievement motive discussed in Chapter 12. That is, he believes that what such training does is help individuals define their own goals for performance, which leads to a realistic level of aspiration, particularly if the teacher aids in the process by assigning tasks of appropriate difficulty for a particular student. Of special importance is orienting the pupils to judging their performance in terms of their own past accomplishments rather than the accomplishments of others (that is, using a social norm standard for evaluating their achievements), for people can improve over their past performance even though they are still doing poorly relative to others. All these procedures increase the student's sense of personal responsibility for setting the goals in the first place, for the performance that follows, for evaluating the performance, and for deciding what to do next. So the student develops internal, as opposed to external, reasons for success and failure, which in turn leads to increased valuing of the self for having been the key factor in the whole achievement process.

All these factors involve cognitive processes that increase the perceived probability of success. That is, if students understand that they are picking the standards for performance in terms of which they will be judged; if, when they learn how well they have done, they can see the outcome as a result of their personal efforts; if they have control over what level of difficulty they will perform at next; and if they are in charge of rewarding themselves for performing well, they will have higher self-esteem. And higher self-esteem translates into a greater perceived probability of success in general, and also a greater perceived probability of success in particular with respect to the tasks they are working on.

Most of the effects of the courses Heckhausen (1980) reviews have been in the cognitive area—that is, the changes observed have been in goal setting, causal attribution, and self-confidence. Longer-range effects on performance in school or in life have seldom been obtained. Heckhausen and Krug (1982) conclude that the reason for the lack of effects of these changes on school performance lies in the way school learning is structured:

> Although children are more achievement motivated after the training program, they are still academic low achievers. They would like to be successful, but they now find that the school situation does not lend itself to satisfying their need to achieve. It may be possible to assume self-responsibility, but setting one's own goals is hardly feasible. Furthermore, assignments are too difficult compared to one's performance standard. Success, if any, is therefore still more likely to be attributed to chance than effort, and there are few opportunities for self-reinforcement or for anticipating positive effects.

So the conclusion might be drawn that cognitive inputs produce cognitive outputs, but that the ultimate effect of changing the cognitions associated with the achievement motive is not well documented. This type of motivation training can be viewed as focusing primarily on the cognitive variables that influence probability of success in the general formula governing the likelihood that a response will occur (summarized in Figure 12.15).

• ACHIEVEMENT MOTIVATION TRAINING FOR ENTREPRENEURS

In the 1960s a motivation training program was developed that was aimed at influencing all the theoretical determinants of performance—namely, motive strength, perceived probability of success, and the incentive value of success. It grew out of the research on the achievement motive (reviewed in Chapters 7 and 11), which showed that people high in *n* Achievement had many of the characteristics needed for successful entrepreneurship and that successful entrepreneurs or small businesspeople were in fact higher in *n* Achievement. Since it had also been demonstrated that countries more oriented around *n* Achievement in popular literature developed more rapidly economically, it seemed reasonable to infer that this came about in part because there were more energetic entrepreneurs in such countries and that therefore one of the ways to promote economic development in a country might be to strengthen the achievement motive among its business entrepreneurs.

So training courses in achievement motivation were provided for small businessmen, particularly in India at the outset, because it was a country that was underdeveloped and needed more successful entrepreneurs outside its great metropolitan centers to create more jobs for unemployed or underemployed workers in smaller cities throughout the country (McClelland & Winter, 1969/1971). After the courses had been successfully offered in a number of cities in India and elsewhere, it was decided to try to have a major impact by this means on economic development in a limited area.

Business activities in two small cities in southeast India were carefully monitored for several years before, during, and after the business leaders in one of the cities received achievement motivation training. The cities were chosen to be as comparable as possible. They were about the same size, with populations of around 100,000; the distribution of the work force in various categories was similar; they consumed equivalent amounts of electricity per capita, indicating approximately equal levels of industrial development; and they were located in the same state, Andhra Pradesh, so the people belonged to the same culture and spoke the same language. One was a seaport and the other, a river port on a major inland waterway. It was hoped that providing achievement motivation training for the businessmen in one city, Kakinada, would stimulate them to outperform the businessmen in the neighboring control city, Rajahmundry, producing in the long run a significant difference in the level of economic development of the two urban areas.

Through speeches at local businessmen's clubs and other recruitment efforts, some fifty-two businessmen from Kakinada were persuaded to leave their businesses and spend two weeks being trained in achievement motivation at the Small Industries Extension Training Institute at Hyderabad, over two hundred miles away. They were trained in four batches of ten to fourteen participants each. The training was intensive, lasting ten or more hours a day, and it was based on all that was known at the time about how to introduce personality change. It was generally believed that it was difficult, if not impossible, to change adults in any very fundamental way such as might be involved in increasing their need to achieve. Certainly the research findings on the effects of prolonged psychotherapy were not very encouraging. It typically involved many more hours of person-to-person contact than was available in a short group training course, and its effects in producing fundamental personality change were in some doubt (Eysenck, 1952). However, religious groups like the Mormons or the Jesuits seemed to be effective in producing personal change through intensive training, so it was decided to make an all-out effort to produce motive change in any way possible, drawing on the experience of religious groups and on whatever scientific information was available.

Training Inputs in Courses for Small Businessmen

Twelve different types of training inputs were devised (McClelland, 1965; McClelland & Winter, 1969/1971). They can be classified according to which determinant of performance output they should affect, as shown in Table 14.1. Great emphasis was placed on increasing motive strength directly by learning how to think, talk, and act like a person high in *n* Achievement. So they wrote

Table 14.1.

TRAINING INPUTS IN COURSES FOR BUSINESS ENTREPRENEURS (after McClelland & Winter, 1969/1971)

Purpose Is to Increase		
Motive Strenth (n Achievement) M ×	*Perceived Probability of Success* P_s ×	*Incentive Value of Being More Entrepreneurial* V
1. Learning the achievement associative network (scoring system)	1. Prestige suggestion that they could change and become more entrepreneurial	1. Realization that chosen occupation requires it
2. Practicing such things as moderate goal setting in action; getting turned on by performance	2. Commitment to concrete goals and plans (increased effort)	2. Realization that chosen occupation fits in with life goals
3. Following behavior of attractive entrepreneurial models (vicarious satisfaction)	3. Keeping track of progress toward goals; using feedback to increase self-confidence	3. Clarification of how this value fits in with other values that might conflict with it
	4. Receiving warmth and respect from trainers during confusion and failure	4. Retreat setting to dramatize importance of life change
	Gaining confidence from experiences in course exercises (see Item 2 in *M* column)	
	Gaining confidence from self-knowledge and from knowing how to change	5. New reference group of trainees to give reminders and reinforcement after training

imaginative stories to pictures, learned to score them for *n* Achievement, and practiced writing stories that scored as high as possible in *n* Achievement. Thus, they learned to think and talk in achievement terms all day long. They learned to act like a person high in *n* Achievement by participating in various games in which they had to set goals for themselves and observe whether they reached them or not. In particular, they participated in a business simulation game in which they had to set production goals for themselves and either made or lost money, depending on whether they attained the goals or not. They observed and discussed their own behavior as compared with the behavior of others in the same situation and compared their performance with the model of the person high in *n* Achievement, who sets moderate goals, takes personal responsibility, uses feedback to modify goals, and takes initiative to find new ways of achieving goals. (See the summary in Chapter 7 of the characteristic behaviors of people high in *n* Achievement.)

The purpose of these games was not only to give people experience in action of behaving in particular ways, but also to provide the positive affect from effective performance that by definition is the basis on which the achievement motive is built. The excitement and enthusiasm generated by the various group activities was considerable and could have been strong enough to help forge new motivational associative networks. Finally, the participants were exposed to attractive models of successful entrepreneurial behavior in the form of visitors who had done well in business and who talked to the group about what they had done. Thus, the trainees could observe for themselves that these successful men in fact did think, talk, and act like the model of the person with high *n* Achievement that they were attempting to emulate in their own behavior.

Several training inputs should have affected the perceived probability of success determinant of performance outcome. Every effort was made to convince the businessmen that they could and should change and become more entrepreneurial and successful. Prestige suggestion has been found by psychologists over and over again to be an important means of introducing attitude change (see Hovland, Janis, & Kelley, 1953). It lies behind such diverse phenomena as the *placebo effect* (Benson & Epstein, 1975), in which a patient gets better just from being given a "sugar pill" by a medical authority, and the *Hawthorne effect,* in which workers in the Hawthorne plant of Western Electric performed better whenever management introduced change, even if the change was back to a previous way of doing things (Roethlisberger & Dickson, 1947). So efforts were made to build the prestige of those offering the training by stressing the fact that they represented a world-famous university, that the training was based on carefully collected scientific evidence, and that it had the backing of an important government-sponsored institution and the Ford Foundation. All these inputs were designed to counteract the prevailing, rather low level of perceived probability of success, since the businessmen were gloomy about their own prospects and about the possibility of economic development in India as a whole.

Of equal importance was the emphasis at the end of the program on getting the businessmen to commit themselves to concrete goals for business activities that were so specific that they could easily keep track over the coming months of how well they were achieving them. Most of them were used to setting goals in general terms like "When I get back I am certainly going to work harder." But they learned that such a goal is not acceptable to a person high in *n* Achievement, because it is not specific: there would be no way to tell whether they had reached it or not, and it is not specific as to *when* it would be achieved. They learned to set more appropriate goals like "Monday after I get back I am going to work out a careful plan showing how the purchase of an air conditioner for my sari shop should increase turnover and profits over a six-month period so that I can pay off the loan to purchase the air conditioner. I am going to take this plan to the Bank of India the next day to get a loan of so many rupees. I expect to get an answer on the loan within one week, to purchase the air conditioner and install it within another week, and to track the increased business over the next six months so that I can calculate at the end of the time whether or not the investment has been worth it." Such plans not only improve business practice; they also create more confidence in people that they know exactly what they are doing and are therefore more likely to succeed.

In the course of the businessmen's learning what their motives were, as revealed in the stories they wrote and as shown in their behavior in discussion or in the business games, many received unpleasant surprises as they realized they had not been behaving in ways consistent with the model of successful entrepreneurial behavior. Self-knowledge is an obvious first step to change, but it can involve strong feelings of failure and confusion. Thus, it was considered very important to generate an atmosphere of warmth and respect for the individual during the training, which helped people remain confident as they underwent the necessary restructuring of their thinking about themselves and their lives. In other words, the trainers were behaving like the experimenters in the studies reported earlier by Heckhausen (1980) and Stamps (1973): they were diminishing fear of failure by reacting to failure either neutrally or as if it were normal under the circumstances, stressing the importance of renewed effort to change the situation, and giving all kinds of positive reinforcement for efforts to understand oneself and to change. As noted at the bottom of the middle column in Table 14.1, self-confidence or the perceived probability of success was also promoted by the experience the men were gaining in performing more successfully in various games throughout the course, as well as by the growing realization that they were understanding themselves better all the time and knew how to do specific things that would change their business behavior for the better. For it increases self-confidence to realize that you know something other people do not know about how to get what you want.

The third set of training inputs affected primarily the incentive value of being more entrepreneurial. Most of the men in the course were already in business, so it was easy to explain to them that if they meant to do well in their chosen occupation, they needed to behave more along the specific lines outlined in the course. The incentive value of being entrepreneurial was bolstered by the simple argument that their occupation required it. If they wanted to do something else, such as be a teacher, an artist, or a sadhu (a religious renunciate), being more entrepreneurial would not be so important; since they had decided to be businessmen, however, it obviously was very important to them.

Raising the question of their occupational goals inevitably stimulated them to think about what their general goals in life were. In one exercise, for example, they were asked to go off by themselves, meditate for an hour, and prepare an inscription they would like to see on their tombstone. This led to a discussion of what each man valued most in life and how that fitted in with the general values held by others around him. The purpose of considering these matters was to see how the incentive value of being more entrepreneurial fitted or failed to fit in with other goals the person might have. For example, a man might have written on his tombstone that he wanted to be remembered as "a generous family man." Discussion might reveal that he often felt a conflict between spending time at work and with his family. Thus, what he might do in the course of discussing this conflict was figure out how his work might contribute to his desire to be viewed as a generous family man. In another instance, a man might realize that he had failed to take some initiative in business, because in India many families operate under the joint family system, in which the oldest competent male—usually the father—is definitely in charge. Thus, it might have seemed completely inappropriate to the man under the prevailing system of Indian values to take an initiative that clearly belonged to another in the family. The purpose of these training inputs was to embed the value of being more entrepreneurial firmly within a network of supporting—or at least nonconflicting—values relating to life goals and the norms of Indian culture.

Requiring that the men leave their home towns for training in a dormitory setting in another place helped to dramatize the importance of the life change the courses were supposed to produce. The effectiveness of religious retreats is based in part on the fact that people withdraw from everyday pursuits and surroundings and seek to create a new self-image or identity, which can be carried back to the old setting. Furthermore, being away with others who are undergoing the same emotional experiences creates a new reference group, and there is considerable evidence that perceived membership in a new reference group helps attitude change to persist (see Berelson & Steiner, 1964). The men in these courses came to know each other very well, since they spent over one hundred hours together discussing their most intimate thoughts and plans. They came to realize that the future economic progress of their community depended on them and, more specifically, on the plans each of them had made for increased business activity. They also knew what each member of the group had committed himself to do when he returned, so they would obviously be in a position to know whether he had done what he said he was going to do or not. All of this served to underline for every participant the great importance of being more entrepreneurial when he returned to contribute to community development and to earn the approval of his many newfound friends, who were part of the same forward movement.

Changes in Business Activity After Motivation Training in India

What were the effects of these intensive efforts to increase achievement motivation and improve entrepreneurial performance? Since the men had been taught the scoring system for n Achievement, it was not possible to determine directly in the usual way whether their achievement motivation had increased, as in the Heckhausen training courses reviewed earlier, which had not employed the TAT as a training device. So attention was focused on developing an index of entrepreneurial behavior or business activity that could apply equally well to people in any line of work (McClelland & Winter, 1969/1971). The men were questioned about all aspects of their business activity during the previous two years at the time they started the training and again six, twelve, eighteen, and twenty-four months after the training was completed. Efforts were made to get information on capital invested, monthly business income, profits, and number of employees, although it was very difficult to get accurate economic figures from many of them, partly because of their reluctance to provide it for fear that tax collectors might find out about it, and partly because many of the businessmen were not very good at keeping such records.

In the end, a very simple coding system was devised for assessing the level of business activity. If, by all signs, business activity had proceeded at about the same pace for the past two years, the subject received a 0. If his business had noticeably declined in income or profitability or if he had gone out of business, he received a -1. He received a $+1$ if he had undertaken some specific plans to improve his business, such as taking a course in accounting, planning a new plant, joining a voluntary business organization, or going to work more often or earlier. A score of $+2$ was given if he had actually started a new business, been responsible for an unusual increase in the firm's income or profitability level, or received an unusual promotion in the firm. To receive a $+2$, a man had to have done something that was clearly visible and obvious to all as representing an improvement in business activity, and that involved a clear financial change. Every attempt was made to check carefully on statements made in interviews about changes. Thus, if a man said he had built a new warehouse, the interviewer would go to make sure it was really there and had been built since the course; if a man said he had hired three new employees to handle increased business, the interviewer would make sure the employees were really present when he visited the man's place of business.

Achievement motivation training was effective in increasing the level of business activity measured in this way, but the effect was much larger for those who had the opportunity to change their behavior. The men were divided into those who were in charge of their businesses and those who worked for someone else. For seventy men in charge who were trained in achievement motivation from various cities in India (including especially Kakinada), the average business activity score in the two years after the training was 1.39, in contrast to an average score of 0.57 for sixty businessmen in charge from the same or similar cities in India (including especially Rajahmundry) who were not trained in achievement motivation. The difference is highly significant. However, the comparable average score for men not in charge who were trained was 0.71, in contrast to an average score of 0.38 for those not trained and not in charge, a difference that does not reach accepted levels of significance. In other words, a change in motivational intent is unlikely to lead to a change in actual behavior unless the opportunity is present, as Figures 6.1 and 12.15 make clear.

For those who were in charge, an effort was made to see whether any particular combination of training inputs was more effective than any other combination. That is, some of the training inputs listed in Table 14.1 were not present in some training courses given in other cities in India. For example, some were given without having a retreat setting or without the extensive follow-up every six months for two years that was carried out for the Kakinada trainees. A total training input score for each course was obtained by assigning a value of 0 for *not present,* 1 for *partly present,* or 2 for *fully present* for each of the twelve training inputs, so the maximum total score would be 24.

Table 14.2 shows the average business activity level scores in the two years before and the two years after training for a representative sample of courses varying in strength of training inputs. The average level of business activity in the two years before the course was about the same for all groups compared. Any kind of achievement motivation training increased business activity levels in the two years after the course as compared with the average level for untrained Indian businessmen in the same two-year period. Beyond this, it appears that the more training inputs that were present in the course, the greater was the increase in activity level afterward. Clearly, the Hyderabad course was less effective than the Kakinada courses, and the Bombay and Barcelona courses fell somewhere in between. The more training inputs that were fully present, the greater was the increase in business activity levels after the training.

Beyond this, we cannot draw any conclusions from the data as to whether particular inputs were essential or more effective than others. No courses were run without the training inputs designed to increase motive strength and focusing, for example, just on the cognitive training inputs designed to increase perceived probability of success, as in the Heckhausen studies previously referred

---

Table 14.2.

BUSINESS ACTIVITY LEVELS OF BUSINESSMEN WITH AND WITHOUT ACHIEVEMENT MOTIVATION TRAINING, FOR MEN IN CHARGE ONLY (after McClelland & Winter, 1969/1971)

Group	Amount of Training Input	N	Mean Activity Scores for Two-Year Period		Percent rated +2 After Training
			Before Training	After Training	
Untrained Indian businessmen (including those in Rajahmundry)	0.0	60	0.58	0.57	28
Training courses in:					
Hyderabad, India	10.0	10	0.60	1.06	40
Bombay, India	15.5	18	0.65	1.39	67
Barcelona, Spain	20.5	19	0.53	1.37	58
Kakinada, India	22.5	21	0.35	1.61	81

to. However, these data also show that the result is not just dependent on some general prestige suggestion effect, for if it were, the men in the Hyderabad course should have gained as much in activity level as those receiving a fuller set of training inputs in the Kakinada courses.

Other measures of the effectiveness of the training were employed. One of the most significant ones was the number of new jobs created per entrepreneur before and after the training, because it could be determined with accuracy and because it represented the contribution the training was making to employment, which was a matter of considerable interest to the Indian government. Figure 14.2 shows that in the two-year period before the training in the two cities directly compared (Kakinada and Rajahmundry), on the average an entrepreneur had created employment for between one and two persons. In the two years after the training had taken place for businessmen in Kakinada, the picture was quite different. The entrepreneurs trained in achievement motivation in Kakinada had hired, on the average, twice as many new employees as the untrained entrepreneurs in the control city of Rajahmundry. The proportion of firms employing more people afterward than before is significantly higher for the trained than the untrained businessmen.

However, we could argue that this effect is not contributing to overall em-

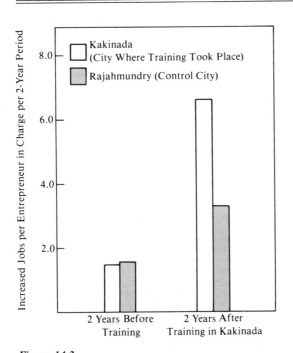

Figure 14.2.

Increased Jobs Created by Entrepreneurs Trained and Untrained in Achievement Motivation (after McClelland & Winter, 1969/1971).

ployment or economic development. Rather, is it not possible that the trained businessmen are simply taking business away from their less-motivated competitors? If a man adds an air conditioner to his sari shop, he may do more business, but shop owners without air conditioners may do less business, so there is no net gain in employment. Case studies suggested that this was not all that happened, because a number of new firms were created where none had existed before. For example, one man created a trucking company, and it got fresh vegetables to market that had simply spoiled previously.

Furthermore, the statistics on overall employment in the two cities show that the efforts of the trained entrepreneurs affected the economy of the area as a whole, as Figure 14.3 shows. When the training was started, the two cities were closely matched in the total number of employees in firms employing ten or more people. Shortly thereafter, there was a general economic depression that affected the east coast of India, which resulted in a significant drop in employment in both cities by the spring of 1967. However, the drop was much larger in Rajahmundry, where no training had taken place, and no recovery in overall

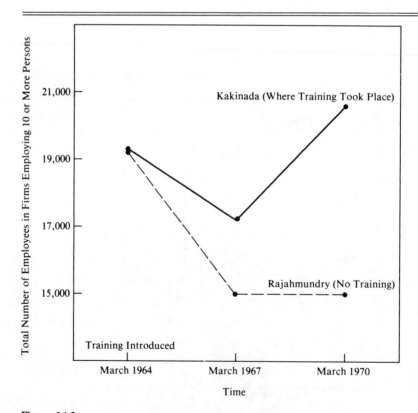

Figure 14.3.

Total Employment over Time in Two Indian Cities Where Entrepreneurial Training Did and Did Not Take Place (after McClelland & Winter, 1969/1971).

employment had occurred in that city by the spring of 1970. However, in Kakinada, where fifty-two key businessmen had been given achievement motivation training, employment rose again considerably so that by 1970 it was somewhat higher than six years earlier. Case studies documented just how and why this increase in employment had taken place as a result of the increased efforts of the businessmen who had undergone motivation training.

McClelland and Winter (1969/1971) also make the point that the cost per new job created through entrepreneurial training is one twentieth of the cost of creating a new job by other methods the government of India had employed. For example, in a government loan program to aid small industry in Andhra Pradesh, actual figures show that the cost per new job created was over 3500 rupees, whereas the cost of motivation training to produce a new job was estimated to be around 183 rupees. Since in terms of local purchasing, a rupee was roughly the equivalent of a dollar at that time, it is clear that motivation training is a comparatively much less expensive way to create employment. Obviously, the application of a little carefully validated psychological knowledge can have far-reaching economic effects.

Factors Affecting the Success of Entrepreneurial Training in India

McClelland and Winter (1969/1971) were interested in finding out what psychological factors might be responsible for the fact that the training was effective for some participants and not others, so they divided the businessmen into those who became active after the course and those who were inactive and compared them on a number of variables. Their first hypothesis was that traditional Indian values might have prevented some men from believing that they could or should be more active and successful. However, they found no significant differences in the way "actives" and "inactives" responded to an extensive questionnaire covering measures of Cautious Fatalism, Respect for Powerful Others, Conformity to Caste Rules, and Submissive Conflict Avoidance. For example, it was thought that inactives might be less willing to take initiative because they subscribed more to sentiments like "It is better to follow the leadership of wise elders than to do what one thinks is best." However, all the businessmen tended to agree somewhat with this statement, and those who changed after the course agreed with it as much as those who did not change. On the whole, the businessmen were not particularly fatalistic or tradition bound, but within these limits the actives were as traditional as the inactives. For example, less than half of the men said they observed Rahukal (a period during the day when they did not conduct any business), but 50 percent of the actives said they followed this tradition as compared with only 20 percent of the inactives. This is even the opposite of what might be expected, although overall there was no significant difference in how much the actives and inactives followed tradition.

One psychological variable that predicted who would not change was the n Power score, as obtained from TATs administered before and after the course and two to three years later. For those in charge who remained inactive, the average n Power score increased from 3.2 before training to 6.8 two to three years later, a highly significant difference. Among the men who were also in charge but became active, the increase in *n* Power score was small and insignificant. A careful analysis showed that those in charge who remained inactive gained more in *n* Power than they did in *n* Achievement, whereas the reverse was true of those in charge who became active. In other words, it looks as if the achievement motivation training had led to an increased desire to have impact or to be recognized as a success for some men, which does not translate into taking the entrepreneurial, moderate-risk steps necessary to improve business performance.

It had been expected that the *n* Achievement scores might also remain higher two to three years after the course for those who were active as compared to those who were inactive, on the grounds that the achievement-related associative network should have remained more salient for those whose behavior showed they were more guided by it. However, results did not confirm this hypothesis. The average *n* Achievement score increased greatly right after training, as would be expected, since the businessmen had been trained specifically to write stories high in *n* Achievement. When the men were retested two to three years later, the average score had declined considerably, showing forgetting, but there were no differences at any testing point in the average *n* Achievement scores of the actives and inactives.

Later Heckhausen (1971, 1980) scored the protocols for his measures of *h* Success and *f* Failure, in which the men had not received specific instruction. He found that for the men in charge, those who were active had declined in *f* Failure from before the course to two or three years later, whereas those who were inactive had increased in *f* Failure. The result is shown most clearly in the Net Hope score, which subtracts the *f* Failure score from the *h* Success score, as shown in Figure 14.4. On the left side of the figure the results for the trained Indian businessmen show that the Net Hope score rose more steeply for those who became active than it did for those who remained inactive. On the right side of the figure are some comparable results obtained by Varga (1977) in a similar evaluation of the effects of achievement motivation training courses in Indonesia, Pakistan, Iran, and Poland. Once again, those who became active after training gained much more in Net Hope than those who stayed inactive.

Heckhausen points out that the difficulty with the Indian results is that it is impossible to know whether lower Net Hope causes inactivity or inactivity causes lower Net Hope, because the retesting was done so much later that the participants would by then have known whether they were going to be successful or not in improving their business. On the other hand, Varga's data are not as open to the same criticism, since the retesting occurred earlier, at a time when the businesspeople would be less certain about how well they were doing. Thus, the most likely conclusion is that achievement motivation training is most effective for increasing business performance for those in whom it succeeds in increasing the Net Hope score.

A somewhat similar result was obtained by applying the scoring system for "efficacy" developed by Pizer (in McClelland & Winter, 1969/1971) to differentiate the story content of those who were active or inactive after an achievement

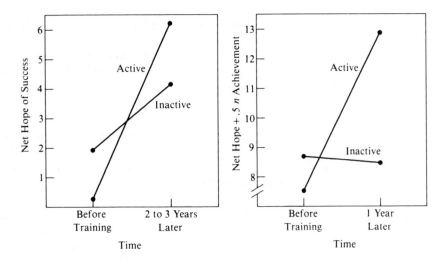

Figure 14.4.

Changes in Values for Net Hope Score Between the First Measure Taken Before Training and Later Measures for Participants Who Were Active or Inactive After Training. (*Left*) Reanalysis of data from the Indian training (McClelland & Winter, 1969/1971) by Heckhausen (1971). (*Right*) Evaluation of courses sponsored by the United Nations Industrial Development Organization (UNIDO) in Indonesia, Pakistan, Iran, and Poland by Varga (1977) (after Heckhausen & Krug, 1982).

training course in Bombay. It scored for whether the main character in the story was doing something or being passive, for whether the hero relied on internal or external resources, and for whether he or she solved or avoided problems. In the stories obtained two to three years after training in Kakinada, it was found that those who had become active had gained much more in efficacy scores as contrasted with those who had remained inactive. In other words, a positive problem-solving approach in the stories after the training—whether it is defined as Net Hope or efficacy—is significantly associated with becoming more active. What is also of interest is that the Pizer efficacy score is very similar in conception to the deCharms Origin-Pawn score, which, as we shall see in a moment, has been found to be related to better performance in school after motivation training.

Entrepreneurial Training for Minority Businesspeople in the United States

Similar achievement motivation training courses have been offered to a number of different groups of businesspeople in the United States, particularly those in underdeveloped areas or from minority groups. As compared with untrained people, a much higher percentage of trained white businesspeople in McAlester,

Oklahoma, or trained black businesspeople in Washington, D.C., showed six or more concrete signs of increased business activity six months after training. Also, the number of new employees hired among the trained businesspeople was approximately double what it was among the untrained businesspeople, in a pattern very similar to what was discovered in India (McClelland & Winter, 1969/1971).

Figure 14.5 summarizes the effects of achievement motivation training for black and Hispanic businesspeople in nine different cities across the United States. In this study it was possible to get better estimates of the financial condition of the firms than in previous research. As the comparisons in Figure 14.5 show, training increased significantly monthly sales, personal income, and profits. In presenting these data, Miron and McClelland (1979) point out that the gains are much larger than could be attributed to general improvement in business conditions at the time, as measured by similar statistics for the country as a whole or for the regions in which the training took place. Overall, the evidence is persuasive that achievement motivation training improves the performance of small businesspeople, as it ought to according to theory.

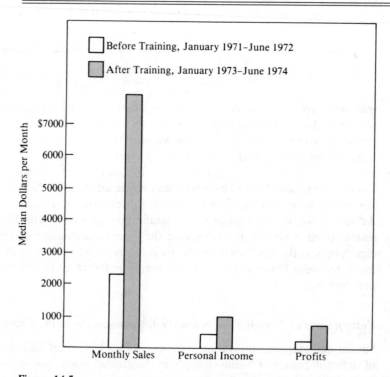

Figure 14.5.

Effects of Achievement Motivation Training for Sixty-seven Minority Entrepreneurs in Nine U.S. Cities on Monthly Sales, Personal Income, and Profits (after Miron & McClelland, 1979).

• ACHIEVEMENT MOTIVATION TRAINING IN SCHOOLS

It was natural to wonder whether achievement motivation training would improve academic performance, although on theoretical grounds it was not altogether clear why it should. For higher *n* Achievement should lead to more entrepreneurial activities—setting moderate goals for oneself, taking initiative, and so on—but it was not at all clear that such activity would lead to better grades. On the contrary, most teachers set the goals for their students and require that the students do the lessons as they are assigned rather than take initiative to do things in their own way, as Heckhausen and Krug (1982) point out. Furthermore, *n* Achievement scores have seldom been shown to be related to getting better grades in school (see Chapters 6 and 7). The Heckhausen studies referred to earlier made more sense theoretically, since they were designed primarily to increase self-confidence or perceived probability of success rather than achievement motive strength per se.

Nevertheless, attempts were made to increase achievement motivation in schoolchildren in the United States (Alschuler, 1973) and India (Mehta, 1969) by adapting the courses used to train businesspeople for application to the school situation. In the United States, intensive courses in *n* Achievement were given in special classes for children run by outside experts rather than their usual teachers (McClelland, 1972). The goal, as in the case of the entrepreneurial training for businesspeople, was to create the maximum pressure for personal change, using most of the training inputs outlined in Table 14.1. That is, the children were taught the scoring system for *n* Achievement and practiced various goal-setting games so that they could learn to think, talk, and act like a person high in *n* Achievement. Efforts were made to dramatize the training by segregating it from regular schoolwork so that they could really believe they could perform better in all sorts of ways, including getting better grades in school.

This kind of training has not generally improved academic performance, although it does appear to increase entrepreneurial activities outside of school (Alschuler, 1973). Mehta (1969) reports that such training in Indian schools was sometimes effective in improving academic performance. Whenever effects were found, they tended to be larger for boys and for performance in quantitative studies like math and science.

Some typical results are summarized in Figure 14.6. In this study, some eighth-graders in San Mateo County, California, received achievement motivation training on four weekends either at school or at a camp in the mountains (Ryals, cited in McClelland, 1972). The question of interest was whether students' grades had gained more or less than would be expected based on their grades in the same subject the previous year. In the measure utilized, students who got just as high a grade as would have been expected from their grade the previous year would end up with a score of 50; if they did better than would have been expected, they would get a score above 50; and if they did worse, they would get a score below 50. As Figure 14.6 shows, those who received achievement motivation training either at school or in the camp did not get bet-

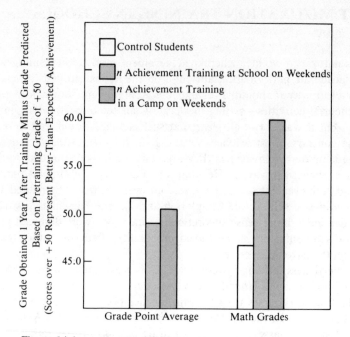

Figure 14.6.

Effects of Achievement Motivation Training on Grades Relative to What Is Expected Based on Past Performance for Eighth-Graders (after Ryals, cited in McClelland, 1972).

ter grades overall than those who had received no such training. However, they did get significantly higher math grades, and the gains were greater for those who had had achievement motivation training in a retreat setting designed to increase the incentive value of change, as shown in Table 14.1. The results could not be due to the fact that teachers would assign higher grades to those they knew had received motivation training, because the same result appeared for an objective test of science knowledge. These courses also differed from earlier ones that were less effective in that they were given by the students' own teachers rather than by outsiders.

Using the students' own teachers to provide the motivation training has the advantage of capitalizing on the Pygmalion effect. The teachers believed the training would increase motivation, and they should therefore have begun to react to the students as if they were better motivated and more capable. This, in turn, should have increased the students' perceived probability of success, which should have facilitated their performance.

As one might expect, this effect is magnified if the motivation training is spread out through the school year and integrated with regular classroom instruction. In Berea, Ohio, nearly all the teachers in the Smith elementary school were given instruction in how to train students in achievement motivation, so the whole school was oriented more toward motivating pupils (McClelland,

1979a). The teachers implemented the general principles of achievement motivation training in various ways in their classrooms, using curricular materials designed to teach the children the achievement problem-solving sequence in thought and in action through games.

All the children in the sixth grade of Smith received achievement motivation training and then graduated to the Roehm junior high school in another part of the city. There they entered the seventh grade with graduates of a comparable elementary school (Fairwood) who had not received achievement motivation training. It was unlikely that the teachers in the junior high school paid much attention to which elementary school their pupils had come from or that they knew that some of their students had received achievement motivation training, so the grades they assigned the seventh-grade students should be relatively unbiased reports of how well the students were performing. All the pupils had taken the Ohio Academic Ability Test, so it was possible to develop an equation to predict from their scores on this test the grade point average they should be receiving in the seventh grade. It was determined on the basis of this prediction equation whether a student was doing better or worse than expected. As the formula for predicting behavior states, performance should be a function of $M \times P_s \times V$. In this instance, the P_s variable is represented by the academic skills measured by the Ohio Academic Ability Test. To test for the effects of increases in motive strength, the influence of ability on performance is removed by simply noting whether students are performing better or worse than would be expected based on their ability.

As Figure 14.7 makes clear, a much higher percentage of the students who had received achievement motivation training were academic overachievers in seventh grade. As compared with pupils from Fairwood, motivation training at Smith increased the proportion of overachievers among students of high, medium, or low academic ability. Overall, 67 percent of the Smith children who had received achievement motivation training were overachievers in the seventh grade, as compared with less than half (44 percent) of the Fairwood children who had not received achievement motivation training (McClelland, 1979a). The difference is highly significant statistically. What is particularly interesting about this result is that the training changed the children in ways that carried over to the next school year in a different school with teachers who had received no special instruction in the field of motivation. So their better performance could no longer be attributed to teacher expectations that they were abler and would do better.

• ORIGIN TRAINING IN THE CLASSROOM

deCharms developed a variant of achievement motivation training that included his Origin-Pawn concept. In his terms,

> An Origin is a person who feels that he is in control of his fate; he feels that the cause for his behavior is within himself. A Pawn feels that he is pushed around, that someone else pulls the strings and he is the puppet. He feels the locus of causality

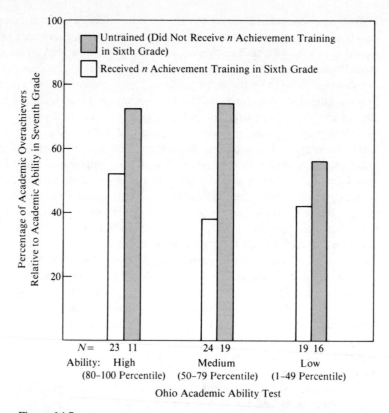

Figure 14.7.

Percentage of Academic Overachievers in Seventh Grade as a Function of Receiving or Not Receiving Achievement Motivation Training in Sixth Grade (after McClelland, 1979a).

for his behavior is external to himself. The motivational effects of these two personal states are extremely important. The Origin is positively motivated, optimistic, confident, accepting of challenge. The Pawn is negatively motivated, defensive, irresolute, avoidant of challenge. The Origin feels potent; the Pawn feels powerless. (deCharms, 1976)

He relates the Origin concept to the feeling of *personal causation,* which is related to Robert White's concept of effectance. As Chapters 5 and 8 pointed out, the power motive probably derives from a sense of effectance, from having impact, or from feeling potent. So one could argue that deCharms introduced some aspects of power motivation into what he called *Origin training.*

The training was tried out in a black inner city school district in St. Louis, where many of the children were underachievers and felt like Pawns. A number of sixth-grade teachers from the district participated in a five-day residential training workshop very much like one used to train entrepreneurs (see Table 14.1). They learned about *n* Achievement, *n* Power, and *n* Affiliation both in theory and in practice; they also were introduced to the Origin-Pawn concept. They experienced Origin-Pawn feelings by playing a game in which they first could construct anything they liked out of Tinker Toys and then were forced to use the same materials in ways precisely and assertively ordered by the instructor. The instructions were purposely exasperating and even contradictory: "Take a spool, connect it to a red rod on the round side of the spool. I did *not* say to put the assembly down. Put the assembly down now. Pick up the assembly. Connect another round spool to the other side of the red rod" (deCharms, 1976). The teachers got some feeling of what it was like to be a Pawn and realized that they could readily create these feelings in their pupils through overly conscientious instruction. So the overall goal of the workshop was not only to inform the teachers on how to develop achievement motivation, but also to help them learn how to treat their pupils like Origins.

deCharms also felt that the teachers should be treated as Origins, so they decided themselves at the end of a workshop how to utilize the information they had been given to set specific goals for changes in what they did in their classrooms in the coming academic year. They decided to focus their efforts in four areas. The first was *achievement thinking.* For example, the children wrote ten weekly essays entitled "My Stories of Achievement." The second area was *self-concept.* The students examined themselves by responding to promptings such as "My favorite daydream . . ." or "If I had three wishes . . ."

Goal setting was the third area. The students were taught how to get pleasure from moderate goal setting by participating in a version of the old-fashioned spelling bee modified to take achievement motivation concepts into account. Modern teachers and students do not like the spelling bee very much, because poor spellers consistently fail in public and drag their team's score down. The students' performance is evaluated in reference to a social norm—how well others spell. But deCharms altered the procedure so that performance could be evaluated in terms of a self-experienced norm—how well the student had spelled previously, as in some of Heckhausen's studies. The teacher determined which words each child could spell at the beginning of each week by testing him or her for the words to be learned that week. Then, as children's turns came in the spelling bee, they were asked whether they wanted to try to spell an easy, moderately difficult, or very difficult word for them, for which they would receive one, two, or three points for success, depending on the word's difficulty for them. This put the poor spellers and the good spellers on the same basis in terms of potentially contributing points to their team's score. Most of the children learned the advantages of picking moderately difficult words to spell, and spelling improved greatly as a result.

The fourth area in which the teachers decided to focus their efforts was *learning to act like an Origin:*

> The children were told that an Origin is someone who takes *personal responsibility, prepares* his work carefully, *plans* his life to help him reach his goals, *practices* his

skills, *persists* in his work, has *patience,* for he knows that some goals take time in reaching, *performs*—he knows he has to do things in order to reach his goals— checks his *progress*—i.e., uses feedback—and moves toward *perfecting* his skills, paying special attention to improvement. (deCharms, 1976)

The teachers practiced behaving like Origins by setting goals for schoolwork and for the weekend, checking on progress, analyzing what they could or could not do, examining the importance of goals in terms of their self-concept, and so on. Much of this training overlaps with training in the achievement motivation problem-solving thought sequence, as summarized in Figure 6.6.

To determine the effects of ten weeks of Origin training, deCharms employed the usual measures of motive strength and moderate goal setting; he also designed a special coding system for stories, which measured whether the children were thinking like an Origin. He was led to do this partly because more traditional self-report measures of whether the children felt they were internally or externally controlled did not sensitively pick up the effects of Origin training.

Despite the repeated emphasis in the training on taking personal control of what they did, those children who had received the training did not score any higher on Rotter's Measure of Internal Control (1966) than those who had not received the training, nor, for that matter, was there a consistent increase in average *n* Achievement scores among the trained as compared with the untrained students. Boys did show a significant increase in *n* Achievement scores after training in the sixth grade, but girls did not, and by the seventh grade the boys' average *n* Achievement score had dropped back to about what it was at the end of the fifth grade. The training did produce an increase in moderate goal setting—in picking what level of difficulty to work at among arithmetic tasks—but the effect was significant only for "externals" (those who, on the Rotter scale, said that the way things turned out depended on outside factors beyond their control). They had tended before the training to pick the most difficult items to work on, and after the training they shifted much more often to choosing moderately difficult tasks.

However, the main effects of Origin training were on the Origin thinking score and on performance on achievement tests. As the graphs in Figure 14.8 show, the mean Origin score rose directly after motivation training, whether it was in the sixth or seventh grade. The higher average Origin score of the trained students fell off somewhat in the eighth grade and still further by the eleventh grade, when no training had occurred since the seventh grade, but it was still significantly higher than for the untrained students (deCharms, 1980). The Origin scoring system gives points for references in the stories to internal control, internal goal setting and choice of acts to pursue the goal, reality perception, personal responsibility, and self-confidence.

For example, the Origin score of the following story is very high:

The boy is thinking of a present to get his mother.

The boy got three job no matter how long and hard to get the money.

he wants her the best present for her.

He will get her something very meanfull and lovely to her. (deCharms, 1980)

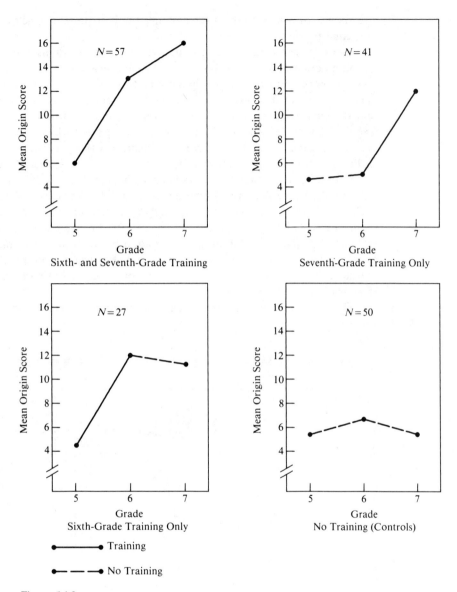

Figure 14.8.

Mean Origin Score Before and After Motivational Training (after deCharms, 1976).

The story is scored for internal control, because there is a completely internally motivated decision, approach, and solution to the problem. The boy internally sets his own goal, takes the instrumental activities necessary to achieve it ("three job"), shows perception of reality in that he has no money, shows personal responsibility for persistence ("no matter how long and hard to get the money"), and shows concern for others ("wants her the best present"); self-confidence is expressed in the last sentence.

The boy acts as an Origin throughout and ends up doing something that has an emotional impact on his mother, which means the story also contains power imagery. But the power thinking is definitely of the socialized type, and one might expect, because of the emphasis on personal responsibility for others, that the Origin score would correlate with the socialized power (*s* Power) score (see Chapter 8). In fact, this is the case. Wittcoff (1980) has shown that Origin training increases the *s* Power score and decreases the personalized power (*p* Power) score from the fifth to the sixth grade. The *s* Power score, it will be recalled from Chapter 8, is associated with high Activity Inhibition and *p* Power, with low Activity Inhibition. In a sample of twenty-one pupils in deCharms's study who were high in Activity Inhibition, the correlation between the *n* Power and Origin scores is .36 ($p < .10$). Among an equal number of pupils low in Activity Inhibition, the correlation between these two measures is only .12. Thus, there is reason to believe that the Origin score taps something of the same characteristic measured by the *s* Power score. Both emphasize having a responsible impact on others.

The effect of Origin training on academic achievement is marked, as Figure 14.9

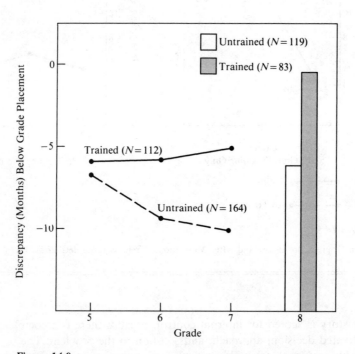

Figure 14.9.

Mean Discrepancy from Grade Placement (Iowa Test of Basic Skills) for Pupils Given or Not Given Origin Training in Sixth and Seventh Grades (after deCharms, 1980).

makes evident. The measure is based on the Iowa Test of Basic Skills, which is designed to show whether children are achieving at the level expected for their grade placement. The untrained students in this district fell farther and farther behind, until by the seventh grade they were, on the average, ten months below the achievement expected at that grade. In contrast, those who received Origin training in the sixth and seventh grade reversed this trend (deCharms, 1980). By the end of the eighth grade—one year after they stopped receiving training —they were, on the average, achieving at the level expected of that grade.

deCharms (1980) also followed up the trained and untrained students some years later to determine what proportion graduated from high school. As Figure 14.10 makes clear, the percentage of pupils graduating from high school tends to be quite low in this district—particularly among boys, only a little over 20 percent of whom graduate from high school if they have not had Origin training (0 years of Origin training in Figure 14.10). Higher percentages of girls graduate from high school, and Origin training does not significantly increase this figure. However, significantly more of the trained boys went on to high-school graduation. Again, this effect is notable because it occurred some five years after the training intervention had taken place. It is also cost effective, since an inexpensive, short-term training input resulted in a gain in the proportion of high-school graduates, which should have a significant impact on the life-long earning streams of those who graduate.

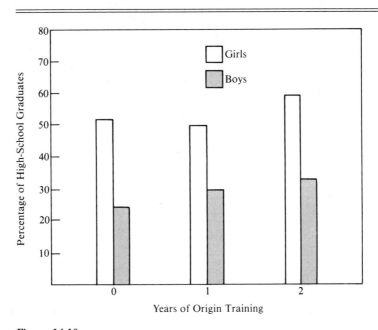

Figure 14.10.

Effects of Amount of Origin Training on High-School Graduation for Girls and Boys (after deCharms, 1980).

As would be expected from these results, those whose Origin scores were high after training did significantly better on the Iowa Test of Basic Skills for their grade than those who resisted the training and whose Origin scores stayed low. The "natural highs"—those whose Origin scores were high even before the training—performed the best, those whose scores changed from low to high scored next best, and those who showed no change performed worst. Even among untrained groups, those whose Origin score was naturally high performed significantly better on the achievement tests than those whose Origin score was naturally low. This seems to establish the fact that Origin thinking mediated the connection between the training and improved academic performance.

deCharms also developed a questionnaire that enabled him to find out whether the pupils in a class perceived the teacher as creating an Origin climate. For example, an item like "The teacher lets us try new ways of doing things" is scored positively for Origin climate; one like "The teacher gets upset when we don't do things her way" is scored negatively. He found that teachers who had received motivation training were perceived by their pupils as having created classrooms with significantly higher Origin climate scores. Finally, there was a significant correlation between the perceived Origin climate scores and the academic performance of the children in the classrooms (deCharms, 1976). All of these relationships that deCharms empirically established are summarized in Figure 14.11. Origin motivation training for teachers led them to sponsor Origin training for their pupils, which improved school learning through getting the children to think more like Origins. Origin training for teachers also helped create classroom climates that were perceived by pupils as encouraging Origin behavior, and this perception was also associated with improved school learning. Some teachers created Origin climates without having had special training, and in these classrooms, too, the children performed better.

While Origin training included elements of achievement thinking and acting, it is doubtful both on theoretical and empirical grounds that it served to improve academic performance through increasing *n* Achievement. As noted at the

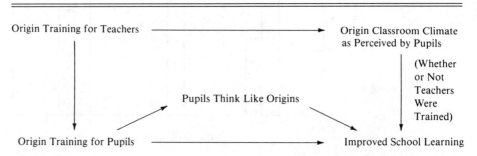

Figure 14.11.

Effects of Origin Training for Teachers and Students on School Learning (after deCharms, 1976).

outset, high *n* Achievement should increase entrepreneurial behavior, which is not usually associated with better academic performance. Furthermore, *n* Achievement scores did not rise consistently in deCharms's studies. Rather, the effectiveness of the training may lie in its influence on the P_s, or self-confidence, variable in the performance equation and also through its effect on the value placed on controlling one's own life through careful planning, goal setting, and evaluation of performance.

Finally, there is the hint that Origin training increases socialized power concerns, which could facilitate better academic performance, since a lot of prestige and recognition goes with getting better grades in school. Remember that one study cited in Chapter 8 found that high *n* Power is associated with getting better grades in school; reference to another such study occurs in the next section. Origin training, as it has so far been delivered, seems to be somewhat more effective for boys, perhaps because the assertive achievement-power complex is more associated at the present time in the United States with male, rather than female, role behavior. It is probable that motivation training for girls would be more effective if it were designed with their needs, realities, and perceptions taken more into account.

Another possible explanation for the effectiveness of Origin training in improving academic achievement lies in the fact that it emphasized the problem-solving aspects of the scoring system for *n* Achievement, which Lasker (1978) found to be related to higher levels of ego development, as measured by Loevinger (1966). (See Figure 7.14.) Thus, it could have improved performance by teaching the children to cope with the world in a more mature way. The only difficulty with this interpretation is that the deCharms group failed to find an increase in Loevinger's measure of ego development after Origin training over and above what occurred naturally between the seventh and ninth grades. Since maximum changes in ego development scores occur at this age, it is possible that the measure is not sensitive enough to pick up additional improvements in maturity possibly introduced by Origin training.

• POWER MOTIVATION TRAINING

Developing Courage in Outward Bound

Fersch (1971) reasoned that Outward Bound training should develop power motivation, because the participants spend time in a wilderness setting carrying out demanding and dangerous physical exploits. They go for long hikes, climb mountains, walk tree trunks high above the ground, escape from being tied and thrown into the water, and spend three days all alone in the woods with no food and very little equipment. The emphasis is on being tough, courageous, and capable of meeting all types of physical challenges (Newman, 1980). The ideology of the Outward Bound movement is captured by the titles of popular articles describing it like "You Will Never Be Afraid to Try" or "Metamorphosis of a Marshmallow."

Fersch studied a group of ninth-graders about fourteen years of age, most of whom were underachieving in school and economically underprivileged, who went for a month's Outward Bound training one summer (mostly on scholarship money). They also participated in a month's Upward Bound training in achievement motivation. He tested them in May before the summer, again when they returned from Outward Bound, and a year later. He had expected that Outward Bound would increase average *n* Power scores but found that this was not the case either for those who stayed for the program or for the substantial number who dropped out after a few days. However, those who scored high in *n* Power before going were significantly more likely to stay rather than drop out of the program, demonstrating that the program provided opportunities for displaying power that would be more appealing to those high in *n* Power.

Furthermore, for those who stayed in the program, the *n* Power score obtained afterward significantly correlated with social competence displayed during the following school year. The social competence measure was made up of gains in grade point average over the previous year plus the number of socialized power and achievement activities the student participated in during the school year. Socialized power activities included assuming leadership positions of various types either in school or outside of school.

Among those who stayed in the Outward Bound program who were from impoverished backgrounds, the gain in the *n* Power score from before to after the training also significantly predicted who would do well academically and socially in the coming year. No other variable significantly predicted increased social competence. That is, neither the *n* Power scores beforehand nor the *n* Achievement scores beforehand or afterward, nor staff ratings of how much they learned from Outward Bound, nor self-image scores predicted improved performance in school. Somehow, the Outward Bound training in meeting physical challenges capably made the *n* Power scores after the course more diagnostic of who would be more likely to behave assertively in a responsible way later. There was an overall significant drop in *n* Power scores for those who stayed for the Outward Bound program. This suggests that so many demands for being powerful and assertive had led through catharsis to a decrease in *n* Power, much as eating satiates the hunger drive. Thus, those whose *n* Power score remained high despite this "satiation effect" would be more likely to be those whose power motive was strongest and most likely to continue to express itself throughout the school year.

Socializing the Power Motive Among Alcoholics

Once it was realized that heavy drinking was a response to a strong impulsive need for power (see Chapter 8), it seemed reasonable to try to help alcoholics through a training program that explained to them why they were drinking and how they might satisfy their power needs in other, less destructive ways. So a course was designed, patterned after the motivation training courses for entrepreneurs, except that it placed primary emphasis on understanding how the power motive affected thought and action (Boyatzis, 1974; Cutter, Boyatzis, & Clancy, 1977).

Participants learned the *n* Power scoring system and participated in games like arm wrestling or leading a person around blindfolded that gave them concrete affective experiences of being powerful or powerless. They learned, in particular, the difference between the drive for personalized power over someone else and socialized power, which involves more self-control and acting powerfully on behalf of others, as when a mother cares for her baby or a father looks after his child. They reviewed the evidence that alcohol increases feelings of power, which is particularly appealing to those with a strong impulsive personalized power need that is blocked from finding satisfaction in other ways.

Toward the end of the course they set concrete goals for how they planned to satisfy their power needs in other ways than through drinking. Thus, they might want to try to improve the respect with which they were regarded by dressing better, by doing better at their jobs, or by helping others, using a technique that Alcoholics Anonymous has found to be useful in rehabilitating alcoholics. In that organization, reformed alcoholics spend a lot of time helping each other whenever they feel like drinking or get in trouble. Concrete goal setting and the realization that they understand their drinking problem both contribute to the perceived probability of success variable, which should lead to improved performance after the course (see Table 14.1). Furthermore, efforts were made to affect the third, or incentive, variable in the response output prediction equation by increasing the value to themselves and to their friends of overcoming alcohol addiction, although most of the participants understood the value quite well but felt they were incapable of doing anything about their problem.

One systematic attempt has been made to study the effectiveness of this type of power motivation training (PMT). The participants were hard-core alcoholics, nearly all male, who were patients living at a Veterans Administration clinic near Boston. All of them were receiving standard treatment for alcoholism, including detoxification, ingestion of Antabuse (which causes nausea and vomiting when alcohol is swallowed), group therapy, participation in Alcoholics Anonymous, and occupational therapy, if desired. Nearly everyone had been an alcoholic for years and been in and out of the hospital many times. Most of them were unable to work consistently because of their drinking problem.

Fifty of the alcoholics were randomly assigned to PMT in groups of eight to ten members meeting approximately three and a half hours a day for ten days, for a total of thirty-five hours of training. They were followed up six and twelve months after the courses to see how they were doing in comparison with a matched group of fifty alcoholics who had received only the standard treatment. The criterion of improved status included both decreased drunkenness and ability to work, except for the few who were retired or physically incapacitated. Total abstinence was not used as a measure of improvement, although it is the most widely used measure, because it did not seem reasonable to classify people as improved who are abstinent but not working or abstinent because they are in jail or back in the hospital undergoing further treatment. So people were regarded as reasonably rehabilitated if they were drunk less than once a month and working five out of the past six months, unless they were unable to work because of age or physical incapacity (McClelland, 1977b).

By this criterion, the standard treatment plus PMT was significantly more effective than the standard treatment alone, as Figure 14.12 shows. After the standard treatment, only about one quarter of the alcoholics could be considered improved a year later, but the percentage doubled for those who had received PMT in addition. The greater effectiveness of PMT in the rehabilitation of alcoholics is not exceeded by any of the other intensive therapies for alcoholics that have been evaluated by Armour, Polich, and Stamboul (1978), although direct comparisons are difficult, because they used a much less rigorous criterion of rehabilitation than the one adopted here.

There were other small signs that the PMT had been helpful. Of those who were not improved in the first six months after discharge, a larger percentage (32 percent) of those receiving PMT showed up as improved after twelve months than was true among those who had received the standard treatment (12 percent). The trend is interesting, because it is the opposite of the general belief in the alcoholism field that once people have started to drink again, they inevitably get worse. Furthermore, five men from among those receiving standard treatment died in the year after discharge, whereas none from the PMT group died (McClelland, 1977b).

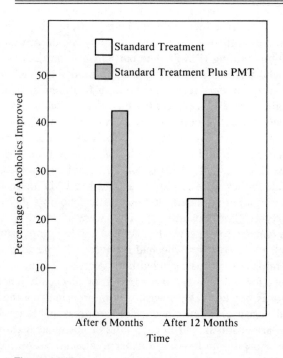

Figure 14.12.

Effects of Power Motivation Training on Improved Functioning of Alcoholics (after McClelland, 1977b).

Empowering the Staff of Community Action Agencies

During the late 1960s and early 1970s, the Office of Economic Opportunity authorized the creation of Community Action Agencies (CAAs), which were to be "developed, conducted, and administered with the maximum, feasible participation of the residents of the areas and members of the groups served" (McClelland et al., 1975). The agencies, which mounted programs to serve the poor, were to be administered as much as possible by the poor themselves. However, it was soon apparent that poor people had had little experience in managing others or in acting powerfully and effectively to serve their interests in the community. So a form of power motivation training was provided for 194 staff members or neighborhood workers from ten different CAAs in Kentucky between January and April of 1970 (McClelland, Rhinesmith, & Kristensen, 1975). The objectives of the workshop were to "explain how socialized power needs have to be developed to promote community change" (McClelland et al., 1975) and to help participants experience ways of strengthening the organization by making others feel strong, by cooperating rather than competing, by confronting and resolving conflicts and difficulties rather than denying them, and by stimulating others to take proactive, strong action rather than be passive.

To implement these objectives, the participants learned the n Power scoring system, participated in a negotiation exercise and the blindfold game, to experience feelings of being powerful or powerless, and also studied cases in which community action had been successful or not. All three types of inputs listed in Table 14.1 were included—namely, increasing power motive strength, improving the perceived probability of success, and emphasizing the great importance of becoming more effective influencers if they were to improve services to the disadvantaged in their communities. All staff members were rated for the degree of their participation in the workshop on a scale of 1 to 4. In two of the agencies, the average level of participation of staff members was significantly lower than for the other eight agencies, indicating that the training had been ineffective, either because the staff members were not interested or because the trainers had failed to put the training across.

Approximately six months after the training, each staff member was contacted and interviewed intensively by a graduate student from the University of Kentucky who had had no contact with the training. The staff members' performance was then rated by the graduate students on a scale of -1 to $+2$ in terms of how effective they had been since the training. The points in the scale were defined as they were for evaluating entrepreneurial behavior, -1 indicating that the person had definitely been performing less well than usual; 0 meaning that the person was performing pretty much as he or she had been all along; $+1$ indicating a definite improvement in performance, including particularly planning better and involving more people in programs; and $+2$ meaning the person had undertaken a new project, had been promoted, or had shown unusual initiative.

According to this method of evaluation, 52 percent of those who had been trained were judged to have improved in performance over how they had behaved previously. But how can such a figure be compared with the proportion who might have improved without training? A base line figure can be estimated from calculating the percentage who improved from the two agencies where the power motivation training was judged at the time to be ineffective or poor. Only 25 percent of the staff members from these two agencies were judged by the interviewers to have improved their performance, although the interviewers, of course, had no way of knowing that the power motivation training in these instances had been judged ineffective. In contrast, 60 percent of the staff members from the remaining agencies were judged by the interviewers to have improved their performance some months after training, a difference that is highly significant statistically. Although the measure of evaluation is crude, it suggests that power motivation training was effective in making staff members of CAAs become more effective organizers and influencers in their communities.

Leadership Training for Managers

The leadership motive pattern (high *n* Power higher than *n* Affiliation, and high self-control or Activity Inhibition) is associated with greater managerial success, as studies reviewed in Chapter 8 demonstrate. So it seemed reasonable to assume that trying to create this motivational pattern in managers would improve their performance. Accordingly, courses have been offered to business managers that provide training in power motivation as a key element in a program designed to improve managerial performance. The courses provide training in the thought characteristics of all three social motives, power- and achievement-related games, self-study, goal setting and planning, and all of the other characteristics usually involved in motivation training courses, as summarized in Table 14.1. More emphasis is given on exercising power in a socialized way to influence others on behalf of the institution, as well as to cases and goal setting specifically related to managerial responsibilities.

An evaluation of the effectiveness of this type of training in a large U.S. corporation was carried out by McClelland and Burnham (1976). In this instance, the men trained were managers of sixteen sales districts in different parts of the country. The first measure of the effectiveness of the training involved a comparison of how the salesmen perceived the organizational climate in their districts before and after their managers were trained. As Figure 14.13 shows, the salesmen, after their managers had been trained, felt a greater sense of responsibility, more organizational clarity, and greater team spirit. The results fit expectation, because the emphasis in the training of the sales managers was on the fact that they were no longer salesmen—individual achievers—but managers of others, whose primary responsibility was to empower others to take more initiative and to create a climate that strengthened and supported the individual salesmen.

The second measure of the effectiveness of the training involved whether it was associated with an increase in sales for the company. The training for the sales managers took place late in 1972; sales at the company were up substantially in 1973 over 1972, and profitability shifted from a $15 million loss in 1972

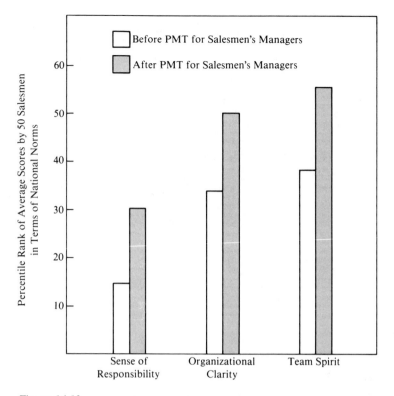

Figure 14.13.

Effects of Power Motivation Training for Managers on Organizational Climate Perceptions of the Salesmen They Managed (after McClelland & Burnham, 1976).

to a $3 million profit in 1973. Of course, many factors other than managerial training could, and probably did, play a role in increasing sales and profitability, but it is significant that increases in sales were most closely associated with increases in the organizational climate dimensions, which had been affected by managerial training. The salesmen filled out the organizational climate questionnaire in the fall of 1972, before their managers were trained, and again in April 1973, some months after their managers had been back on the job. Figure 14.14 shows that it was precisely those sales districts whose climate morale scores were highest in April 1973 that turned in the best gains in sales for the whole year of 1973. It seems unlikely that the higher morale scores in April could be attributed entirely to sales gains already made early in the year, so it seems reasonable to infer that power motivation training for managers was associated with higher morale scores among those who worked for them, who in turn produced higher gains in sales. The managers were using their knowledge of their own and others' motives to behave in ways that created a climate that empowered their salesmen to do better.

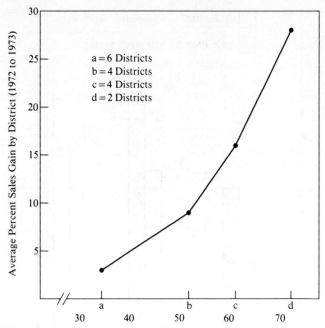

Figure 14.14.

Relationship of Perceived Organizational Climate to Subsequent Gains in Sales (after McClelland & Burnham, 1976).

Research on power motivation training has not been nearly as extensive as research on achievement motivation training, but such as it is, it appears to be reasonably effective and for much the same reasons. That is, it affects motive strength, probability of success, and the value placed on the particular kind of successful outcome being emphasized in the training. Much more research is needed to find out which training inputs are most effective in what combinations. But what is known is that power and achievement motivation training courses are effective in changing the way people think, talk, and act, which in turn leads to socially important outcomes, such as better performance in school, small business success, more frequent recovery from alcoholism, and more effective organizational performance for managers.

NOTES AND QUERIES

1. Why do you think the teacher in the fifth grade in Figure 14.1 had so much less of an effect on pupil test performance than the teacher in the third grade? Formulate a hypothesis to explain this difference based on deCharms's research on the Origin-Pawn dimension, reviewed later in the chapter, and explain how you would test the hypothesis.

2. Explain the relative failure of increasing perceived probability of success in improving academic performance in terms of the findings presented in Chapter 13 on the interactive effects on performance of the M, P_s, and V variables.

3. In Chapter 8, some findings are reported that suggest that perceived probability of success in performing is not as important in determining the behavior of individuals high in n Power as it is for individuals high in n Achievement. If the power motive turns out to be the major motive behind academic success, could this explain why increasing perceived probability of success by training has weak long-term effects on school grades?

4. Do you believe training programs for small businesspeople would increase their performance if training omitted teaching n Achievement but included inputs related to the probability of success (P_s) and the incentive value of success (V). Justify your answer in terms of theory and research evidence. Review the literature on the effects of skills training on the performance of small businesspeople (see Miron & McClelland, 1979).

5. In terms of the model for predicting operant behavior reviewed in Chapter 13, list as many reasons as you can that might explain why blacks and women in the United States have until recently seldom been successful entrepreneurs.

6. Indians outside of India (for example, in East Africa) often appear to be more successful businesspeople than Indians in India. Give several alternative theoretical explanations for this phenomenon. How would you test each one?

7. In terms of findings reported in Chapters 6 and 7, make a list of the kinds of classroom situations in which pupils receiving training in achievement motivation would not be expected to do better.

8. If Origin training improves school performance, why is it not being used in school systems today? Try to frame your answer in terms of the dominant motives and goals of the main actors in the school system—teachers, pupils, parents, and administrators.

9. Suppose achievement motivation training were really effective in the schools. Can you think of any possible negative consequences of such an eventuality?

10. There is some evidence (Ellingstad & Struckman-Johnson, 1978) that power motivation training for individuals picked up for drunken driving is not particularly effective in reducing drunken driving behavior. Try to explain this result in theoretical terms.

11. In Chapter 7 it is reported that a strong emphasis on toilet training in childhood is associated with high n Achievement in adulthood. Try to account for this result in terms of the model used in this chapter to explain the effectiveness of various training inputs. Use the model also to explain

the association between permissiveness about sex and aggression in early childhood and high *n* Power in adulthood.

12. According to the theory presented in this book (see especially Chapters 4 and 5), motives are built on the affect associated with natural incentives. Explain in terms of such a theory how motives could be acquired or strengthened in the types of training programs described in this chapter. What natural incentives are experienced? How have they been modified by cognitive growth? What affect is experienced at what points? Does this help explain why nearly all training programs of this type employ games?

13. Is there any solid evidence in the chapter that a *motive disposition* has been strengthened by training, or do you believe all the results obtained can be explained by changes in the other determinants of response output or by changes in the way an existing motive expresses itself?

14. Design an experiment to show that training definitely increased motive strength rather than changed some other variable. If, after achievement motivation training, students responded differently to homogeneous and heterogeneous classrooms (see Chapter 7), would that be firm evidence that the overall *n* Achievement level had been raised?

15

Milestones in the Progress Toward a Scientific Understanding of Human Motivation

$\mathbf{M}$otivation has always fascinated people and will continue to fascinate them so long as there are people around to wonder why human beings and animals behave as they do. Nearly everyone develops an explicit or implicit theory of motivation. We think we know why our parents are sometimes disagreeable and try to continue to control what we do: they want the pleasure of continuing to dominate us. Or we think we know why our girlfriend or boyfriend has abandoned us: he or she prefers to be with someone with greater prestige or more possessions than we have. Or we think we know why we cannot seem to study very hard: we have a low need to achieve. Authors, philosophers, economists, politicians, and the people next door have all operated in terms of theories of motivation. Shakespeare vividly portrayed the lust for power in *MacBeth* and the longings of love in his *Sonnets.* Plato explored the nature of love in the *Symposium.* Economists think in terms of the desire to acquire possessions, and they write of the importance of the profit motive. Political observers from Machiavelli to the present have stressed the importance of the desire for power in human affairs.

What have psychologists added to this parade of observations and theories about human motivation? It is time to review what has been accomplished and what remains to be discovered. The mass of detail in individual chapters may obscure the broad outline of progress that has been made. So let us take a look at the big picture without bothering to cite evidence to support the generalizations made. It can be found in previous chapters. What follows is a brief natural history of developments in the field of motivation, with an emphasis on psychology's accomplishments and on matters that need further clarification.

• MEASURING MOTIVES

To begin with, psychologists have tried to be more systematic than others interested in motivation. They have sought to define what constitutes a motive carefully and to arrive at lists of the most important motives, as McDougall and Murray did for normal behavior, or Freud and the psychoanalysts did for abnormal behavior. But the key to progress in science lies not only in theoretical clarification, but also in adequate measurement. Consequently, Murray and Cattell devised methods of measuring the various motives that psychologists and others had found to be necessary to explain behavioral outcomes as diverse as neurosis, creativity, or animal learning.

They succeeded only to a limited extent, in part because the measures they developed were composites that did not distinguish clearly enough between motives and other personal characteristics. In Murray's studies, judges pooled their observations of many different behaviors into a final estimate of the strength of a particular motive, but such judgments were strongly influenced by other characteristics the person was thought to have, so the motive measure was impure. Although Cattell pooled many different measures statistically, the same difficulty arose: the items making up the factor score for a particular motive contained responses that reflected other personal characteristics like traits as well as motives.

And inventories of self-reports of desires, wishes, and needs developed by many psychologists proved to have the same drawback: they too reflected important nonmotivational characteristics, such as the response bias to present oneself in a favorable light.

Another attempt to measure motives grew out of the behaviorist tradition represented by Hull, which considered tension, or strong stimulation, as the ultimate wellspring of human and animal action. Organisms were conceived as seeking to reduce the tension caused by deprivation of substances like food and water needed for survival. An elaborate theory was constructed that explained how secondary motives and rewards were acquired through association with a primary drive like hunger and its relief through eating.

Since the theory was applied deductively to explain human behavior, it did not result in further investigation of complex human motives until Spence, Taylor, and their associates realized that individual differences in drive strength might be measured by a Manifest Anxiety questionnaire, as explained in Chapter 3. That is, according to behaviorist theory, an organism would soon learn, in the course of trying to reduce the tension of biological needs, that certain cues would be associated with a lack of the rewards needed to reduce the tension. The discomfort or upset caused by the anticipation of the lack of something needed could readily be conceptualized as anxiety. So people manifesting more anxiety could be understood as being under greater tension or as having greater drive strength. The use of various questionnaires to measure the strength of the anxiety motive led to the accumulation of much information about how this motive functions to facilitate some behaviors and to inhibit others, as outlined in Chapters 3 and 12. Research using this approach to measuring anxiety led to important developments, not only in the understanding of factors governing efficiency of performance, but also those underlying neurosis (Eysenck, 1957a).

However, the approach has important limitations in extending our understanding of human motivation. It is based on a greatly oversimplified theoretical notion that all motives can be traced to a single master motive, namely, anxiety. Furthermore, the measure of anxiety obtained from self-reports on questionnaires is impure, because some of the items refer more to traits or styles of responding than to motives in themselves, and because such self-reports are influenced by response biases—like the desire to gain sympathy or avoid disapproval —that have nothing to do with the strength of the anxiety itself. Finally, the approach is weak because it does not deal carefully with what it is a person is anxious about or with the negative state the person is trying to avoid. From clinical studies of individuals it is clear that a distinction must be made between different types of anxiety, such as anxiety over failure and anxiety over possible rejection. Later work with another method of measurement has differentiated a variety of avoidance motives, including fear of failure, fear of rejection, fear of success, fear of power, fear of intimacy, and so forth (see Chapter 10). Empirical progress in this area has been limited, but it has been sufficient to show that these different fears have very different effects on behavior, so it is not possible to think in terms of one master anxiety motive. For example, whereas those high in fear of failure generally avoid competition (Table 10.5), there is no evidence that those high in *f* Power do; in fact, they report that they get into arguments more frequently than those low in *f* Power (see Table 10.9).

An important step in the methodology of measuring human motives was taken when it was decided to arouse motives experimentally and examine their effects on all types of behavior (Chapter 6). Arousing the hunger motive in human subjects established that its effects were most sensitively reflected in fantasy or associative thought, thus confirming an important insight Freud had reached fifty years earlier. He too found that motivational factors could be most readily identified in dreams and free associations. Other types of behavior, such as self-reports of motive states, percepts, or action trends, reflect motive arousal less sensitively, because they are more influenced by nonmotivational factors such as response bias, objective stimulus properties of the external environment, or opportunities for action in the environment.

Because of these drawbacks, the effects of arousing various motives on associative thought were carefully identified and worked into coding systems that could be objectively and reliably scored. It was then reasoned that if a person produced under neutral testing conditions many of the thoughts characteristic of people in whom the motive was aroused, then that person could be presumed to be thinking characteristically as if he or she were regularly in a state of arousal so far as that motive was concerned. For example, if a man thinks like hungry people when he is not hungry (that is, when he has just eaten), then it could be presumed that he has a characteristically high level of concern about hunger or eating (that is, he has a strong hunger motive).

One important advantage of this method is that motive definitions do not depend on a priori conceptions of how a motive *should* show itself in thought or on dictionary definitions of characteristics supposedly typical of a given motive. Rather, the coding system that makes up the definition of a motive is empirically determined by the effects of arousing the motive on associative thought. This method of measuring human motives has been successful in producing coding systems that identified several major motive systems, the effects of which have been extensively studied for the past generation.

• DEFINITION OF A MOTIVE

This method also led to a working definition of a motive as *a recurrent concern for a goal state based on a natural incentive—a concern that energizes, orients, and selects behavior.* Explaining the key terms in this definition should help clarify and summarize what psychologists have learned about human motivation as covered in this book. Basically, a *motive disposition* refers to thinking about a goal state frequently—to a *recurrent* concern. It does not refer to fleeting or occasional thoughts, since nearly every eventuality occurs to everyone once in a while. A person who has just eaten may once in a while think about being without food, but it is only the person who thinks about being without food frequently when he or she is not hungry whom we would want to characterize as having a strong hunger motive. Similarly, it is people who think about doing things well when there is no stimulus to do so whom we would characterize as high in *n* Achievement.

The fact that the concern is about a *goal state* has the important implication that the means of getting to the goal is not part of the definition of a motive. The goal state may be defined in terms of the outcome of certain acts, such as doing something better (for the achievement motive), or having impact (for the power motive), but the particular acts that lead to such outcomes are not part of the definition. This is an important distinction, because many theorists identify motives in terms of certain acts or behavioral trends that define them. For example, psychologists often speak of an aggressive drive. But aggression is a type of activity that is highly controlled in human society, so it would be hazardous to attempt to infer the strength of the aggressive urge or drive from the number of aggressive acts a person commits. It is better to define the motive behind aggressive acts in terms of their intended effect as determined from thoughts about goal states, which research suggests can be more broadly defined as "having impact." Then intended injury to someone, which defines *aggression* for many psychologists, becomes one type of having impact, and attaining higher status becomes another way of having impact. Or aggression can be seen as one means of having impact and accumulating prestige as another. This is why the concern to have impact is defined as the power motive rather than the aggression motive, since the latter defines the *means* of having impact too narrowly.

The goal states involved in motivational concerns are presumably based on and derived from natural incentives, which innately give rise to various emotions. The chief theoretical advantage of basing motives on natural incentives is that it explains why there should be relatively few major motive systems, why they have such a pervasive effect on behavior, and why motives are so intimately connected with emotional states. If it were not for the grounding of major motive systems in something, it would be hard to differentiate a purely cognitive wish like "I want to know how this story turns out" from pervasive major motive systems. We may think of such cognitive desires as being for a subgoal in the service of some ultimate goal, such as the need to achieve, which has been shown to lead people to try to finish incompleted tasks (Chapter 7); however, what is it that makes a goal state like wanting to do something better (as in the achievement motive) more basic or pervasive than any simple cognitive desire? If a natural incentive is not responsible for this difference, then some other, as yet undiscovered, factor must be responsible.

The insistence on the importance of natural incentives has another advantage. It accounts for the phenomenon of intrinsic motivation, or the tendency of people to engage in activities that seem to be satisfying in themselves like whistling, chewing gum, dancing, jogging, or playing with Rubik's cube. It stretched belief to figure out how such activities could be in the service of major motive systems like *n* Achievement or *n* Power. Furthermore, arousing these other motive systems interferes with carrying out such intrinsically satisfying activities (Deci, 1975). Thus, it seems better conceptually to think of such activities as incentive driven. That is, the natural incentives continue to produce the primitive

behaviors that define them, quite apart from whether they have become organized into major motive systems for an individual. Thus, chewing gum or hitting
a nail with a hammer may continue to give impact satisfaction if occasion provides the opportunity, whether or not such activities have become organized into
a major power motive system for a person.

The use of the word *concern* in the motive definition refers directly to the
fact that motives are best measured by coding concerns in associative thought or
fantasy. The measurement implication of the definition is important, because
without it, the definition would not represent much of an advance over previous
definitions provided by McDougall, Cattell, Freud, or Maslow. The term *concern* is used because it does not imply the conscious goal-directed striving that
is part of many definitions of motives, for all the empirical work on motives
identified through coding associative thought indicates that motives are not necessarily part of the person's conscious self-image. Thus, another of Freud's insights has been confirmed—namely, that some important motives are not conscious. In contrast, not all people are not conscious of the strength of their
major motive systems, as Freud seems to suggest at times. Some are and some
are not. This is the inference to be drawn from the empirical fact that the conscious value placed on achievement, affiliation, and power is essentially uncorrelated with the *n* Achievement, *n* Power, and *n* Affiliation scores as determined
by coding the content of associative thought. For this reason it is essential to
distinguish between values, which are part of the self-picture, and motives,
which are not. The ideas people have about what is important in life or to them
have a strong influence on what they choose to do, but in the scheme presented
here, they are determinants of behavior that are essentially independent of motive systems. Thus, choices in many situations, particularly those in which the
alternatives are cognitively understood, are determined primarily by values, and
motives play little part in determining what people do in such situations (see
Chapter 13).

The influence of values, skills, and opportunities on conscious choices and
actions explains why it is so difficult to assess motive strength from what people
say and do. They may say over and over again in a questionnaire that they want
to achieve, but that is because the items explicitly tap the value they and their
culture place on achievement. It is not evidence that they have a recurrent concern about the goal state of doing things better. Or they may greet a number of
guests effusively at a cocktail party, but that is not a sure indication that they
have high *n* Affiliation. They may be acting that way because of social norms
governing the behavior of hosts at such a party and because they have an image
of themselves as good hosts. Or even if they are high in *n* Affiliation, they may
fail to show affiliative behavior in the presence of superiors, because social
norms they have interiorized dictate that they should not be affiliative to such
people.

So motivational concerns are best measured in associative thought where the
influence of values, skills, and opportunities is less marked. Technically, of
course, it should be possible to measure the strength of a motivational concern
from its behavioral effects, if those effects are relatively uninfluenced by values,

skills, and opportunities or if the effect of these other determinants of behavior is controlled or standardized. A typical example is the "doodling" index of *n* Achievement devised by Aronson (1958) and described in Chapter 7. People high in *n* Achievement doodle differently from those low in *n* Achievement. Since there are no conscious values affecting how a person should doodle, since it requires no particular skill, and since situational influences are slight, the doodling index of *n* Achievement is reasonably valid. That is, it is influenced primarily by the motivational concern and not by other determinants of behavior. In similar fashion, we could attempt to devise an index of the strength of a person's power motive from its behavioral correlates as summarized in Chapter 8, such as, in the case of men, the frequency of getting into arguments, playing competitive sports, drinking alcohol, and accumulating prestige supplies. Such attempts have been made, but they have limited value because the outlets for the power drive vary so much as a function of sex, age, level of maturity, and social class.

The only motivational concerns that can be estimated with reasonable validity from conscious choices are those that involve negative incentives. Thus, an avoidance motive like fear of failure can be measured fairly adequately by a Test Anxiety questionnaire, although even here the direct measure of the concern over failure in associative thought appears to be somewhat more valid (Chapter 10). The explanation for the greater validity of self-report measures of an avoidance motive like the fear of failure may lie in the fact that the source of the negative incentive is often external, in contrast to a positive incentive like doing better or having impact, which can only be observed internally. Thus, fear of failure develops out of threats from external authorities such as teachers or parents, which people can readily identify. Furthermore, there is no strong value against admitting test anxiety, at least among most students, so conscious reports can reflect the avoidance motive reasonably accurately. In contrast, values may interfere with admitting to fear of weakness or fear of success, so it is a matter for further investigation to discover whether self-report measures can substitute for the more direct measures of avoidance motives in associative thought.

The term *concern* also signifies that a motive is more general than an intent. An intent is, by definition, more specific and limited in time. Thus, Freud uncovered unconscious intents that led to the forgetting of a name or dreaming that one could not give a dinner party. But the intents were in the service of more general motivational concerns. Conscious intents, in contrast, are the product not only of motives, but also of other determinants of behavior such as the value people place on performing an act or their estimate of the probability that it can be performed.

The measures of motivational concerns derived from coding associative thought have proved to satisfy for the most part the requirements for good measurement. They reflect sensitively known differences in motivational states when aroused experimentally. They signify differences in motive strength more uniquely than other behaviors that are more influenced by nonmotivational determinants such as values, skills, and opportunities. They are valid in the sense that they satisfy the requirements of the functional definition of a motive, which states that it energizes, orients, and selects behavior. That is, people who score high on one of these motive measures, such as *n* Affiliation, behave as they should if they were in fact more motivated for affiliation. They behave more energetically in an affiliative manner; that is, they perform affiliative acts more frequently. They perceive affiliative cues in the environment more readily, and they learn affiliative networks more quickly. Other reported measures of motive dispositions have not been shown to satisfy these requirements for distinguishing between a more and less motivated person in a particular area.

The chief difficulty with the associative thought measures of motive strength has been their presumed unreliability. The motive scores people obtained on one occasion have generally not agreed very well with the scores they obtained on a second occasion, nor have the scores obtained from one group of stories agreed very well with the scores obtained from another group of stories, even when all the stories are obtained on the same occasion. In psychometric terms, the internal consistency and test-retest reliability of the measures have been so low that many psychologists have felt the measures could not be taken seriously.

What can a person's *n* Achievement level really be if estimates of its strength vary so much from one occasion to another? Two recent developments—one theoretical and the other practical—suggest that the reliability of the measures is not nearly as low as it has been estimated to be. Both developments rely on the fact that once a thought has been expressed spontaneously, it tends to be used up, so to speak, so different thoughts are more likely to be expressed next. If a person tells an achievement-related story first, he or she is less likely to tell an achievement-related story next. Thus, there is little consistency in the amount of achievement imagery expressed on two occasions.

Atkinson and Birch (1978) have built a theoretical model questioning the common assumption that variations in scores represent "error" in estimating a true score and demonstrating that there can be consistency in levels of *n* Achievement expressed over long periods of time even though there is moment-to-moment inconsistency, which is in fact predicted by their theory and therefore cannot be considered "error" (see Chapter 6). At a practical level, Winter and Stewart (1977) have demonstrated that test-retest reliability increases greatly if the subjects' set to be creative and to vary the type of story told is broken by telling them that they can tell the same or a different story, depending on how they feel at the moment. Under these instructions, the estimates of motive strength from coding associative thought are satisfactorily stable. Now that substantial progress has been made in establishing the reliability of these measures, investigation of other motive systems should proceed more rapidly.

Nevertheless, associative measures of motive strength are easily influenced by situational factors that constrain the spontaneity with which a person thinks and writes. If subjects feel threatened or anxious, their thought processes are no longer spontaneous, and motive scores derived from them are no longer valid. Lundy (1981a) has developed a method for scoring stories that estimates the extent to which they are spontaneous so that the investigator can determine whether the motive scores derived from them are likely to be valid (see Chapter 6).

• ACCUMULATED KNOWLEDGE ABOUT THREE IMPORTANT HUMAN MOTIVE SYSTEMS

The Achievement Motive

Gains in knowledge about what motives are and how they can be measured have led to substantial progress in the accumulation of knowledge about three important motive systems that govern human behavior. Historically, the first of these to be intensively investigated was the achievement motive, or *n* Achievement. As work on it progressed, it became apparent that it might better have been named the *efficiency motive,* because it represents a recurrent concern about the goal state of doing something better. Doing something better implies some standard of comparison—either internal or external—and it is perhaps best conceived in terms of efficiency or an input/output ratio. Doing better or improving means getting the same output for less work; getting greater output for the same work; or, best of all, getting greater output for less work. So people high in *n* Achievement are attracted primarily to situations where there is some possibility for improvement of this kind. They are not attracted to, and do not work harder in, situations where there is no possibility of improvement—that is, where tasks are very easy or very difficult—or where external rewards such as money or recognition are provided. In order to know whether they are doing better, they prefer situations in which they have personal responsibility for the outcome and that give them feedback on how well they are doing.

What proved particularly important was the realization that people with these characteristics should make good entrepreneurs, as well as the demonstration that successful entrepreneurs did, in fact, have higher *n* Achievement. This, in turn, led to an extensive investigation linking high levels of *n* Achievement in individuals and in countries to increases in entrepreneurial behavior and more rapid rates of economic growth. It turned out that the achievement motive has been a major factor in the economic rise and fall of ancient and modern civilizations. In fact, since efficient business activity is a key element in the economic success of individuals and nations, it is not stretching the evidence too far to suggest that the achievement motive has a lot to do with wealth and poverty or the standards of living people enjoy.

Early studies indicated that high *n* Achievement might be fostered in middle childhood by parents who set higher standards of performance for their children, often because they belonged to reform groups that stressed that their beliefs or ways of doing things were better than traditional ways. In this manner, higher *n* Achievement levels could be explained among certain minority groups, among Protestants in the early days of the Reformation, or in countries where the Communist reformation first occurred (see Chapter 11). More recent research has found that parental insistence on high standards of performance in the first years of life for controlling involuntary functions like eating or elimination is associated with higher levels of adult *n* Achievement. The finding is of great theoretical importance, because it supports the notion that motivational concerns can be formed very early in life, before infants have developed much self-consciousness or the cognitive capacity to evaluate their own performance.

This also helps explain why conscious values, which are formed much later in life, after cognitive development, can be quite different from motivational concerns based on very early affective learnings.

The Power Motive

The need for power as coded in associative thought represents a recurrent concern to have impact certainly on people, and perhaps on things as well. The latter possibility has not been extensively investigated, although McAdams (1982a) has shown that peak experiences, involving feelings of physical or psychological strength, were more likely to be recollected by individuals high in *n* Power. High *n* Power is associated with many competitive and assertive activities and with an interest in attaining and preserving prestige and reputation.

However, since competitive and particularly aggressive activities are highly controlled by society because of their potentially disruptive effects, the outlets for the power motive vary greatly according to the norms the person has interiorized as to what is acceptable behavior. Thus, sex typing has an important effect. The behavioral outlets of high *n* Power in men and women are different. The power motive leads to more openly competitive and assertive behavior among men than women, and also more often to accumulating resources as a means of exerting influence among traditional women than among men. Social class also makes a difference. Lower-class men high in *n* Power tend to be more openly aggressive than middle-class men at the same level of *n* Power. Level of maturity also shunts the power drive in one direction or another. If people high in *n* Power are at the oral intake stage (Stage I), they tend to engage more in power-oriented reading; if they are at the stage of autonomy or self-control (Stage II), they tend to bottle up much anger; if they are at the assertive stage (Stage III), they express their anger more openly in assertive and competitive activities; and if they are at the stage of mutuality (Stage IV), they tend to share more secret information with their intimates and to assume responsible positions in voluntary organizations.

From reviewing this research, one gets the impression that the power motive is something like a hydra-headed monster that shows very different faces depending on other variables. Sometimes it leads to dominance, as in Stage III people who are oriented around assertiveness. And sometimes it leads to submissiveness, as in Stage I people who are oriented around gaining power from following leaders from whom they take in strength.

Nowhere is this variability more obvious than when high *n* Power is either associated with a high or low degree of internal inhibition. If men are high in *n* Power and low in inhibition, they tend to think in terms of personally dominating others. They drink too much. They are Don Juans trying to seduce as many women as possible. They lie, trick, and deceive. They are socially irresponsible. In short, they have some of the characteristics of the image of Satan. In contrast, men high in *n* Power and high in inhibition have some of the characteristics of the image of God. They think in terms of exercising their power on behalf of others; they engage in less impulsive self-indulgent behavior like drinking; they assume positions of leadership in voluntary organizations; they believe in centralized authority, hard work, self-sacrifice, and charity. In short, they are responsible citizens. They make good husbands and good managers in business organizations, particularly if they are also low in *n* Affiliation. People with this motivational profile (high *n* Power higher than *n* Affiliation, and high in Activity Inhibition), variously called the imperial power motive syndrome or the leadership motive syndrome, tend to be empire builders, and countries with the same profile in their popular literature tend also to be imperial: they collect more of their gross national income in taxes; spend more of it on military preparations; and, at least in the case of the United States, tend more often to go to war. Just as the achievement motive appears to lie at the base of economic growth, the power motive, if it is disciplined, lies behind the effective governing of people, which can lead to the organizational success of great civilizations like the Roman Empire.

The chief weakness of people with the leadership motive syndrome is that they are particularly prone to illness if they are stressed or frustrated. They are more likely to develop high blood pressure under such conditions and to fall prey to illnesses resulting from a weakening of the body's immune defense system, for the inhibition of a strong power motive in combination with low interest in affiliation appears to result in hormonal changes that damage the lymphocytes that function to maintain the body's immune defenses.

Less is known about the sources of the power motive in society and in childhood, but what is known follows the pattern discovered for the achievement motive, which suggests that how parents treat their children makes a difference. Parents who have lost power and been oppressed, like the Jews in Nazi Germany or unemployed black males in the United States, tend to develop a strong power motive, perhaps in retaliation. They are also probably more permissive in allowing their children to express power. The one solid piece of evidence we have is that parents who are permissive about expressions of sex and aggression in early childhood tend to have children who as adults have a higher *n* Power. It is also true that children of Jewish parents who were particularly persecuted in Germany had higher average levels of *n* Power than children of other Jewish parents who had left Germany but who had not been so oppressed. And there is evidence that the particularly oppressed and stressed parents placed more emphasis on the assertion of Jewish identity in order to insure survival, from which it may be inferred that they were also more permissive about early assertiveness in their children.

The Affiliative Motives

Less is known about the affiliative motives than about the achievement or power motives. The recurrent concern involved is for the goal state of *being with* another, but it is not certain what the natural incentive for this goal state is. Does love, or the desire to be with others, develop primarily out of sexual contact gratifications, as suggested by Freud and Plato, or is it connected with the "good vibes" identified by Condon as characterizing harmonious relations between two persons? (See Chapter 9.) Are the sexual motive and the affiliative motives connected at all, for that matter? No one knows for sure, because it has proved very difficult to develop a measure of the strength of the sexual motive by arousing and coding fantasy changes in the usual way. The reason is that anxiety, inhibition, or some other factor blocks the direct expression of sexual thoughts following sexual arousal, just as Freud discovered years ago. Some tentative attempts have been made to derive an indirect or symbolic measure of the strength of the sexual motive, but they need much further elaboration.

Coding systems for two affiliative motives have been developed and investigated. One, the *n* Affiliation score, is associated somewhat with fear of rejection and with more active efforts to be with people as if one fears being left alone. The other, the intimacy motive, is more of a "being" as opposed to a "doing" motive. Those who score high in it take pleasure in intimate sharing with others and are perceived to be natural, warm, sincere, appreciative, and loving. They are interested in establishing and maintaining warm interpersonal relationships, but they are not anxious in the absence of others. In contrast, those high in *n* Affiliation, while having some of the same interest in interpersonal relationships, are more often anxious about whether they are liked or not, so that often they are not very popular.

The affiliative motives are of central importance for mental and physical health and a sense of well-being, just as Plato argued centuries ago. College men who scored high in the intimacy motive were judged to have made a happier, better adjustment to life by a psychiatrist who interviewed them regularly over a period of years without knowledge of their scores. And several studies have shown that a strong *n* Affiliation or intimacy motive, particularly if it is accompanied by low inhibition, is associated with a stronger immune defense system against disease (see Chapter 9). The reason for this relationship is not known, although presumably it involves some reduction in the stress hormones that damage lymphocyte function. At any rate, the data, so far as they go, support the folk psychological notion that love is good for your health.

Little is known about the origins of the affiliative motives in society or in childhood. In an extensive study, no parent training practices in the early years of life turned out to be significantly and consistently associated with adult *n* Affiliation scores. The reason may be that the investigators focused more on what the parents *did* than on the nature of the relationship between parent and child, which may have had more to do with the formation of the affiliative motives. Certainly the matter cries out for further investigation using modern techniques for coding the relationships between parents and children.

• UNDERSTANDING HOW MOTIVES COMBINE WITH OTHER CHARACTERISTICS TO DETERMINE ACTION

Psychologists have had a great and abiding interest in building theories or models to predict choices or action tendencies. They have nearly always in recent years assumed that motive strength was one of the determinants of choice. A significant step forward was taken by Atkinson when, building on earlier work of Lewin and Hull, he proposed that an approach tendency was jointly determined by motive strength (M_s), probability of success (P_s), and the incentive value of success (I_s). He assumed further that the incentive value of success was a simple linear function of difficulty or the reciprocal of the probability of success ($1 - P_s$), and that multiplying the three determinants by each other produced the best prediction of an approach tendency. The model proved to be quite useful in predicting the level of difficulty at which people would choose to work as a function of the strength of their *n* Achievement, the probability of success, and the incentive value of success defined as $1 - P_s$. Subsequently, psychologists have spent a great deal of time trying to clarify and expand the meaning of the model. Atkinson himself, in collaboration with Birch (Atkinson & Birch, 1978), developed a more abstract definition of the variables in the model and their interrelationships that, when formulated in terms of a computer model, permitted the deduction of what behaviors one could expect under various circumstances.

Others worked to clarify the meaning of the original model. As a first step, it seems desirable not to use the term *motivation* as Atkinson has to describe the impulse or tendency to act that is a product of all the determinants of action, because it is confusing to think of the cognitive and skill determinants of the impulse to act as motivational in nature. Furthermore, we must distinguish between motive as a disposition and the arousal of the motive at a particular time and place, which is best conceived as a *state* of motivation. But if the term *motivation* is used to describe an aroused motive, it cannot also be used to describe the outcome of all the determinants of action. Much confusion in the interpretation of experiments has arisen from using the term *motivation* in these two different senses.

Also, the meaning of the *probability of success* term in the model has come in for considerable expansion. It covers the perceived probability of success at a task, and also the demonstrated skill at the task, which affects the probability of success in actuality. It refers to one's general level of self-confidence or feeling of efficacy, and also to the confidence one feels in reference to a particular task. It includes the feeling of whether one has voluntarily chosen to do something or whether one has control over the situation or not. And much work has been done on the causal explanations for success or failure, which either increase or decrease the perceived probability of success. For example, if people ascribe failure to lack of effort, they are likely to have a higher perceived probability of success on the next trial than if they perceive failure as having been due to lack of ability. All these variables contribute to the perceived probability of success, which is an important determinant of the impulse to act.

As for the incentive value in the model, attention has shifted from difficulty as the only or the major determinant of the outcome to other values that influence the impulse to act in different ways. The importance of the action or whether it is necessary to get to subsequent goals are both important contributors to its incentive value. Other values relating to whether the action is appropriate for one's sex, age, or culture also influence the strength of the incentive to perform the task in one way or another. For example, the incentive value of working in groups is apparently much greater for native Hawaiians than it is for other U.S. citizens. What is needed is a much more systematic classification of the values that enter into influencing the outcome of various equations designed to predict one kind of performance or another from motives, probability of success, and incentive values. At the present time psychologists have pretty much limited their efforts to demonstrating that different values, in combination with different motives and probabilities of success, *can* produce different behavioral outcomes.

Finally, the model has been in great need of empirical testing outside the achievement area in connection with motives and outcomes other than approach tendencies to tasks of different difficulty levels. In Chapter 13 we demonstrated that the model had considerable utility in predicting performance success on a laboratory task and also the frequency with which college students were found to be interacting with another person. In both cases, motive strength (as represented by either *n* Achievement or *n* Affiliation scores) predicted the outcome, but the incentive value placed on achievement or affiliation did not. And in both instances, the motive level multiplied by the skill level (either actual skill or perceived social skill) predicted the action outcomes over and beyond what could be predicted from either variable alone. Skill contributed to more of a certain kind of performance only when a person was highly motivated. In contrast, multiplying aroused motive strength (*n* Achievement) times the incentive value placed on achievement (*v* Achievement) improved performance, whereas multiplying *n* Affiliation times the value placed on affiliation did not increase the frequency with which students performed affiliative acts. What accounts for this difference? Under what circumstances does incentive value multiply with motive strength to increase the probability of a response, and under what circumstances does it not? Many more multivariate studies of this type need to be carried out to test the general applicability of the model of the multiple determinants of the impulse to act.

What is suggested by these preliminary investigations is that (1) the three variables do appear to give the best prediction of an action tendency if they are multiplied as the model assumes; (2) motive dispositions are more powerful predictors of operant or spontaneous acts, whereas incentive values are better predictors of cognitive choices; and (3) a better prediction of operant outcomes can be made if competing motivational dispositions are taken into account. All of these conclusions have great significance for further research in the field of motivation, for psychologists need to test the assumption that the determinants of action multiply with each other outside the area of choosing tasks of different difficulty.

Furthermore, psychologists have not usually made the distinction between trying to predict cognitively based choices as compared with operant actions. And even though Atkinson (1980) has insisted on the theoretical importance of taking motive ratios into account, he has apparently never done so in an empirical test as to whether this gives a better prediction of outcomes. In fact, if the ratio of *n* Affiliation to other motives present in the individual is combined with perceived social skill, and with the value placed on affiliation and their interactions, over 75 percent of the variation in the frequency with which students are found to be relating to others at random moments can be accounted for from the three predictors. The remaining variation appears largely due to the environmental conditions that made interaction impossible. Such a result may be a fluke, since it suggests a much higher degree of predictability for human behavior than has been thought possible, but it serves to underline the importance of doing many more such multivariate studies if one is seriously interested in accounting for the variability in human behavior. Psychologists have expended far too much of their energies studying one variable at a time.

What these studies also indicate is that whereas the values people espouse may be slightly influenced by motive dispositions, they are essentially independent determinants of action outcomes, just as probability of success is. Value and motive measures are not highly correlated, and they predict different action outcomes singly or in combination with other variables.

• SOME ISSUES NEEDING FURTHER CLARIFICATION

While some theoretical and factual progress has been made in our understanding of human motivation, much more remains to be made. As we have reviewed milestones in what has been learned about various aspects of motivation, we have often concluded by observing that we need to know more about this matter. Certainly there will continue to be refinements in the way motives are defined and measured and in our understanding of how they influence behavior, but it is also useful to call attention to major gaps in our knowledge and to speculate about matters that should engage the attention of psychologists increasingly in the future. What are some of the major issues that especially need clarification?

Examining the Biological Basis of Major Motive Systems

We have repeatedly argued on theoretical and empirical grounds that motives are based on natural incentives, specific to the human species, which innately arouse or "turn on" the individual in different ways, as reflected in a limited number of types of emotions. Yet the evidence for such a proposition is not as direct or conclusive as it ought to be. Most of it is circumstantial or indirect, based on inferences from such diverse phenomena as language learning in children, intrinsically satisfying activities, what produces smiling in infants, the universality of a few human emotions, and the involvement of older parts of the brain in emotion and motivation, as summarized in Chapters 4 and 5.

Furthermore, in a few cases the evidence for innate biological involvement in a motive system is quite direct. This is true for the hunger motive, in which hypothalamic arousal occurs directly in response to lowered available blood sugar or to the sight or smell of tasty food. It is also true for the sexual motive, in which the production of sex hormones at puberty clearly provides the biological basis for a type of affective arousal in connection with sexual stimuli that makes learnings associated with it much stronger and more basic than they would be if they had a purely cognitive basis. And there is some beginning evidence, as noted in Chapter 8, that the catecholamine hormonal system, particularly brain norepinephrine turnover, provides the biological substrate that produces the affect associated with the impact or power incentive.

What is exciting about this type of evidence is that it suggests that the biological aspect of different motive systems may be quite specific. Nearly all earlier theories of motivation involved some type of physiological or cortical arousal, but it was conceived in very general terms. Thus, drive—whether as tension or anxiety—was thought to result in general psychophysiological arousal, and different emotions seemed to have more or less the same physiological effects. But newer, more sensitive techniques of biochemical analysis have begun to produce evidence that the effects of different motivational or emotional states on hormones may be quite different. So it could turn out that each of the major motive systems is based on a different natural incentive, as demonstrated by uniquely different hormonal effects of each natural incentive.

Clearly, what is needed is a much better way of determining what natural incentives exist for the human species, how they produce different types of affective arousal represented by varying profiles of hormone release, and how specific types of affective arousal form the basis for developing major motive systems through cognitive development and associative learning. Working out these relationships is a problem of the greatest importance to understanding the nature of human motives and will require great ingenuity to solve.

Defining and Measuring Other Major Motive Systems

Progress in understanding the achievement, power, affiliative, and avoidance motives has been considerable, but it inevitably raises several questions. Why have these motives been studied and not others? Are they the most important motives? What other motives need study? Such questions cannot be answered with any certainty.

Work on the achievement motive began because of a historical accident: psychologists at the time had had some experience in influencing performance through what they then called *ego-involving instructions*. It was soon realized that these instructions set higher achievement goals for the subjects and produced changes in associative thought that came to be called the *achievement motive*. Yet if one were to imagine coding all the thoughts that all the people in the world are having at this moment, or have had over time, the frequency of achievement-related thoughts would certainly be lower than the frequency of thoughts related to power or affiliation. Empirical evidence for this conclusion is to be found in the scoring of hundreds of pages of fiction, children's textbooks, and hymns throughout the history of the United States (McClelland, 1975). Power-related thoughts were the most common; affiliation-related thoughts, next in frequency; and achievement-related thoughts, least frequent. To come at it from a different angle, if one were to code the imagery in great legends or sacred texts like the *Bhagavad Gita* or the Bible, one would find that they are primarily about power and love. Achievement concerns play a minor role. This is not to say that achievement concerns are unimportant: they seem to be a key factor in technological and economical progress, but they are of lesser interest to most people most of the time than power and affiliative concerns.

What about other motives? There are a number crying out for investigation, such as the need to nurture or be nurtured, curiosity, or simply the need to maintain consistency and avoid dissonance. In the last instance, psychologists have identified what appears to be a strong natural incentive but have not developed a measure of individual differences in motive strength centered on this incentive.

There is no lack of motives to be investigated. What has inhibited people from investigating them by the methods proposed here are doubts about the reliability of the measures, which have only recently been put to rest; the effort required to develop a motive scoring system through arousal experiments, which must then be validated behaviorally; and the training and time needed to get reliable coding of associative thought, as compared to the minimal effort needed to score responses on questionnaires, which can be coded instantly by machine. Yet the great expenditure of time and effort that developing coding systems for associative thought requires appears to be fully justified in terms of the greater theoretical and practical value of the measures of motive strength obtained in this way.

Determining What Collective Motive Levels Mean

A surprising virtue of measuring motive systems by coding thought turned out to be that applying the same codes to the popular literature (that is, the thoughts produced by a society) appears to give a useful estimate of motive levels among cultures or nations. Although questionnaires and other tests cannot be administered to individuals from long past historical periods to measure the strength of their motives, the cultures in which they lived have left behind songs, stories, legends, literary documents, and even designs on vases that can and have been scored for motivational systems in the same way records from individuals living at the present time have been scored. What is surprising is that nations whose records score high in a particular motive behave like individuals whose records score high on the same motive. The parallels are striking. Individuals whose stories score high in *n* Achievement show the characteristics of successful entrepreneurs, and small businesses headed by people higher in *n* Achievement grow faster. A high level of *n* Achievement in the folk tales of preliterate cultures signifies the presence of more entrepreneurs in those cultures than in cultures whose folk tales score low in *n* Achievement. Furthermore, nations whose children's stories score higher in *n* Achievement tend to grow more rapidly economically, and in several countries, rates of economic growth were greater after historical periods when *n* Achievement levels were high in popular literature than they were when *n* Achievement levels were low.

Men who write stories high in *n* Power and low in Activity Inhibition tend to drink more heavily, and drinking tends also to be heavier in cultures whose folk tales score high in *n* Power and low in Activity Inhibition. Individuals scoring high in *n* Power and high in Activity Inhibition tend to make good managers of large, complex organizations, and countries with the same motivational pattern show signs of being better organized in several ways. People scoring high in *n* Affiliation like people and show signs of being in better health. Countries scoring high in *n* Affiliation show signs of respecting the rights of individuals more, and their public health figures indicate a lower incidence of several physical illnesses.

What do these parallels mean? Can we think in terms of a group mind that has motivational characteristics analogous to those possessed by an individual? Or are estimates of national motive levels obtained from group literary products a useful approximation of average motive levels that would be obtained from national representative sample surveys of individuals in the countries concerned? Or is the ideational content of popular literature somehow responsible for levels of individual motivation in the country? These are all questions that need further investigation.

The important point is that the method of measuring individual motive strength is applicable to group products and therefore opens up the possibility of all sorts of historical and cross-sectional studies of the influence of levels of motivational ideology on the behavior of a country or groups within a country. Different types of literature are read by different segments of a society, so it should be possible to estimate motive levels of these different segments by coding literature that is popular in each segment. Would, for example, levels of motivation in men's and women's magazines in 1957 and again in 1976 parallel the average levels of motive strength among men and women at the two time periods, as determined by scoring individual protocols in the national sample surveys conducted at these two time periods? Would the motivational content of songs popular for different generations in the United States predict what that generation would spend its money on, how many children it would have on the average, or how susceptible it would prove to be to death from various illnesses? The possibilities of this type of analysis appear almost limitless. Psychology has made available to historians and sociologists a new tool that can measure motivational levels in the past or in various segments of society, which can be used to interpret what happens in a country in much the same way as economic statistics were used by social scientists when they became available to explain social developments.

Improving the Theoretical and Practical Understanding of How to Develop Motives

Motives are learned, although they are based on natural incentives, which have an innate component. If they are learned, what kinds of teaching or learning promote their development? Some evidence points to the importance of the emphasis parents place on certain behaviors in early childhood or, in the case of the achievement motive, in middle childhood. In that instance, if the parents set high standards for performance and the father does not direct too closely the child's effort to achieve these goals, the development of the achievement motive is facilitated.

This only raises two further questions. If parents are in effect developing motives or teaching them unconsciously by what they do, why do some parents behave that way and others do not? The answer to the question is by no means well worked out, but it seems to involve special experiences the parents have had as members of minority groups or reformist groups that have provided them with an ideology that leads them to emphasize one aspect of child training over another. However, the connection is by no means obvious or straightforward. Because parents want their child to have achievement motivation, they may insist that the child do well at all tasks early, but this does not automatically result in a higher level of adult *n* Achievement. The child training of importance may appear to be quite unrelated to achieving and involve scheduling feeding and severe toilet training. If so—if the development of a motive depends on such chancy matters as the exposure of a parent to reformist ideology or the unavailability of disposable diapers, which makes severe toilet training more desirable, why leave the matter to chance? Why not teach the motives directly? Can they be taught?

Many efforts have been made to teach motivation, with varying degrees of success. Generally speaking, German psychologists have concentrated on the cognitive aspects of achievement motivation, teaching students to set moderate goals and to attribute failure to lack of effort, so as generally to build self-confidence or the perceived probability of success variable in the formula for predicting performance outcomes. They did not include the associative thought measure of *n* Achievement as part of the instruction, partly because they wanted to reserve it to determine whether motive strength had in fact been increased, and partly because the cognitive aspects of behavior change were easier to introduce into the schoolroom. In general, they found significant changes in the cognitive variables they were trying to influence, and at times they also produced an increase in achievement motive strength. However, the long-term effects of the motivation training on performance in school were seldom significant, and they attributed this to the fact that school does not provide opportunities for the proper exercise of the achievement motive.

Another possible explanation for the result is that by concentrating on cognitive changes, the German psychologists were influencing situation-dependent, or respondent, behavior, whereas if they had concentrated more on changing the motive itself, they might have influenced spontaneous, nonsituation-dependent (or operant) behaviors, which in the long run might have made more of a difference in school performance. To put the matter simply, if pupils have learned to set moderate goals, it is necessary that their teacher provide them with opportunities to choose moderate goals if the acquired behavior is to result in an improvement in performance. But since teachers do not regularly do this, learning to set moderate goals may have little effect. In contrast, if pupils are taught achievement thinking, or Origin thinking, they may spontaneously think of moderate goals they can set without being given the opportunity by the teacher. The evidence for such an inference is by no means conclusive, since much achievement motivation training in the United States, as well as in Germany, has been unsuccessful in improving academic performance. The matter cries out for further investigation.

For the most part, U.S. psychologists started motivation training courses by teaching participants the scoring system for the various motives so that they could learn to think in appropriate ways. The cognitive and value aspects of the motivation-action sequence were also taught, as in Germany. The courses in achievement motivation were successful in improving entrepreneurial behavior for small businesspeople in a number of different countries around the world and among minority businesspeople in the United States. The improvement seems to be due to a shift from the fear of failure to the hope of success aspect of achievement motivation, and also to strengthening the other determinants of an action outcome—namely, the perceived probability of success and the value placed on business improvement. Effects of achievement motivation training on academic performance have sometimes been successful and sometimes not, perhaps because schools do not provide opportunities to exercise the achievement motive, as the German psychologists argue, or perhaps because doing well in school is more in the service of the power motive than the achievement motive. The most successful type of motivation training for improving academic performance is Origin training, as developed by deCharms (1976), and it contains an element of power motivation training.

Power motivation training has also shown some preliminary success in changing individuals for whom the power motive is a key element in their performance. Since high *n* Power and low inhibition is associated with heavy drinking in men, it was reasoned that training emphasizing inhibition or socializing the power motive would help male alcoholics recover, and this turned out to be the case. And since people high in *n* Power and high in Activity Inhibition tend to make better managers, motivation training emphasizing this motive syndrome ought to improve managerial behavior. This also turned out to be the case. But the findings are preliminary and greatly in need of further confirmation.

The fact is that despite a great deal of effort and experience, we still do not know whether psychologists have succeeded in developing motives, although they have certainly changed behavior. Nor do we know precisely how motives are most easily developed, probably because we do not yet have a clear grasp of the natural course of development of motives as children grow up. Further research in the area of motive development is greatly needed.

• THE RELATIONSHIP OF PROGRESS IN PSYCHOLOGY TO ITS ROLE IN SOCIETY

Psychologists who have attempted to develop motives have encountered many difficulties, both of a theoretical and a practical nature. Their experience highlights the relationship of progress in psychology to its role in society. On the theoretical side, the pressure, for example, to produce improved performance in school has at times been so great that it has clouded the issue of whether the training is developing motives. Or the interest in getting results in improved performance has diverted attention from the theoretical issues of just what educational inputs are producing the changes. On the practical side, ethical questions have been raised as to whether it is proper to try to influence children's motives, and there has been some confusion as to who should be in charge of motivation training programs. Furthermore, psychologists may be interested in developing training programs but not be particularly skilled at or interested in continuing to deliver them. Even when training has shown promise, it is not clear what agents or institutions should provide the training. If power motivation training continues to show promise in rehabilitating alcoholics, who will provide it? Alcoholism in our society is defined as a disease, and therefore doctors usually provide treatment for alcoholism. But doctors do not think of themselves as educators or trainers and are rarely willing to prepare themselves to offer motivation training.

The problem has been most evident in the case of achievement motivation training for small business entrepreneurs, which has been demonstrated over and over again in different countries to be effective so far as the participants are concerned, and also very probably so far as the community is concerned in which they work, and ultimately so far as the nation is concerned of which the community is a part. Despite all this evidence, achievement motivation training for entrepreneurs is seldom offered on a regular basis anywhere in the world today. Dozens of individuals in the public and private sector have been trained to give the courses and have given them successfully in many different countries. Typically, they continue to offer the courses only so long as a special research grant is available to pay for their services.

The training is of obvious benefit to the entrepreneurs, but not necessarily to an educational institution that provides it, particularly since the training courses are short and not part of the regular curriculum the institution provides. So the courses are discontinued. Or the trainers have become upwardly mobile because of their greater achievement orientation, and they get promoted to better jobs and stop training. The small businesspeople themselves cannot afford to pay the amount of money it would take to provide the courses without a research subsidy. Banks or public agencies supposedly fostering small business have failed to provide the training, partly because they do not think of themselves as educators and partly because psychological interventions simply do not seem as important or as easily made as economic changes brought about by the infusion of more capital, a decrease in the tax rate, an improvement in the terms of trade, or the exploitation of a new natural resource.

This story provides a case study in the relationship of psychology to society. Ultimately, progress in psychology depends on the extent to which it is valued and used by society. It has not always been regarded as a worthwhile field of scientific endeavor and in fact is so regarded in only a few countries in the world today, including the English-speaking countries, Scandinavia, The Netherlands, West Germany, Japan, and India. With the support it has received in these countries, the psychology of motivation has made real progress in the last generation. People in this field have discovered much new knowledge, some of it of practical use to society. If society can accept such contributions as valuable, the promise of psychology will appear even greater, and the field will get the financial and institutional support and the commitment from individual investigators it needs to study the many questions about human motivation that still need answers.

For, while some progress has been made in measuring a few human motives and in understanding their origins and effects on behavior, much remains to be discovered and clarified. The scientific study of human motives is still at an early stage.

Bibliography

Abelson, R. P. Psychological status of the script concept. *American Psychologist,* 1981, *36,* 715–729.

Ach, N. *Über die Willensakt und das Temperament.* Leipzig: Quelle and Meyer, 1910.

Adams, W. I., Lorens, S. A., & Mitchell, C. L. Morphine enhances lateral hypothalamic self-stimulation in the rat. *Proceedings of the Society for Experimental Biology,* 1972, *140,* 770–771.

Adler, A. *Neurotic constitution.* New York: Moffat, Ward, 1917.

Adorno, T. W., Frenkel-Brunswik, E., Levinson, D. J., & Sanford, R. N. *The authoritarian personality.* New York: Harper, 1950.

Ainsworth, M. D. S. The development of the infant-mother attachment. In B. M. Caldwell & H. N. Ricciuti (Eds.), *Review of child development research* (Vol. 3). Chicago: University of Chicago Press, 1973.

Alexander, C. N. *Ego development, personality, and behavioral change in inmates practicing the transcendental meditation technique: A cross-sectional and longitudinal study.* Unpublished doctoral dissertation, Harvard University, 1982.

Allen, G. J., & Condon, T. J. Whither subliminal psychodynamic activation studies? *Journal of Abnormal Psychology,* 1982, *91,* 126–130.

Allport, G. W. *Personality: A psychological interpretation.* New York: Holt, 1937.

Allport, G. W. Effect: A secondary principle of learning. *Psychological Review,* 1946, *53,* 335–347.

Allport, G. W. The trend in motivational theory. *Journal of Orthopsychiatry,* 1953, *23,* 107–119.

Alschuler, A. S. *Developing achievement motivation in adolescents.* Englewood Cliffs, N.J.: Educational Technology Publications, 1973.

Amoroso, D. M., Brown, M., Pruesse, M., Ware, E. E., & Pilkey, D. W. An investigation of behavioral and psychological reactions to pornographic stimuli. In *Technical report of the Commission on Obscenity and Pornography* (Vol. 8). Washington, D.C.: U.S. Government Printing Office, 1971.

Andrews, G. R., & Debus, R. L. Persistence and the causal perception of failure: Modifying cognitive attributions. *Journal of Educational Psychology,* 1978, *70,* 154–166.

Andrews, J. D. W. *The achievement motive in lifestyle among Harvard freshmen.* Unpublished doctoral dissertation, Harvard University, Department of Social Relations, 1966.

Andrews, J. D. W. The achievement motive in two types of organizations. *Journal of Personality and Social Psychology,* 1967, *6,* 163–168.

Angelini, A. L. Studies in projective measurement of achievement motivation of Brazilian students, males and females: Proceedings of the 15th International Congress of Psychology, Brussels, 1957. *Acta Psychologica,* 1959, *15,* 359–360.

Argyle, M., & Cook, M. *Gaze and mutual gaze.* Cambridge, England: Cambridge University Press, 1976.

Armour, D. J., Polich, J. M., & Stamboul, H. B. *Alcoholism and treatment.* New York: Wiley, 1978.

Aronoff, J. *Psychological needs and cultural systems.* New York: Van Nostrand, 1967.

Aronoff, J. The cane-cutters of St. Kitts. *Psychology Today,* August 1971, pp. 53–55.

Aronson, E. The need for achievement as measured in graphic expression. In J. W. Atkinson (Ed.), *Motives in fantasy, action, and society.* Princeton, N.J.: Van Nostrand, 1958.

Asch, S. E. Effects of group pressure upon the modification and distortion of judgments. In H. Guetzkow (Ed.), *Groups, leadership, and men.* Pittsburgh: Carnegie Press, 1951.

Atkinson, J. W. The achievement motive and recall of interrupted and completed tasks. In D. C. McClelland (Ed.), *Studies in motivation.* New York: Appleton-Century-Crofts, 1955.

Atkinson, J. W. Motivational determinants of risk-taking behavior. *Psychological Review,* 1957, *64,* 359–372.

Atkinson, J. W. Towards experimental analysis of human motivation in terms of motives, expectancies, and incentives. In J. W. Atkinson (Ed.), *Motives in fantasy, action, and society.* Princeton, N.J.: Van Nostrand, 1958.

Atkinson, J. W. *Introduction to motivation.* New York: Van Nostrand, 1964.

Atkinson, J. W. Thematic apperceptive measurement of motivation in 1950 and 1980. In G. d'Ydevalle & W. Lens (Eds.), *Cognition in human motivation and learning.* Hillsdale, N.J.: Erlbaum, 1980.

Atkinson, J. W., & Birch, D. *The dynamics of action.* New York: Wiley, 1970.

Atkinson, J. W., & Birch, D. *Introduction to motivation* (2nd ed.). New York: Van Nostrand, 1978.

Atkinson, J. W., Bongort, K., & Price, L. H. Explorations using computer simulation to comprehend TAT measurement of motivation. *Motivation and emotion,* 1977, *1,* 1–27.

Atkinson, J. W., Heyns, R. W., & Veroff, J. The effect of experimental arousal of the affiliation motive on thematic apperception. *Journal of Abnormal and Social Psychology,* 1954, *49,* 405–410.

Atkinson, J. W., & Litwin, G. H. Achievement motive and test anxiety conceived as motive to approach success and motive to avoid failure. *Journal of Abnormal and Social Psychology,* 1960, *60,* 52–63.

Atkinson, J. W., & McClelland, D. C. The effects of different intensities of the hunger drive on thematic apperception. *Journal of Experimental Psychology,* 1948, *38,* 643–658.

Atkinson, J. W., & O'Connor, P. Neglected factors in studies of achievement-oriented performance: Social approval as an incentive and performance decrement. In J. W. Atkinson & N. T. Feather (Eds.), *A theory of achievement motivation.* New York: Wiley, 1966.

Atkinson, J. W., & Raphelson, A. C. Individual differences in motivation and behavior in particular situations. *Journal of Personality,* 1956, *24,* 351–363.

Atkinson, J. W., & Reitman, W. R. Performance as a function of motive strength and expectancy of goal attainment. *Journal of Abnormal and Social Psychology,* 1956, *53,* 361–366.

Atkinson, J. W., & Walker, E. L. The affiliation motive in perceptual sensitivity to faces. *Journal of Abnormal and Social Psychology,* 1956, *53,* 38–41.

Axelrod, J. Neurotransmitters. *Scientific American,* 1974, *230*(6), 59–71.

Bakan, D. *Sigmund Freud and the Jewish mystical tradition.* New York: Van Nostrand, 1958.

Bakan, D. *The duality of human existence.* Boston: Beacon Press, 1966.

Bakan, P. Two streams of consciousness: A typological approach. In K. S. Pope & J. L. Singer (Eds.), *The stream of consciousness.* New York: Plenum, 1978.

Bales, R. F., & Cohen, S. P. *SYMLOG: A system for the multiple level observation of groups.* New York: Free Press, 1979.

Bandura, A. Self-efficacy mechanism in human agency. *American Psychologist,* 1982, *37,* 122–147.

Barclay, A. M. The effect of hostility on physiological and fantasy responses. *Journal of Personality,* 1969, *37,* 651–667.

Barclay, A. M. Linking of sexual and aggressive motives: Contributions of "irrelevant" arousals. *Journal of Personality,* 1971, *39,* 481–492.

Barclay, A. M., & Haber, R. N. The relation of aggression to sexual motivation. *Journal of Personality,* 1965, *33,* 462–475.

Baron, J. Menstrual hormone changes and instinctual tendencies in dreams. *Motivation and Emotion,* 1977, *1,* 273–282.

Barrett, G. V., & Franke, R. H. Psychogenic death: A reappraisal. *Science,* 1970, *167,* 304–306.

Bartmann, T. *Denkerziehung im Programmierten Unterricht.* Munich: Manz, 1965.

Beardslee, D. C., & Fogelson, R. Sex differences in sexual imagery aroused by musical stimulation. In J. W. Atkinson (Ed.), *Motives in fantasy, action, and society.* Princeton, N. J.: Van Nostrand, 1958.

Bell, A. P., Weinberg, M. S., & Hammersmith, S. K. *Sexual preference: Its development in men and women.* Bloomington, Ind.: Indiana University Press, 1981.

Benesh, M., & Weiner, B. On emotion and motivation: From the notebooks of Fritz Heider. *American Psychologist,* 1982, *37,* 887–895.

Benson, H. *The relaxation response.* New York: Morrow, 1975.

Benson, H., & Epstein, M. D. The placebo effect: A neglected asset in the care of patients. *Journal of the American Medical Association,* 1975, *232,* 1225–1227.

Berelson, B., & Steiner, G. A. *Human behavior: An inventory of scientific findings.* New York: Harcourt, Brace and World, 1964.

Berlew, D. E. *The achievement motive and the growth of Greek civilization.* Unpublished honors thesis, Wesleyan University, 1956.

Berlew, D. E. *A study of interpersonal sensitivity.* Unpublished doctoral dissertation, Harvard University, 1959.

Berlew, D. E., & Williams, A. F. Interpersonal sensitivity under motive arousing conditions. *Journal of Abnormal and Social Psychology,* 1964, *68,* 150–159.

Berlyne, D. E. Arousal and reinforcement. In D. Levine (Ed.), *Nebraska Symposium on Motivation: 1967.* Lincoln: University of Nebraska Press, 1967.

Berlyne, D. E., & Madsen, K. B. *Pleasure, reward, preference.* New York: Academic Press, 1973.

Beswick, D. G. *Theory and measurement of human curiosity.* Unpublished doctoral dissertation, Harvard University, 1965.

Bieber, I., Dain, H. J., Dince, P. R., Drellich, M. G., Grand, H. G., Gundlach, R. H., Kremer, M. W., Rifkin, A. H., Wilbur, C. B., & Bieber, T. B. *Homosexuality: A psychoanalytic study.* New York: Basic, 1962.

Birch, H. G. The role of motivational factors in insightful problem-solving. *Journal of Comparative Psychology,* 1945, *38,* 295–317.

Birk, L., Huddleston, W., Millers, E., & Cohler, B. Avoidance conditioning for homosexuality. *Archives of General Psychiatry,* 1971, *25,* 314–323.

Birney, R. C., Burdick, H., & Teevan, R. C. *Fear of failure motivation.* New York: Van Nostrand, 1969.

Blehar, M. C., Lieberman, A. F., & Ainsworth, M. D. S. Early face-to-face interaction and its relationship to later mother-infant attachment. *Child Development,* 1977, *48,* 182–194.

Blodgett, H. C. The effect of the introduction of reward upon the maze performance of rats. *University of California Publications in Psychology,* 1929, *4*(8), 113–134.

Borg, S., Kvande, H., & Sedvall, G. Central norepinephrine metabolism during alcohol intoxication in addicts and healthy volunteers. *Science,* 1981, *213,* 1135–1137.

Bowlby, J. *Attachment and loss* (Vol. 1), *Attachment.* New York: Basic, 1969.

Boyatzis, R. E. *A two factor theory of affiliation motivation.* Unpublished doctoral dissertation, Harvard University, 1972.

Boyatzis, R. E. Affiliation motivation. In D. C. McClelland & R. S. Steele (Eds.), *Human motivation: A book of readings.* Morristown, N.J.: General Learning Press, 1973.

Boyatzis, R. E. *Power motivation training workbook.* Boston: McBer and Company, 1974.

Boyatzis, R. E. *The competent manager: A model for effective performance.* New York: Wiley, 1982.

Bradburn, N. M., & Berlew, D. E. Need for achievement in English economic growth. *Economic Development and Cultural Change,* 1961, *10,* 8–20.

Bramante, M. *Sex differences in fantasy patterns: A replication and elaboration.* Unpublished doctoral dissertation, City University of New York, 1970.

Bray, D. W., Campbell, R. J., & Grant, D. L. *Formative years in business: A long term study of managerial lives.* New York: Wiley, 1974.

Brazelton, T. B., Koslowski, B., & Main, M. The origins of reciprocity: The early mother-infant interaction. In M. Lewis & L. A. Rosenblum (Eds.), *The effect of the infant on the caregiver.* New York: Wiley, 1974.

Breit, S. Arousal of achievement motivation with causal attributions. *Psychological Reports,* 1969, *25,* 539–542.

Bremer, J. *Asexualization.* New York: Macmillan, 1959.

Briddell, D. W., Rimm, D. C., Caddy, G. R., Krawitz, G., Sholis, D., & Wunderlin, R. J. Effects of alcohol and cognitive set on sexual arousal. *Journal of Abnormal Psychology,* 1978, *87,* 418–430.

Brophy, J. E., & Good, T. L. Teacher's communication of differential expressions for children's classroom performance: Some behavioral data. *Journal of Educational Psychology,* 1970, *61,* 365–374.

Broverman, D., Klaiber, E. L., Kobayashi, Y., & Vogel, W. Roles of activation and inhibition in sex differences in cognitive abilities. *Psychological Review,* 1968, *75,* 23–50.

Broverman, D. M., Klaiber, E. L., Vogel, W., & Kobayashi, Y. Short-term versus long-term effects of adrenal hormones on behaviors. *Psychological Bulletin,* 1974, *81,* 672–694.

Brown, J. S. Gradients of approach and avoidance responses and their relation to level of motivation. *Journal of Comparative and Physiological Psychology,* 1948, *41,* 450–465.

Brown, J. S. *The motivation of behavior.* New York: McGraw-Hill, 1961.

Brown, N. O. *Life against death.* Middletown, Conn.: Wesleyan University Press, 1959.

Brown, R. *A first language: The early stages.* Cambridge, Mass.: Harvard University Press, 1973.

Bruner, J. S., & Goodman, C. C. Value and need as organizing factors in perception. *Journal of Abnormal and Social Psychology,* 1947, *42,* 33–44.

Bruner, J. S., Matter, J., & Papanek, M. Breadth of learning as function of drive level and mechanization. *Psychological Review,* 1955, *62,* 1–10.

Brunswik, E., & Reiter, L. Eindruckscharaktere schematisierter Gesichter. *Zeitschrift für Psychologie,* 1938, *142,* 67–134.

Buber, M. *Between man and man.* New York: Macmillan, 1965.

Buber, M. *I and thou.* New York: Scribner, 1970.

Burdick, H. A., & Burnes, A. J. A test of "strain towards symmetry" theories. *Journal of Abnormal and Social Psychology,* 1958, *57,* 367–370.

Bursztajn, H., Feinbloom, R. I., Hamm, R. M., & Brodsky, A. *Medical choices, medical chances: How patients, families, and physicians can cope with uncertainty.* New York: Delacorte, 1981.

Burton, M. J., Mora, F., & Rolls, E. T. Visual and taste neurons in the lateral hypothalamus and substantia innominata: Modulation of responsiveness by hunger. *Journal of Physiology,* 1975, *252,* 50–51.

Burwen, L. S., & Campbell, D. T. The generality of attitudes toward authority and non-authority figures. *Journal of Abnormal and Social Psychology,* 1957, *54,* 24–31.

Butler, R. A. Incentive conditions which influence visual exploration. *Journal of Experimental Psychology,* 1954, *48,* 19–23.

Byrne, D. Anxiety and the experimental arousal of affiliation need. *Journal of Abnormal and Social Psychology,* 1961, *63,* 660–662. (a)

Byrne, D. Interpersonal attraction as a function of affiliation need and attitude similarity. *Human Relations,* 1961, *14,* 283–289. (b)

Byrne, D. Response to attitude similarity-dissimilarity as a function of affiliation need. *Journal of Personality,* 1962, *30,* 164–177.

Byrne, D., McDonald, R. D., & Mikawa, J. Approach and avoidance affiliation motives. *Journal of Personality,* 1963, *31,* 21–37.

Cannon, W. B. *Bodily changes in pain, hunger, fear, and rage: An account of recent researches into the function of emotional excitement.* New York: Appleton-Century-Crofts, 1915.

Cannon, W. B., & Washburn, A. L. An explanation of hunger. *American Journal of Psychology,* 1912, *29,* 441–454.

Capote, T. *In cold blood: A true account of a multiple murder and its consequences.* New York: Random, 1965.

Carlson, N. R. *Physiology of behavior.* Boston: Allyn and Bacon, 1977.

Cattell, R. B. *Personality and motivation: Structure and measurement.* Yonkers, N.Y.: World Book, 1957.

Cattell, R. B. *The scientific analysis of personality.* Baltimore, Md.: Penguin, 1965.

Cattell, R. B., Kawash, G. F., & DeYoung, G. E. Validation of objective measures of ergic tension: Response of the sex urge to visual stimulation. *Journal of Experimental Research on Personality,* 1972, *6,* 76–83.

Ceranski, D. S., Teevan, R., & Kalle, R. J. A comparison of three measures of the motive to avoid failure: Hostile press, test anxiety, and resultant achievement motivation. *Motivation and Emotion,* 1979, *3,* 395–404.

Chanowitz, B., & Langer, E. Knowing more (or less) than you can show: Understanding control through the mindlessness/mindfulness distinction. In M. E. P. Seligman & J. Garber (Eds.), *Human helplessness.* New York: Academic Press, 1982.

Chapin, M., & Dyck, D. G. Persistence in children's reading behavior as a function of N length and attribution retraining. *Journal of Abnormal Psychology,* 1976, *85,* 511–515.

Child, I. L., Frank, K. F., & Storm, T. Self-ratings and TAT: Their relations to each other and to adulthood background. *Journal of Personality,* 1956, *25,* 96–114.

Cicchetti, D., & Sroufe, L. A. The relationship between affective and cognitive development in Down's syndrome infants. *Child Development,* 1976, *47,* 920–929.

Clark, R. A. The projective measurement of experimentally induced levels of sexual motivation. *Journal of Experimental Psychology, 1952, 44,* 391–399.

Clark, R. A. The effects of sexual motivation on phantasy. In D. C. McClelland (Ed.), *Studies in motivation.* New York: Appleton-Century-Crofts, 1955.

Clark, R. A., & McClelland, D. C. A factor analytic integration of imaginative and performance measures of the need for Achievement. *Journal of General Psychology, 1956, 55,* 73–83.

Cofer, C. N. *Motivation and emotion.* Glenview, Ill.: Scott, Foresman, 1972.

Combs, A. W. A comparative study of motivations as revealed in Thematic Apperception stories and autobiography. *Journal of Clinical Psychology, 1947, 3,* 65–75.

Comfort, A. *The joy of sex.* New York: Simon and Schuster, 1974.

Condon, W. S. An analysis of behavioral organization. In S. Weitz (Ed.), *Non-verbal communication: Readings with commentary* (2nd ed.). New York: Oxford University Press, 1979.

Conners, C. K. *Needs for affiliation and response to social influence.* Unpublished doctoral dissertation, Harvard University, 1961.

Constantian, C. A. *Motives and dimensions as predictors of behavior in a small group.* Unpublished manuscript, Harvard University, Department of Psychology and Social Relations, 1978.

Constantian, C. A. *Attitudes, beliefs, and behavior in regard to spending time alone.* Unpublished doctoral dissertation, Harvard University, Department of Psychology and Social Relations, 1981.

Corbett, D., La Ferriere, A., & Miliver, P. M. Plasticity of the medial prefrontal cortex: Facilitated acquisition of intracranial self-stimulation by pretraining self-stimulation. *Physiology and Behavior, 1982, 28,* 531–534.

Cortés, J. B. The achievement motive in the Spanish economy between the 13th and 18th centuries. *Economic Development and Cultural Change, 1960, 9,* 144–163.

Cortés, J. B., & Gatti, F. M. *Delinquency and crime: A biopsychosocial approach.* New York: Seminar Press, 1972.

Costa, P., & McClelland, D. C. *Predicting rank in class from motivational, social class, and intelligence measures.* Unpublished manuscript, Harvard University, Department of Psychology and Social Relations, 1971.

Cottrell, N. B. Social facilitation. In C. G. McClintock (Ed.), *Experimental social psychology.* New York: Holt, Rinehart and Winston, 1972.

Cottrell, N. B., Wack, D. L., Sekerak, G. J., & Rittle, R. Social facilitation of dominant responses by the presence of an audience and the mere presence of others. *Journal of Personality and Social Psychology, 1968, 9,* 245–250.

Couch, A. S., & Keniston, K. Yea-sayers and nay-sayers: Agreeing response set as a personality variable. *Journal of Abnormal and Social Psychology, 1960, 60,* 151–174.

Courts, F. A. Relations between experimentally induced muscular tension and memorization. *Journal of Experimental Psychology, 1939, 25,* 235–256.

Cramer, P., & Hogan, K. Sex differences in verbal and play fantasy. *Developmental Psychology, 1975, 11,* 145–154.

Crespi, L. P. Quantitative variation of incentive and performance in the white rat. *American Journal of Psychology, 1942, 55,* 467–517.

Crockett, H. J., Jr. The achievement motive and differential occupational mobility in the United States. *American Sociological Review, 1962, 27,* 191–204.

Cronbach, L. J., & Meehl, P. E. Construct validity in psychological tests. *Psychological Bulletin, 1955, 52,* 281–302.

Crowne, D. P., & Marlowe, D. *The approval motive.* New York: Wiley, 1964.

Csikszentmihalyi, M. *Beyond boredom and anxiety.* San Francisco: Jossey-Bass, 1975.

Cutter, H. S. G., Boyatzis, R. E., & Clancy, D. D. The effectiveness of power motivation training for rehabilitating alcoholics. *Journal of Studies in Alcohol,* 1977, *38*(1), 131–141.

Cytowic, R. E. The long ordeal of James Brady. *New York Times Magazine,* September 27, 1981.

D'Andrade, R. G., Dart, J. *The interpretation of* r *versus* r². Unpublished manuscript, University of California at Irvine, Department of Anthropology, 1982.

Darley, J. M., & Batson, C. D. "From Jerusalem to Jericho": A study of situational and dispositional variables in helping behavior. *Journal of Abnormal and Social Psychology,* 1973, *27,* 100–108.

Davidson, R. J., Saron, C., & McClelland, D. C. Effects of personality and semantic content of stimuli on augmenting and reducing in the event-related potential. *Biological Psychology,* 1980, *11,* 249–255.

Davies, E. This is the way that Crete went–Not with a bang but a simper. *Psychology Today,* June 1969, pp. 43–47.

deCharms, R. Affiliation motivation and productivity in small groups. *Journal of Abnormal and Social Psychology,* 1957, *55,* 222–226.

deCharms, R. *Personal causation.* New York: Academic Press, 1968.

deCharms, R. *Enhancing motivation: Change in the classroom.* New York: Irvington, 1976.

deCharms, R. The origins of competence and achievement motivation in personal causation. In L. J. Fyans, Jr. (Ed.), *Achievement motivation: Recent trends in theory and research.* New York: Plenum, 1980.

deCharms, R. That's not psychology! The implications of McClelland's approach to motivation. In A. J. Stewart (Ed.), *Motivation and society.* San Francisco: Jossey-Bass, 1982.

deCharms, R., & Carpenter, V. Measuring motivation in culturally disadvantaged school children. In H. J. Klausmeirer & G. T. O'Hearn (Eds.), *Research and development toward the improvement of education.* Madison, Wis.: Educational Research Services, 1968.

deCharms, R., & Davé, P. N. Hope of success, fear of failure, subjective probability, and risk-taking behavior. *Journal of Personality and Social Psychology,* 1965, *1,* 558–568.

deCharms, R., & Moeller, G. H. Values expressed in American children's readers: 1800–1950. *Journal of Abnormal and Social Psychology,* 1962, *64,* 136–142.

deCharms, R., Morrison, H. W., Reitman, W. R., & McClelland, D. C. Behavioral correlates of directly and indirectly measured achievement motivation. In D. C. McClelland (Ed.), *Studies in motivation.* New York: Appleton-Century-Crofts, 1955.

deCharms, R., & Muir, M. S. Motivation: Social approaches. *Annual Review of Psychology,* 1978, *29,* 91–113.

Deci, E. L. *Intrinsic motivation.* New York: Plenum, 1975.

Decke, E. Effects of taste on the eating behavior of obese and normal persons. In S. Schachter (Ed.), *Emotion, obesity and crime.* New York: Academic Press, 1971.

Dember, W. N., Earl, R. W., & Paradise, N. Response of rats to differential stimulus complexity. *Journal of Comparative and Physiological Psychology,* 1957, *50,* 514–518.

Diaz, A. J. *An empirical study of the effect of CEO motives on intra-industry performance with examples drawn from US and Japanese auto manufacturers.* Unpublished Bachelor of Arts thesis, Harvard College, Department of Psychology and Social Relations and Economics, 1982.

Dienstbier, R. A. Emotion-attribution theory: Establishing roots and exploring future perspectives. In H. E. Howe, Jr. (Ed.), *Nebraska Symposium on Motivation: 1978.* Lincoln: University of Nebraska Press, 1979.

Doherty, M. A., & Walker, R. E. The relationship of personality characteristics, awareness and attitude in a verbal conditioning situation. *Journal of Personality,* 1966, *34,* 504–516.

Dollard, J., Doob, L. W., Miller, N. E., Mowrer, O. H., & Sears, R. R. *Frustration and aggression.* New Haven, Conn.: Yale University Press, 1939.

Donley, R. E., & Winter, D. G. Measuring the motives of public officials at a distance: An exploratory study of American presidents. *Behavioral Science,* 1970, *15,* 227–236.

Douvan, E. Social status and success strivings. *Journal of Abnormal and Social Psychology,* 1956, *52,* 219–223.

Duda, J. L. Achievement motivation among Navajo students: A conceptual analysis with preliminary data. *Ethos,* 1980, 316–331.

Duffy, E. *Activation and behavior.* New York: Wiley, 1962.

Duncan, O. D., Featherman, D. L., & Duncan, B. *Socio-economic background and achievement.* New York: Harcourt Brace, 1972.

Dutton, D. G., & Aron, A. P. Some evidence for heightened sexual attraction under conditions of high anxiety. *Journal of Personality and Social Psychology,* 1974, *30,* 510–517.

Dweck, C. S. The role of expectations and attributions in the alleviation of learned helplessness. *Journal of Personality and Social Psychology,* 1975, *31,* 674–685.

Dweck, C. S., & Wortman, C. B. Learned helplessness, anxiety and achievement motivation: Neglected parallels in cognitive, affective and coping responses. In H. W. Krohne & L. Laux (Eds.), *Achievement, stress, and anxiety.* Washington, D.C.: Hemisphere Publishing, 1982.

Easterlin, R. A. *Population, labor force and long swings in economic growth: The American experience.* New York: Columbia University Press, 1968.

Edwards, A. L. *The social desirability variable in personality assessment and research.* New York: Dryden Press, 1957.

Eibl-Eibesfeldt, I. *Ethology: The biology of behavior.* New York: Holt, Rinehart and Winston, 1970.

Ekman, P. Universal and cultural differences in facial expressions of emotion. In J. K. Cole (Ed.), *Nebraska Symposium on Motivation: 1971.* Lincoln: University of Nebraska Press, 1972.

Elashoff, J. D., & Snow, R. E. *A case study in statistical inference: Reconstruction of the Rosenthal-Jacobson data on teacher expectancy.* (Tech. Rep. 15). Stanford, Calif.: Stanford Center for Research and Development in Teaching, School of Education, Stanford University, 1970.

Ellingstad, U. S., & Struckman-Johnson, D. L. *Short term rehabilitation study: 12 month analyses.* Vermillion: University of South Dakota, Human Factors Laboratory, 1978.

Ellis, H. *The psychology of sex.* New York: New American Library, 1954.

Endler, N. S. Persons, situations, and their interactions. In A. I. Rabin, J. Aronoff, A. M. Barclay, & R. A. Zucker (Eds.), *Further explorations in personality.* New York: Wiley, 1981.

Entin, E. E. *The relationship between the theory of achievement motivation and performance on a simple and a complex task.* Unpublished doctoral dissertation, University of Michigan, 1968.

Entin, E. E., & Feather, N. T. Attribution to success and failure in contingent and noncontingent paths. In J. O. Raynor & E. E. Entin (Eds.), *Motivation, career striving, and aging.* New York: Hemisphere Publishing Corp., 1982.

Entin, E. E., & Raynor, J. O. Effects of contingent future orientation and achievement motivation on performance in two kinds of tasks. *Journal of Experimental Research in Personality,* 1973, *6,* 134–320.

Entin, E. E., & Raynor, J. O. Success versus moving on in contingent paths. In J. O. Raynor and E. E. Entin (Eds.), *Motivation, career striving, and aging.* New York: Hemisphere Publishing Corp., 1982.

Entwisle, D. R. To dispel fantasies about fantasy-based measures of achievement motivation. *Psychological Bulletin,* 1972, *77,* 377–391.

Epstein, S. The measurement of drive and conflict in humans: Theory and experiment. In M. R. Jones (Ed.), *Nebraska Symposium on Motivation: 1962.* Lincoln: University of Nebraska Press, 1962.

Erikson, E. H. *Childhood and society* (2nd ed.). New York: Norton, 1963. (Originally published, 1950).

Erikson, E. H. Sex differences—The play configuration of pre-adolescents. *American Journal of Orthopsychiatry,* 1951, *21,* 667–692.

Erikson, E. H. *Insight and responsibility.* New York: Norton, 1964.

Estes, W. K. Generalization of secondary reinforcement from the primary drive. *Journal of Comparative and Physiological Psychology,* 1949, *42,* 286–295.

Estes, W. K. Stimulus response theory of drive. In M. R. Jones (Ed.), *Nebraska Symposium on Motivation: 1958.* Lincoln: University of Nebraska Press, 1958.

Ewing, J. A., Rouse, B. A., & Pellizzari, E. D. Alcohol sensitivity and ethnic background. *American Journal of Psychiatry,* 1974, *131,* 206–210.

Exline, R. V. Need affiliation and initial communication behavior in problem solving groups characterized by low interpersonal visibility. *Psychological Reports,* 1962, *10,* 79–89.

Eysenck, H. J. *Dimensions of personality.* London: Routledge and Kegan Paul, 1947.

Eysenck, H. J. The effects of psychotherapy: An evaluation. *Journal of Consulting Psychology,* 1952, *16,* 319–324.

Eysenck, H. J. *The dynamics of anxiety and hysteria.* New York: Praeger, 1957. (a)

Eysenck, H. J. *Sense and nonsense in psychology.* Harmondsworth, England: Penguin, 1957. (b)

Eysenck, H. J. *Fact and fiction in psychology.* Harmondsworth, England: Penguin, 1965.

Eysenck, H. J. *Eysenck on extroversion.* New York: Wiley/Halsted, 1973.

Falbo, T., & Beck, R. C. Naive psychology and the attributional model of achievement. *Journal of Personality,* 1979, *47,* 185–195.

Farber, I. E. Anxiety as a drive state. In M. R. Jones (Ed.), *Nebraska Symposium on Motivation: 1954.* Lincoln: University of Nebraska Press, 1954.

Feather, N. T. The relationship of persistence at a task to expectation of success and achievement related motives. *Journal of Abnormal and Social Psychology,* 1961, *63,* 552–561.

Feather, N. T. Persistence at a difficult task with alternative tasks of intermediate difficulty. *Journal of Abnormal and Social Psychology,* 1963, *66,* 604–609.

Feather, N. T. *Values in education and society.* New York: Free Press, 1975.

Feather, N. T., & Simon, J. G. Fear of success and causal attribution for outcome. *Journal of Personality,* 1973, *41*(4), 525–542.

Feij, J. A. Debilitating anxiety, facilitating anxiety, and general anxiety. In C. D. Spielberger & I. G. Sarason (Eds.), *Stress and anxiety* (Vol. 1). New York: Wiley, 1975.

Feierabend, I. K., & Feierabend, R. L. Aggressive behaviors within politics, 1947–62: A cross-national study. *Journal of Conflict Resolution,* 1966, *10,* 249–271.

Fersch, E. A., Jr. *Inward bound: The motivational impact of a combined Outward Bound-Upward Bound program on adolescents from poverty families.* Unpublished doctoral dissertation, Harvard University, 1971.

Feshbach, S. The drive-reducing function of fantasy behavior. *Journal of Abnormal and Social Psychology,* 1955, *50,* 3–11.

Feshbach, S. The stimulating versus cathartic effects of a vicarious aggressive activity. *Journal of Abnormal and Social Psychology,* 1961, *63,* 381–385.

Feshbach, S. Aggression. In P. H. Mussen (Ed.), *Carmichael's manual of child psychology.* New York: Wiley, 1970.

Festinger, L. Development of differential appetite in the rat. *Journal of Experimental Psychology,* 1943, *32,* 226–234.

Festinger, L., & Carlsmith, J. M. Cognitive consequences of forced compliance. *Journal of Abnormal and Social Psychology,* 1959, *58,* 203–210.

Fishman, D. B. Need and expectancy as determinants of affiliative behavior in small groups. *Journal of Personality and Social Psychology,* 1966, *4,* 155–164.

Fiske, D. W., & Maddi, S. R. *The functions of varied experience.* Homewood, Ill.: Dorsey, 1961.

Fleming, J. *Approach and avoidance motivation in interpersonal competition: A study of black male and female college students.* Unpublished doctoral dissertation, Harvard University, Department of Psychology and Social Relations, 1974.

Fleming, J. *Fear of success as a motivational construct: A functional interpretation.* Unpublished manuscript, Radcliffe Institute, 1975. (a)

Fleming, J. *Fear of success in black college students: Its assessment and functional significance.* Unpublished manuscript, Radcliffe Institute, 1975. (b)

Fleming, J. *The impact of college environments on black students.* San Francisco: Jossey-Bass, 1983.

Fodor, E. M., & Farrow, D. L. The power motive as an influence on the use of power. *Journal of Personality and Social Psychology,* 1979, *37,* 2091–2097.

Fodor, E. M., & Smith, T. The power motive as an influence on group decision making. *Journal of Personality and Social Psychology,* 1982, *42,* 178–185.

Foss, G. The influence of androgens on sexuality in women. *Lancet,* 1951, *260,* 667–669.

Frankenhaeuser, M. Psychoneuroendocrine approaches to the study of emotion as related to stress and coping. In H. E. Howe, Jr. (Ed.), *Nebraska Symposium on Motivation: 1978.* Lincoln: University of Nebraska Press, 1978.

Frankenhaeuser, M., Dunne, E., & Lundberg, U. Sex differences in sympathetic-adrenal medullary reactions induced by different stressors. *Psychopharmacology,* 1976, *47,* 1–5.

French, E. G. Some characteristics of achievement motivation. *Journal of Experimental Psychology,* 1955, *50,* 232–236.

French, E. G. Motivation as a variable and work partner selection. *Journal of Abnormal and Social Psychology,* 1956, *53,* 96–99.

French, E. G. Development of a measure of complex motivation. In J. W. Atkinson (Ed.), *Motives in fantasy, action, and society.* Princeton, N.J.: Van Nostrand, 1958. (a)

French, E. G. Effects of the interaction of motivation and feedback on task performance. In J. W. Atkinson (Ed.), *Motives in fantasy, action, and society.* Princeton, N.J.: Van Nostrand, 1958. (b)

French, E. G., & Chadwick, I. Some characteristics of affiliation motivation. *Journal of Abnormal and Social Psychology,* 1956, *52,* 296–300.

French, E. G., & Lesser, G. S. Some characteristics of the achievement motive in women. *Journal of Abnormal and Social Psychology,* 1964, *68,* 119–128.

French, E. G., & Thomas, F. H. The relationship of achievement motivation to problem-solving effectiveness. *Journal of Abnormal and Social Psychology,* 1958, *56,* 45–48.

Freud, S. [Interpretation of dreams.] In A. A. Brill (Ed. and trans.), *The basic writings of Sigmund Freud.* New York: Random House, 1938. (Originally published, 1900.)

Freud, S. [Psychopathology of everyday life.] In A. A. Brill (Ed. and trans.), *The basic writings of Sigmund Freud.* New York: Random House, 1938. (Originally published, 1901.)

Freud, S. [Three contributions to the theory of sex.] In A. A. Brill (Ed. and trans.), *The basic writings of Sigmund Freud.* New York: Random House, 1938. (Originally published, 1905.)

Freud, S. [The history of the psychoanalytic movement.] In A. A. Brill (Ed. and trans.), *The basic writings of Sigmund Freud.* New York: Random House, 1938. (Originally published, 1910.)

Freud, S. [Totem and taboo.] In A. A. Brill (Ed. and trans.), *The basic writings of Sigmund Freud.* New York: Random House, 1938. (Originally published, 1918.)

Freud, S. [*The ego and the id*] (J. Riviere, trans.). London: Hogarth, 1927. (Originally published, 1923.)

Freud, S. [*The future of an illusion*] (W. D. Robson-Scott, trans.). New York: Doubleday, 1957. (Originally published, 1927.)

Freud, S. [*Civilization and its discontents*] (J. Riviere, trans.). New York: Doubleday, 1958. (Originally published, 1930.)

Friedman, M., & Rosenman, R. H. *Type A behavior and your heart.* New York: Fawcett, 1974.

Frieze, I. H., & Weiner, B. Cue utilization and attributional judgments for success and failure. *Journal of Personality,* 1971, *39,* 591–606.

Fromm, E. *Man for himself.* New York: Rinehart, 1947.

Galbraith, J. K. *The new industrial state.* Boston: Houghton Mifflin, 1967.

Gallimore, R. Affiliation, social context, industriousness and achievement. In R. H. Munroe, R. L. Munroe, & B. B. Whiting (Eds.), *Handbook of cross-cultural human development.* New York: Garland STPM, 1981.

Gallimore, R., Boggs, J. W., & Jordan, C. *Culture, behavior and Education: A study of Hawaiian-Americans.* Beverly Hills, Calif.: Sage, 1974.

Garcia, J., Hankins, W. G., & Rusiniak, K. W. Behavioral regulation of the milieu interne in man and rat. *Science,* 1974, *185,* 824–831.

Garcia, J., & Koelling, R. A. Relation of cue to consequence in avoidance learning. *Psychonomic Science,* 1966, *4,* 123–124.

Geen, R. G., & Gange, J. J. Drive theory of social facilitation: Twelve years of theory and research. *Psychological Bulletin,* 1977, *84,* 1267–1288.

Gesell, A., & Ilg, F. L. *Infant and child in the culture of today.* New York: Harper, 1943.

Giese, H., & Schmidt, A. *Studenten Sexualität.* Hamburg: Rowohlt, 1968.

Giliberto, S. M. *Motivation and the Methodist revival period.* Unpublished honors thesis, Harvard University, Department of Psychology and Social Relations, 1972.

Gilligan, C., & Pollak, S. *The vulnerable and invulnerable physician.* Unpublished manuscript, Bunting Institute of Radcliffe College, 1982.

Glass, D. C., & Wood, J. D. The control of aggression by self-esteem and dissonance. In P. G. Zimbardo (Ed.), *The cognitive control of motivation.* Glenview, Ill.: Scott, Foresman, 1969.

Goleman, D. Jason and Medea's love story. *Psychology Today,* April 1976.

Gombrich, R. F. *Precept and practice: Traditional Buddhism in the rural highlands of Ceylon.* London: Oxford University Press, 1971.

Gough, H. G., & Heilbrun, A. B., Jr. *The adjective checklist manual.* Palo Alto, Calif.: Consulting Psychologists Press, 1975.

Grant, E. C. G., & Myers, E. Mental effects of oral contraceptives. *Lancet,* 1967, *2,* 945–946.

Greene, D. L., & Winter, D. G. Motives, involvements in leadership among black college students. *Journal of Personality,* 1971, *39,* 319–332.

Greenstein, F. I. *Personality in politics.* New York: Markham, 1969.

Grinker, J. The control of classical conditioning by cognitive manipulation. In P. G. Zimbardo (Ed.), *The cognitive control of motivation.* Glenview, Ill.: Scott, Foresman, 1969.

Grossman, S. P. Eating or drinking elicited by direct adrenergic or cholinergic stimulation of hypothalamus. *Science,* 1960, *132,* 301–302.

Grunt, J. A., & Young, W. C. Differential reactivity of individuals and the response of the male guinea pig to testosterone proprionate. *Endocrinology,* 1952, *51,* 237–248.

Gur, R. C., & Gur, R. E., Handedness, sex, and eyedness as moderating variables in the relation between hypnotic susceptibility and functional brain asymmetry. *Journal of Abnormal Psychology,* 1974, *83,* 635–643.

Gutheil, E. A. *The language of the dream.* New York: Macmillan, 1939.

Guthrie, E. R. *The psychology of learning.* New York: Harper & Row, 1935.

Haber, R. N. Discrepancy from adaptation level as a source of affect. *Journal of Experimental Psychology,* 1958, *56,* 370–375.

Hagen, E. E. *On the theory of social change.* New York: Dorsey, 1962.

Halisch, F., & Heckhausen, H. Search for feedback information and effort regulation during task performance. *Journal of Personality and Social Psychology,* 1977, *35,* 724–733.

Hall, C. S. A cognitive theory of dream symbols. *Journal of General Psychology,* 1953, *48,* 169–186.

Hall, C. S., & Lindzey, G. *Theories of personality.* New York: Wiley, 1957.

Hamburg, D. A., Hamburg, B. A., & Barchas, J. D. Anger and depression in perspective of behavioral biology. In L. Levi (Ed.), *Emotions: Their parameters and measurement.* New York: Raven, 1975.

Hancock, J. G., & Teevan, R. C. Fear of failure and risk-taking behavior. *Journal of Personality,* 1964, *32,* 200–209.

Haner, C. F., & Brown, J. S. Clarification of the instigation to action concept in the frustration-aggression hypothesis. *Journal of Abnormal and Social Psychology,* 1955, *51,* 204–206.

Hardy, K. R. Determinants of conformity and attitude change. *Journal of Abnormal and Social Psychology,* 1957, *54,* 289–294.

Harlow, H. F. *Learning to love.* San Francisco: Albion, 1971.

Harlow, H. F., Harlow, M. K., & Meyer, D. R. Learning motivated by a manipulation drive. *Journal of Experimental Psychology,* 1950, *40,* 228–234.

Harlow, H. F., Harlow, M. K., & Suomi, J. J. From thought to therapy: Lessons from a primate laboratory. *American Scientist,* 1971, *59,* 538–549.

Harlow, H. F., & Zimmerman, R. R. Affectual responses in the infant monkey. *Science,* 1959, *130,* 421–432.

Harris, H. *An experimental model of the effectiveness of project management offices.* Unpublished master's dissertation, Massachusetts Institute of Technology, 1969.

Hassan, M. K., Enayatullah, & Khalique, A. A study of anxiety in school children as related to child-rearing attitude and some personality traits of parents. *Indian Journal of Psychiatric Social Work,* July 1977, pp. 1–7.

Hawke, C. C. Castration and sex crimes. *American Journal of Mental Deficiency,* 1950, *55,* 220–226.

Hayashi, T., & Habu, K. A research on achievement motive: An experimental test of the "thought sampling" method by using Japanese students. *Japanese Psychological Research,* 1962, *4,* 30–42.

Hayashi, T., & Yamaushi, K. The relation of children's need for achievement to their parents' home discipline in regard to independence and mastery. *Bulletin Kyoto Gakugei University* (Series A). 1964, *25,* 31–40.

Heathers, G. L. The avoidance of repetition of a maze reaction in the rat as a function of the time interval between trials. *Journal of Psychology,* 1940, *10,* 350–380.

Heckhausen, H. *Hoffnung und Furcht in der Leistungsmotivation.* Meisenheim, West Germany: Hain, 1963.

Heckhausen, H. *The anatomy of achievement motivation.* New York: Academic Press, 1967.

Heckhausen, H. Trainings-kurse zur Erhöhung der Leistungsmotivation und der unternehmerischen Aktivität in einem Entwicklungsland: Eine nachträgliche Analyse des erzielten Motivwandels. *Zeitschrift für und Entwicklungspsychologie und Pädagogische Psychologie,* 1971, *3,* 253–268.

Heckhausen, H. Intervening cognitions in motivation. In D. E. Berlyne & K. B. Madsen (Eds.), *Pleasure, reward, preference.* New York: Academic Press, 1973.

Heckhausen, H. *How to improve poor motivation in students.* Paper presented at the 18th International Congress of Applied Psychology, Montreal, 1974.

Heckhausen, H. *Effort expenditure, aspiration level and self-evaluation before and after unexpected performance shifts.* Mimeographed lectures at the Universities of Bergen and Oslo, Norway, 1975. (a)

Heckhausen, H. *Perceived ability, achievement motive and information choice: A study by Meyer reanalyzed and supplemented.* Unpublished manuscript, Ruhr University at Bochum, West Germany, 1975. (b)

Heckhausen, H. *Motivation und Handeln.* New York: Springer-Verlag, 1980.

Heckhausen, H. Task-irrelevant cognitions during an exam: Incidence and effects. In H. W. Krohne & L. Laux (Eds.), *Achievement, stress, and anxiety.* Washington, D.C.: Hemisphere Publishing, 1982.

Heckhausen, H., & Krug, S. Motive modification. In A. J. Stewart (Ed.), *Motivation and society.* San Francisco: Jossey-Bass, 1982.

Heider, F. *The psychology of interpersonal relations.* New York: Wiley, 1958.

Heilbrun, K. S. Reply to Silverman. *Journal of Abnormal Psychology,* 1982, *91,* 134–135.

Heiman, J. R. The psychology of erotica: Women's sexual arousal. *Psychology Today,* August 1975, pp. 90–94.

Heller, D. *Children of holocaust survivors: The second generation effect.* Unpublished Bachelor of Arts thesis, Harvard College, Department of Psychology and Social Relations, 1979.

Henley, N. M. Power, sex, and nonverbal communication. In Z. Rubin (Ed.), *Doing unto others.* Englewood Cliffs, N.J.: Prentice-Hall, 1974.

Hermann, M. G. Assessing the personalities of Soviet politburo members. *Personality and Social Psychology Bulletin,* 1980, *6,* 332–352.

Heyns, R. W., Veroff, J., & Atkinson, J. W. A scoring manual for the affiliation motive. In J. W. Atkinson (Ed.), *Motives in fantasy, action, and society.* Princeton, N.J.: Van Nostrand, 1958.

Hill, C. T., Rubin, Z., & Peplau, L. Breakups before marriage: The end of 103 affairs. *Journal of Social Issues,* 1976, *32,* 147–168.

Hoffman, L. W. Fear of success in 1965 and 1972. *Journal of Consulting and Clinical Psychology,* 1974, *42,* 353–358.

Hopkins, J. R., Zelazo, P. R., Jacobson, S. W., & Kagan, J. Infant reactivity to stimulus-schema discrepancy. *Genetic Psychology Monographs,* 1976, *93,* 27–62.

Horner, M. S. *Sex differences in achievement motivation and performance in competitive and non-competitive situations.* Unpublished doctoral dissertation, University of Michigan, 1968.

Horner, M. S. A psychological barrier to achievement in women: The motive to avoid success. In D. C. McClelland & R. S. Steele (Eds.), *Human motivation: A book of readings.* Morristown, N.J.: General Learning Press, 1973.

Horner, M. S., Tresemer, D. W., Berens, A. F., & Watson, R. I., Jr. *Scoring manual for an empirically-derived scoring system for motive to avoid success.* Unpublished manuscript, Harvard University, Department of Psychology and Social Relations, 1973.

Horney, K. *Our inner conflicts.* New York: Norton, 1945.

Horowitz, R. A. N *Achievement correlates and the executive role.* Unpublished Bachelor of Arts thesis, Harvard University, Department of Social Relations, 1961.

Hovland, C. I., Janis, I. L., & Kelley, H. H. *Communication and persuasion: Psychological studies of opinion change.* New Haven, Conn.: Yale University Press, 1953.

Hoyos, C. Motivationspsychologie Untersuchungen von Kraftfahrern mit dem TAT nach McClelland, *Archiv für die gesamte Psychologie,* 1965. (Supplementary Vol. 7)

Hudson, L. *Contrary imaginations.* London: Methuen, 1966.

Hull, C. L. *Principles of behavior.* New York: Appleton-Century-Crofts, 1943.

Hull, C. L. *A behavior system.* New Haven, Conn.: Yale University Press, 1952.

Hurley, J. R. The Iowa Picture Interpretation Test: A multiple-choice variation of the TAT. *Journal of Consulting Psychology, 1955, 19,* 372–376.

Inkeles, A., & Levinson, D. J. National character: The study of modal personality and sociocultural systems. In *Handbook of social psychology (Vol. 2), Special fields in applications.* Cambridge, Mass.: Addison-Wesley, 1954.

Izard, C. E. Emotions as motivations: An evolutionary-developmental perspective. In H. E. Howe, Jr. (Ed.), *Nebraska Symposium on Motivation: 1978.* Lincoln: University of Nebraska Press, 1979.

Jackaway, R., & Teevan, R. Fear of failure and fear of success: Two dimensions of the same motive. *Sex Roles, 1976, 2,* 283–293.

Jackson, D. N. A modern strategy for personality assessment: The personality research form. *Research Bulletin No. 33c.* London, Canada: University of Western Ontario, Department of Psychology, 1966.

Jemmott, J. B., III. *Psychosocial stress, social motives and disease susceptibility.* Unpublished doctoral dissertation, Harvard University, 1982.

Jenkins, J. G. Instruction as a factor in "incidental" learning. *American Journal of Psychology, 1933, 45,* 471–477.

Johnston, R. A. A methodological analysis of several revised forms of the Iowa Picture Interpretation Test. *Journal of Personality, 1957, 25,* 283–293.

Jones, D. F. *The need for power as a predictor of leadership and exploitation in a variety of small group settings.* Unpublished Bachelor of Arts thesis, Wesleyan University, 1969.

Jones, E. E., & Davis, K. E. From acts to dispositions: The attribution process in person perception. In L. Berkowitz (Ed.), *Advances in experimental social psychology* (Vol. 2). New York: Academic Press, 1965.

Jones, M. C. The elimination of children's fears. *Journal of Experimental Psychology, 1924, 7,* 383–390.

Jones, M. R. (Ed.), *Nebraska Symposium on Motivation: 1955.* Lincoln: University of Nebraska Press, 1955.

Jopt, U. J., & Ermshaus, W. Wie generalisiert ist das Selbstkonzept eigener Fähigkeit? *Zeitschrift für experimentelle und angewandte Psychologie, 1977, 24,* 578–601.

Jopt, U. J., & Ermshaus, W. Motivspezifizität des Zusammenhangs Zwischen Selbstbelohnung und Kausalattribierung nach Erfolg und Misserfolg. *Archiv für Psychologie, 1978, 130,* 53–68.

Jung, C. G. [*Memories, dreams, reflections.*] (A. Jaffé, Ed.; R. Winston & C. Winston, trans.). New York: Random, 1961.

Kagan, J., Kearsley, R. B., & Zelazo, P. R. *Infancy: Its place in human development.* Cambridge, Mass.: Harvard University Press, 1978.

Kagan, J., & Moss, H. A. *Birth to maturity.* New York: Wiley, 1962.

Kalin, R. Social drinking in different settings. In D. C. McClelland, W. N. Davis, R. Kalin, & E. Wanner, *The drinking man: Alcohol and human motivation.* New York: Free Press, 1972.

Kalin, R., Kahn, M., & McClelland, D. C. The effects of male social drinking on fantasy. *Journal of Personality and Social Psychology, 1965, 1,* 441–452.

Kaltenbach, J. E., & McClelland, D. C. Achievement and social status in three small communities. In D. C. McClelland, A. L. Baldwin, U. Bronfenbrenner, & F. L. Strodtbeck (Eds.), *Talent and society.* Princeton, N.J.: Van Nostrand, 1958.

Karabenick, S. Fear of success, achievement and affiliation dispositions, and the performance of men and of women under individual competitive conditions. *Journal of Personality, 1977, 45,* 117–149.

Karabenick, S. A., & Yousseff, Z. I. Performance as a function of achievement level and perceived difficulty. *Journal of Personality and Social Psychology,* 1968, *10,* 414–419.

Kardiner, A. (Ed.). *Psychological frontiers of society.* New York: Columbia University Press, 1945.

Kawamura-Reynolds, M. Motivational effects of an audience in the content of imaginative thought. *Journal of Personality and Social Psychology,* 1977, *35,* 912–919.

Keister, M. Behavior of young children in failure. In R. Updegraff (Ed.), *Studies in pre-school education.* Iowa City, Iowa: University of Iowa Studies in Child Welfare, 1938.

Kelly, G. *The psychology of personal constructs.* New York: Norton, 1955.

Keshock, J. D. *An investigation of the effects of the expectancy phenomenon upon the intelligence, achievement and motivation of inner city elementary school children.* Unpublished doctoral dissertation, Case Western Reserve University, 1970.

Kinsey, A., Pomeroy, W. B., & Martin, C. E. *Sexual behavior in the human male.* Philadelphia: Saunders, 1948.

Kintsch, W. *Memory and cognition.* New York: Wiley, 1977.

Kirshnit, C. E., & McClelland, D. C. *Short term shifts in immunocompetence in response to emotion-arousing films.* Unpublished manuscript, Harvard University, Department of Psychology and Social Relations, 1983.

Klaiber, E. L., Broverman, D. M., & Kobayashi, Y. The automatization cognitive style, androgens, and monoamine oxidase. *Psychopharmacologia,* 1967, *11*(4), 320–336.

Klein, S. B. *Motivation: Biosocial approaches.* New York: McGraw-Hill, 1982.

Kleinbeck, U., & Schmidt, K. H. Aufgabenwahl im Ernstfall einer betrieblichen Ausbildung: Instrumentalitäts-theoretische Ergänzung aum Risikowahlmodell. *Zeitschrift für Entwicklungspsychologie und Pädagogische Psychologie,* 1979, *11,* 1–11.

Kleininna, P. R., Jr., & Kleininna, A. M. A categorized list of motivation definitions, with a suggestion for a consensual definition. *Motivation and Emotion,* 1981, *5,* 263–291.

Kline, P. *Fact and fantasy in Freudian theory* (2nd ed.). London: Methuen, 1981.

Klinger, E. Short-term stability and concurrent validity of TAT need scores: Achievement, affiliation and hostile press. *Proceedings of the 76th Annual Convention of the American Psychological Association, American Psychologist,* 1968, *23,* 878.

Klinger, E. *Meaning and void.* Minneapolis: University of Minnesota Press, 1977.

Klinger, E., Barta, S. G., & Maxeiner, M. E. Motivational correlates of thought content frequency and commitment. *Journal of Personality and Social Psychology,* 1980, *39,* 1222–1237.

Kock, S. W. [*Management and motivation.*] English summary of a doctoral dissertation presented at the Swedish School of Economics, Helsinki, Finland, 1965.

Kohlberg, L. Stage and sequence: The cognitive-developmental approach to socialization. In D. Goslin (Ed.), *Handbook of socialization theory and research.* Chicago: Rand McNally, 1969.

Kolb, D. A. Achievement motivation training for underachieving high school boys. *Journal of Personality and Social Psychology,* 1965, *2,* 783–792.

Kolb, D. A., & Boyatzis, R. E. On the dynamics of the helping relationship. *Journal of Applied Behavioral Science,* 1970, *6,* 267–289.

Kolp, P. *Navaho economic change.* Unpublished doctoral dissertation, Massachusetts Institute of Technology, 1965.

Konečni, V. J. The mediation of aggressive behavior: Arousal level versus anger and cognitive labelling. *Journal of Personality and Social Psychology,* 1975, *32,* 706–712.

Korman, A. *The psychology of motivation.* New York: Prentice-Hall, 1974.

Lacey, J. I. Somatic response patterning and stress: Some revisions of activation theory. In M. H. Appley & R. Trumbull (Eds.), *Psychological stress.* New York: McGraw-Hill, 1967.

Langer, E. J., & Rodin, J. The effects of choice and enhanced personal responsibility for the aged: A field experiment in an institutional setting. *Journal of Personality and Social Psychology,* 1976, *34,* 191–198.

Lansing, J. B., & Heyns, R. W. Need affiliation and frequency of four types of communication. *Journal of Abnormal and Social Psychology,* 1959, *58,* 365–372.

Lansky, D., & Wilson, G. T. Alcohol, expectations, and sexual arousal in males: An information processing analysis. *Journal of Abnormal Psychology,* 1981, *90,* 35–45.

Larson, R., & Csikszentmihalyi, M. Experiential correlates of time alone in adolescence. *Journal of Personality,* 1978, *46,* 677–693.

Lasker, H. M. *Ego development and motivation: A cross-cultural cognitive-developmental analysis of n Achievement.* Unpublished doctoral dissertation, University of Chicago, Department of Sociology, 1978.

Laufen, A. *Validierungsschlüssel des TAT Verfahrens zur Erhebung der Anschlussmotivation.* Unpublished diploma dissertation, Psychological Institute of the Ruhr University at Bochum, West Germany, 1967.

Lawrence, P. R., & Lorsch, J. W. New management job: The integrator. *Harvard Business Review,* 1967, *45*(6), 142–151.

Lazarus, R. S., & Alfert, E. The short-circuiting of threat by experimentally altering cognitive appraisal. *Journal of Abnormal Psychology and Social Psychology,* 1964, *69,* 195–205.

Le Magnen, J. Hyperphagie provoquée chez le rat blanc par altération du mécanisme de satiété périphérique. *Comptes Rendus des Séances de la Société de Biologie,* 1956, *150,* 32.

LeVine, R. *Dreams and deeds: Achievement motivation in Nigeria.* Chicago: University of Chicago Press, 1966.

Levy, D. M. Oppositional syndromes and oppositional behavior. In P. H. Hoch and J. Zubin (Eds.), *Psychopathology of childhood.* New York: Grune and Stratton, 1955.

Lewin, K. *A dynamic theory of personality.* New York: McGraw-Hill, 1935.

Lewin, K., Dembo, T., Festinger, L., & Sears, P. S. Level of aspiration. In J. M. Hunt (Ed.), *Personality and the behavior disorders* (Vol. 1). New York: Ronald Press, 1944.

Ley, R. G., & Bryden, M. P. A dissociation of right and left hemispheric effects for recognizing emotional tone and verbal content. *Brain and Cognition,* 1982, *1,* 3–9.

Lichter, S. R., & Rothman, S. Jewish ethnicity and radical culture: A social psychological study of political activists. *Political Psychology,* 1982, *3*(1–2), 116–157.

Linton, R. *The cultural background of personality.* New York: Appleton-Century, 1945.

Lipman-Blumen, J., Leavitt, H. J., Patterson, K. J., Bies, R. J., & Handley-Isaksen, A. A model of direct and relational achieving styles. In L. J. Fyans, Jr. (Ed.), *Achievement motivation: Recent trends in theory and research.* New York: Plenum, 1980.

Littig, L. W. Effects of motivation on probability preferences. *Journal of Personality,* 1963, *31,* 417–427.

Littig, L. W., & Williams, C. E. Need for affiliation, self-esteem, and social distance of black Americans. *Motivation and Emotion,* 1978, *2,* 369–373.

Litwin, G. H. *Motives and expectancy as determinants of preference for degrees of risk.* Unpublished Bachelor of Arts thesis, University of Michigan, Department of Psychology, 1958.

Litwin, G. H., & Siebrecht, A. *Integrators and entrepreneurs: Their motivation and effect on management.* St. Louis: Hospital Progress, 1967.

Locke, E. A. Toward a theory of task motivation and incentives. *Organizational Behavioral and Human Performance,* 1968, *3,* 157–189.

Locke, E. A. Personnel attitudes and motivation. *Annual Review of Psychology,* 1975, *26,* 457–480.

Locke, E. A., & Bryan, J. F. Grade goals as determinants of academic achievement. *Journal of General Psychology,* 1968, *79,* 219–228.

Locke, E. A., Shaw, K. N., Saari, L. M., & Latham, G. P. *Goal setting and task performance: 1969–1980* (Tech. Rep. for the Organizational Effectiveness Research Program). Washington, D.C.: Office of Naval Research, 1980.

Loehlin, J. C., & Nichols, R. C. *Heredity, environment and personality.* Austin: University of Texas Press, 1976.

Loevinger, J. The meaning and measurement of ego development. *American Psychologist,* 1966, *21,* 195–206.

Loevinger, J. *Ego development: Conceptions and theories.* San Francisco: Jossey-Bass, 1976.

Lohr, S. The efficiency of Japanese management. *New York Times,* February 27, 1982, p. 29.

Lorenz, K. The past twelve years in the comparative study of behavior. In C. H. Schiller (Ed.), *Instinctive behavior.* New York: International Universities Press, 1952.

Lorenz, K. *On aggression.* New York: Harcourt Brace Jovanovich, 1966.

Luborsky, L., & Sargent, H. D. The psychotherapy research project, V: Sample use of method. *Bulletin of the Menninger Clinic,* 1956, *20,* 263–276.

Lundy, A. C. *Conditions of test administration and TAT validity.* Unpublished manuscript, Harvard University, Department of Psychology and Social Relations, 1980.

Lundy, A. C. *Situationally evoked schema sets in TAT-based research: A cognitive explanation for differential TAT validity.* Unpublished doctoral dissertation, Harvard University, 1981. (a)

Lundy, A. C. *The reliability of the Thematic Apperception Test.* Unpublished manuscript, Harvard University, Department of Psychology and Social Relations, 1981. (b)

Lynn, R. An achievement motivation questionnaire. *British Journal of Psychology,* 1969, *60,* 529–534.

Maas, J. W., Hattox, S. E., Greene, N. M., & Landis, P. H. 3-methoxy-4-hydroxy-phenylglycol production by human brain in vivo. *Science,* 1979, *205,* 1025–1027.

Maccoby, E. E., & Jacklin, C. N. *The psychology of sex differences.* Stanford, Calif.: Stanford University Press, 1974.

Mace, C. A. *Incentives: Some experimental studies* (Rep. No. 72). London: Industrial Health Research Board (Great Britain), 1935.

MacKintosh, J. H., & Grant, E. C. The effect of olfactory stimuli on agonistic behavior of laboratory mice. *Zeitschrift für Tierpsychologie,* 1966, *23,* 584–587.

MacLean, P. D. Sensory and perceptive factors in emotional functions of the triune brain. In L. Levi (Ed.), *Emotions: Their parameters and measurement.* New York: Raven, 1975.

Maddi, S. R. Affective tone during environmental regularity and change. *Journal of Abnormal and Social Psychology,* 1961, *62,* 338–345.

Maddi, S. R., Charlens, A. M., Maddi, D., & Smith, A. J. Effects of monotony and novelty on imaginative productions. *Journal of Personality,* 1962, *30,* 513–527.

Maehr, M. L. Culture and achievement motivation. *American Psychologist,* 1974, *29,* 887–896.

Maehr, M. L., & Kleiber, D. A. The graying of achievement motivation. *American Psychologist,* 1981, *36,* 787–793.

Magnusson, D. The person and the situation in an interactional model of behavior. *Scandinavian Journal of Psychology,* 1976, *17,* 253–271.

Mahone, C. H. Fear of failure and unrealistic vocational aspiration. *Journal of Abnormal and Social Psychology,* 1960, *60,* 253–261.

Mandler, G., & Sarason, S. B. A study of anxiety and learning. *Journal of Abnormal and Social Psychology,* 1952, *47,* 166–173.

Mandler, J. M. Effect of early food deprivation on adult behavior in the rat. *Journal of Comparative and Physiological Psychology,* 1958, *51,* 513–517.

Mann, J., Berkowitz, L., Sidman, J., Starr, S., & West, S. Satiation of the transient stimulating effect of erotic films. *Journal of Personality and Social Psychology,* 1974, *30,* 729–735.

Mansson, H. H. The relation of dissonance reduction to cognitive, perceptual, consummatory, and learning measures of thirst. In P. G. Zimbardo (Ed.), *The cognitive control of motivation.* Glenview, Ill.: Scott, Foresman, 1969.

Maranell, G. M. The evaluation of presidents: An extension of the Schlesinger poll. *Journal of American History,* 1970, *57,* 104–113.

Marquis, D. P. Learning in the neonate: The modification of behavior under three feeding schedules. *Journal of Experimental Psychology,* 1941, *29,* 263–282.

Marshall, G. D., & Zimbardo, P. G. Affective consequences of inadequately explained physiological arousal. *Journal of Personality and Social Psychology,* 1979, *37,* 970–988.

Martindale, C. *Romantic progression: The psychology of literary history.* Washington, D.C.: Hemisphere Publishing, 1975.

Martindale, C. *The role of poet, styles, and sinusoidal patterns of regression.* Unpublished manuscript, University of Maine, Department of Psychology, 1977.

Maslow, A. *Motivation and personality.* New York: Harper & Row, 1954.

Maslow, A. H. A theory of metamotivation: The biological rooting of the value life. *Journal of Humanistic Psychology,* 1967, *7,* 93–127.

Maslow, A. *Toward a psychology of being.* New York: Van Nostrand, 1968.

Mason, J. W. Emotion as reflected in patterns of endocrine integration. In L. Levi (Ed.), *Emotions: Their parameters and measurement,* New York: Raven, 1975.

Masters, W., & Johnson, V. *Human sexual response.* Boston: Little, Brown, 1966.

Matthews, K. A., & Saal, F. E. Relationship of the type A coronary-prone behavior pattern to achievement, power, and affiliation motives. *Psychosomatic Medicine,* 1978, *40,* 631–636.

May, R. *Sex and fantasy.* New York: Norton, 1980.

Mayer, J. Regulation of energy intake and body weight: The glucostatic theory and the lipostatic hypothesis. *Annals of the New York Academy of Science,* 1955, *63,* 15–43.

Mayer, J., & Marshall, N. B. Specificity of gold-thio glucose for ventromedial hypothalamic lesions and obesity. *Nature,* 1956, *178,* 1399–1400.

McAdams, D. P. *Validation of a thematic coding system for the intimacy motive.* Unpublished doctoral dissertation, Harvard University, 1979.

McAdams, D. P. A thematic coding system for the intimacy motive. *Journal of Research in Personality,* 1980, *14,* 413–432.

McAdams, D. P. Intimacy motivation. In A. J. Stewart (Ed.), *Motivation and society.* San Francisco: Jossey-Bass, 1982. (a)

McAdams, D. P. Experiences of intimacy and power: Relationships between social motives and autobiographical memory. *Journal of Personality and Social Psychology,* 1982, *42,* 292–302. (b)

McAdams, D. P., & Constantian, C. A. *Intimacy and affiliation motives in daily living: An experience sampling analysis.* Unpublished manuscript, Loyola University, 1982.

McAdams, D. P., Healey, S., & Krause, S. *Relationships between social motives and patterns of friendship.* Unpublished manuscript, Loyola University, Department of Psychology, 1982.

McAdams, D. P., & Losoff, M. *Friendship motivation in fourth and sixth graders: A thematic analysis.* Unpublished manuscript, Loyola University, Department of Psychology, 1982.

McAdams, D. P., & McClelland, D. C. *Social motives and memory.* Unpublished manuscript, Harvard University, Department of Psychology and Social Relations, 1983.

McAdams, D. P., & Powers, J. Themes of intimacy in behavior and thought. *Journal of Personality and Social Psychology,* 1981, *40,* 573–587.

McAdams, D. P., & Vaillant, G. E. Intimacy motivation and psychosocial adaptation: A longitudinal study. *Journal of Personality Assessment,* 1982, *46,* 586–593.

McClelland, D. C. Functional autonomy of motives as an extinction phenomenon. *Psychological Review,* 1942, *49,* 272–283.

McClelland, D. C. *Personality.* New York: Sloane, 1951.

McClelland, D. C. Some social consequences of achievement motivation. In M. R. Jones (Ed.), *Nebraska Symposium on Motivation: 1955.* Lincoln: University of Nebraska Press, 1955.

McClelland, D. C. Methods of measuring human motivation. In J. W. Atkinson (Ed.), *Motives in fantasy, action, and society.* Princeton, N.J.: Van Nostrand, 1958. (a)

McClelland, D. C. The use of measures of human motivation in the study of society. In J. W. Atkinson (Ed.), *Motives in fantasy, action, and society.* Princeton, N. J.: Van Nostrand, 1958. (b)

McClelland, D. C. *The achieving society.* Princeton, N. J.: Van Nostrand, 1961. (Reissued with a new preface, New York: Irvington, 1976.)

McClelland, D. C. The harlequin complex. In R. W. White (Ed.), *The study of lives.* New York: Atherton Press, 1963.

McClelland, D. C. Toward a theory of motive acquisition. *American Psychologist,* 1965, *20,* 321–333. (a)

McClelland, D. C. *N* Achievement and entrepreneurship: A longitudinal study. *Journal of Personality and Social Psychology,* 1965, *1,* 389–392. (b)

McClelland, D. C. Does education accelerate economic growth? *Economic Development and Cultural Change,* 1966, *14,* 257–278.

McClelland, D. C. Money as a motivator: Some research insights. *McKinsey Quarterly,* 1967, *4,* 10–21.

McClelland, D. C. What is the effect of achievement motivation training in the schools? *Teachers College Record,* 1972, *74,* 129–145.

McClelland, D. C. *Power: The inner experience.* New York: Irvington, 1975.

McClelland, D. C. Sources of stress in the drive for power. In G. Serban (Ed.), *Psychopathology of human adaptation.* New York: Plenum Press, 1976.

McClelland, D. C. The psychological causes and consequences of modernization: An Ethiopian case study. *Economic Development and Cultural Change,* 1977, *25* (Suppl.), 43–66. (a)

McClelland, D. C. The impact of power motivation training on alcoholics. *Journal of Studies on Alcohol,* 1977, *38*(1), 142–144. (b)

McClelland, D. C. Inhibited power motivation and high blood pressure in men. *Journal of Abnormal Psychology,* 1979, *88,* 182–190. (a)

McClelland, D. C. *Increasing achievement motivation* (Mimeographed report). Boston: McBer and Company, 1979. (b)

McClelland, D. C. Motive dispositions: The merits of operant and respondent measures. In L. Wheeler (Ed.), *Review of personality and social psychology* (Vol. 1). Beverly Hills, Calif.: Sage, 1980.

McClelland, D. C. Is personality consistent? In A. I. Rabin, J. Aronoff, A. M. Barclay, & R. A. Zucker (Eds.), *Further explorations in personality.* New York: Wiley, 1981. (a)

McClelland, D. C. Comment on Lord Vaizey's paper on psychological factors in economic growth. In H. Giersch (Ed.), *Towards an explanation of economic growth.* Tübingen, West Germany: Mohr, 1981. (b)

McClelland, D. C. The need for power, sympathetic activation and illness. *Motivation and Emotion,* 1982, *6*(1), 31–41.

McClelland, D. C., Alexander, C., & Marks, E. The need for power, stress, immune function and illness among male prisoners. *Journal of Abnormal Psychology,* 1982, *91*(1), 61–70.

McClelland, D. C., & Apicella, F. S. A functional classification of verbal reactions to experimentally induced failure. *Journal of Abnormal and Social Psychology,* 1945, *40,* 376–390.

McClelland, D. C., & Atkinson, J. W. The projective expression of needs, I: The effect of different intensities of the hunger drive on perception. *Journal of Psychology,* 1948, *25,* 205–222.

McClelland, D. C., Atkinson, J. W., Clark, R. A., & Lowell, E. L. *The achievement motive.* New York: Appleton-Century-Crofts, 1953.

McClelland, D. C., Baldwin, A. L., Bronfenbrenner, U., & Strodtbeck, F. L. *Talent and society.* Princeton, N. J.: Van Nostrand, 1958.

McClelland, D. C., & Boyatzis, R. E. The leadership motive pattern and long term success in management. *Journal of Applied Psychology,* 1982, *67*(6), 737–743.

McClelland, D. C., & Burnham, D. H. Power is the great motivator. *Harvard Business Review,* March–April 1976, pp. 100–110; 159–166.

McClelland, D. C., Colman, C., Finn, K., & Winter, D. G. Motivation and maturity patterns in marital success. *Social Behavior and Personality,* 1978, *6,* 163–171.

McClelland, D. C., Constantian, C., Pilon, D., & Stone, C. Effects of child-rearing practices on adult maturity. In D. C. McClelland (Ed.), *The development of social maturity.* New York: Irvington, 1982.

McClelland, D. C., Davidson, R. J., Floor, E., & Saron, C. Stressed power motivation, sympathetic activation, immune function and illness. *Journal of Human Stress,* 1980, *6*(2), 11–19.

McClelland, D. C., Davidson, R. J., & Saron, C. *Evoked potential indicators of the impact of the need for power on perception and learning.* Unpublished manuscript, Harvard University, 1979.

McClelland, D. C., Davidson, R., Saron, C., & Floor, E. The need for power, brain norepinephrine turnover and learning. *Biological Psychology,* 1980, *10,* 93–102.

McClelland, D. C., Davis, W. B., Kalin, R., & Wanner, E. *The drinking man: Alcohol and human motivation.* New York: Free Press, 1972.

McClelland, D. C., & Friedman, G. A. Child-rearing practices and the achievement motivation appearing in folktales. In T. M. Newcomb, E. L. Hartley, & G. E. Swanson (Eds.), *Readings in social psychology* (2nd ed.). New York: Holt, Rinehart and Winston, 1952.

McClelland, D. C., & Jemmott, J. B., III. Power motivation, stress and physical illness. *Journal of Human Stress,* 1980, *6*(4), 6–15.

McClelland, D. C., & Kirshnit, C. *Effects of motivational arousal on immune function.* Unpublished manuscript, Harvard University, Department of Psychology and Social Relations, 1982.

McClelland, D. C., & Klemp, G. *Validation of the human service worker test.* Unpublished manuscript, 1974. (Available from McBer and Co., Boston, Mass.)

McClelland, D. C., & Liberman, A. M. The effect of need for achievement on recognition of need-related words. *Journal of Personality,* 1949, *18,* 236–251.

McClelland, D. C., Locke, S. E., Williams, R. M., & Hurst, M. W. *Power motivation, distress and immune function.* Unpublished manuscript, Harvard University, 1982.

McClelland, D. C., & Maddocks, A. *The effects of films on arousing motives in individuals with different motive dispositions.* Unpublished manuscript, Harvard University, Department of Psychology and Social Relations, 1983.

McClelland, D. C. & Maddocks, A. *The joint effect of* n *Power and brain norepinephrine turnover on recall: A replication.* Unpublished manuscript, Harvard University, Department of Psychology and Social Relations, 1984.

McClelland, D. C., & Pilon, D. A. Sources of adult motives in patterns of parent behavior in early childhood. *Journal of Personality and Social Psychology,* 1983, *44*(3), 564–574.

McClelland, D. C., Rhinesmith, S., & Kristensen, R. The effects of power training on community action agencies. *Journal of Applied Behavioral Science,* 1975, *11,* 92–115.

McClelland, D. C., Rindlisbacher, A., and deCharms, R. C. Religious and other sources of parental attitudes toward independence training. In D. C. McClelland (Ed.), *Studies in motivation.* New York: Appleton-Century-Crofts, 1955.

McClelland, D. C., & Teague, G. Predicting risk preferences among power-related tasks. *Journal of Personality,* 1975, *43,* 266–285.

McClelland, D. C., & Watson, R. I., Jr. Power motivation and risk-taking behavior. *Journal of Personality,* 1973, *41,* 121–139.

McClelland, D. C., & Watt, N. F. Sex-role alienation in schizophrenia. *Journal of Abnormal Psychology,* 1968, *73,* 226–239.

McClelland, D. C., & Winter, D. G. *Motivating economic achievement.* New York: Free Press, 1969. (Afterword to the paperback edition, 1971.)

McDougall, W. *An introduction to social psychology.* London: Methuen, 1908.

McDougall, W. *The energies of men.* London: Methuen, 1932.

McKeachie, W. J. Motivation, teaching methods, and college learning. In M. R. Jones (Ed.), *Nebraska Symposium on Motivation: 1961.* Lincoln: University of Nebraska Press, 1961.

McKenna, R. J. Some effects of anxiety level and food cues on the eating behavior of obese and normal subjects. *Journal of Personality and Social Psychology,* 1972, *22,* 311–319.

McMurray, G. A. Experimental study of a case of insensitivity to pain. Reprinted with additions from the *Archives of Neurology and Psychiatry,* 1950, *64,* 650–667.

Mehrabian, A. Measures of achieving tendency. *Educational and Psychological Measurement,* 1969, *29,* 445–451.

Mehrabian, A. The development and validation of measures of affiliative tendency and sensitivity to rejection. *Educational and Psychological Measurement,* 1970, *30,* 417–428.

Mehrabian, A., & Ksionzky, S. *A theory of affiliation.* Lexington, Mass.: Heath, 1974.

Mehta, P. *The achievement motive in high school boys.* New Delhi: National Council of Educational Research and Training, 1969.

Melton, A. W. Learning. In W. S. Monroe (Ed.), *Encyclopedia of Educational Research.* New York: Macmillan, 1941.

Meyer, J. P. Causal attributions for success and failure: A multivariate investigation of dimensionality, formation, and consequences. *Journal of Personality and Social Psychology,* 1980, *38,* 704–718.

Meyer, W. U. *Leistungsmotiv und Ursachenerklärung von Erfolg und Misserfolg.* Stuttgart: Klett, 1973.

Meyer, W. U. [*Perceived ability and informational choice.*] Unpublished manuscript, Psychological Institute of the Ruhr University at Bochum, West Germany, 1975.

Meyer-Bahlburg, H. F. L. Sex hormones in male homosexuality in comparative perspective. *Archives of Sexual Behavior,* 1977, *6,* 297–325.

Milgram, S. Behavioral study of obedience. *Journal of Abnormal and Social Psychology,* 1963, *67,* 371–378.

Milgram, S. Some conditions of obedience and disobedience to authority. *Human Relations,* 1965, *18,* 57–76.

Miller, N. E. Fear as motivation and fear-reduction as reinforcement in the learning of new responses. *Journal of Experimental Psychology,* 1948, *38,* 89–101.

Miller, N. E. Comments on theoretical models illustrated by the development of the theory of conflict. *Journal of Personality,* 1951, *20,* 82–100.

Miller, N., & Dollard, J. *Social learning and imitation,* New Haven, Conn.: Yale University Press, 1941.

Miron, D., & McClelland, D. C. The impact of achievement motivation training on small business performance. *California Management Review,* 1979, *21*(4), 13–28.

Mischel, W. *Personality and assessment.* New York: Wiley, 1968.

Mischel, W., & Gilligan, C. Delay of gratification, motivation for the prohibited gratification and responses to temptation. *Journal of Abnormal and Social Psychology,* 1964, *69,* 411–417.

Money, J., & Ehrhardt, A. *Man and woman, boy and girl.* Baltimore: Johns Hopkins University Press, 1972.

Montgomery, K. S., & Segall, M. Discrimination learning based on exploratory drive. *Journal of Comparative and Physiological Psychology,* 1955, *48,* 225–228.

Morris, D. *The naked ape.* London: Constable, 1967.

Moulton, R. W. Notes for a projective measure of fear of failure. In J. W. Atkinson (Ed.), *Motives in fantasy, action, and society.* Princeton, N. J.: Van Nostrand, 1958.

Moulton, R. W., Raphelson, A. C., Kristofferson, A. B. & Atkinson, J. W. The achievement motive and perceptual sensitivity under two conditions of motive-arousal. In J. W. Atkinson (Ed.), *Motives in fantasy, action, and society.* Princeton, N. J.: Van Nostrand, 1958.

Mowrer, O. H. *Learning theory and personality dynamics.* New York: Ronald Press, 1950.

Moyer, K. E. *The psychobiology of aggression.* New York: Harper & Row, 1976.

Mücher, H., & Heckhausen, H. Influence of mental activity and achievement motivation on skeletal muscle toneness. *Perceptual and Motor Skills,* 1962, *14,* 217–218.

Mueller, S. C. *Motivation and reactions to the work role among female performers and music teachers.* Unpublished doctoral dissertation. University of Michigan, 1975.

Murray, E. J. *Sleep, dreams, and arousal.* New York: Appleton-Century-Crofts, 1965.

Murray, H. A. *Explorations in personality.* New York: Oxford University Press, 1938.

Murray, H. A. American Icarus. In A. Burton, and R. E. Harris (Eds.), *Clinical studies of personality.* New York: Harper and Row, 1955.

Mussen, P. H., & Jones, M. C. Self-conceptions, motivations and interpersonal attitudes of late- and early-maturing boys. *Child Development,* 1957, *28,* 243–256.

Mussen, P. H., & Scodel, A. The effects of sexual stimulation under varying conditions on TAT sexual responsiveness. *Journal of Consulting Psychology,* 1955, *19,* 90.

Nakamura, J. *Achievement motivation in developmental perspective.* Unpublished manuscript, University of Chicago, Department of Sociology, 1981.

Neihardt, J. C. *Black Elk speaks: Being a life story of a holy man of the Oglala Sioux.* New York: Simon and Schuster, 1972. (Originally published, 1932.)

Newman, R. S. Alleviating learned helplessness in a wilderness setting: An application of attribution theory to Outward Bound. In L. J. Fyans, Jr. (Ed), *Achievement motivation: Recent trends in theory and research.* New York: Plenum, 1980.

Nicholls, J. G. The development of the concepts of effort and ability, perception of academic attainment, and the understanding that difficult tasks require more ability. *Child Development,* 1978, *49,* 800–814.

Noujaim, K. *Some motivation determinants of effort allocation and performance.* Unpublished doctoral dissertation, Massachusetts Institute of Technology, 1968.

Nuttall, R. L. Some correlates of high need for achievement among urban Negroes. *Journal of Abnormal and Social Psychology,* 1964, *68,* 593–600.

O'Connor, P. A., Atkinson, J. W., & Horner, M. Motivational implications of ability grouping in schools. In J. W. Atkinson & N. T. Feather (Eds.), *A theory of achievement motivation.* New York: Wiley, 1966.

Ogilvie, D. *Psychodynamics of fantasized flight: A study of people in folk tales.* Unpublished doctoral dissertation, Harvard University, 1967.

Oke, A., Keller, R., Mefford, I., & Adams, R. N. Lateralization of norepinephrine in human thalamus. *Science,* 1978, *200,* 1411–1413.

Olds, J. A physiological study of reward. In D. C. McClelland (Ed.), *Studies in motivation.* New York: Appleton-Century-Crofts, 1955.

Olds, J. *Drives and reinforcements: Behavioral studies of hypothalamic functions.* New York: Raven, 1977.

Olds, J., & Milner, P. Positive reinforcement produced by electrical stimulation of the septal area and other regions of the rat brain. *Journal of Comparative and Physiological Psychology.* 1954, *47,* 419–427.

Olson, G. A., Olson, R. D., Kastin, A. J., & Coy, D. H. Endogenous opiates: 1979. *Peptides,* 1980, *1,* 365–379.

Orne, M. T. On the social psychology of the psychological experiment: With particular reference to demand characteristics and their implications. *American Psychologist,* 1962, *17,* 776–783.

Panksepp, J. Aggression elicited by electrical stimulation of the hypothalamus in albino rats. *Physiology and Behavior,* 1971, *6,* 321–329.

Papanek, G. S. The development of entrepreneurship. *American Economic Review,* 1962, *52,* 46–58.

Parsons, J. E., & Goff, S. B. Achievement motivation and values: An alternative perspective. In L. J. Fyans, Jr. (Ed.), *Achievement motivation: Recent trends in theory and research.* New York: Plenum, 1980.

Passer, M. W. *Perceiving the causes of success and failure revisited: A multidimensional scaling approach.* Unpublished doctoral dissertation, University of California, Los Angeles, 1977.

Patrick, J. R. Studies in rational behavior and emotional excitement, II: The effect of emotional excitement on rational behavior of human subjects. *Journal of Comparative Psychology,* 1934, *18,* 153–195.

Patten, R. L., & White, L. A. Independent effects of achievement motivation and overt attribution on achievement behavior. *Motivation and Emotion,* 1977, *1,* 39–59.

Patterson, M. L. An arousal model of interpersonal intimacy. *Psychological Review,* 1976, *83,* 235–245.

Pearlson, H. B. Effects of temporal distance from a goal and number of tasks required for goal attainment on achievement-related behavior. In J. O. Raynor & E. E. Entin (Eds.), *Motivation, career striving, and aging.* New York: Hemisphere Publishing Corp., 1982.

Pearlson, H. B., & Raynor, J. O. Motivational analysis of the future plans of college men: Imagery used to describe future plans and goals. In J. O. Raynor & E. E. Entin (Eds.), *Motivation, career striving, and aging.* New York: Hemisphere Publishing Corp., 1982.

Peplau, L. A., Rubin, Z., & Hill, C. The sexual balance of power. *Psychology Today,* November 1976, pp. 142–151.

Perlmuter, L. C., Scharff, K., Karsh, R., & Monty, R. A. Perceived control: A generalized state of motivation. *Motivation and Emotion,* 1980, *4,* 35–45.

Phillips, A. G., Carter, D. A., & Fibiger, H. C. Differential effects of para-chlorophenyl alanine on self-stimulation in eaudate putamen and lateral hypothalamus. *Psychopharmacology,* 1976, *49,* 23–27.

Piaget, J. *The moral judgement of the child.* New York: Harcourt Brace, 1932.

Pilon, D. A., Jr. *The effect of personality needs and motives on political values and attitudes.* Unpublished doctoral dissertation, Harvard University, 1981.

Plutchik, R. *Emotion: A psychoevolutionary synthesis.* New York: Harper & Row, 1980.

Pottharst, B. C. *The achievement motive and level of aspiration after experimentally induced success and failure.* Unpublished doctoral dissertation, University of Michigan, 1955.

Rabin, A. I., Aronoff, J., Barclay, A. M., & Zucker, R. A. *Further explorations in personality.* New York: Wiley, 1981.

Rachman, S. Sexual fetishism: An experimental analogue. *Psychological Record,* 1966, *16,* 293–296.

Radnitzky, G. *Contemporary schools of metascience.* Chicago: Regnery, 1973.

Raphelson, A. C. The relationships among imaginative, direct verbal, and physiological measures of anxiety in an achievement situation. *Journal of Abnormal and Social Psychology,* 1957, *54,* 13–18.

Raynor, J. O. *The relationship between distant future goals and achievement motivation.* Unpublished doctoral dissertation, University of Michigan, 1968.

Raynor, J. O. A theory of personality functioning and change. In J. O. Raynor & E. E. Entin (Eds.), *Motivation, career striving, and aging.* New York: Hemisphere Publishing Corp., 1982.

Raynor, J. O., & Entin, E. E. *Motivation, career striving, and aging.* New York: Hemisphere Publishing Corp., 1982. (a)

Raynor, J. O., & Entin, E. E. Future orientation and achievement motivation. In J. O. Raynor and E. E. Entin (Eds.), *Motivation, career striving, and aging.* New York: Hemisphere NY, 1982. (b)

Raynor, J. O., & Harris, V. A. Performance in decreasing and increasing probability contingent paths. Unpublished data, 1973. Summarized in J. O. Raynor & E. E. Entin (Eds.), *Motivation, career striving, and aging.* New York: Hemisphere Publishing Corp., 1982.

Raynor, J. O., & Smith, C. P. Achievement-related motives and risk-taking in games of skill and chance. *Journal of Personality,* 1966, *34,* 176–198.

Raynor, J. O., & Teitelbaum, R. C. Time-linked sense of self and the *n* Achievement score. In J. O. Raynor and E. E. Entin (Eds.), *Motivation, career striving, and aging.* New York: Hemisphere Publishing Corp., 1982.

Richter, C. P. Animal behavior and internal drives. *Quarterly Review of Biology,* 1927, *2,* 307–343.

Robinson, R. G. Differential behavioral and biochemical effects of right and left hemispheric cerebral infarction in the rat. *Science,* 1979, *105,* 707–710.

Roethlisberger, F. J., & Dickson, W. J. *Management and the worker.* Cambridge, Mass.: Harvard University Press, 1947.

Rogers, C. R. *Counselling and psychotherapy.* New York: Houghton Mifflin, 1942.

Rogers, C. R. *Client-centered therapy: Its current practice, implications, and theory.* Boston: Houghton Mifflin, 1951.

Rogers, E. M., & Neill, R. E. *Achievement motivation among Colombian peasants.* East Lansing: Michigan State University, 1966.

Rogers, E. M., & Svenning, L. *Modernization among peasants: The impact of communication.* New York: Holt, Rinehart and Winston, 1969.

Rokeach, M. *The nature of human values.* New York: Free Press, 1973.

Rose, R. M., Holaday, J. W., & Bernstein, I. S. Plasma testosterone, dominance rank, and aggressive behavior in male rhesus monkeys. *Nature,* 1971, *231,* 366–368.

Rosen, B. C. The achievement syndrome. *American Sociological Review,* 1956, *21,* 203–211.

Rosen, B. C. Race, ethnicity and the achievement syndrome. *American Sociological Review,* 1959, *24,* 47–60.

Rosen, B. C., & D'Andrade, R. G. The psychological origins of achievement motivation. *Sociometry,* 1959, *22,* 185–218.

Rosen, D. H. *Lesbianism: A study of female homosexuality.* Springfield, Ill.: Charles C Thomas, 1974.

Rosenbaum, G. Stimulus generalization as a function of level of experimentally induced anxiety. *Journal of Experimental Psychology,* 1953, *45,* 35–43.

Rosenfeld, H. M., & Franklin, S. S. Arousal of need for affiliation in women. *Journal of Personality and Social Psychology,* 1966, *3,* 245–248.

Rosenthal, R. *Experimenter effects in behavioral research.* New York: Appleton-Century-Crofts, 1966.

Rosenthal, R. (Ed.), *Skill in nonverbal communication.* Cambridge, Mass.: Oelgeschlager, 1979.

Rosenthal, R., & Jacobson, L. *Pygmalion in the classroom.* New York: Holt, Rinehart and Winston, 1968.

Rosenthal, R., & Rubin, D. B. Interpersonal expectancy effects: The first 345 studies. *The Behavioral and Brain Sciences,* 1978, *3,* 377–415.

Ross, H. L., & Glaser, E. M. *A study of successful persons from seriously disadvantaged backgrounds.* Los Angeles: Human Interaction Institute, 1970.

Rothman, S. *Radical Christians, radical Jews.* New York: Oxford University Press, 1981.

Rothman, S., et al. Ethnic variations in student radicalism: Some new perspectives. In S. Bialer & S. Sluzar (Eds.), *Radicalism in the contemporary age: Sources of contemporary radicalism* (Vol. 1). Boulder, Colorado: Westview, 1977.

Rothman, S., & Lichter, S. R. Power, politics and personality in "Post-industrial society." *Journal of Politics,* 1978, *40,* 675–707.

Rotter, J. B. Generalized expectancies for internal versus external control of reinforcement. *Psychological Monographs,* 1966, Whole No. *80.*

Rowland, N. E., & Antelman, S. M. Stress-induced hyperphagia and obesity in rats: A possible model for understanding human obesity. *Science,* 1976, *191,* 310–312.

Rubin, Z. *Doing unto others.* New York: Prentice-Hall, 1974.

Rubinstein, E., & Sprafkin, J. N. Television: A channel to social values. In D. C. McClelland (Ed.), *The development of social maturity.* New York: Irvington, 1982.

Russett, B. M., et al. *World handbook of political and social indicators.* New Haven, Conn.: Yale University Press, 1964.

Ryan, T. A. *Intentional behavior.* New York: Ronald Press, 1970.

Salter, C. A., Meunier, J. L., & Triplett, W. M. Multiple measurement of anxiety and its effects on complex verbal learning. *Psychological Reports,* 1976, *38,* 691–694.

Samelson, F. The relation of achievement and affiliation motives to conforming behavior in two conditions of conflict with a majority. In J. W. Atkinson (Ed.), *Motives in fantasy, action, and society.* Princeton, N.J.: Van Nostrand, 1958.

Sanford, R. N. The effects of abstinence from food upon imaginal processes: A further experiment. *Journal of Psychology,* 1937, *3,* 145–159.

Sarason, I. G. Experimental approaches to test anxiety: Attention and the uses of information. In C. D. Spielberger (Ed.), *Anxiety and behavior* (Vol. 2). New York: Academic Press, 1971.

Sarason, S. B., & Mandler, G. Some correlates of test anxiety. *Journal of Abnormal and Social Psychology,* 1952, *47,* 810–817.

Sarason, S. B., Mandler, G., & Craighill, P. G. The effect of differential instructions on anxiety and learning. *Journal of Abnormal and Social Psychology,* 1952, *47,* 561–565.

Sawchenko, P. E., & Swanson, L. W. Central noradrenergic pathways for the integration of hypothalamic neuroendocrine and autonomic responses. *Science,* 1981, *214,* 685–687.

Schachter, S. *The psychology of affiliation.* Stanford, Calif.: Stanford University Press, 1959.

Schachter, S. Some extraordinary facts about obese humans and rats. *American Psychologist,* 1971, *26,* 129–144. (a)

Schachter, S. *Emotion, obesity, and crime.* New York: Academic Press, 1971. (b)

Schachter, S., Goldman, R., & Gordon, A. Effects of fear, food deprivation, and obesity on eating. *Journal of Personality and Social Psychology,* 1968, *10,* 91–97.

Schachter, S., & Singer, J. E. Cognitive, social, and physiological determinants of emotional state. *Psychological Review,* 1962, *69,* 379–399.

Schein, M. W., & Hale, E. B. Stimuli eliciting sexual behavior. In F. A. Beach (Ed.), *Sex and behavior.* New York: Wiley, 1965.

Schmalt, H. D. *Die Messung des Leistungsmotiv.* Göttingen, West Germany: Hogrefe, 1976.

Schnackers, U., & Kleinbeck, U. Machtmotiv und machtthematisches Verhalten in einem Verhandlungsspiel. *Archiv für Psychologie,* 1975, *127,* 300–319.

Schneider, K. Leistungsmotive, Kausalerklärungen für Erfolg und Misserfolg und erlebte Affekte Nach Erfolg und Misserfolg. *Zeitschrift für experimentelle und angewandte Psychologie,* 1977, *24,* 613–637.

Schneider, K. Atkinson's "risk preference" model: Should it be revised? *Motivation and Emotion,* 1978, *2,* 333–344.

Schneider, K., & Kreuz, A. Die Effekte unterschiedlicher Anstrengung auf die Mengen und Güteleistung bei einer einfachen und schweren Zahlensymbolaufgabe. *Psychologie und Praxis,* 1979, *23,* 34–42.

Scholem, G. G. *Major trends in Jewish mysticism.* Jerusalem: Schocken, 1941.

Scholem, G. G. *La kabbala et sa symbolique.* Paris: Payot, 1966.

Sears, R. R. *Survey of objective status of psychoanalytic concepts.* New York: Social Science Research Council, 1943.

Sears, R. R., Maccoby, E. E., & Levin, H. *Patterns of child rearing.* Evanston, Ill.: Row Peterson, 1957.

Sears, R. R., Rau, L., & Alpert, R. *Identification and child rearing.* Stanford, Calif.: Stanford University Press, 1965.

Seligman, M. E. P. *Helplessness: On depression, development, and death.* San Francisco: Freeman, 1975.

Selye, H. *The stress of life.* New York: McGraw-Hill, 1956.

Sheffield, F. D., & Roby, T. B. Reward value of a non-nutritive sweet taste. *Journal of Comparative and Physiological Psychology,* 1950, *43,* 471–481.

Sheffield, F. D., Wolff, J. J., & Backer, R. Reward value of copulation without sex drive reduction. *Journal of Comparative and Physiological Psychology,* 1951, *44,* 3–8.

Sheldon, W. H. (with the collaboration of S. S. Stevens). *The varieties of temperament: A psychology of constitutional differences.* New York: Harper, 1942.

Sheppard, H. L., & Belitsky, A. H. *The job hunt.* Baltimore: Johns Hopkins University Press, 1966.

Sherif, M. *An outline of social psychology.* New York: Harper, 1948.

Shinn, M. *Secondary school coeducation and the fears of success and failure.* Unpublished honors thesis, Harvard University, Department of Psychology and Social Relations, 1973.

Shiomi, K. Relations of pain threshold and pain tolerance in cold water with scores on the Maudsley Personality Inventory and Manifest Anxiety Scale. *Perceptual and Motor Skills,* 1978, *47,* 1155–1158.

Shipley, T. E., Jr., & Veroff, J. A projective measure of need for affiliation. *Journal of Experimental Psychology,* 1952, *43,* 349–356.

Shrable, K., & Moulton, R. W. Achievement fantasy as a function of variations in self-rated competence. *Perceptual and Motor Skills,* 1968, *27,* 515–528.

Silverman, L. H. Psychoanalytic theory: "The reports of my death are greatly exaggerated." *American Psychologist,* 1976, *31,* 621–637.

Silverman, L. H., Bronstein, A., & Mendelsohn, E. The further use of the subliminal psychodynamic actuation method for the clinical theory of psychoanalysis. *Psychotherapy: Theory, Research, and Practice,* 1976, *13,* 2–16.

Silverman, L. H., Klinger, H., Lustbader, L., Farrell, J., & Martin, A. The effect of subliminal drive stimulation on the speech of stutterers. *Journal of Abnormal Psychology*, 1972, *155*, 14–21.

Silverman, L. H., Kwawer, J. S., Wolitzky, C., & Coran, M. An experimental study of aspects of the psychoanalytic theory of male homosexuality. *Journal of Abnormal Psychology*, 1973, *82*, 178–188.

Sinha, B. P., & Mehta, P. Farmers' need for achievement and change-proneness in acquisition of information from a farm telecast. *Rural Sociology*, 1972, *37*, 417–427.

Skinner, B. F. *The behavior of organisms*. New York: Appleton-Century-Crofts, 1938.

Skinner, B. F. *Science and human behavior*. New York: Macmillan, 1953.

Skinner, B. F. *The behavior of organisms*. New York: Prentice-Hall, 1966, preface to the 7th ed.

Smetana, J. G., & Adler, N. E. Fishbein's value $\times$ expectancy model: An examination of some assumptions. *Personality and Social Psychology Bulletin*, 1980, *6*, 89–96.

Smith, C. P. *Achievement-related motives in children*. New York: Russell Sage, 1969.

Solomon, R. L. The opponent-process theory of acquired motivation: The costs of pleasure and the benefits of pain. *American Psychologist*, 1980, *35*, 691–712.

Sonnenfeld, J. *It's time to break for a station identification: A motivational analysis of a college radio station as a voluntary organization*. Unpublished manuscript, Harvard University, Department of Psychology and Social Relations, 1975.

Sorrentino, R. M. Extending theory of achievement motivation to the study of group processes. In J. W. Atkinson & J. O. Reynor (Eds.), *Motivation and achievement*. Washington, D.C.: Hemisphere Publishing, 1974.

Sorrentino, R. M., & Sheppard, B. H. Effects of affiliation-related motives on swimmers in individual versus group competition: A field experiment. *Journal of Personality and Social Psychology*, 1978, *36*, 704–714.

Southwood, K. E. *Some sources of political disorder: A cross-national analysis*. Unpublished doctoral dissertation, University of Michigan, 1969.

Spelke, E., Zelazo, P., Kagan, J., & Kotelchuck, M. Father interaction and separation protest. *Developmental Psychology*, 1973, *9*(1), 83–90.

Spence, K. W. *Behavior theory and conditioning*. New Haven, Conn.: Yale University Press, 1956.

Spence, K. W. Behavior theory and selective learning. In M. R. Jones (Ed.), *Nebraska Symposium on Motivation: 1958*. Lincoln: University of Nebraska Press, 1958. (a)

Spence, K. W. A theory of emotionally based drive (D) and its relation to performance in simple learning situations. *American Psychologist*, 1958, *13*, 131–141. (b)

Spence, K. W., Farber, I. E., & McFann, H. H. The relation of anxiety (drive) level to performance in competitional and noncompetitional paired-associates learning. *Journal of Experimental Psychology*, 1956, *52*, 296–305.

Spielberger, C. D. (Ed.). *Anxiety and behavior*. New York: Academic Press, 1966.

Spielberger, C. D., Gorsuch, R. L., & Lushene, R. E., *STAI manual for the state-trait anxiety inventory*. Palo Alto, Calif.: Consulting Psychologists Press, 1970.

Spitz, R. A., & Wolf, K. M. The smiling response: A contribution to the ontogenesis of social relations. *Genetic Psychology Monographs*, 1946, *34*, 57–125.

Spitz, R. A., & Wolf, K. M. Autoerotism during the first year of life. *Psychoanalytic study of the child*, 1949, *3/4*, 85–120.

Sroufe, L. A., & Waters, A. The ontogenesis of smiling and laughter: A perspective on the organization of development of infancy. *Psychological Review*, 1976, *83*, 173–183.

Sroufe, A., & Waters, E. Attachment as an organizational construct. *Child Development*, 1977, *48*, 1184–1199.

Stamps, L. The effects of intervention techniques on children's fear of failure behavior. *Journal of Genetic Psychology,* 1973, *123,* 85–97.

Steele, R. S. *The physiological concomitants of psychogenic motive arousal in college males.* Unpublished doctoral dissertation, Harvard University, 1973.

Steele, R. S. Power motivation, activation, and inspirational speeches. *Journal of Personality,* 1977, *45,* 53–64.

Steele, R. S. Psychoanalysis and hermeneutics. *International Review of Psychoanalysis,* 1979, *6,* 389–411.

Stein, L. Norepinephrine reward pathways: Role in self-stimulation, memory consolidation, and schizophrenia. In J. K. Cole & T. B. Sonderegger (Eds.), *Nebraska Symposium on Motivation: 1974.* Lincoln: University of Nebraska Press, 1975.

Stennet, R. G. The relationship of performance level to level of arousal. *Journal of Experimental Psychology,* 1957, *54,* 54–61.

Stewart, A. J. *Scoring system for stages of psychological development.* Unpublished manuscript, Harvard University, Department of Psychology and Social Relations, 1973.

Stewart, A. J. *Longitudinal prediction from personality to life outcomes among college-educated women.* Unpublished doctoral dissertation, Harvard University, Department of Psychology and Social Relations, 1975.

Stewart, A. J. *The study of experience-induced affective development.* Unpublished manuscript, Boston University, Department of Psychology, 1978.

Stewart, A. J. (Ed.). *Motivation and society.* San Francisco: Jossey-Bass, 1982.

Stewart, A. J., & Chester, N. L. Sex differences in human social motives: Achievement, affiliation and power. In A. J. Stewart (Ed.), *Motivation and society.* San Francisco: Jossey-Bass, 1982.

Stewart, A. J., & Rubin, Z. Power motivation in the dating couple. *Journal of Personality and Social Psychology,* 1976, *34,* 305–309.

Stone, A. *The effect of sanctioned overt aggression on total instigation to aggressive responses.* Unpublished honor's thesis, Harvard University, Department of Psychology and Social Relations, 1950.

Storms, M. D. A theory of erotic orientation development. *Psychological Review,* 1981, *88,* 340–353.

Sullivan, H. S. *The interpersonal theory of psychiatry.* New York: Norton, 1953.

Sulloway, F. *Freud: Biologist of the mind.* New York: Basic, 1979.

Swanson, G. E. *Religion and regime.* Ann Arbor: University of Michigan Press, 1967.

Taylor, J. A. The relationship of anxiety to the conditioned eyelid response. *Journal of Experimental Psychology,* 1951, *41,* 81–92.

Taylor, J. A. A personality scale of manifest anxiety. *Journal of Abnormal and Social Psychology,* 1953, *48,* 285–290.

Teevan, R. C., Burdick, H., & Stoddard, N. Relationship between incentive and expectations of success. *Psychological Reports,* 1976, *39,* 411–419.

Telford, C. W. The refractory phase of voluntary and associative processes. *Journal of Experimental Psychology,* 1931, *14,* 1–36.

Tennyson, R. D., & Woolley, F. R. Interaction of anxiety with performance on two levels of task difficulty. *Journal of Educational Psychology,* 1971, *62,* 463–467.

Terhune, K. W. Motives, situation and interpersonal conflict within prisoners' dilemma. *Journal of Personality and Social Psychology,* 1968, *8*(3), Part 2. (Monograph Suppl.) (a)

Terhune, K. W. Studies of motives, cooperation and conflict within laboratory microcosms. In G. H. Snyder (Ed.), *Studies in international conflict.* Buffalo, N.Y.: University of Buffalo Studies, 1968, *4*(1), 29–58. (b)

Tessler, M. A., O'Barr, W. M., & Spain, D. H. *Tradition and identity in changing Africa.* New York: Harper & Row, 1973.

Thayer, R. E. Measurement of activation through self-report. *Psychological Reports,* 1967, *20,* 663–678.

Thompson, D. A., & Campbell, R. G. Hunger in humans induced by 2-deoxy-D-glucose: Glucoprivic control of taste preference and food intake. *Science,* 1977, *198,* 1065–1068.

Thorndike, E. L. *The associative processes in animals.* Boston: Ginn and Company, 1899.

Thorndike, E. L. *Animal intelligence.* New York: Macmillan, 1911.

Thurstone, L. L. Ability, motivation, and speed. *Psychometrika,* 1937, *2,* 249–254.

Tinbergen, N. *The study of instinct.* London: Oxford University Press, 1951.

Tolman, E. C. *Purposive behavior in animals and men.* New York: Appleton-Century-Crofts, 1932.

Tomkins, S. S. *Affect, imagery, consciousness: The positive affects* (Vol. 1). New York: Springer, 1962.

Tomkins, S. S. *Affect, imagery, consciousness: The negative affects* (Vol. 2). New York: Springer, 1963.

Toynbee, A. J. *A study of history.* New York: Oxford University Press, 1947.

Trevelyan, G. M. *English social history.* New York: Longmans, Green, 1942.

Trope, Y. Seeking information about one's ability as a determinant of choice among tasks. *Journal of Personality and Social Psychology,* 1975, *32,* 1004–1013.

Udry, J. R., & Morris, N. M. Distribution of coitus in the menstrual cycle. *Nature,* 1968, *220,* 593–596.

Uleman, J. S. *A new TAT measure of the need for power.* Unpublished doctoral dissertation, Harvard University, 1966.

Uleman, J. S. The need for influence: Development and validation of a measure, in comparison with a need for power. *Genetic Psychology Monographs,* 1972, *85,* 157–214.

Underwood, B., Moore, B. S., & Rosenhan, D. Affect and self-gratification. *Developmental Psychology,* 1972, *8,* 209–214.

Valins, S. Cognitive effects of false heart-rate feedback. *Journal of Personality and Social Psychology,* 1966, *4,* 400–408.

Vander, A. J., Sherman, J. H., & Luciano, D. S. *Human physiology: The mechanisms of body function.* New York: McGraw-Hill, 1975.

Varga, K. Who gains from achievement motivation training? *Vikalpa (The Journal for Decision Makers),* 1977, *2,* 187–200. (Available from the Indian Institute of Management, Ahmadabad, India.)

Veroff, J. Development and validation of a projective measure of power motivation. *Journal of Abnormal and Social Psychology,* 1957, *54,* 1–8.

Veroff, J. Social comparison and the development of achievement motivation. In C. P. Smith (Ed.), *Achievement related motives in children.* New York: Russell Sage, 1969.

Veroff, J. Assertive motivations: Achievement versus power. In D. G. Winter & A. J. Stewart (Eds.), *Motivation and society.* San Francisco: Jossey-Bass, 1982.

Veroff, J., Atkinson, J. W., Feld, S. C., & Gurin, G. The use of thematic apperception to assess motivation in a nationwide interview study. *Psychological Monographs,* 1960, *74*(12, Whole No. 499).

Veroff, J., Depner, C., Kulka, R., & Douvan, E. Comparison of American motives: 1957 versus 1976. *Journal of Personality and Social Psychology,* 1980, *39,* 1249–1262.

Veroff, J., Douvan, E., & Kulka, R. *The American experience.* Basic, 1982.

Veroff, J., & Veroff, J. P. B. Reconsideration of a measure of power motivation. *Psychological Bulletin,* 1972, *78,* 279–291.

Vogel, W., Baker, R. W., & Lazarus, R. S. The role of motivation in psychological stress. *Journal of Abnormal and Social Psychology,* 1958, *56,* 105–112.

Waelder, R. *Basic theory of psychoanalysis.* New York: International University Press, 1960.

Wainer, H. A., & Rubin, I. M. Motivation of research and development entrepreneurs. *Journal of Applied Psychology,* 1969, *53,* 178–184.

Walker, E. L. Psychological complexity as a basis for a theory of motivation and choice. In D. Levine (Ed.), *Nebraska Symposium on Motivation: 1964.* Lincoln: University of Nebraska Press, 1964.

Walker, E. L. Psychological complexity and preference: A hedge-hog theory of behavior. In D. E. Berlyne & K. B. Madsen (Eds.), *Pleasure, reward, preference.* New York: Academic Press, 1973.

Walker, E. L., & Atkinson, J. W. The expression of fear-related motivation in thematic apperception as a function of proximity to an atomic explosion. In J. W. Atkinson (Ed.), *Motives in fantasy, action, and society.* Princeton, N.J.: Van Nostrand, 1958.

Walker, E. L., & Heyns, R. W. *An anatomy for conformity.* Englewood Cliffs, N.J.: Prentice-Hall, 1962.

Walker, W. I. Escape, exploratory, and food seeking responses of rats in a novel situation. *Journal of Comparative and Physiological Psychology,* 1959, *52,* 106–111.

Walster, E., Walster, G. W., & Berscheid, E. *Equity theory and research.* Boston: Allyn and Bacon, 1978.

Ward, L., & Wilson, J. P. Motivation and moral judgment as determinants of behavioral acquiescence and moral action. *Journal of Social Psychology,* 1980, *112*(2), 271–286.

Warden, C. J. *Animal motivation: Experimental studies on the albino rat.* New York: Columbia University Press, 1931.

Watson, R. I., Jr. *Motivational and sex differences in aggressive behavior.* Unpublished doctoral dissertation, Harvard University, 1974.

Weber, M. [*The Protestant ethic and the spirit of capitalism*] (T. Parsons, trans.). New York: Scribner, 1930. (Originally published, 1904.)

Weiner, B. Role of success and failure in the learning of easy and complex tasks. *Journal of Personality and Social Psychology,* 1966, *3,* 339–344.

Weiner, B. A theory of motivation for some classroom experiences. *Journal of Educational Psychology,* 1979, *71,* 3–25.

Weiner, B. *Human motivation.* New York: Holt, Rinehart and Winston, 1980. (a)

Weiner, B. A cognitive (attribution)-emotion-action model of motivated behavior: An analysis of judgments of help-giving. *Journal of Personality and Social Psychology,* 1980, *39,* 186–200. (b)

Weiner, B. *The emotional consequences of causal ascriptions.* Unpublished manuscript, University of California, Los Angeles, Department of Psychology, 1981.

Weiner, B., Frieze, I., Kukla, A., Reed, L., Rest, S., & Rosenbaum, R. M. Perceiving the causes of success and failure. In E. E. Jones, D. E. Kanouse, H. H. Kelley, R. E. Nisbett, S. Valins, & B. Weiner (Eds.), *Attribution: Perceiving the causes of behavior.* Morristown, N.J.: General Learning Press, 1971.

Weiner, B., Heckhausen, H., Meyer, W. U., & Cook, R. E. Causal ascriptions and achievement behavior. *Journal of Personality and Social Behavior,* 1972, *21,* 239–248.

Weiner, B., & Kukla, A. An attributional analysis of achievement motivation. *Journal of Personality and Social Psychology,* 1970, *15,* 1–20.

Weiner, B., & Potepan, P. A. Personality characteristics and affective reactions toward exams of superior and failing college students. *Journal of Educational Psychology,* 1970, *61,* 144–151.

Weiner, B., Russell, D., & Lerman, D. The cognition-emotion process in achievement-related context. *Journal of Personality and Social Psychology,* 1979, *37,* 1211–1220.

Weiss, J. M., Stone, E. A., & Harrell, N. Coping behavior and brain norepinephrine in rats. *Journal of Comparative and Physiological Psychology,* 1970, *72,* 153–160.

Weitzner, M. Manifest anxiety, amphetamine, and performance. *Journal of Psychology,* 1965, *60,* 71–79.

Wendt, H. W. Motivation, effort and performance. In D. C. McClelland (Ed.), *Studies in motivation.* New York: Appleton-Century-Crofts, 1955.

Wendt, H. W. Risk-taking as a function of pre-verbal 'imprinting'? Some data and speculations. *Archiv für die gesamte Psychologie,* 1961, *113,* 325–350.

Wendt, H. W. Early circannual rhythms and adult human behavior: Components of a chronobehavioural theory, and critique of persistent artifacts. *International Journal of Chronobiology,* 1974, *2,* 57–86.

White, R. W. Competence and the psychosexual stages of development. In M. R. Jones (Ed.), *Nebraska Symposium on Motivation: 1960.* Lincoln: University of Nebraska Press, 1960.

Whiting, B. B. Sex identity conflict and physical violence: A comparative study. *American Anthropologist,* 1965, *67,* 123–140.

Whiting, B. B., & Whiting, J. W. M. *Children of six cultures: A psycho-cultural analysis.* Cambridge, Mass.: Harvard University Press, 1975.

Wilsnack, S. C. The effects of social drinking on women's fantasy. *Journal of Personality,* 1974, *42,* 43–61; 243–261.

Wilson, G. T., & Lawson, D. M. Expectancies, alcohol, and sexual arousal in male social drinkers. *Journal of Abnormal Psychology,* 1976, *85,* 587–594. (a)

Wilson, G. T., & Lawson, D. M. The effects of alcohol on sexual arousal in women. *Journal of Abnormal Psychology,* 1976, *85,* 489–497. (b)

Wilson, G. T., & Lawson, D. M. Expectancies, alcohol, and sexual arousal in women. *Journal of Abnormal Psychology,* 1978, *87,* 358–367.

Winter, D. G. *Power motivation in thought and action.* Unpu'.lished doctoral dissertation, Harvard University, 1967.

Winter, D. G. *The power motive.* New York: Free Press, 1973.

Winter, D. G. *The power motive in women.* Unpublished manuscript, Wesleyan University, Department of Psychology, 1982.

Winter, D. G., & Healy, J. M., Jr. *An integrated system for scoring motives in running text: Reliability, validity, and convergence* (Paper presented at the American Psychological Association, Los Angeles, 1981). Department of Psychology, Wesleyan University, 1982.

Winter, D. G., McClelland, D. C., & Stewart, A. J. *A new defense of the liberal arts.* San Francisco: Jossey-Bass, 1982.

Winter, D. G., & Stewart, A. J. Power motive reliability as a function of retest instructions. *Journal of Consulting and Clinical Psychology,* 1977, *45,* 436–440.

Winter, D. G., & Stewart, A. J. Power motivation. In H. London and J. Exner (Eds.), *Dimensions of personality.* New York: Wiley, 1978.

Winter, D. G., Stewart, A. J., & McClelland, D. C. Husband's motives and wife's career level. *Journal of Personality and Social Psychology,* 1977, *35,* 159–166.

Winter, S. Characteristics of fantasy while nursing. *Journal of Personality,* 1969, *37,* 58–72.

Winterbottom, M. R. The relation of need for achievement to learning experiences in independence and mastery. In J. W. Atkinson (Ed.), *Motives in fantasy, action, and society.* Princeton, N. J.: Van Nostrand, 1958.

Wise, R. A. Action of drugs of abuse on brain reward systems. *Pharmacology, Biochemistry and Behavior,* 1980, *13* (Suppl. 1), 213–223.

Wittcoff, C. *Power motivation in the schools.* Unpublished manuscript, Washington University, Graduate Institute of Education, 1980.

Wolfe, J. B. Effectiveness of token-rewards for chimpanzees. *Comparative Psychology Monographs,* 1936, *12* (No. 60).

Wolfenstein, M., & Leites, N. *The movies: A psychological study.* New York: Free Press, 1950.

Woodworth, R. S. *Experimental psychology.* New York: Holt, 1938.

Wormley, W. *Portfolio manager preference in an investment decision-making situation: A psychophysical study.* Unpublished doctoral dissertation, Harvard University, 1976.

Wortman, C. B., & Brehm, J. W. Responses to uncontrollable outcomes: An integration of reactance theory and the learned helplessness model. *Advances in Experimental Social Psychology,* 1975, *8,* 277–336.

Wundt, W. *Grundzüge der physiologischen Psychologie.* Leipzig: Engelmann, 1874.

Yerkes, R. M., & Dodson, J. D. The relation of strength of stimulus to rapidity of habit formation. *Journal of Comparative and Neurological Psychology,* 1908, *18,* 459–482.

Young, P. T. *Motivation and emotion.* New York: Wiley, 1961.

Youngleson, M. L. The need to affiliate and self-esteem in institutionalized children. *Journal of Personality and Social Psychology,* 1973, *26,* 280–286.

Zajonc, R. B. Social facilitation. *Science,* 1965, *149,* 269–274.

Zajonc, R. B. Feeling and thinking: Preferences need no inferences. *American Psychologist.* 1980, *35,* 151–175.

Zajonc, R. B., & Sales, S. M. Social facilitation of dominant and subordinate responses. *Journal of Experimental and Social Psychology,* 1966, *2,* 160–168.

Zanna, M. P., & Cooper, J. Dissonance and the pill: An attribution approach to studying the arousal properties of dissonance. *Journal of Personality and Social Psychology,* 1974, *29,* 703–709.

Zeigarnik, B. Über das Behalten von erledigten und unerledigten Handlungen. *Psychologische Forschung,* 1927, *9,* 1–85.

Zimbardo, P. G. The human choice: Individuation, reason, and order versus deindividuation, impulse, and chaos. In W. J. Arnold & D. Levine (Eds.), *Nebraska Symposium on Motivation: 1969.* Lincoln: University of Nebraska Press, 1970.

Zimbardo, P. G. *Psychology and life.* Glenview, Ill.: Scott, Foresman, 1979.

Zuckerman, M. The sensation seeking motive. *Progress in Experimental Personality Research,* 1974, *7,* 80–148.

Zuckerman, M. General and situation-specific traits and states: New approaches to assessment of anxiety and other instincts. In M. Zuckerman & C. D. Spielberger (Eds.), *Emotions and anxiety.* Hillsdale, N.J.: Erlbaum, 1976.

Zuckerman, M., & Wheeler, L. To dispel fantasies about the fantasy-based measure of fear of success. *Psychological Bulletin,* 1975, *82,* 932–946.

Zumkley, H. *Aggression und Katharsis.* Göttingen, West Germany: Hogrefe, 1978.

Acknowledgments ===

The following figures are used by permission or adapted from the sources cited.

1.1   From N.E. Miller, "Comments on theoretical models illustrated by the development of the theory of conflict," *Journal of Personality,* 1951, Vol. 20, pp. 82–100. Copyright 1951 Duke University Press. Reprinted by permission of Duke University Press, Durham, N.C.

1.4   R.C. Clark in D.C. McClelland (Ed.) *Studies In Motivation,* 1955, p. 52. Reprinted by permission of Irvington Publishers, New York.

3.1   From C.J. Warden, *Animal Motivation: Experimental Studies on the Albino Rat.* Copyright 1931. Reprinted by permission of Columbia University Press.

3.4   From H.C. Blodgett, "The effect of the introduction of regard upon the maze performance of rats," *University of California Publications in Psychology,* 1929, Vol. 4, No. 8, pp. 113–134. Copyright 1929 University of California Press.

3.5   From L.P. Crespi, "Quantitative variation of incentive and performance in the white rat," *American Journal of Psychology,* 1942, vol. 55, pp. 467–517. Copyright © 1942, 1980 by the Board of Trustees of the University of Illinois.

3.6   K.W. Spence, "A theory of emotionally based drive (D) and its relation to performance in simple learning situations," *American Psychologist,* 1958, *13,* p. 134. Copyright © 1958 by The American Psychological Association. Reprinted by permission of the publisher.

3.7   From K.W. Spence, et al., "The relation of anxiety (drive) level to performance in competitional and non-competitional paired-associates learning," *Journal of Experimental Psychology,* 1956, Vol. 52, pp. 296–305. Copyright 1956 by the American Psychological Association. Adapted by permission of the author.

3.8   From R.B. Zajonc and S.M. Sales, "Social facilitation of dominant and subordinate responses," *Journal of Experimental and Social Psychology,* Vol. 2, pp. 160–168. Copyright 1966 by the American Psychological Association. Adapted by permission of the author.

4.1   From *Experimental Psychology* by Robert S. Woodworth. Copyright 1938 by Henry Holt & Co. Copyright Renewed 1966. Reprinted by permission of Holt, Rinehart & Winston, CBS College Publishing.

4.2   D.C. McClelland, J.W. Atkinson, R.A. Clark, and E.L. Lowell, *The Achievement Motive,* 1953, p. 43. Reprinted with permission from Irvington Publishers, New York.

4.3   From P.D. MacLean, "Sensory and perceptive factors in emotional functions of the triune brain," in L. Levi (Ed.) *Emotions: Their Parameters and Measurement,* 1975, p. 75. Reprinted by permission of Raven Press, New York.

4.4 (both photos) Reprinted from C.E. Izard's contribution to the 1978 *Nebraska Symposium on Motivation,* by permission of University of Nebraska Press. Copyright © 1979 by the University of Nebraska Press.

5.3, 5.4 From S.R. Maddi, "Affective tone during environmental regularity and change," *Journal of Abnormal and Social Psychology,* Vol. 62, pp. 338–345. Copyright 1961 by the American Psychological Association. Reprinted by permission of the publisher and the author.

5.5, 5.6 Figure 1, page 35, and Figure 3, page 43, from "Infant reactivity to stimulus-schema discrepancy," by J. Roy Hopkins, Philip R. Zelazo, Sandra W. Jacobson, and Jerome Kagan, which appeared in *Genetic Psychology Monographs,* 1975, Vol. 93, pp. 27–62.

5.7 *Archives of General Psychiatry,* Vol. 15, 1966. Copyright © 1966, American Medical Association.

6.4 From *The Achievement Motive: with a new preface by J.W. ATKINSON.* David C. McClelland et al. 1980. Reprinted with permission from Irvington Publishers, New York.

6.6 D.C. McClelland, J.W. Atkinson, R.A. Clark, E.L. Lowell, *The Achievement Motive,* 1953, p. 231. Reprinted with permission from Irvington Publishers, New York.

6.8 H. Heckhausen, "Achievement Motive Research: Current Problems and . . .", in *Nebraska Symposium on Motivation* (1968) p. 149. From *The Anatomy of Achievement Motivation.* Copyright 1967. Reprinted by permission of Academic Press and the author.

6.9 From L. Luborsky and H.D. Sargent, "The Psychotherapy research project, V. Sample use of method," Menninger Clinic Bulletin, 1956, vol. 20, pp. 263–276. Copyright 1956 the Menninger Clinic.

6.10 From A.C. Lundy, "Situationally evoked schema sets in TAT-based research: A cognitive explanation for differential TAT validity." *Unpublished doctoral dissertation,* 1981.

6.11 J.W. Atkinson, Thematic appreceptive measurement of motivation in 1950 and 1980, in G. d'Ydewalle and W. Lens (Eds.), *Cognition in Human Motivation and Learning.* Copyright 1980. Reprinted by permission of Lawrence Erlbaum Associates, Inc.

6.12 From J.W. Atkinson, et al., "Explorations using computer simulation to comprehend TAT measurement of motivation," *Motivation and Emotion,* Vol. 1, pp. 1–27. Copyright 1977 Plenum Publishing Corporation.

6.13 D.C. McClelland, J.W. Atkinson, R.A. Clark, and E.L. Lowell, *The Achievement Motive,* 1953, p. 207. Reprinted with permission from Irvington Publishers, New York.

7.1 From R. deCharms and V. Carpenter, "Measuring Motivation in Culturally Disadvantaged School Children," in H.J. Klausmeirer and G.T. O'Hern (Eds.), *Research and Development Toward the Improvement of Education,* 1968, p. 40. Reprinted by permission of the author.

7.3 From H. Heckhausen, "How to improve poor motivation in students." *Paper given at the 18th International Congress of Applied Psychology,* Montreal, 1974.

7.4 From J.O. Raynor and E.E. Entin, *Motivation, Career Striving, and Aging,* p. 107. Copyright 1982 Hemisphere Publishing Corporation.

7.5 From *Motives in Fantasy, Action, and Society* by John W. Atkinson, ed. Copyright © 1958 by D. Van Nostrand Company, Inc. Reprinted by permission of Wadsworth Publishing Company, Belmont, California 94002.

7.6 From N.T. Feather, "The relationship of persistence at a task to expectation of success and achievement related motives," *Journal of Abnormal and Social Psychology,* Vol. 63, pp. 552–561. Copyright 1961 by the American Psychological Association. Reprinted by permission of the author.

7.7 From J.W. Atkinson and D. Birch, *Introduction to Motivation,* 2nd Ed., p. 152. Copyright 1978 Wadsworth Publications Inc.

7.8 R.M. Sorrentino, "Extending theory of achievement motivation to the study of group processes," in J.W. Atkinson and J.O. Raynor (Eds.), *Motivation and Achievement,* p. 28. Copyright © 1974. Reprinted by permission of Hemisphere Publishing Corporation.

7.12   D.C. McClelland, J.W. Atkinson, R.A. Clark, and E.L. Lowell, *The Achievement Motive,* 1953, p. 300. Reprinted with permission from Irvington Publishers, New York.

7.13   From B.C. Rosen and R.G. D'Andrade, "The psychological origins of achievement motivation," *Sociometry,* 1959, Vol. 22, pp. 185–218. Copyright by D.C. McClelland, *The Achieving Society,* Van Nostrand Reinhold, 1961, re-issued with a new preface by Irvington Publishers Inc. Reprinted with permission from Irvington Publishers, Inc., New York.

8.1   From R.S. Steele, "Power motivation, activation, and inspiration speeches," *Journal of Personality,* 1977, vol. 45, pp. 53–64. Copyright 1977 Duke University Press. Reprinted by permission of Duke University Press, Durham, N.C.

8.2   From R.J. Davidson, et al., "Effects of personality and semantic content of stimuli on augmenting and reducing in the event-related potential," *Biological Psychology,* 1980, Vol. 11, pp. 249–255. Copyright 1980 North-Holland Publishing Company.

8.3   From D.C. McClelland, et al., "The need for power, brain norepinephrine turnover and learning," *Biological Psychology,* 1980, Vol. 10, pp. 93–102. Copyright 1980 North-Holland Publishing Company.

8.4   From U. Schnackers and U. Kleinbeck, "Machtmotiv und machtthematisches Verhalten," *Archiv für Psychologie,* 1975, Vol. 127, pp. 300–319. Copyright 1975 Archiv für Psychologie.

8.5   From D.C. McClelland and R.I. Watson, Jr., "Power motivation and risk-taking behavior," *Journal of Personality,* Vol. 41, pp. 121–139. Copyright 1973 Duke University Press.

8.6, 8.7   Reprinted with permission of The Free Press, a Division of MacMillan, Inc. from *The Drinking Man* by David C. McClelland, William N. Davis, Rudolph Kalin and Eric Wanner. Copyright © 1971 the authors.

8.8   Reprinted with permission of Macmillan Publishing Company from *The Drinking Man: Alcohol and Human Motivation* by David C. McClelland, William N. Davis, Rudolph Kalin, Eric Wanner. Copyright © 1970 by David C. McClelland, William N. Davis, Rudolph Kalin, Eric Wanner.

8.9   From D.C. McClelland and R.E. Boyatzis, "The leadership motive pattern and long term success in management," *Journal of Applied Psychology,* Vol. 67, No. 6, pp. 737–743. Copyright 1982 by the American Psychological Association. Reprinted by permission of the author.

8.11   From D.C. McClelland, et al., "The need for power, stress, immune function and illness among male prisoners," *Journal of Psychology,* Vol. 91, No. 1, pp. 61–70. Copyright 1982 by the American Psychological Association. Adapted by permission of the author.

9.2   Adapted from 1961 *Nebraska Symposium on Motivation* edited by Marshall R. Jones, by permission of University of Nebraska Press. Copyright © 1961 by the University of Nebraska Press.

9.3   From J.B. Jemmott, et al., "Academic stress, power motivation, and immunity." *Unpublished paper,* 1982, Princeton University.

9.4   From D.C. McClelland and C. Kirshnit, "Effects of motivational arousal on immune function." *Unpublished paper,* 1982.

10.2   J. Aronoff, *Psychological Needs and Cultural Systems,* pp. 62–63; 72, 76. Copyright 1967. Reprinted by permission of Wadsworth Publishing Co.

10.3   Figure adapted from data in "Motivation and moral development as determinants of behavioral acquiescence and moral action," by Laetitia Ward and John P. Wilson, which appeared in *Journal of Social Psychology,* 1980, 112, 271–286.

10.4   K. Schneider, "Atkinson's risk preference model: should it be revised?" *Motivation and Emotion,* Vol. 2, pp. 333–334, 1978 Plenum Publishing Corporation.

10.5   R.C. Birney, H. Burdick, and R.C. Teeven, *Fear of Failure Motivation,* p. 92. Reprinted by permission of the authors.

10.6   From R.M. Sorrentino and B.H. Sheppard, "Effects of affiliation-related motives on swimmers in individual versus group competition: A field experiment," *Journal of Personality and Social Psychology,* 1978, Vol. 36, pp. 704–714. Copyright 1978 by the American Psychological Association. Adapted by permission of the author.

10.7 From A. Mehrabian, "Verbal and nonverbal interaction of strangers in a waiting room," *Journal of Experimental Research in Personality,* 1971, 5, p. 133. Copyright 1971 by the American Psychological Association. Reprinted by permission of the author.

11.2 (both photos): Fitzwilliam Museum, Cambridge.

11.4 From N.M. Bradburn and D.E. Berlew, "Need for achievement in English economic growth," *Economic Development and Cultural Change,* 1961, vol. 10, pp. 8–20. Copyright 1961 University of Chicago Press.

11.6 Reprinted with the permission of The Free Press, a Division of Macmillan, Inc. from *The Drinking Man* by David C. McClelland, William N. Davis, Rudolf Kalin and Eric Wanner. Copyright © 1971 by the authors.

11.10 From R. deCharms and G.H. Moeller, "Values expressed in American children's readers: 1800–1950," *Journal of Abnormal and Social Psychology,* Vol. 64, pp. 136–142. Copyright 1962 by the American Psychological Association. Reprinted by permission of the author.

11.11, 11.12, 11.13 From A.J. Diaz, "An Empirical Analysis of the Effect of CEO Motives on Intra-Industry Performance in the American and Japanese Automobile Markets." *Unpublished A.B. thesis,* Harvard College, 1982.

12.1 From H. Heckhausen, "Effort expenditure, aspiration level and self-evaluation before and after unexpected performance shifts." Mimeographed lectures at the University of Bergen and Oslo, Norway, 1975.

12.2 From *Human Motivation* by Bernard Weiner. Copyright © 1980 by Holt, Rinehart & Winston. Reprinted by permission of Holt, Rinehart & Winston, CBS College Publishing. Adapted from Lazarus and Alpert, *Journal of Abnormal and Social Psychology,* 1964, Vol. 69, pp. 195–205.

12.3 J.O. Raynor and R.C. Teitelbaum, "Time-linked sense of self and the *n* Achievement score," in J.O. Raynor and E.E. Entin (Eds.), *Motivation, Career Striving and Aging,* p. 304. Copyright © 1982. Reprinted by permission of Hemisphere Publishing Corporation.

12.4 From S. Valins, "Cognitive effects of false heart-rate feedback," *Journal of Personality and Social Psychology,* Vol. 4, pp. 400–408. Copyright 1966 by the American Psychological Association. Reprinted by permission of the author.

12.5 From S. Schachter and J.E. Singer, "Cognitive, social, and physiological determinants of emotional state," *Psychological Review,* Vol. 69, pp. 379–399. Copyright 1962 by the American Psychological Association. Reprinted by permission of the author.

12.6 From M.P. Zanna and J. Cooper, "Dissonance and the pill: An attribution approach to studying the arousal properties of dissonance," *Journal of Personality and Social Psychology,* Vol. 29, pp. 703–709. Copyright 1974 by the American Psychological Association. Reprinted by permission of the author.

12.8 W. Meyer, *Leistungsmotive und Ursachenerklärung von Erfolg und Misserfolg.* Published by Ernst Klett Verlag, 1973. Reprinted by permission.

12.9 From H. Heckhausen, *Motivation und Handeln,* p. 524. Copyright 1980 Springer-Verlag New York, Inc.

12.10 From H. Heckhausen, "Effort expenditure, aspiration level and self-evaluation before and after unexpected performance shifts." Mimeographed lectures at the University of Bergen and Oslo, Norway, 1975.

12.11 From F. Halisch and H. Heckhausen, "Search for feedback information and effort regulation during task performance," *Journal of Personality and Social Psychology,* Vol. 35, pp. 724–733. Copyright 1977 by the American Psychological Association. Reprinted by permission of the author.

12.12 From H. Heckhausen, "Perceived ability, achievement, motive and information choice: A study by Meyer reanalyzed and supplemented." Unpublished paper, Ruhr University, 1975.

12.13 J.O. Raynor and E.E. Entin, *Motivation, Career Striving and Aging,* p. 25. Copyright © 1982. Reprinted by permission of Hemisphere Publishing Corporation.

12.14 From E.E. Entin and J.O. Raynor, "Effects of contingent future orientation and achievement motivation on performance in two kinds of tasks," *Journal of Experimental Research in Personality,* 1973, Vol. 6, pp. 134–320. Copyright © 1973 Academic Press, Inc.

12.16 From A. Bandura, "Self-efficacy mechanism in human agency," *American Psychologist,* Vol. 37, pp. 122–147. Copyright 1982 by the American Psychological Association. Reprinted by permission of the author.

13.1, 13.2 R.L. Patten and L.A. White, "Independent effect of achievement motivation and overt attribution on achievement behavior," *Motivation and Emotion,* Vol. 1, pp. 39–59, 1977 Plenum Publishing Corporation.

14.1 From R. Rosenthal and D.B. Rubin, "Interpersonal expectancy effects; the first 345 studies," *The Behavioral and Brain Science,* 1978, Vol. 3, pp. 377–415. Copyright 1978 Cambridge University Press.

14.2 Adapted with permission of Macmillan Publishing Company from *Motivating Economic Achievement* by David C. McClelland and David G. Winter. Copyright © 1969 by David C. McClelland and David G. Winter.

14.3 Reprinted with permission of The Free Press, a Division of Macmillan, Inc. from *Motivating Economic Achievement* by David C. McClelland and David G. Winter. Copyright © 1969 by the authors.

14.4 From H. Heckhausen and S. Krug, "Motive Modification," in A.J. Stewart, *Motivation and Society,* p. 277. Copyright 1982 Jossey-Bass, Inc.

14.5 © 1979 by the Regents of the University of California. Reprinted from *California Management Review,* Volume XXI, no. 4, pp. 13 to 28 by permission of the Regents.

14.8 R. deCharms, *Enhancing Motivation: Change in the Classroom,* 1976, p. 137. Reprinted with permission from Irvington Publishers, N.Y.

14.9, 14.10 From R. deCharms, "The origins of competence and achievement motivation in personal causation" in L.J. Fyans, Jr. (Ed.) *Achievement Motivation: Recent Trends in Theory and Research.* Copyright © 1980 Plenum Publishing Corporation.

14.11 R. de Charms, *Enhancing Motivation: Change in the Classroom,* 1976. Reprinted with permission from Irvington Publishers, N.Y.

14.13, 14.14 Reprinted by permission of the *Harvard Business Review.* Two exhibits from "Power is The Great Motivator" by David C. McClelland and David H. Burnham (March/April 1976). Copyright © 1976 by the President and Fellows of Harvard College; all rights reserved.

The following tables are used by permission or adapted from the sources cited.

1.2 From A.W. Combs, "A comparative study of motivations as revealed in Thematic Apperception stories and autobiography," *Journal of Clinical Psychology,* 1947, Vol. 3, pp. 65–75. Copyright © 1947 Clinical Psychology Publishing Co., Inc.

2.1 From W. McDougall, *The Energies of Men,* 1932, pp. 97–98. Reprinted by permission of the publishers, Methuen & Co.

2.2 Data based on Hierarchy of Needs in "A Theory of Human Motivation" in *Motivation and Personality,* 2nd Edition, by Abraham H. Maslow. Copyright © 1978 by Abraham H. Maslow. By permission of Harper & Row, Publishers, Inc.

2.3   From C.S. Hall and G. Lindzey, *Theories of Personality,* 1957, pp. 218–219. Reprinted by permission of John Wiley & Sons, Inc.

2.4   Reprinted from *Insight and Responsibility* by Erik H. Erikson, by permission of W.W. Norton & Company, Inc. Copyright © 1964 by Erik H. Erikson.

3.2   From B. Weiner, "Role of success and failure in the learning of easy and complex tasks," *Journal of Personality and Social Psychology,* 1966, vol. 3., pp. 339–344. Copyright 1966 by the American Psychological Association. Adapted by permission of the author.

3.3   From K. Kawamura-Reynolds, *Journal of Personality and Social Psychology,* Vol. 35, pp. 912–919. Copyright 1977 by the American Psychological Association. Reprinted by permission of the publisher and author.

4.1   From R.L. Solomon, "The opponent-process theory of acquired motivation: The costs of pleasure and the benefits of pain," *American Psychologist,* Vol. 35, pp. 691–712. Copyright 1980 by the American Psychological Association. Reprinted by permission of the author.

4.2   Information adapted from P. Ekman, in J.K. Cole (Ed.) *Nebraska Symposium on Motivation,* 1971.

5.2   Reprinted with permission of Macmillan Publishing Company from *The Drinking Man: Alcohol and Human Motivation* by David C. McClelland, William N. Davis, Rudolf Kalin, Eric Wanner. Copyright © 1970 by David C. McClelland, William N. Davis, Rudolf Kalin, Eric Wanner.

5.3   From D.C. Beardslee and R. Fogelson, "Sex differences in sexual imagery aroused by musical stimulation," in J.W. Atkinson (Ed.) *Motives in Fantasy, Action, and Society,* 1958, p. 136. Reprinted by permission of Wadsworth Publishing Co.

5.4, 5.5   Reprinted by permission of Macmillan, Inc. from *The Nature of Human Values* by Milton Rokeach. Copyright © 1973 by The Free Press, a Division of Macmillan Publishing Co., Inc.

6.2, 6.3   From S. Schacter, *Emotion, Obesity and Crime,* p. 110. Copyright © 1971. Reprinted by permission of Academic Press, Inc. and the author.

6.4   D.C. McClelland, J.W. Atkinson, R.A. Clark, E.L. Lowell (Eds.), *The Achievement Motive,* 1953, p. 141. Reprinted with permission from Irvington Publishers, New York.

6.7   From J.W. Atkinson and G.H. Litwin, "Achievement motive and test anxiety conceived as motive to approach success and motive to avoid failure," *Journal of Abnormal and Social Psychology,* Vol. 60, pp. 52–63. Copyright 1960 by the American Psychological Association. Reprinted by permission of the author.

7.4   From P.A. O'Connor, J.W. Atkinson, M. Horner, "Motivational Implications of Ability Grouping in Schools," in J.W. Atkinson and N.T. Feather (Eds.) *A Theory of Achievement Motivation,* 1966, p. 105. Reprinted by permission of John Wiley & Sons, Inc.

7.5   From D.C. McClelland and P.A. Pilon, "Sources of adult motives in patterns of parent behavior in early childhood," *Journal of Personality and Social Psychology,* Vol. 44, No. 3, pp. 564–574. Copyright 1983 by the American Psychological Association. Reprinted by permission of the author.

8.1   From D.G. Winter and A.J. Stewart, "Power Motivation," in H. London and J. Exner (Eds.) *Dimensions of Personality,* p. 399. Reprinted by permission of John Wiley & Sons, Inc.

8.2   From R.S. Steele, "The physiological concomitants of psychogenic motive arousal in college males." *Unpublished Ph.D. thesis,* 1973.

8.4   Adapted with permission of Macmillan Publishing Company from *The Power Motive* by David G. Winter. Copyright © 1973 by David G. Winter.

8.8   From D.G. Winter and A.J. Stewart, "Power Motivation," in H. London and J. Exner (Eds.) *Dimensions of Personality,* 1978, p. 416.

8.10   From D.C. McClelland and J.B. Jemott, IIII, "Power motivation, stress and physical illness,"

Journal of Human Stress, 1980, Vol. 6, No. 4, pp. 6–15. Copyright 1980 Opinion Publications, Inc.

8.11 R.R. Sears, E.E. Maccoby, H. Levin (Eds.), *Patterns of Child Rearing,* Copyright 1957, p. 570. Reprinted by permission of Stanford University Press.

9.1 Giese and Schmidt, from *Eysenck on Extroversion* by H.J. Eysenck. Copyright 1973, p. 80. Reprinted by permission of Granada Publishing Limited.

9.2 Reprinted from the book, *Sex and Fantasy* by Robert May, published by W.W. Norton and Co. Copyright © 1980 by Robert May. Used by permission of W.W. Norton and Co. and John Brockman Associates, Inc.

9.3 From J.W. Atkinson and P. O'Connor, "Neglected Factors in Studies of Achievement-Oriented Performance: Social Approval as an Incentive and Performance Decrement," in J.W. Atkinson and N.T. Feather (Eds.) *A Theory of Achievement Motivation,* pp. 314, 316. Reprinted by permission of John Wiley & Sons, Inc.

9.4 From D.B. Fishman, "Need and expectancy as determinants of affiliative behavior in small groups," *Journal of Personality and Social Psychology,* Vol. 4, pp. 155–164. Copyright 1966 by the American Psychological Association. Reprinted by permission of the author.

9.5 From R.E. Boyatzis, "A Two Factor Theory of Affiliation Motivation," *unpublished doctoral dissertation,* Harvard University 1972, pp. 144–164.

9.6, 9.7 From D.P. McAdams, "A thematic coding system for the intimacy motive," *Journal of Research in Personality,* 1980, Vol. 14, pp. 413–432. Copyright 1980 Academic Press, Inc.

9.9 From D.P. McAdams and J. Powers, "Themes of intimacy in behavior and thought," *Journal of Personality and Social Psychology,* Vol. 40, pp. 573–587. Copyright 1981 by the American Psychological Association. Reprinted by permission of the author.

10.1 Adapted from *Motives in Fantasy, Action, and Society* by John W. Atkinson, ed. Copyright © 1958 by D. Van Nostrand Company, Inc. Reprinted by permission of Wadsworth Publishing Company, Belmont, California 94002.

10.2 From J.W. Atkinson, "Motivational determinants of risk-taking behavior," *Psychological Review,* Vol. 64, pp. 359–372. Copyright 1957 by the American Psychological Association. Adapted by permission of the author.

10.3 From C.H. Mohone, "Fear of failure and unrealistic vocational aspiration," *Journal of Abnormal and Social Psychology,* pp. 253–261. Copyright 1960 by the American Psychological Association. Adapted by permission of the publisher.

10.4 From I.G. Sarason, "Experimental approaches to test anxiety: attention and the uses of information," in C.D. Spielberger (Ed.), *Anxiety and Behavior,* Vol. II, Copyright 1971. Reprinted by permission of Academic Press, Inc. and the author.

10.5 R.C. Birney, H. Burdick, and R.C. Teevan, *Fear of Failure Motivation,* 1969. Reprinted by permission of the authors.

10.6 D.S. Ceranski, et al., "A comparison of three measures of the motive to avoid failure: Hostile press, test anxiety, and sesultant achievement motivation," *Motivation and Emotion,* Vol. 3, pp. 395–404, 1979 Plenum Publishing Corporation.

10.8 From J. Fleming, *The Impact of College Environments on Black Students* (in press). Reprinted by permission of Jossey-Bass, Inc., Publishers and Jacqueline Fleming.

10.10 From J. Veroff, "Assertive Motivations," in D.G. Winter and A.J. Stewart (Eds.) *Motivation and Society: Essays in Honor of David C. McClelland,* 1982, p. 121. Reprinted by permission of Jossey-Bass, Inc., Publishers.

11.1 From E. Davies, "This is the way that Crete went, not with a bang but a simper," *Psychology Today,* 1969, Vol. 3, no. 6, pp. 43–47. Reprinted from Psychology Today Magazine. Copyright © 1969 American Psychological Association.

11.5 Reprinted with permission of The Free Press, a Division of Macmillan, Inc. from *The*

Index